OXYGEN TRANSPORT
TO TISSUE VII

ADVANCES IN EXPERIMENTAL MEDICINE AND BIOLOGY

Recent Volumes in this Series

A Continuation Order Plan is available for this series. A continuation order will bring delivery of each new volume immediately upon publication. Volumes are billed only upon actual shipment. For further information please contact the publisher.

OXYGEN TRANSPORT TO TISSUE VII

Edited by

F. Kreuzer

University of Nijmegen
Nijmegen, The Netherlands

S. M. Cain

University of Alabama at Birmingham
Birmingham, Alabama

Z. Turek

University of Nijmegen
Nijmegen, The Netherlands

and

T. K. Goldstick

Northwestern University
Evanston, Illinois

PLENUM PRESS • NEW YORK AND LONDON

Library of Congress Cataloging in Publication Data

International Symposium on Oxygen Transport to Tissue (8th: 1984: Nijmegen, Netherlands)
  Oxygen transport to tissue VII.

  (Advances in experimental medicine and biology; v. 191)
  "Proceedings of the 8th International Symposium on Oxygen Transport to Tissue, held August 26–30, 1984, in Nijmegen, the Netherlands" — T.p. verso.
  Includes bibliographies and index.
  1. Oxygen transport (Physiology) — Congresses. 2. Oxygen in the body — Congresses. I. Kreuzer, F (Ferdinand), 1919-   . II. Title. III. Title: Oxygen transport to tissue —7. IV. Series. [DNLM: 1. Biological Transport — congresses. 2. Oxygen — blood — congresses. 3. Oxygen — metabolism — congresses. 4. Oxygen Consumption — congresses. W1 AD559 v.191/QV 312 I613 1984o]
  QP99.3.O9I54   1984   599′.011   85-24424

ISBN-13: 978-1-4684-3293-0   e-ISBN-13: 978-1-4684-3291-6
DOI: 10.1007/978-1-4684-3291-6

Proceedings of the 8th International Symposium on Oxygen Transport to Tissue, held August 26–30, 1984, in Nijmegen, The Netherlands

© 1985 Plenum Press, New York

softcover reprint of the hardcover 1st edition 1985

A Division of Plenum Publishing Corporation
233 Spring Street, New York, N.Y. 10013

THE NIJMEGEN MEETING 1984 HAS BEEN SUPPORTED BY GENEROUS GIFTS FROM:

Sustaining member of ISOTT:

AVL AG, Schaffhausen, Switzerland

SPONSORS:

Organon Teknika N.V., Turnhout, Belgium

F. Hoffmann-La Roche & Co., AG, Basel, Switzerland

Royal Netherlands Academy of Arts and Sciences, Amsterdam,
    The Netherlands

KLM, Royal Dutch Airlines, Schiphol/Amsterdam, The Netherlands

Laméris Laboratorium B.V., Breukelen, The Netherlands

Orange Medical Instruments, High Wycombe, Bucks, United Kingdom

Draegerwerk AG, Lübeck, West Germany

Janssen Pharmaceutics B.V., Goirle, The Netherlands

Boehringer Mannheim GmbH, Mannheim, West-Germany

Glaxo B.V., Nieuwegein, The Netherlands

Salm and Kipp, Breukelen, The Netherlands

Springer-Verlag, Berlin-Heidelberg - New York-Tokyo

Hewlett Packard Nederland B.V., Amsterdam, The Netherlands

Science Trading GmbH, Frankfurt am Main, West-Germany

ISOTT OFFICERS AND COMMITTEES, 1984

Officers:
President: F. Kreuzer, Nijmegen, The Netherlands
President-Elect: I. Longmuir, Raleigh, NC, USA
Past-President: D. Bruley, Ruston, LA, USA
Treasurer: I. Silver, Bristol, United Kingdom
Secretary: T. Goldstick, Evanston, IL, USA

Executive Committee:
R. Bourgain, Brussels, Belgium
D. Bruley, Ruston, LA, USA
S. Cain, Birmingham, AL, USA
E. Dóra, Budapest, Hungary
W. Erdmann, Rotterdam, The Netherlands
T. Goldstick, Evanston, IL, USA
J. Grote, Bonn, West-Germany
C. Honig, Rochester, NY, USA
F. Kreuzer, Nijmegen, The Netherlands
I. Longmuir, Raleigh, NC, USA
N. Mitagvaria, Tbilisi, USSR
M. Mochizuki, Yamagata, Japan
I. Silver, Bristol, United Kingdom
D. Wilson, Philadelphia, PA, USA

Organizing Committee:
R. Bourgain, Brussels, Belgium
D. Bruley, Ruston, LA, USA
T. Goldstick, Evanston, IL, USA
J. Grote, Bonn, West-Germany
F. Kreuzer, Nijmegen, The Netherlands
D. Lübbers, Dortmund, West-Germany
K. Rakusan, Ottawa, Ontario, Canada
I. Silver, Bristol, United Kingdom

Program Committe:
S. Cain, Birmingham, AL, USA, and Nijmegen, The Netherlands
R. Goris, Nijmegen, The Netherlands
L. Hoofd, Nijmegen, The Netherlands
H. Kimmich, Nijmegen, The Netherlands
F. Kreuzer, Nijmegen, The Netherlands
J. van Namen-Vrijenhoek, Nijmegen, The Netherlands
Z. Turek, Nijmegen, The Netherlands

Advisory and executive assistance of the Congress Office,
    Public Relations Department, University of Nijmegen,
    Nijmegen, The Netherlands

Secretariat by A. Minke, Nijmegen, The Netherlands

PREFACE

Since there are many different tissues and organs in the body, a study of oxygen transport to tissue necessarily involves a great diversity of bodily functions. Furthermore, these tissue functions can be approached from the viewpoint of several disciplines. Eventually, however, all of these approaches must be combined to arrive at a comprehensive picture. This multidisciplinary effort, though imperative, has been implemented slowly because traditional biological science has been largely organ- or discipline oriented. Initiatives to realize an effective international multidisciplinary collaboration have assumed increasing momentum for the past 20 years. These include meetings held in Bad Oeynhausen in 1965 (book in 1968, edited by D.W. Lübbers, U.C. Luft, G. Thews and E. Witzleb), in Nijmegen in 1968 (book in 1969, edited by F. Kreuzer), in Vancouver in 1970 (J. Strauss), and in Dortmund in 1971; this last was in connection with the 25th International Physiological Congress in Munich (book in 1973, edited by M. Kessler, D.F. Bruley, L.C. Clark, Jr., D.W. Lübbers, I.A. Silver and J. Strauss). This increasing international cooperation called for a more formal organization of these individual initiatives.

The credit for taking this decisive step goes to H.I. Bicher and D.F. Bruley from the U.S.A. and D.W. Lübbers and M. Kessler from Germany, who got together in 1972 to plan a large-scale international meeting and to organize an international society. The first meeting that originated from this combined effort was held in Clemson-Charleston, South Carolina, in 1973 (M.H. Knisely, D.F. Bruley, H.I. Bicher). Here the International Society on Oxygen Transport to Tissue (ISOTT) was founded and it was decided to convene yearly meetings alternating between the U.S.A. and Europe. The proceedings of this first ISOTT meeting were edited by H.I. Bicher and D.F. Bruley and published in two volumes in 1973 in the Advances in Experimental Medicine and Biology by Plenum Press which was to publish also all the following ISOTT volumes labeled by Roman numerals.

The next meeting in 1974 was organized by H.I. Bicher and incorporated into the FASEB program in Atlantic City; the abstracts were published in Federation Proceedings in the session on Oxygen

Transport to Tissue. The third meeting, which was the first in Europe, took place in Mainz in 1975 under the leadership of G. Thews, J. Grote and D.D. Reneau (book ISOTT-II, edited by J. Grote, D. Reneau and G. Thews). Yearly meetings followed: 1976 by B. Chance in Anaheim in conjunction with FASEB (two sessions on Oxygen Transport to Tissue in Federation Proceedings); 1977 in Cambridge, England, by I.A. Silver (book ISOTT-III, 1978, edited by I.A. Silver, M. Erecińska and H.I. Bicher); 1978 in Atlantic City again with FASEB (abstracts under code ISOTT in Federation Proceedings); 1979 in La Jolla by J. Strauss (abstracts); 1980 in Budapest as a Satellite Symposium of the 28th International Congress of Physiological Sciences by A.G.B. Kovách (book Vol. 25 of Advances in Physiological Sciences, 1981, edited by A.G.B. Kovách, E. Dóra, M. Kessler and I.A. Silver); 1981 in Detroit by H.I. Bicher (book ISOTT-IV, 1983, edited by H.I. Bicher and D.F. Bruley); 1982 in Dortmund by D.W. Lübbers (book ISOTT-V, 1984, edited by D.W. Lübbers, H. Acker, E. Leniger-Follert and T.K. Goldstick); 1983 in Ruston by D.F. Bruley (book ISOTT-VI, 1984, edited by D.F. Bruley, H.I. Bicher and D.D. Reneau).

After 12 years we are happy to report that ISOTT has prospered and has become a society of primary importance to workers in the broad field of oxygen transport to tissue. The meetings have united workers in physiology, biophysics, biochemistry, biology, anatomy, pharmacology, biomedical and chemical engineering, mathematics, clinical sciences, and industrial applications. A concerted effort has emerged in a multidisciplinary experimental, theoretical and clinical approach to the complex problems of oxygen transport to tissue. There were, at these meetings, regularly about 150 participants from all over the world, and the books of proceedings have included 100 or more papers in each volume. May an old student wish also hold for ISOTT: "Vivat, crescat, floreat"!

At the Nijmegen Meeting of 1984, we have tried to expand the scope of ISOTT somewhat by adding the topic of central gas exchange in the lungs so that the entire oxygen transport chain from ambient air to the mitochondria is covered. Our editorial practices have followed a middle course between rigorous reviewing and simple publishing the papers as submitted. Each paper was reviewed by at least one of the Editors, many by two, and a few by three of them, depending on the problems met. Reviewing concentrated on intelligibility, presentation and format whereas much liberty was granted with respect to the general message of the papers. Our main concern was on speed of publication, hopefully within one year after the Meeting. Because proceedings of a symposium often include works in progress, they are most helpful if published without too much delay. Discussions have been omitted because experience has shown that they often are rather arbitrary and of differing impact, and are often difficult to present in a consistent and useful way. The Book starts with five Minireviews covering important fields of oxygen transport to tissue. The other papers are arranged according to main topics or, in some cases are grouped if they emanated from the same laboratory.

We wish to thank sincerely all the participants and contributors to the Nijmegen Meeting as well as the sponsors who are listed separately. The help of D.W. Lübbers and M. Kessler in preparing a short survey of the history of ISOTT is greatly appreciated. Our thanks are due to Mrs. Annemieke Minke for her secretarial help in the final preparation of the manuscripts.

F. Kreuzer
S.M. Cain
Z. Turek
T.K. Goldstick

CONTENTS

HEART

SKELETAL MUSCLE

METHODS

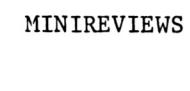MINIREVIEWS

OXYGEN SUPPLY AND MICROCIRCULATION OF THE BRAIN CORTEX[*]

Elfriede Leniger-Follert

Max-Planck-Institut für Systemphysiologie
Rheinlanddamm 201, 4600 Dortmund 1, FRG

INTRODUCTION

The actual oxygen supply of the brain is, as in other organs, dependent on the arterial oxygen capacity, the rate of local blood flow, the diffusion conditions within the organ and the oxygen consumption of the tissue. All these parameters may change under different physiological or pathological conditions and thus influence the O_2 supply of the brain. In the following minireview I will focus on the following points.
1. Brain oxygen supply under normal physiological conditions
2. Oxygen supply during changes in mean arterial blood pressure (MABP)
3. Fluidity of the blood and tissue Po_2
4. Cerebral microflow and tissue Po_2 during changes in functional activity and metabolism
5. Effect of deprived glucose concentration and of ammonia intoxication on oxygen supply.

1. The oxygen supply of the individual organs is mirrored by the tissue oxygen pressure fields as stated by Lübbers (1977, 1981). Theoretical calculations of Krogh (1918/1919), Thews (1960), Bruley et al. (1971), Metzger (1973), and Grunewald and Sowa (1977) with different model assumptions have shown that a three-dimensional O_2 pressure field should exist. After the construction of appropriate Po_2 electrodes it was possible to directly measure the O_2 pressures quantitatively on the surface of the organs and within the tissues (Clark (1956), Silver (1965), Kessler and Lübbers (1966), Whalen (1967), and Baumgärtl and Lübbers (1973)). The representation of the measured Po_2 frequency distribution in so-called "Po_2 histograms" showed that most of the measured values in the

[*]with support of Deutsche Forschungsgemeinschaft Le 517/1-1

brain and also in other organs of different animals were below the venous Po_2, see for example Whalen et al. (1970), Erdmann et al. (1973), Leniger et al. (1975), Lübbers (1977, 1981), Smith et al. (1977), Wiernsperger et al. (1978), Metzger et al. (1980), Grote et al. (1981), and Cahn and Leniger (1983). (For review of other organs see Kessler (1974), and Lübbers (1977, 1981)).

However, in recent investigations we have found in cats with light N_2O anaesthesia that under normal physiological conditions the majority of Po_2 values were above the central venous Po_2 or the Po_2 in the sinus sagittalis as shown in the first figure. Measurements on the human brain cortex during neurosurgical operation confirmed that the tissue Po_2 histogram of the normal brain tissue was shifted more to the right, to higher Po_2 values, in comparison to the above cited investigations, as demonstrated in Fig. 2. (Wüllenweber, Schultheiss, Assad, Leniger-Follert, Pfeiffer, Wassmann: unpublished results)

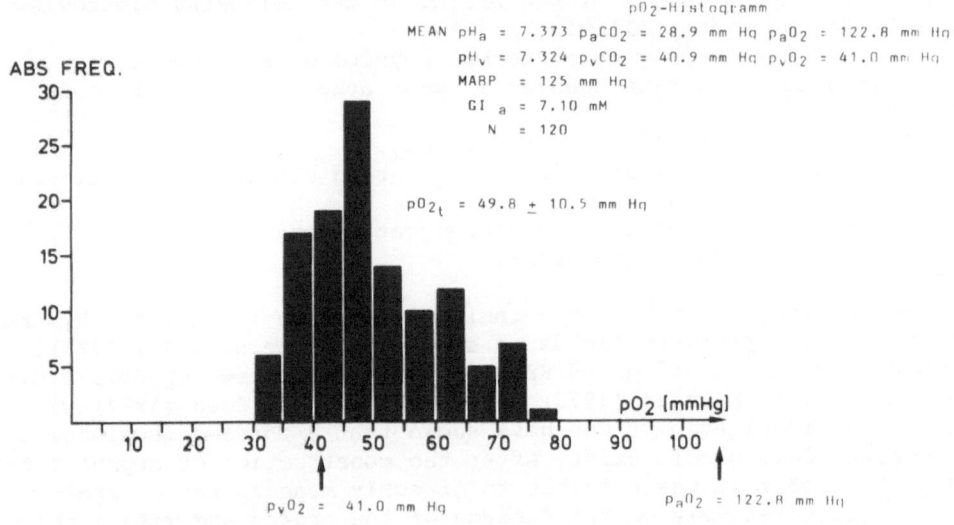

Fig. 1. Po_2 histogram of the cat brain cortex (gyrus supra-sylvius) during N_2O anaesthesia. Note that the majority of Po_2 values is above the central venous Po_2 (Leniger-Follert and Hufnagel, unpublished results)

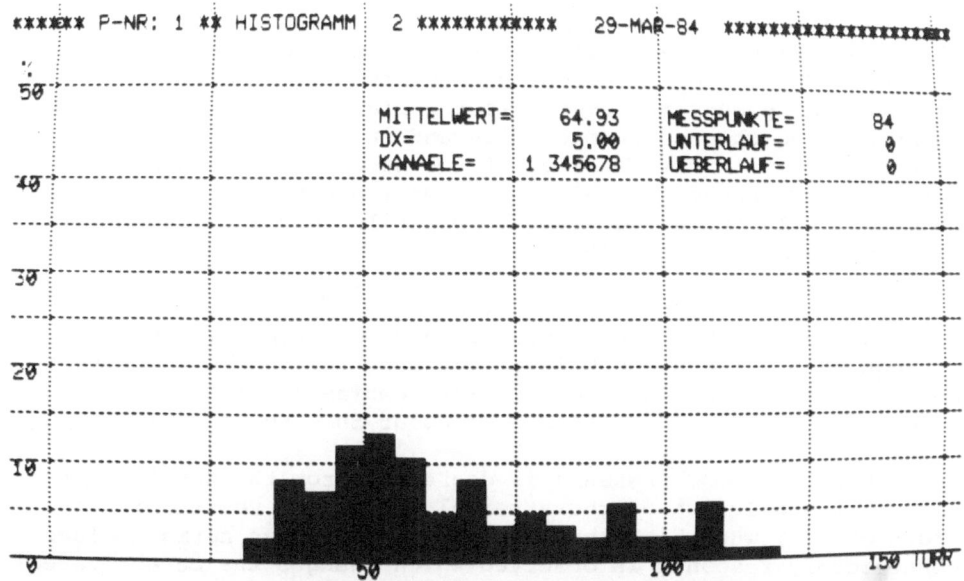

Fig. 2. Po_2 histogram of the normal human brain cortex during neurolept anaesthesia. $P_aO_2 = 167$ mm Hg, $P_aCO_2 = 33$ mm Hg. (Wüllenweber et al. (unpublished results.)

The main reason responsible for this obvious discrepancy seems to be the choice of anaesthesia. In nearly all the above cited investigations pentobarbital was used, which is known to depress functional electrical activity and oxygen consumption of the brain tissue as well as cerebral blood flow. As I will show in the latter part of my presentation, a higher functional activity of the brain causes, in addition to the increased cerebral metabolism, also an increase in cerebral blood flow and in tissue Po_2. Thus, it is possible that the cylinder model of Krogh, primarily developed for the oxygen supply conditions of the skeletal muscle, is valid also for the oxygen supply of the brain under normal functional activation conditions, as this model predicts that only a small fraction of the Po_2 values may be below the venous Po_2.

When, instead of Po_2 histograms with changing positions of the electrodes, the dynamic behavior of Po_2 is measured at the same locations, then fluctuations and waves are sometimes found. These fluctuations were described previously by Clark (1956) and Silver (1965) and later on by numerous authors. They may be caused by two different mechanisms: a) By waves of blood pressure which continue even into the microvessels and thus induce corresponding changes in microflow and in tissue Po_2; or b) By changes in functional activity of the nerve cells which can be estimated by changes in the electrocorticogram. The changes in functional electrical activity secondarily induce changes in the flow in the microcirculatory range.

2. Flow autoregulation and tissue pO_2 in the brain.
As is known from the fundamental studies of Harper (1966) and subsequent studies by many investigators (for review see Kuschinsky and Wahl, 1978), cerebral blood flow remains constant in the mean arterial blood pressure range from about 50 - 60 up to 160 mm Hg.

When the blood pressure is decreased from the normal control value a vasodilation of the arterial resistance vessels in the brain occurs; when blood pressure is raised above normal values a constrictory response is observed which changes the cerebrovascular

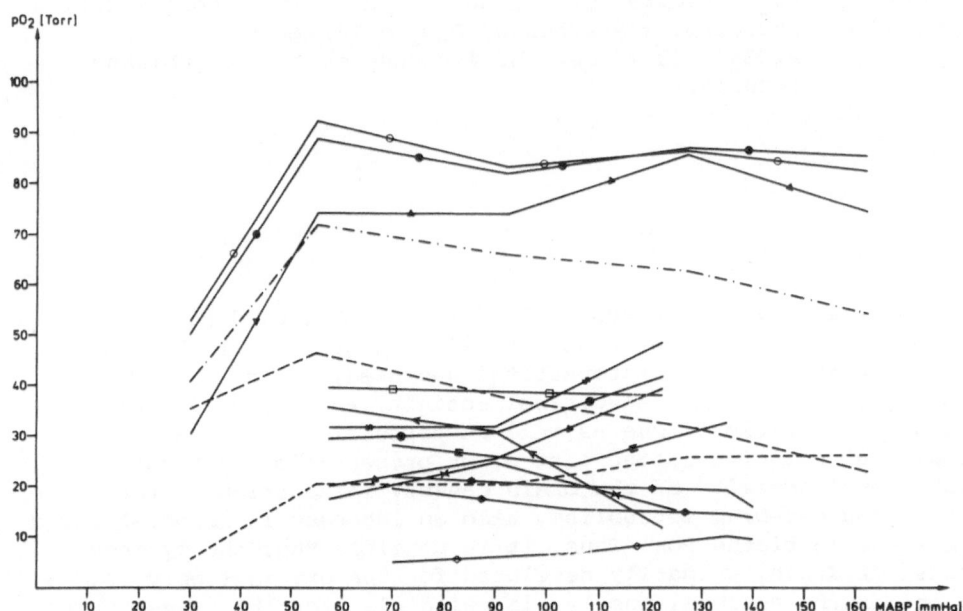

Fig. 3.   Brain tissue Po_2 (cat cortex) in dependence on mean arterial blood pressure (MABP). Note that Po_2 remains in most cases constant in the MABP range from 50 to 160 mm Hg: Below 50 mm Hg tissue Po_2 decreases parallel to the decrease in MAPB
(Leniger-Follert and Gronczewski, unpublished results)

resistance and thus counteracts the changes in MABP. Below the lower limit of the so-called autoregulatory range a decrease in flow occurs in parallel to the decrease in MABP. Fig. 3 shows the behavior of tissue Po_2 at different locations in the cat brain during stepwise changes in MABP induced by the procedure of Katsaros (1965). It can be seen that under normal conditions tissue Po_2 in the cat brain also remained fairly constant in the MABP range of about 50 to 150 mm Hg. Below values of 50 to 55 mm Hg Po_2 decreased drastically. Simultaneous measurements of ECoG and analysis of the power of ECoG clearly revealed that, in addition to the above parameters, functional activity also did not change in the autoregulatory range. As extracellular H^+ and K^+ activities did not change either (own unpublished results, Wahl and Kuschinsky (1979)), we may conclude that the predominant mechanism for the effect of flow autoregulation is a myogenic one, as already suggested by Bayliss long ago.

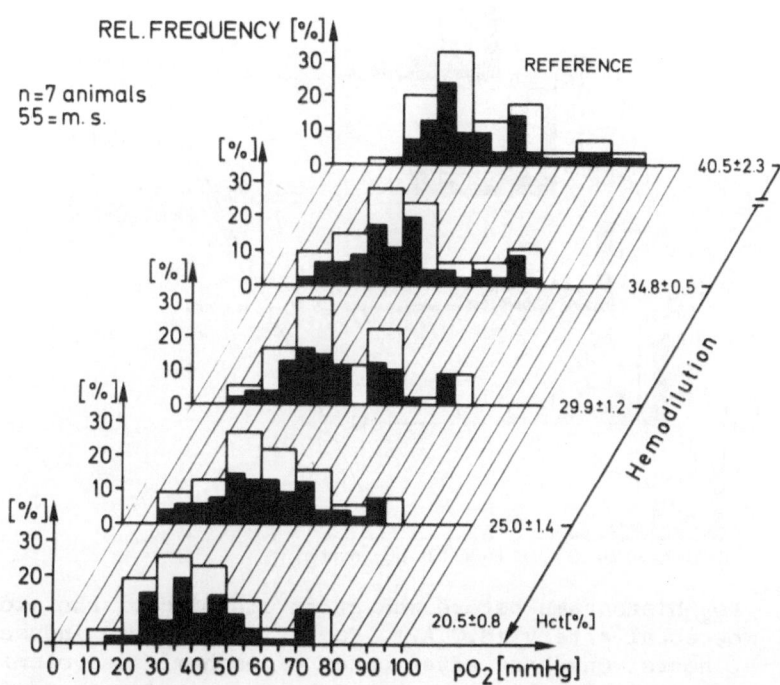

Fig. 4. Po_2 histograms of the normal brain tissue (cat anaesthetized with pentobarbital), at different arterial hematocrit. The histograms are not shifted to hypoxic values. Mean tissue Po_2 amounted in the control period to 42.1 mm Hg with hct of 40.5%, 40.3 mm Hg at 34.8%, 41.1 mm Hg at 29.9%, 41.4 mm Hg at 25.0%, 42.7 mm Hg at 20.5% (From Cahn and Leniger-Follert, Int. J. Microcirc. Clin Exp. 2:297-313(1983))

7

This conclusion may be supported by the fact that the steepness of the pressure changes is important, that is, that autoregulation is immediately seen when blood pressure is changed more slowly and gradually whereas very sudden changes in blood pressure delay the autoregulatory process. Under pathological conditions, for example during hypoxia, brain ischemia, hypoglycemia and severe ammonia intoxication, the flow autoregulation is abolished. In these cases, cerebral blood flow follows passively the changes in the effective perfusion pressure according to the law of

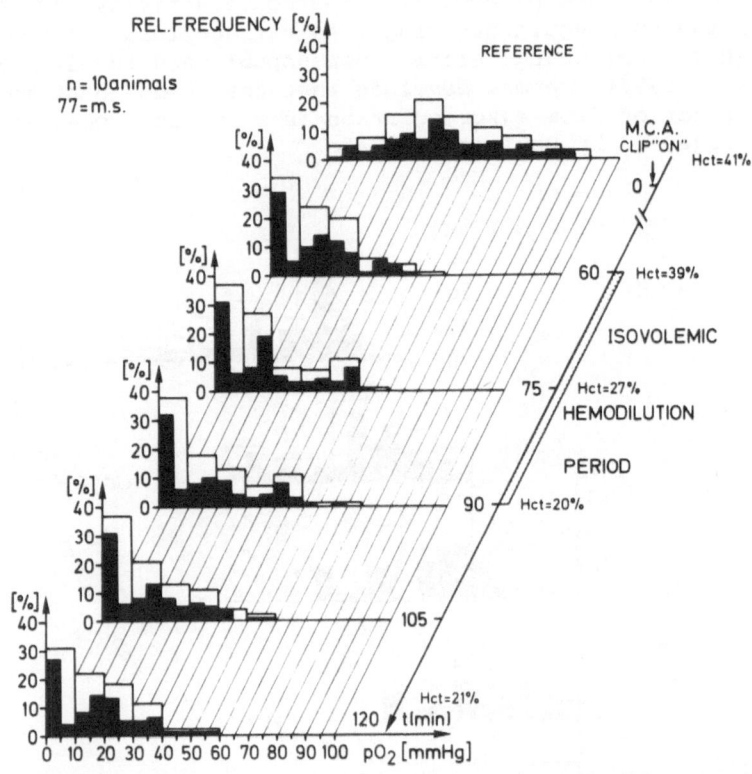

Fig. 5. Po$_2$ histograms before and after clamping of the middle cerebral artery (M.C.A.). Focal ischemia was induced for 2 hours. One hour after onset of ischemia isovolemic hemodilution was induced and hematocrit decreased from 39% to 20%. Mean tissue Po$_2$ 40.7 mm Hg at hct 41% with control state.
60 min after occlusion of MCA Po$_2$ 17.1 at hct 39%.
75 min   "   "   "   "   17.4 at hct 27%.
90 min   "   "   "   "   18.8 at hct 20%.
120 min   "   "   "   "   18.7 at hct 21%.
(From Cahn and Leniger-Follert, Int. J. Microcirc. Clin Exp. 2:297-313 (1983))

Hagen-Poiseuille. Parallel to the flow, brain Po_2 changes in the same direction.

3. Another important factor which influences cerebral blood flow and hence oxygen supply of the brain tissue is the fluidity of the blood. Hämodilution clearly reduces the viscosity and hence increases the blood flow according to the law of Hagen-Poiseuille. This has been proven for the brain as well as for other organs.

Regarding the O_2 supply of the brain the problem remains whether the decreased oxygen capacity of the arterial blood can completely be compensated by the increase in cerebral flow. We investigated this problem together with R. Cahn and induced isovolemic hemodilution with Dextran 40 in anaesthetized cats. Oxygen pressures and ECoG were measured in the normal and ischemic brain. The next figs. show a summary of our results (Cahn and Leniger, 1983). Mean Po_2 values and histograms were not significantly changed in the normal brain cortex when hematocrit was decreased from about 40% to 20% as shown in fig. 4. When focal ischemia was produced in another series of cat experiments tissue Po_2 and ECoG decreased, as was expected, and hypoxia clearly developed (Fig. 5). Hemodilution introduced in the second hour with persistent clamping of the middle cerebral artery did not further reduce the brain oxygen supply. On the other hand, no improvement of the oxygen partial pressures and the ECoG were observed. However, it should be considered that the improved microflow, which we could directly measure, ameliorates the so called "Spülfunktion". Thus, the situation is better for the brain in comparison to the reduced flow without hemodilution. Furthermore, it is possible to increase the low Po_2 in the hypoxic and also in the normal tissue if the oxygen content of the inspired gas is increased and thus arterial Po_2 is elevated (Leniger-Follert, unpublished results). Under the conditions of hemodilution and hypoxia the small constrictory effect of O_2, which normally occurs at the cerebral arterial vessels, is obviously overruled. Thus, a combination of hemodilution and of increased O_2 inspiration may be helpful in certain clinical situations.

4. Numerous investigations have shown that regional cerebral blood flow increases during activation of the corresponding tissue volume. We were able to show that flow in the microcirculatory range also increases in parallel to the increase in functional activity caused by direct electrical or by indirect physiological activation, or by generalized seizures. (Leniger-Follert and Lübbers 1976; Leniger-Follert and Hossmann, 1979; Leniger-Follert, 1984).

Fig. 6 shows a characteristic example of the tight coupling of functional activity and microflow behavior during seizures induced by bicuculline administration. Microflow increased immediately when the first signs of seizure activity appeared.

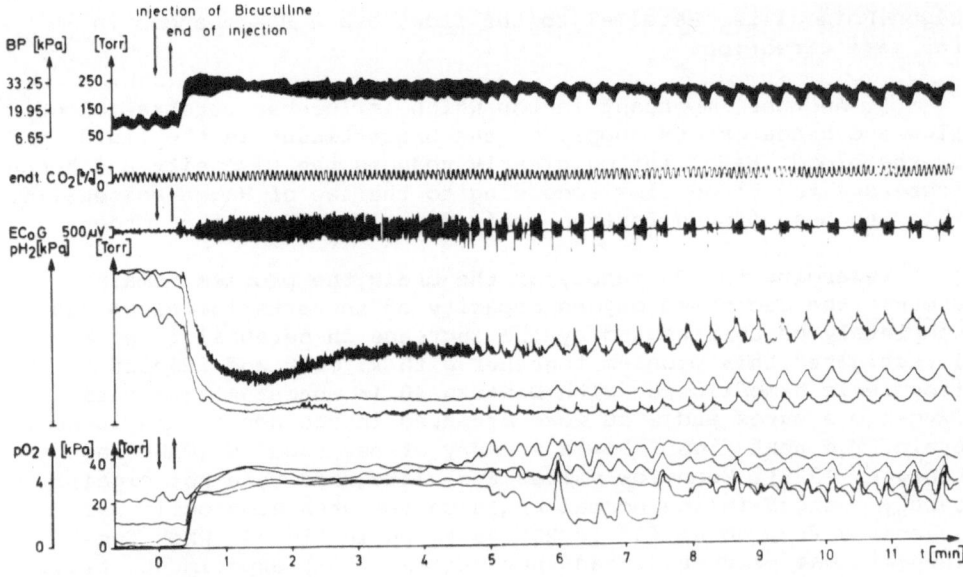

Fig. 6. Original simultaneous recording of blood pressure (BP),
end-tidal CO_2 content (endt. CO_2), electrocorticogram
(ECoG), microflow, and local tissue Po_2 before and
after the injection of bicuculline. A decrease in PH_2
means an increase in microflow. With the onset of seizures, microflow and tissue Po_2 distinctly increase.
During the periods of oscillating electrical activity,
microflow oscillates in parallel with the functional
activity, whereas Po_2 shows a more heterogeneous
behaviour. (From Leniger-Follert, J. Cereb. Blood Flow
Metabol., Vol 4(2) 1984, pp. 150-165)

During the period of oscillating functional activity the close
parallelism was especially distinct. Simultaneous Po_2 measurements showed that no initial hypoxia occured, which could elicit
the increase in flow, but on the contrary, Po_2 values increased
distinctly and later also showed some rhythmic oscillations. These
oscillations were, however, not homogeneous: some Po_2 values
increased during the silent phases, other Po_2 values decreased
simultaneously. The different behavior of Po_2 at different
locations may explain the controversial results reported in the
literature by different authors. However, no doubt exists that
anoxia or hypoxia does not develop during increased activity of
the nerve cells provided the arterial Po_2 is not decreased.

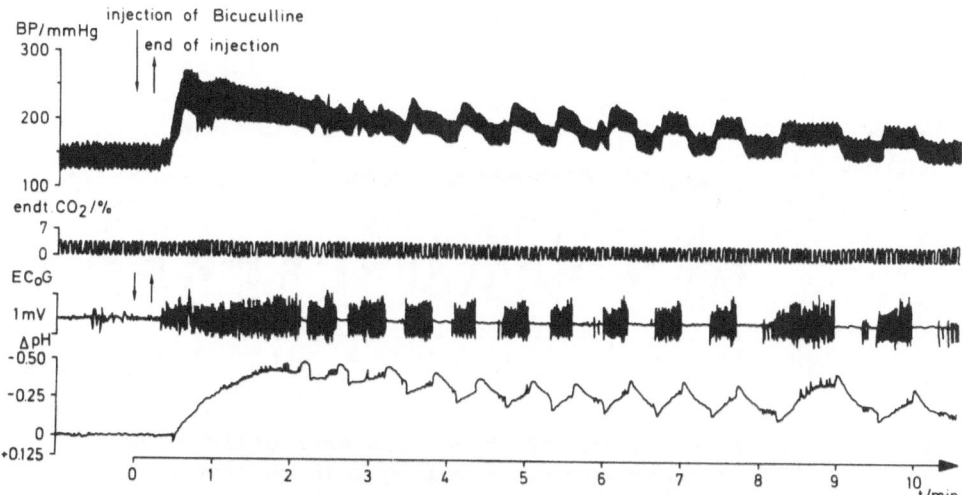

Fig. 7. Original recording of changes in local pH, electrocorticogram (ECoG), end-tidal CO_2 content (endt. CO_2), and
arterial blood pressure (BP). Note that pH changes in an
acidotic direction some seconds after the onset of
changes in ECoG without an initial alkaline shift. During
the period of repetitive short silent and active phases,
pH also oscillates. (From Leniger-Follert, J. Cereb.
Blood Flow Metabol., Vol 4(2) 1984, pp. 150-165)

Measurements of extracellular H^+ activity demonstrated that H^+
activity also cannot be the trigger mechanism for the flow increase
as $[H^+]_O$ increases some seconds <u>after</u> the increase in spike
activity and in microflow. However, in the later course of seizures
$[H^+]_O$ may contribute to the flow regulation, as a considerable
acidotic pH occurs and as H^+ activity oscillates in parallel to
the ECoG activity during the period of silent and non-silent
phases.

As already shown by numerous neurophysiological studies
extracellular K^+ activity increases within milliseconds when the
nerve cells are activated. Fig. 8 very clearly shows the tight
functional parallelism of functional activity and $[K^+]_O$
(Leniger-Follert, 1984), as measured in this case by a valinomycin
surface electrode according to Kessler et al. (1974). As microapplication studies of Wahl et al. (1970), Kuschinsky et al. (1972), and
Betz et al. (1973, 1978) have clearly established that the
pial and intraparenchymal arterial vessels dilate with increasing
acidity and with increasing K^+ activity in the range of 3 to 10 mM,
the conclusion may be drawn that $[K^+]_O$ is a <u>main</u> coupling factor

11

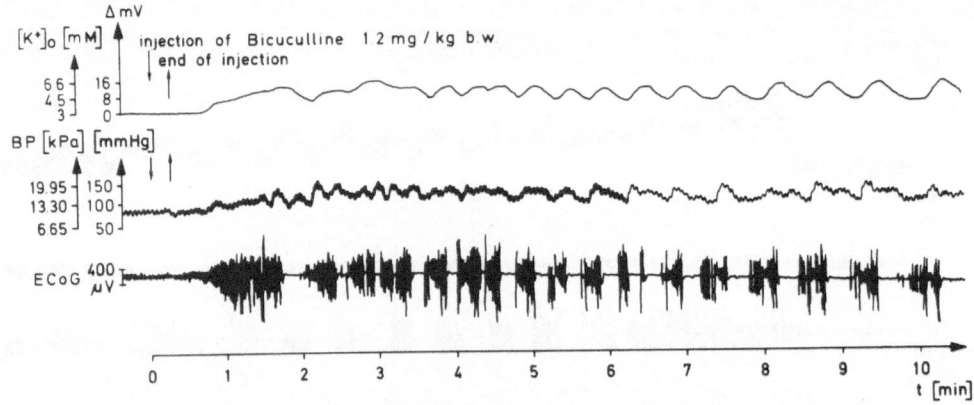

Fig. 8.   Original recording of changes in extracellular K^+
activity measured with a valinomycin surface electrode
and of changes in blood pressure (BP) and electrocorticogram (ECoG). Note the increase in K^+ activity with the
onset of seizures and the oscillations of K^+ activity
parallel to the oscillating functional activity
(From Leniger-Follert, J. Cereb. Blood Flow
Metabol., Vol 4(2) 1984, pp. 150-165)

between the functional activity of the nerve cells and the
cerebral blood flow, and that H^+ activity additionally contributes to the flow increase under extreme activation conditions,
for example under seizures and direct electrical activation.
However, under normal indirect physiological activation $[H^+]_O$
does not change in the activated area, whereas $[K^+]_O$ and
microflow show the same temporal relationship as we have already
reported (Leniger-Follert and Danz, 1981).

     5. Another situation when brain hypoxia is not the cause for
the increase in cerebral blood flow is severe hypoglycemia. In
rats, Norberg and Siesjö (1976) have demonstrated an increase in
blood flow in severe hypoglycemia and in isoelectric coma. Krolicki
and Leniger-Follert (1980) reported that Po_2 in rat brain begins
to increase at a mean arterial glucose concentration of about 1.39
mM and that during isoelectricity Po_2 is strongly elevated in
comparison to control conditions and early hypoglycemia. In cats,
anaesthetized with pentobarbital or with N_2O anaesthesia,
we also found an increase in tissue Po_2 during severe hypoglycemia
although functional activity strongly decreased as shown in
fig. 9 (Leniger et al., 1984).

12

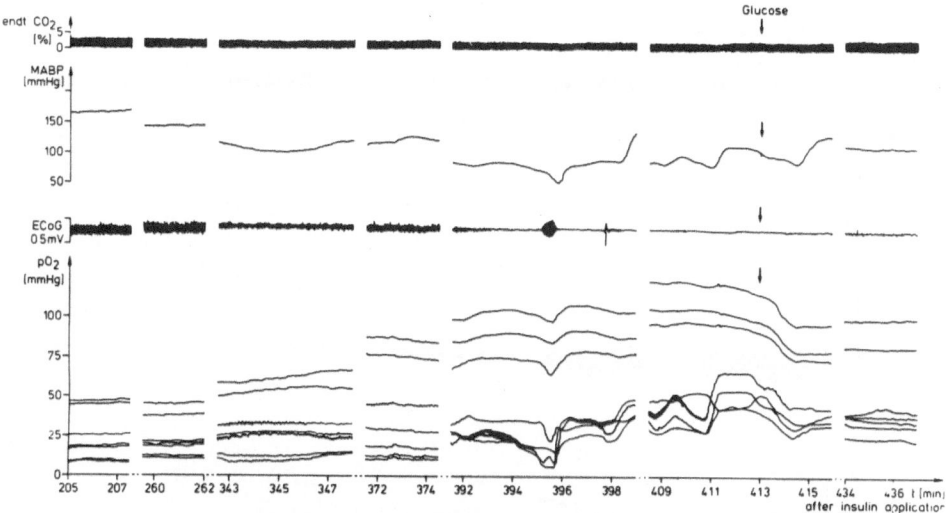

Fig. 9. Original registration of brain Po_2 in the cat during
different states of hypoglycemia. Note the start of
increase in tissue Po_2 at about 340 min after insulin
application although electrical activity decreased.
During isoelectricity Po_2 values are the strongest.
After glucose Po_2 decreases
(Leniger-Follert and Hufnagel, unpublished results)

However, the increase in tissue Po_2 in cats seems to
be less pronounced than the Po_2 increase in rats. When glucose
is administered after a short period of isoelectricity tissue
Po_2 decreases again. A complicating factor which must be considered
in this context is that flow autoregulation is abolished in severe
hypoglycemia. Thus, changes in MABP superimpose on the behavior of
cerebral blood flow and tissue Po_2.

We assume that the cause for the flow increase and Po_2
increase in rats and cats during severe hypoglycemia is the
increased ammonia production which occurs when amino acids
are metabolized instead of the missing glucose. Increased brain
ammonia leads firstly to an increase in cerebral microflow and
tissue Po_2 (Gronczewski and Leniger-Follert, 1984).

Fig. 10 shows an original registration of tissue
Po_2 during different phases of infusion of ammonium acetate.
Ammonium acetate, pH 7.4, was infused at a dose of 100 µM/kgxmin

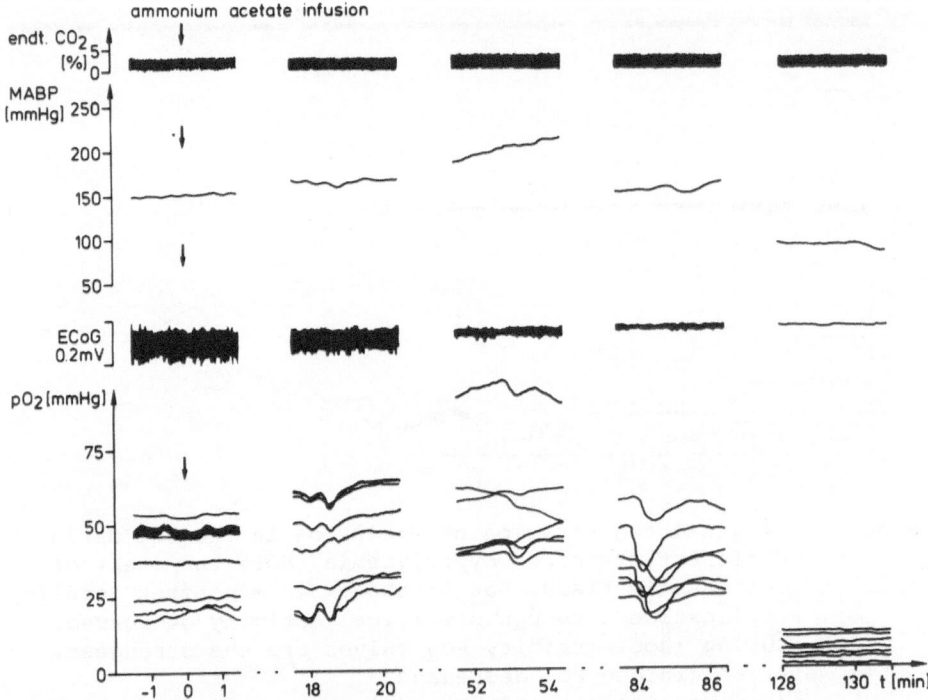

Fig. 10. Original registration of brain Po_2 in the cat during different phases of infusion of ammonium acetate (dose 100 μM/kgxmin). Note the initial increase in Po_2 with simultaneous decrease in ECoG. In the later phase, Po_2 decreases again. At isoelectricity a strong hypoxia or anoxia is present. (Gronczewski and Leniger-Follert, unpublished results)

until isoelectricity of ECoG. It can be clearly seen that Po_2 increased some time after the onset of infusion. Po_2 reached a maximal value and afterwards declined below control values. At isoelectricity hypoxia respectively anoxia developed. Parallel measurements of microflow in another experimental study showed that microflow increased some time after onset of infusion, reached a maximal value and then drastically declined. Fig. 11 shows the Po_2 histograms of different phases of ammonium acetate infusion. A clear shift to the right was seen some time during infusion. At the onset of isoelectricity a hypoxic histogram was observed (Gronczewski and Leniger-Follert, unpublished results).

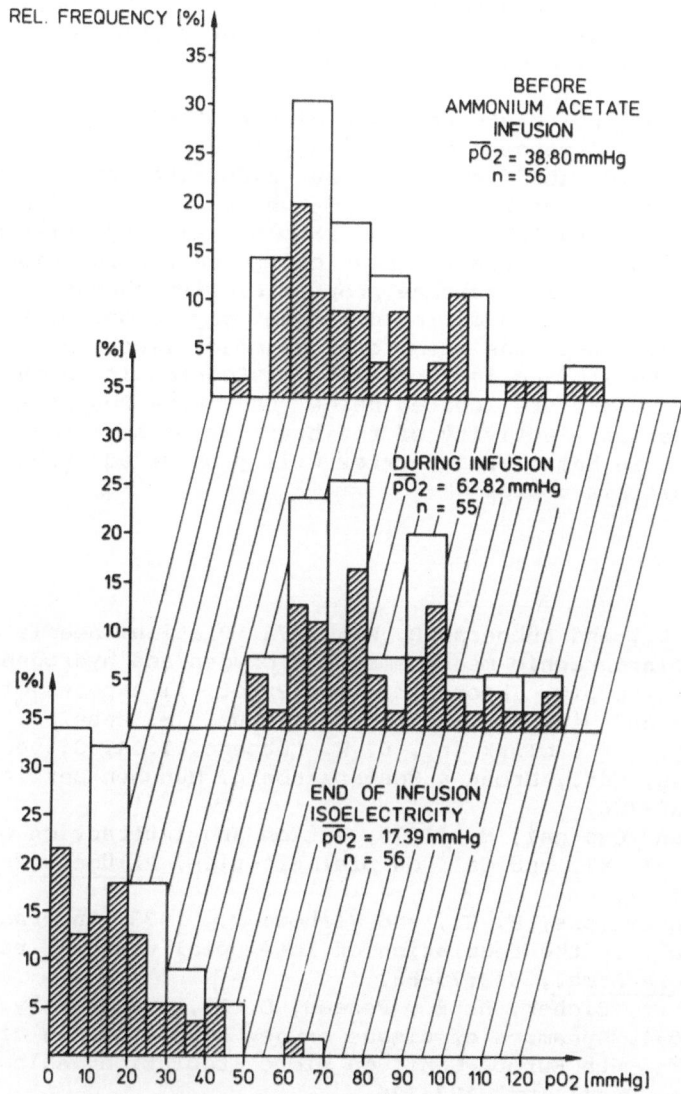

Fig. 11. Po$_2$ histograms at different phases of infusion of ammonium acetate. Note the increase in mean tissue Po$_2$ and the shift of the histogram to the right during infusion. At isoelectricity hypoxia or anoxia is present. (Gronczewski and Leniger-Follert, unpublished results)

With this I come to the end of my presentation. In summary, measurements of microflow, functional activity and of tissue Po$_2$ in the brain have clearly demonstrated that the oxygen supply of the brain changes under different physiological and pathophysiological conditions.

The actual Po$_2$ histogram as a mirror of the oxygen supply of the brain is dependent on a variety of factors arising from the arterial side and from the tissue side. The arterial factors are, beside MABP, the P$_a$CO$_2$ and P$_a$O$_2$ which were not discussed in this minireview. Furthermore, the rheological properties of the blood are important. From the side of tissue the functional activity and the changes in membrane properties with changes in extracellular ion activities during different physiological and pathophysiological conditions seem to be of major importance. A further question to be studied is if the Po$_2$ histograms in which the majority of Po$_2$ values are located below the venous Po$_2$ indicate a reduced functional activity of the brain as we have found. Further measurements in human brain cortex will provide additional information about this topic.

REFERENCES

Baumgärtl, H., and Lübbers, D. W., 1973, Platinum needle electrode for polarographic measurement of oxygen and hydrogen, in: "Oxygen Supply, Theoretical and Practical Aspects of Oxygen Supply and Microcirculation of Tissue," M. Kessler, D. F. Bruley, L. C. Clark jr., D. W. Lübbers, I. A. Silver, J. Strauss, eds., Urban & Schwarzenberg, München-Berlin-Wien, pp. 130-136.

Betz, E., and Czornai, M., 1978, Action and interaction of perivascular H$^+$, K$^+$, and Ca^{++} on pial arteries, Pflügers Arch., 374:67-72.

Betz, E., Enzenross, H. G., and Vlahow, V., 1973, Interaction of H$^+$ and Ca^{++} in the regulation of local pial vascular resistance, Pflügers Arch., 343:79-88.

Bruley, D. F., Bicher, H. E., Reneau, D. D., and Knisely, M. H., 1971, Dynamics of tissue oxygen supply during circulatory failure, 6th Europ. Conf. on Microcirculation, Aalborg 1970, Karger, Basel, pp. 193-196.

Cahn, R., and Leniger-Follert, E., 1983, Effect of isovolemic hemodilution on oxygen supply and electrocorticogram in cat brain during focal ischemia and in normal tissue, Int. J. Microcirc.: Clin. Exp., 2:297-313.

Clark, L. C. jr., 1956, Monitor and control of blood tissue oxygen tension, Trans. Soc. Art. Int. Organs, 2:41.

Erdmann, W., Kunke, St., and Krell, W., 1973, Tissue pO$_2$ and cell function - an experimental study with multimicroelectrodes in the rat brain, in: "Oxygen Supply, Theoretical and Practical

Aspects of Oxygen Supply and Microcirculation of Tissue," M. Kessler, D. F. Bruley, L. C. Clark jr., D. W. Lübbers, I. A. Silver, J. Strauss, eds., Urban & Schwarzenberg, München-Berlin-Wien, pp. 169-174.

Gronczewski, J., and Leniger-Follert, E., 1984, Relationship between microflow, local tissue pO_2 and extracellular activities of potassium and hydrogen ions in the cat brain during intraarterial infusion of ammonium acetate, Adv. Exp. Med. Biol., 169:291-296.

Grote, J., Zimmer, K., and Schubert, R., 1981, Effects of severe arterial hypocapnia on regional blood flow regulation, tissue pO_2 and metabolism in the brain cortex of cats, Pflügers Arch., 391: 195-199.

Grunewald, W., and Sowa, W., 1977, Capillary structures and O_2 supply to tissue. An analysis with a digital diffusion model applied to the skeletal muscle. Rev. Physiol. Biochem. Pharmacol., 77:149-209.

Harper, A. M., 1966, Autoregulation of cerebral blood flow: influence of the arterial blood pressure on the blood flow through the cerebral cortex, J. Neurol. Neurosurg. Psychiat., 29:398-403.

Katsaros, B., 1965, Der Effekt der Durchtrennung der Sinusnerven auf die Atmung der narkotisierten Katze bei konstant gehaltenem arteriellen Druck und seine Abhängigkeit vom CO_2-Druck, Pflügers Arch., 282:179-185.

Kessler, M., Höper, J., and Simon, W., 1974, Methodology and application of multiple ion selective surface electrode (pH, pK, pNa, pCa, pCl) for tissue measurements, Fed. Proc., 33: 279.

Kessler, M., 1974, Lebenserhaltende Mechanismen bei Sauerstoffmangel und bei Störungen der Organdurchblutung. Mitteilg. Max-Planck-Ges. 444-463.

Kessler, M., Lübbers, D.W., 1966, Aufbau und Anwendungsmöglichkeit verschiedener pO_2-Elektroden, Pflügers Arch., 291:82.

Krogh, A., 1918/1919, The rate of diffusion of gases through animal tissues with some remarks on the coefficient of invasion. J. Physiol., 52:391-408.

Krolicki, L., and Leniger-Follert, E., 1980, Oxygen supply of the brain cortex (rat) during severe hypoglycemia, Pflügers Arch., 387:121-126.

Kuschinsky, W., and Wahl, M., 1978, Local chemical and neurogenic regulation of cerebral vascular resistance, Physiol. Rev., 58: 656-689.

Kuschinsky, W., Wahl, M., Bosse, O., and Thurau, K., 1972, Perivascular potassium and pH as determinants of local pial arterial diameter in cats. A microapplication study, Circ. Res., 31: 240-247.

Leniger-Follert, E., 1984, Mechanisms of regulation of cerebral microflow during bicuculline-induced seizures in anaesthetized cats, J. Cereb. Blood Flow Metab., 4:150-165.

Leniger-Follert, E., and Danz, C., 1981, The role of extracellular potassium and hydrogen activities in the brain cortex for regulation of cerebral microcirculation in the cat during generalized seizures and specific sensory stimulation, in: "Progress in Enzyme and Ion-Selective Electrodes," D. W. Lübbers, H. Acker, R. P. Buck, G. Eisenman, M. Kessler and W. Simon, eds., Springer-Verlag, Berlin-Heidelberg-New York, pp. 100-105.

Leniger-Follert, E., Gronczewski, J., and Danz, C., 1984, Regulation of microflow in the cat brain during insulin induced hypoglycemia, Adv. Exp. Med. Biol., 169:297-303.

Leniger-Follert, E., and Hossmann, K.-A., 1979, Simultaneous measurements of microflow and evoked potentials in the somatomotor cortex of the cat brain during specific sensory activation, Pflügers Arch., 380:85-89.

Leniger-Follert, E., and Lübbers, D. W., 1976, Behavior of microflow and local pO_2 of the brain cortex during and after direct electrical stimulation. A contribution to the problem of metabolic regulation of microcirculation in the brain, Pflügers Arch.,366:39-44.

Leniger-Follert, E., Lübbers, D. W., Wrabetz, W., 1975, Regulation of local tissue pO_2 of the brain cortex at different arterial O_2 pressures, Pflügers Arch., 359:81-95.

Lübbers, D. W., 1977, Die Bedeutung des lokalen Gewebesauerstoffdruckes und des pO_2-Histogrammes für die Beurteilung der Sauerstoffversorgung eines Organes, Prak. Anästhesie. Wiederbelebung und Intensivtherapie, 12:183-193.

Lübbers, D. W., 1981, Grundlagen und Bedeutung der lokalen Sauerstoffdruckmessung und des pO_2-Histogramms für die Beurteilung der Sauerstoffversorgung der Organe und des Organismus, in: "Messung des Gewebesauerstoffdruckes bei Patienten," A. M. Ehrly, ed., Gerhard Witzstrock, Baden-Baden-Köln-New York, pp. 11-21.

Metzger, H., 1973, pO_2 histograms of threedimensional systems with homogeneous and inhomogeneous microcirculation - a digital computer study, in: "Oxygen Supply, Theoretical and Practical Aspects of Oxygen Supply and Microcirculation of Tissue," M. Kessler, D. F. Bruley, L. C. Clark jr., D. W. Lübbers, I. A. Silver, J. Strauss, eds., Urban & Schwarzenberg, München-Berlin-Wien, pp. 18-24.

Metzger, H., Heuber-Metzger, S., Steinacker, A., and Strüber, J., 1980, Staining pO_2 measurement sites in the rat brain cortex and quantitative morphometry of the surrounding capillaries, Pflügers Arch., 388:21-27.

Norberg, K., and Siesjö, B. K., 1976, Oxidative metabolism of the cerebral cortex of the rat in severe insulin-induced hypoglycemia, J. Neurochem., 26:345-352.

Silver, I. A., 1965, Some observations on the cerebral cortex with an ultramicro, membrane-covered oxygen electrode, Med. Electron. Biol. Engng., 3:377-387.

Smith, R. H., Guilbeau, E. J., and Reneau, D. D., 1977, The oxygen tension field within a discrete volume of cerebral cortex, Microvasc. Res., 13:233–240.

Thews, G., 1960, Die Sauerstoffdiffusion im Gehirn, Pflügers Arch., 271:197–226.

Wahl, M., Deetjen, P., Thurau, K., Ingvar, D. H., and Lassen, N. A., 1970, Micropuncture evaluation of the importance of perivascular pH for the arteriolar diameter on the brain surface, Pflügers Arch., 316:152–163.

Wahl, M., and Kuschinsky, W., 1979, Unimportance of perivascular H^+ and K^+ activities for the adjustment of pial artery diameter during changes in arterial blood flow pressure in cats, Pflügers Arch., 382:203–208.

Whalen, W. F., Canfield, R., and Nair, P., 1970, Effects of breathing O_2 or $O_2 + CO_2$ and of the injection of neurohumors on the Po_2 of cat cerebral cortex, Stroke, 1:194–200.

Whalen, W. F., Riley, J., and Nair, P., 1967, A microelectrode for measuring intracellular Po_2, J. Appl. Physiol., 23:798–801.

Wiernsperger, N., Gygax, P., and Meier-Ruge, W., 1978, Changes in cerebrocortical pO_2 distribution, rCBF and EEG during hypovolemic shock, Adv. Exp. Med. Biol., 94:605–610.

MYOCARDIAL OXYGEN PRESSURE: MIRROR OF OXYGEN SUPPLY

S. Schuchhardt

Institut für Physiologie
Freie Universität Berlin
Berlin (West)

The supply of oxygen to the tissues of warm-blooded animals follows a common underlying principle. Within it, each organ has its own particular properties. This has just been shown very impressively for the brain by Leniger-Follert (this volume). The heart, also, has its special aspects of oxygen supply: periodic interruption of blood flow due to the heart action, low oxygen content in the coronary veins, continuous changes in the oxygen requirements and so on.

Which oxygen pressures are present in the myocardium?

In the past 20 years, numerous research groups have measured oxygen pressure values or complete histograms under physiologic conditions; or better: under conditions as physiological as possible, i.e.: in the beating heart in situ of an anaesthetized artificially ventilated thoracotomized animal - or in humans during cardiac surgery. Almost all of these pO_2 values were registered using platinum electrodes, particularly needle electrodes; in recent years, surface electrodes have found increasing use.

Both types of electrodes have their advantages and disadvantages. Needle electrodes have the following disadvantages: 1. they are highly susceptible to disturbances; 2. they may destroy tissue and reduce the blood circulation; 3. preparing a histogram requires considerable time. Their advantage is the ability to reach deeper layers of an organ. Surface electrodes have the disadvantage of registering only the outermost layer of an organ, e.g. in the case of the heart, only the epicardium and a bit of the myocardium. They have the following advantages: 1. they permit very stable measurements - being Clark-electrodes; 2. they leave tissues and blood circulation intact; 3. the histogram may be recorded quickly. Be-

cause of these advantages, surface electrodes are greatly superior
to needle electrodes, particularly for practical clinical application. - Both types of electrodes are generally too slow to measure
pO_2 changes during heart cycle; they integrate over these periodic
fluctuations. - I would only like to mention that it is possible to
measure the oxygen pressure on the inside of the ventricles using
catheter electrodes.

Before turning to a historical review of the results, I should
like to remind you of the typical features of a pO_2 histogram of the
heart muscle. I will show a histogram recorded by my group in the
recent past (Fig. 1). Values are shown as a bar diagram and in cumulative form. The tip diameter of the electrodes applied in these
experiments is about 100 µm; now we use thinner electrodes with a
mean diameter of 20 µm. Dog hearts were used with typical penetration
depths of 2-5 mm. The median value is 20 mm Hg, i.e.: approximately
half of all tissue values were below the coronary venous pO_2. This
is similar for all organs as Leniger-Follert has already mentioned
and has many causes: capillary structure, inhomogeneities in blood
flow, uneven distributions of red cells and plasma, possibly a
certain contribution due to shunt diffusion. The contour of this
type of histogram varies considerably under physiological conditions.

All of the factors which influence the oxygen distribution in
the tissues make themselves felt in some form in the histogram, but
in such a summary fashion, that they cannot be analysed in detail.
I will refer to that later on. - In the following table I should
like to give you a review of various measured pO_2 histograms in the
heart muscle as promised (Tab. 1). The mean or median values are set
out in the column "pO_2 histogram". We consider the values of Lösse
et al., which we published 1975, to be somewhat too low; our electrodes had at that time not been systematically tested during the
measurement in the heart. Particularly interesting are determinations
using other methods, e.g. Brantigan et al. (1972) with mass spectrometry and Grunewald and Lübbers (1975) by means of cryophotometric
determinations of the capillary hemoglobin saturation. Both studies
show values within the range of the other measurements. This range
has a mean for needle electrodes of about 20 mm Hg. The mean for
surface electrodes is clearly higher. In a few cases, e.g. Kessler
et al. (1984) and Hauss et al. (1984), the lowest values for tissue
are about 30 mm Hg, i.e. considerably higher than for the coronary
venous pO_2. This, however, is not possible; the lowest values must
be at least somewhat below the venous pO_2. Thus, the corresponding
venous pO_2 value for these pO_2-distributions must be considerably
higher than that of the coronary sinus. It is possible, that the
supply to these outer layers of the heart is better than in the
remaining myocardium.

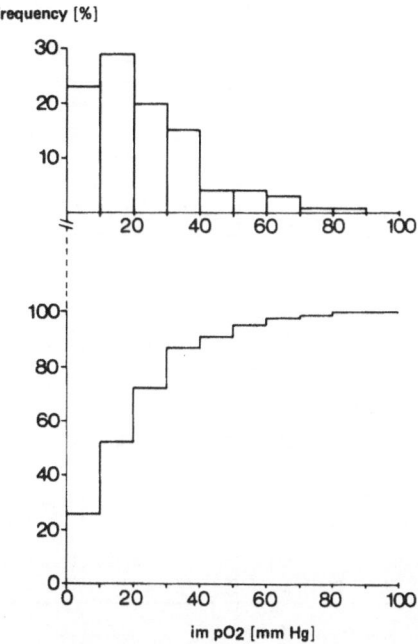

Fig. 1. Frequency distribution of intramyocardial oxygen pressure (im pO_2) plotted as column and cumulative histogram; measured with needle electrodes in the dog heart left ventricle. n=115. Arterial pO_2 60-90 mm Hg; mean coronary venous pO_2 19 mm Hg.

Until now it has not been possible to standardize histograms; they still depend too much on the respective method. - I have not included measurements on human hearts in this list, since in this case the arterial pO_2 scatters over a very large range. Gardner and co-workers (1971) measured oxygen pressures in human hearts using mass spectrometry. Mendler et al. (1973) studied four patients during heart surgery with needle electrodes; the resulting histogram is very similar to those from warm-blooded experimental animals.

Table 1. Review of measured pO_2 histograms in heart muscle.

publication	animal	region left ventricle	method	pO2 histogram (or values) mean	median [mm Hg]	n	remarks	Fi O2	pO2 art. coron.ven. [mm Hg]	
Kadatz	1969 dog	intramyoc.	Pt needle electr.;tip diamet. 15–25μm	24		29		0.21		
Winbury et al.	1971 dog	intramyoc.	double Pt needle electr.;tip diamet. 177μm	21		15	no histogram	0.21		
Whalen	1971 cat	intramyoc.(right and left ventricle)	needle electr.,gold plated;tip diamet. 1–3μm	7		104	suction device for electr.	0.21		
Brantigan et al.	1972 dog	intramyoc.	mass spectrometry;tip diamet. 1.5 mm	18		10	no histogram	0.21		
Lösse et al.	1975 dog	intramyoc.	Pt needle electr.;tip diamet. 35–275μm	19	14	151		0.21	64	19
Grunewald et al.	1975 rabbit	intramyoc.	intracap. Hb-saturat; pO2 calculated	22	22	119		0.21		18
v.d. Laarse et al.	1975 dog	intramyoc.	10 fold Pt-electr. tip diamet. 200μm	32		113		0.21	100 120	
Skolasinska et al.	1978 cat	surface	multiwire Pt Clark type electr.		31	182		0.21		
Schuchhardt et al.	1978 dog	intramyoc.	Pt needle electr.;tip diamet. 100μm	28	25	61		0.21	60 90	19
Kessler et al.	1984 dog	surface	multiwire Pt Clark type electr.	50;59;59 28;49;32		104		0.50 0.21		
Hauss et al.	1984 dog	surface	multiwire Pt Clark type electr.	49		766		0.21	74	

One final point concerning the mean oxygen pressure in the various layers between the endo- and the epicardium: there exist contradictory findings in the literature. Some authors measured lower values in the subendocardial layer, e.g. Moss (1968), Winbury et al. (1971), Weiss (1974) and Yokoyama et al. (1978). Others found no differences. Schuster et al. (1979) and Breull et al. (1981) have studied this question and found no differences in the mean pO_2 in the different layers.

The local oxygen pressure once established in the myocardium remains rather constant if not influenced by experimental interventions and so on.

How does myocardial oxygen pressure vary due to a change in the oxygen supply or in cardiac activity?

There exist only a few investigations about this topic in the beating heart in situ. I would like to begin with our own studies about hypoxia and to show you the behaviour of local ("local" as a relative term) pO_2 registered with needle electrodes during temporary decrease of arterial pO_2 in the dog (Fig. 2). The oxygen pressure is measured at two points in the myocardium; at one point (upper trace) pO_2 is between 35 and 40 mm Hg; at the other one it is between 10 and 15 mm Hg. Furthermore, coronary blood flow and arterial blood pressure are recorded. (The lowest trace are blood gas analyses which need not concern us here.) At the point of the first arrow the dog breathes 10% oxygen for about 7 minutes. The arterial pO_2 during this time is 33 mm Hg. The tissue pO_2 decreases noticeably at both measurement points, the higher value more strongly than the lower. The coronary blood flow increases, but not sufficiently to compensate the decrease in pO_2, which would have been quite possible. It may be easily demonstrated that a large blood flow reserve exists in this case (Fig. 3). In this case, pO_2 was measured in one location only. Up to the vertical arrow, the course of the experiment is the same as before. Then dipyridamole was injected intravenously. The blood flow increases strongly, but pO_2 only marginally, an indication, that the greatest part of the blood flow increase fails to reach the location, where pO_2 is measured. Dipyridamole in about half of the cases enlarges the inhomogeneity of blood flow.

The relationship between intramyocardial oxygen pressure and coronary blood flow during hypoxia is shown graphically by Fig. 4. The arterial oxygen saturation and the corresponding oxygen pressure are plotted on the abscissa (assuming as simplification, that the oxygen binding curve did not shift during the experiments), while the ordinate shows coronary blood flow and intramyocardial pO_2. For an arterial pO_2 of 53 mm Hg, the mean tissue pO_2 has dropped from 22 to 16 mm Hg; the coronary blood flow has increased by only a small amount. Two experiments with 10% O_2 respiration (corresponding mean arterial pO_2 33 mm Hg) we saw in Figs. 2 and 3. Quite on the

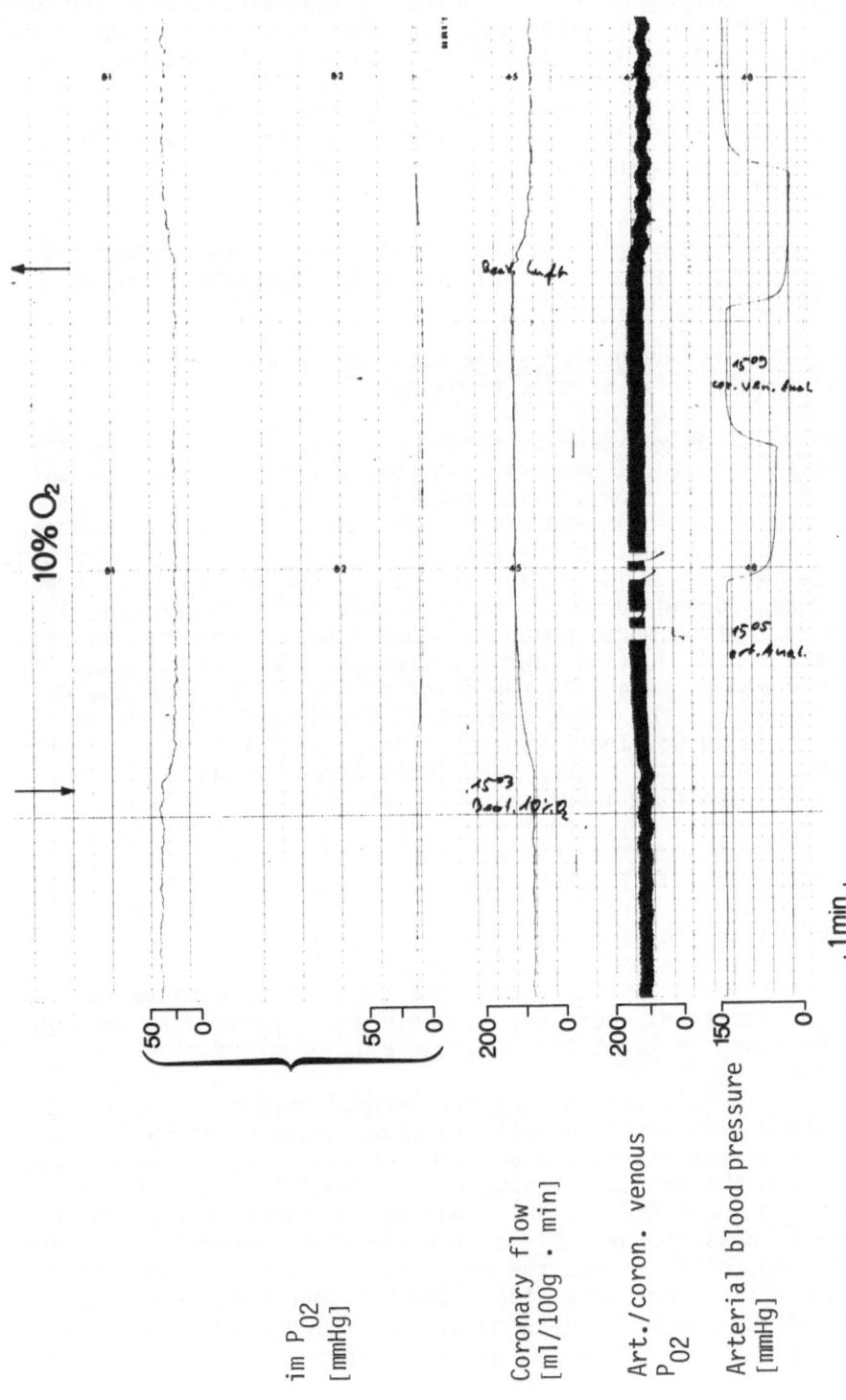

Fig. 2. Recording of intramyocardial oxygen pressure (impO_2) measured at two sites in the dog myocardium, coronary flow and arterial blood pressure during temporary respiration with 10% O_2 (lowest trace: recording of analyses of arterial and coronary venous pO_2).

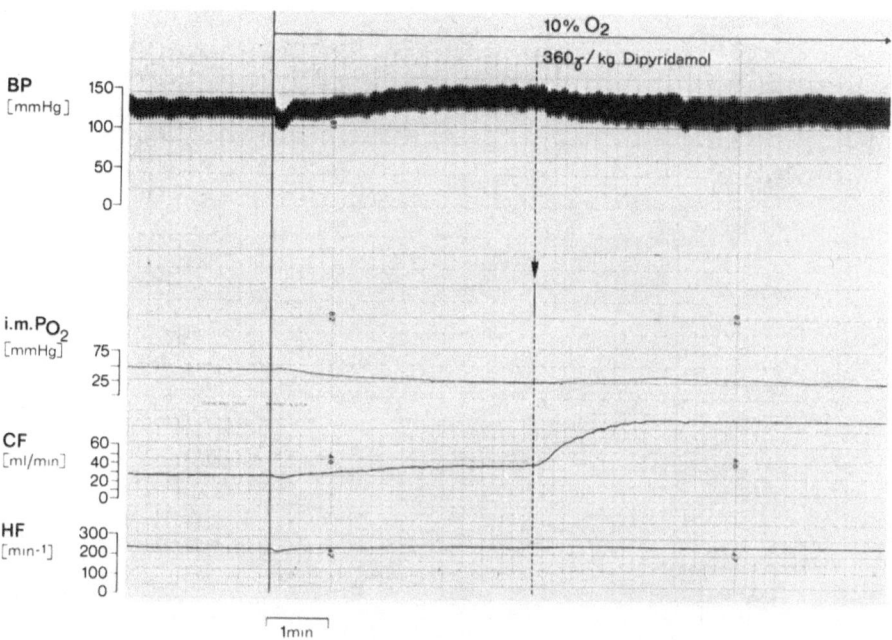

Fig. 3. Recording of arterial blood pressure (BP), intramyocardial
         oxygen pressure (im pO_2), coronary blood flow (CF) and
         heart frequency (HF) in the dog during respiration with
         10% O_2 and administration of dipyridamole.

left side of the figure we have a temporary anoxia, the coronary
blood flow increases by nearly a factor of 6 from the initial value.
Skolasinska et al. (1978) have found very similar results with
surface electrodes on the beating rabbit heart (Fig. 5). A and C are
normal histograms. B is the hypoxia with 10% O_2, the arterial pO_2 is
33 mm Hg, exactly the same value as in our experiments - so to say
the German standard hypoxia. The pO_2 distribution is shifted to the
left. D is an extreme shift to the left during an arterial pO_2 of
19 mm Hg.

    Now, however, I should like to lead you out of the gloomy cave
of anoxia into the realm of hyperoxia. Menke et al. (1984) have investigated the influence of an elevated arterial pO_2 on the tissue
pO_2. Fig. 6 shows an example of temporary respiration of 100% O_2.
The upper trace is the intramyocardial pO_2, measured with needle
electrodes, tip diameter 20 μm. Below it the coronary blood flow,
then blood pressure and heart rate are recorded. In this series of
experiments we carried out test occlusions, in order to determine
the amount of reactive hyperaemia; I shall not discuss this point
further. At the arrow at the bottom the respiration was switched to
100% O_2. pO_2 rises rapidly to a value above 100 mm Hg; such a rise

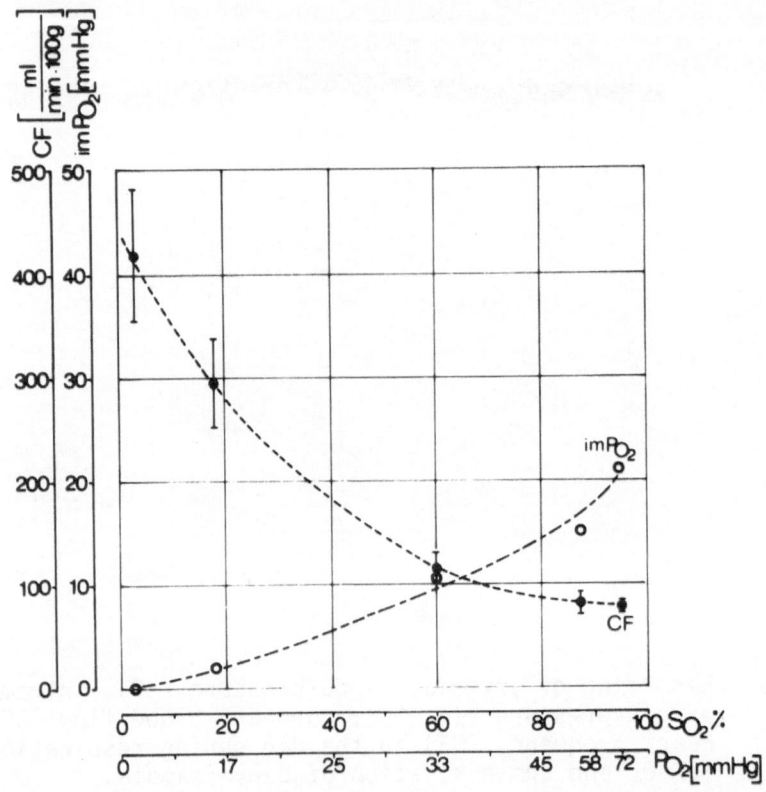

Fig. 4.   Intramyocardial oxygen pressure (im pO_2; median values) and coronary flow (CF; means ± SE) in dependency upon arterial oxygen saturation (SO_2) and arterial oxygen pressure (pO_2) in the dog.

above the binding region of hemoglobin is rarely found in the myocardium, in this series in 6% of the cases. In 20% of the cases the tissue pO_2 does not increase at all. We never found a decrease of pO_2. Fig. 7 shows the shift of the histogram during oxygen respiration. We have here corresponding measurements taken with the same electrode inserted in the tissue, the distribution of the initial values is dotted, the values of O_2-respiration are the full lines. The mean tissue pO_2 increases from 22 to 46 mm Hg. There is a certain relation between the level of the initial pO_2 and the height of the increase; for high initial values, the increase is for the most part larger. This means that with sufficiently thin electrodes a certain differentiation of the pO_2 field in the microregion of the myocardium is possible. Furthermore, the result is an indication of the incompleteness of the regulation. This reaction to pure oxygen is indeed something which nature has not experienced for millions of years; perhaps it has to be relearned. During hyperoxia, the coronary venous

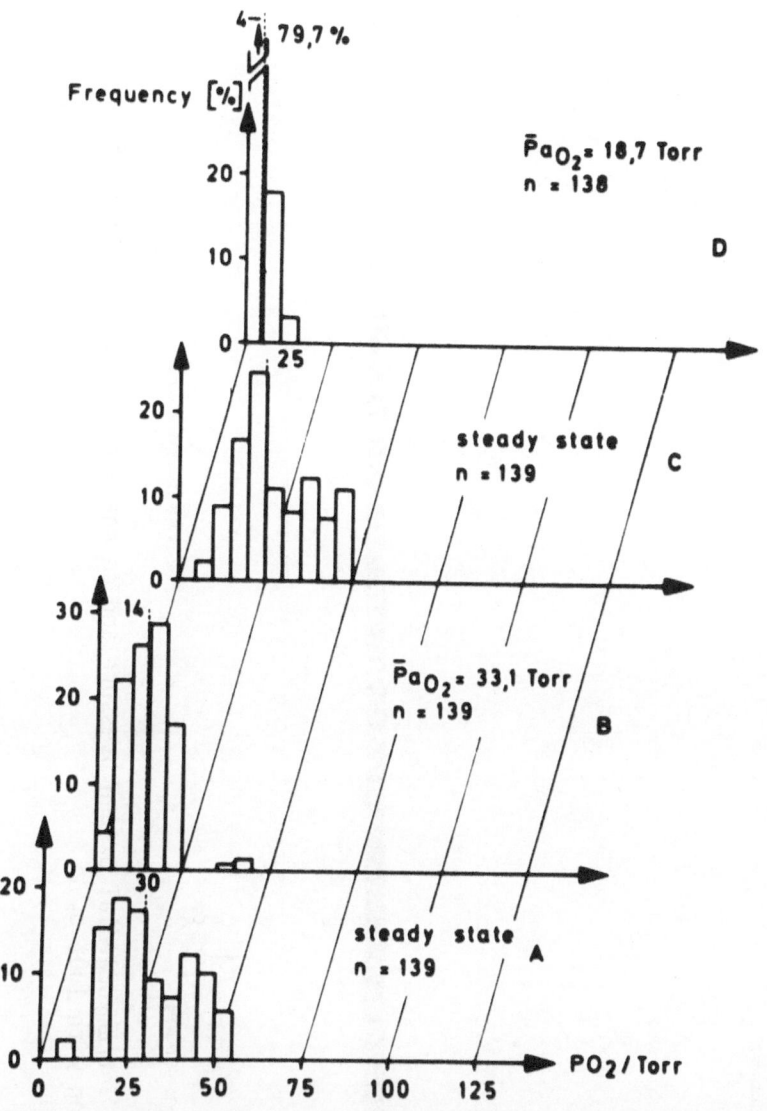

Fig. 5. pO$_2$ distribution on the surface of the beating rabbit heart in situ at normoxia (A, C) and hypoxia (B, D); for further details see text.
From Skolasinska et al. (1978).

pO$_2$ shows only small changes. In the case of hypoxia, as well, the reaction of coronary pO$_2$ is delayed when compared to the tissue pO$_2$. The latter is thus a considerably better mirror of the actual oxygen supply to the myocardium.

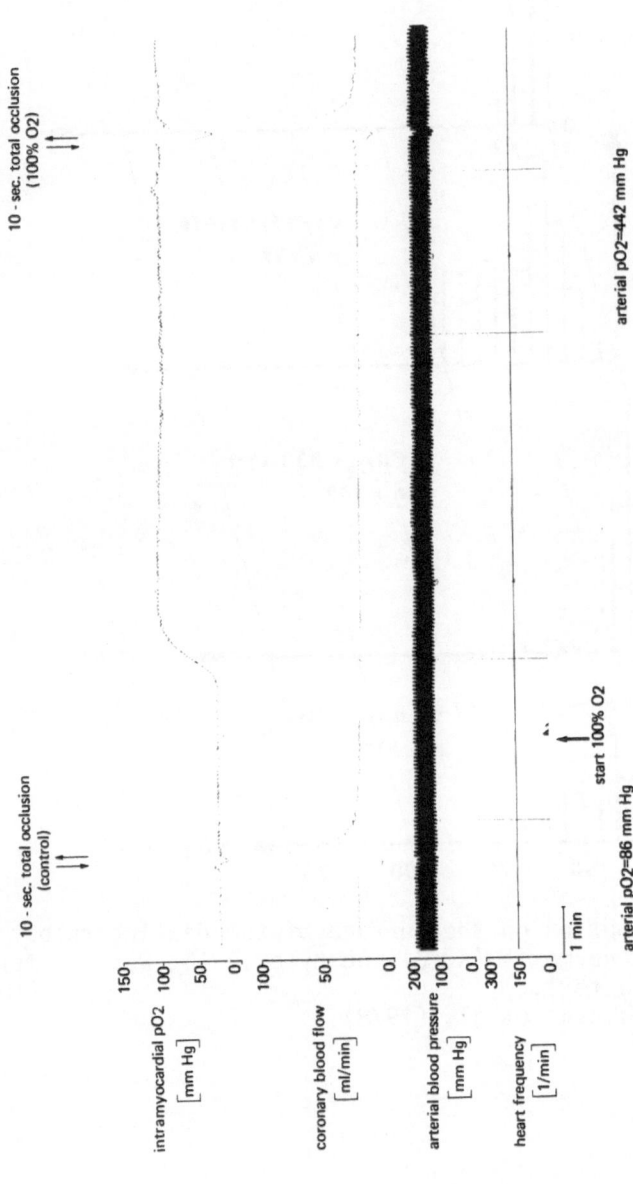

Fig. 6. Recording of intramyocardial oxygen pressure and coronary blood flow in response to ventilation with 100% O_2.

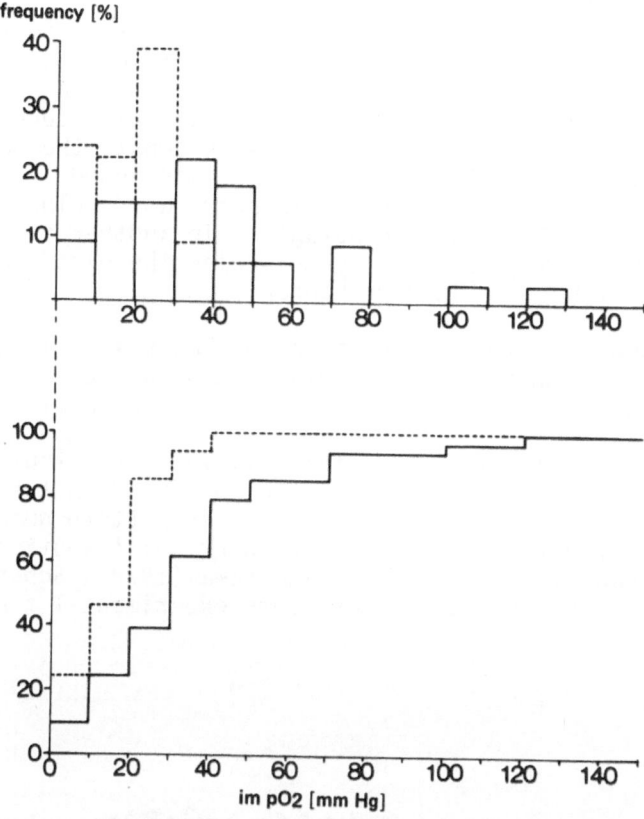

Fig. 7. Oxygen pressure histogram (column and cumulative form) of
dog myocardium (im pO_2) during respiration with air (dotted
line, arterial pO_2 60-90 mm Hg) and pure oxygen (solid
line, mean arterial pO_2 440 mm Hg); measured with needle
electrodes. n=33.

Our second question had been:

How does the oxygen pressure vary due to a change in cardiac work?

This is the most important and almost the only physiologically
relevant case of influence on the heart, which indeed occurs frequently in daily life. We were interested above all in the question
as to whether, at the beginning of changed cardiac work, a temporary
fluctuation in pO_2 occurs, which could trigger the regulation of

blood flow. In dogs, we lowered the cardiac work by cooling the sinus node. In 15 experiments using 6 dogs, pO_2 remained constant 13 times, twice it increased only slightly. In Fig. 8, such an experiment is shown. During the period of cooling the heart rate decreases by one half; the coronary blood flow decreases somewhat; the pO_2 increases slightly, this is one of the exceptions I mentioned. After the cooling, there is a temporary increase in heart work: blood flow increases, but the pO_2 remains constant. - In another series with rats the cardiac work was increased by enlarging the blood volume; here, too, myocardial pO_2 remained unchanged.

Thus answering our two questions we can state: 1. on changing cardiac work no changes in myocardial pO_2 occur; 2. on changing oxygen supply pO_2 is changed and adjusted to a new level.

Finally I should like to refer briefly to the topic I mentioned at the beginning, the formation of the pO_2 field in the microstructure of the myocardium. Concerning the capillary pattern numerous models have been constructed and the resulting pO_2 distributions computed, e.g. by Rakusan (1971), Grunewald and Sowa (1978), Schubert et al. (1983) and others. In recent years some experimental findings were

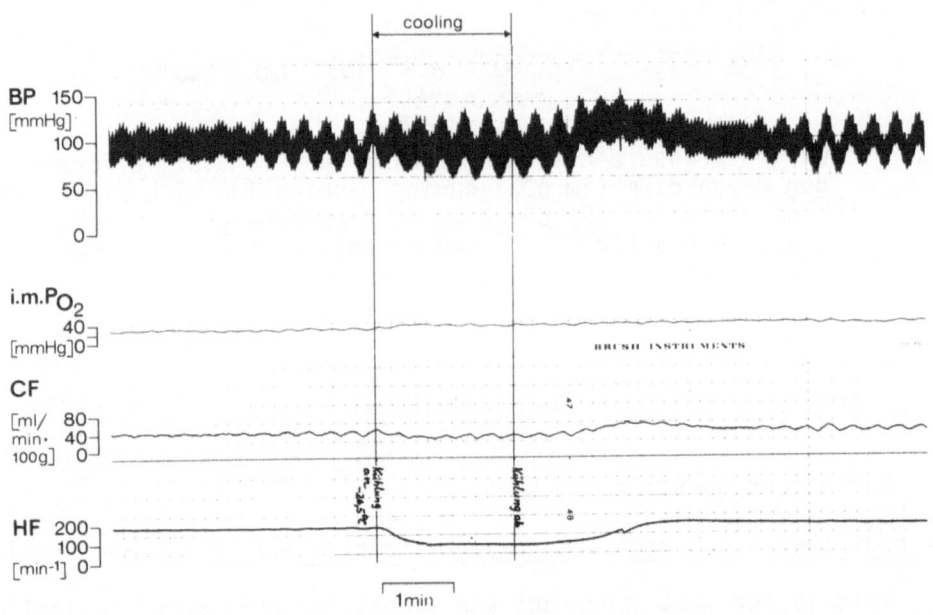

Fig. 8. Recording of arterial blood pressure (BP), intramyocardial oxygen pressure (im pO_2), coronary flow (CF) and heart frequency (HF) in the dog during temporary decrease of the heart rate by cooling the sinus node.

used to develop new concepts concerning the oxygen supply to skeletal muscle. They might in part also be important for the myocardium. Potter and Groom found that on contraction of skeletal muscles, the capillaries were wound up around the muscle fibres, thereby increasing their exchange surface area. In the heart such an improved oxygen exchange would damp the pO_2 decrease during systole. But the application of this model seems to be restricted because the extent of shortening of the heart muscle fibres is considerably less than assumed for skeletal muscles by Potter and Groom (1983).

I mentioned that concerning the measuring of oxygen distributions in the tissue at present we still have to dispense with a correlation of these measured values to microstructure of tissue. Maybe the method of cryomicrophotometry will have the greatest success in attacking this experimental problem. Two years ago Honig et al. (1984) introduced the following picture of oxygen supply to the skeletal muscle fibre based on cryomicrophotometric results. In the muscle fibres themselves there exist uniformly very low oxygen pressures in the range of 1-3 mm Hg. Therefore a diffusion resistance has to be assumed between capillary and muscle fibre. Due to this resistance the velocity of the red cells in the capillaries becomes a decisive quantity in determining oxygen delivery. What is the degree of mean myoglobin saturation in the beating heart? - Coburn et al. some years earlier (1973) measured saturations in the beating dog heart and calculated pO_2 values of 4-6 mm Hg. Figulla et al. (1983) found a nearly full saturation of the myoglobin in the isolated working guinea-pig heart. If there is a diffusion resistance in the capillary domain, the question arises where it is localized exactly. If it is inside the capillary - e.g. the oxygen delivery from the hemoglobin - then indeed the cell velocity can become a limiting factor. If it is outside, the capillary could be regarded as homogeneous oxygen source in its cross-section; in this case an increase of the red cell velocity could have the opposite effect, an increase of the O_2 gradient to the muscle fibre. At present this problem of red cell velocity, I think, is not quite clear and needs further investigation.

I would at the end like to express my thanks to Professor Lübbers; he has patiently discussed numerous questions which have occupied me, and has given me very useful suggestions concerning this lecture.

REFERENCES

Brantigan, J.W., Perna, A.M., Gardner, T.J., and Gott, V.L., 1972, Intramyocardial gas tensions in the canine heart during anoxic cardiac arrest, Surgery, Gynecology and Obstetrics, 134:67-72.
Breull, W., Flohr, H., Schuchhardt, S., and Dohm, H., 1981, Transmural gradients in myocardial metabolic rate, Basic Res.

Cardiol., 76:399-403.

Coburn, R.F., Ploegmakers, F., Gondrie, P., and Abboud, R., 1973, Myocardial myoglobin oxygen tension, Am. J. Physiol., 224: 870-876.

Figulla, H.R., Hoffmann, J., and Lübbers, D.W., 1983, Coronary conductivity and tissue oxygenation as measured by the myoglobin O_2 saturation and the cytochrome aa_3 redox state in the Langendorff guinea pig heart preparation, in: "Oxygen Transport to Tissue - IV", H.I. Bicher and D.F. Bruley, eds., Adv. Exper. Med. Biol., Vol. 159, Plenum Press, New York and London, pp. 579-585.

Gardner, T.J., Brantigan, J.W., Perna, A.M., Bender, H.W., Brawley, R.K., and Gott, V.L., 1971, Intramyocardial gas tensions in the human heart during coronary artery saphenous vein bypass, J. Thorac. Cardiovasc. Surg., 62:844.

Grunewald, W.A., and Lübbers, D.W., 1975, Die Bestimmung der intra-capillären HbO_2-Sättigung mit einer kryo-mikrofotometrischen Methode angewandt am Myocard des Kaninchens, Pflügers Arch., 353:255-273.

Grunewald, W.A., and Sowa, W., 1978, Distribution of the myocardial tissue pO_2 in the rat and the inhomogeneity of the coronary bed, Pflügers Arch., 374:57-66.

Hauss, J., Spiegel, H.-U., and Schönleben, K., 1984, Steady state condition - what does it mean during investigation of oxygen supply?, in: "Oxygen Transport to Tissue - V", D.W. Lübbers, H. Acker, E. Leniger-Follert and T.K. Goldstick, eds., Adv. Exper. Med. Biol., Vol. 169, Plenum Press, New York and London, pp. 887-897.

Honig, C.R., Gayeski, T.E.J., Federspiel, W., Clark, A., jr., and Clark, P., 1984, Muscle O_2 gradients from hemoglobin to cytochrome; new concepts, new complexities, in: "Oxygen Transport to Tissue - V", D.W. Lübbers, H. Acker, E. Leniger-Follert and T.K. Goldstick, eds., Adv. Exper. Med. Biol., Vol. 169, Plenum Press, New York and London, pp. 23-38.

Kadatz, R., 1969, Sauerstoffdruck und Durchblutung im gesunden und koronarinsuffizienten Myocard des Hundes und ihre Beeinflussung durch koronarerweiternde Pharmaka, Arch. Kreislaufforschung, 58:263-293.

Kessler, M., Höper, J., Harrison, D.K., Skolasinska, K., Klövekorn, W.P., Sebening, F., Volkholz, H.J., Beier, I., Kernbach, C., Rettig, V., and Richter, H., 1984, Tissue supply under normal and pathological conditions, in: "Oxygen Transport to Tissue - V", D.W. Lübbers, H. Acker, E. Leniger-Follert and T.K. Goldstick, eds., Adv. Exper. Med. Biol., Vol. 169, Plenum Press, New York and London, pp. 69-80.

Laarse, van der, A., and Freud, G.E., 1975, Multiple measurement of intramural myocardial oxygen tension, in: "Recent Advances in Studies on Cardiac Structure and Metabolism, Vol. V", A. Fleckenstein, and N.S. Dhalla, eds., University Park Press, Baltimore, pp. 441-447.

Lösse, B., Schuchhardt, S., and Niederle, N., 1975, The oxygen pressure histogram in the left ventricular myocardium of the dog, Pflügers Arch., 356:121-132.

Mendler, N., Schuchhardt, S., and Sebening, F., 1973, Measurement of intramyocardial oxygen tension during cardiac surgery in man, Res. Exp. Med., 159:231-238.

Menke, W., Schuchhardt, S., Escher, M., and Fritz, H., 1984, Intra-myocardial oxygen pressure and reactive hyperaemia in response to arterial hyperoxia (Abstract), Pflügers Arch., 400, Suppl., R4.

Moss, A.J., 1968, Intramyocardial oxygen tension, Cardiovasc. Res., 2:314-318.

Potter, R.F., and Groom, A.C., 1983, Capillary diameter and geometry in cardiac and skeletal muscle studied by means of corrosion casts, Microvasc. Res., 25:68-84.

Rakusan, K., 1971, "Oxygen in the Heart Muscle", Thomas, Springfield, Illinois.

Schubert, R.W., Fletcher, J.E., and Reneau, D.D., An analytical model for axial diffusion in the Krogh cylinger, ISOTT, Ruston, Louisiana (1983), in press.

Schuchhardt, S., Schuster, J., and Ryzlewicz, Th., 1978, "Untersuchungen zur Sauerstoffversorgung des Warmblütermyocards mit Platin-Nadel-Elektroden", Westdeutscher Verlag, Opladen.

Schuster, J., Schuchhardt, S., and Fehren, I., 1979, Beeinflussung des pO_2 in verschiedenen Herzmuskelschichten durch Blockade α- u. β-adrenerger Receptoren (Abstract), Z. Kardiol., 68: 259.

Skolasinska, K., Harbig, K., Lübbers, D.W., and Wodick, R., 1978, PO_2 and microflow histograms of the beating heart in response to changes in arterial PO_2, Basic Res. Cardiol., 73:307-319.

Whalen, W., 1971, PO_2 in heart and skeletal muscle, The Physiologist, 14:69-82.

Weiss, H.R., 1974, Control of myocardial oxygenation - effect of atrial pacing, Microvasc. Res., 8:362-376.

Winbury, M.M., Howe, B.B., and Weiss, H.R., 1971, Effect of nitro-glycerin and dipyridamole on epicardial and endocardial oxygen tension - further evidence for redistribution of myocardial blood flow, J. Pharmacol. Exp. Therap., 176:184-199.

Yokoyama, M., Maokawa, K., Katada, Y., Ishikawa, Y., Azumi, T., Mizutani, T., Fukuzaki, H., and Tomomatsu, T., 1978, Effects of graded coronary constriction on regional oxygen and carbon dioxide tensions in outer and inner layers of canine myo-cardium, Japan. Circ. J., 42:701-709.

SKELETAL AND CARDIAC MUSCLE OXYGENATION

Niels Lund

Department of Anesthesiology
University Hospital
S-581 85 Linköping
Sweden

Tissue oxygenation is accomplished through a long chain of complex, interrelated factors. The end result is heterogeneity (in time and space) of local oxygen pressures (see e.g. Duling 1981, Longmuir 1981, Silver 1981).

Table 1. Factors influencing tissue pO_2

EXPERIMENTAL
Species studied
Type of anesthesia
Measurement technique used

SYSTEMIC
Lung ventilation and perfusion
Systemic circulation
Oxygen carrying capacity of blood (hemoglobin)

LOCAL
Capillary geometry
Capillary blood flow distribution
Rheology
Oxygen diffusion across capillary walls
Oxygen diffusion through the tissue
Oxygen utilization in the tissue
Myoglobin (when present)

Table 2. Some examples of polarographically measured tissue
         oxygen pressures (p_tO_2) in striated muscles. All
         pO_2 values are in mm Hg.

Author	Species	Muscle	Mean p_tO_2	Range
Kunze 1969	Man	Tib ant	38	1-110
Lund 1980	Rat	Quadr fem	33	0-100
Lund 1980	Man	Brachiorad	16	6-63
Saborowski 1983	Man	Gastrocn	20	0-55
Thorborg 1984	Rabbit	Vastus med	35	18-41
Kirk & Honig 1964	Dog	Heart	41	
Moss 1968	Dog	Heart	18	7-34
Skolasinska 1978	Cat	Heart	31	5-65
v d Laarse 1978	Dog	Heart	26	0-100
Wiener 1982	Man	Heart	25	
Walfridsson 1984	Pig	Heart	45	29-72

In this space it is impossible to discuss all the above
mentioned factors, therefore only some will be considered.

Type of anesthesia

Anesthetics influence central hemodynamics, peripheral circulation and respiration to various degrees (Longnecker and Harris
1980). In a study on the influences of anesthesia or decerebration
on central and regional hemodynamics in normovolemic and hemor-
rhaged rats, Seyde et al found that pentobarbital was associated
with the most deviations from the awake state in terms of hemodynamics, lactate/pyruvate ratio and arterial blood gases. Decerebration altered central and regional hemodynamics the least, and
the response to hemorrhage in those rats resembled most closely
that in awake rats. Chloralose-urethane altered central hemodynamics and responses to hemorrhage. These problems have, e.g., also
been studied by Faber et al (1982) who compared the effects of
decerebration and chloralose-urethane anesthesia on muscle microcirculation in rats and concluded that brainstem transsection was
less depressant to the microcirculation.

These and other studies thus indicate that many studies on
tissue oxygenation may have been influenced by the anesthetic
agent.

Measurement techniques

Many different techniques have been employed. For "direct"
measurement of tissue oxygen pressures two measurement techniques

dominate the literature: polarography and mass spectrometry. Mass
spectrometry was, e.g., used by Wilson et al (1973) who inserted
a sampling catheter with a diameter of 1.39 mm to a depth of 2-4
mm in ventricular myocardium. The polarographic probes vary very
much in size and shape. They range from intracellular needles to
large surface electrodes. In hamsters, whose plasma was labeled
with albumin conjugated to DTAF Lund, Damon and Duling (unpublished
results) have observed how the tissue and the capillaries were
compressed and displaced during the insertion of a Whalen-type
needle electrode (diameter 2-3 microns) into the cremaster muscle.
All capillary flow stopped within seconds and the perivascular pO_2
fell rapidly. The situation was improved, but not totally allevia-
ted, when the technique for electrode insertion as described by
Kanabus et al (1980) was used. Moss (1968) and van der Laarse
(1978) have published histologic pictures of needle electrode
trauma. Thus, polarographic needles and spectrometer probes inserted
into tissue may, through compression and tissue damage, result in
too low pO_2's.

Studies on myocardial pO_2 have resulted in very different
oxygen pressures. The results obtained with needle electrodes (see
e.g. Moss 1968, van der Laarse 1978) are usually lower than those
obtained with surface-type electrodes (see e.g. Skolasinska et al
1978, Walfridsson et al 1984). As discussed above, the needle
electrode oxygen values may be too low due to tissue damage. However, the higher values obtained with surface electrodes are not
quite consistent with a normal coronary sinus pO_2 of 20 mm Hg.
These discrepancies have not yet been satisfactorily explained.

Hemoglobin

Theoretical considerations indicate that whereas increased
hemoglobin-oxygen affinity may impair oxygen delivery in normoxia
it is beneficial in hypoxic hypoxia (Turek et al 1973). Experimental evidence in normoxia is, however, contradictory and conclusions
have often been drawn from changes in venous pO_2. Nylander et al
(1983) used the MDO electrode to study the effects of increased
blood oxygen affinity on skeletal muscle oxygenation in rats, and
the same technique was used by Wranne et al (1983) to study a human
subject with high hemoglobin affinity. The rat study showed that
muscle oxygenation was not impaired by a chronic left shift on the
oxygen dissociation curve, neither did the left shifted curve improve muscle oxygenation in hypoxic hypoxia. The human subject tolerated an FIO_2 of 0.14 with only a small increase of low tissue
oxygen pressure values.

Capillary geometry

In 1982 Bloch and Iberall proposed that capillaries in striated
muscle are grouped in repeating functional units. Several authors

have studied the morphology of skeletal and cardiac muscle in two dimensions (e.g. Hammersen 1968, Eriksson & Myrhage 1972, Plyley et al 1976, Steinhausen et al 1978, Vetterlein et al 1982). Only a few studies have been done on three-dimensional microvascular geometry, e.g. Potter & Groom (1983).

Many factors influence the number of capillaries that are observed, e.g. arterial and/or tissue oxygen pressure (Honig & Bourdeau-Martini 1974, Duling 1978, Lindbom 1980, Jackson & Duling 1983), and arterial pCO_2 and pH (Bourdeau-Martini & Honig 1973).

In an effort to elucidate the three-dimensional vascular geometry in striated muscle Lund, Damon and Duling (unpublished results) used in vivo epifluorescent microscopy to analyze the anterior tibialis muscle in the golden hamster. DTAF-labeled albumin (Damon & Duling 1984) was injected via a femoral venous cannula, and up to eight overlapping microscopic fields (538x700 μm each) were videotaped at successive 10 μm depths to a total of 160-180 μm. Vascular patterns were traced onto acetate overlays, which were then stacked in a frame to produce a three-dimensional array. They found microvascular modules consisting of 12-20 capillaries most of which were supplied by one common arteriole and drained into one common venule. The modules were staggered both longitudinally and vertically, thus making them difficult to detect without detailed reconstruction of the anatomy and flow patterns in the living muscle. This technique should also make it possible to correlate MDO oxygen electrode measurements with microvascular geometry and blood flow to enable detailed analysis of different tissue oxygen pressure histogram types.

Capillary blood flow distribution

In the same study by Lund, Damon & Duling the direction of flow both within and among modules was carefully assessed because of the importance of countercurrent flow in understanding tissue oxygenation. Within a unit the majority of the capillaries showed concurrent flow. Most countercurrent flow was attributable to either capillaries in adjacent units or to a complex capillary geometry usually found at the ends of units. Few interconnections and therefore little flow exchange was observed between adjacent modules. The effects of capillary flow patterns and the ratio of concurrent to countercurrent flow on tissue oxygenation has been analyzed by e.g. Grunewald & Sowa (1977) and Wieringa et al (1982).

In cardiac muscle the questions of capillary geometry and capillary blood flow distribution has important clinical implications. It has long been discussed whether ischemic border zones exist or not (see e.g. Hearse & Yellon 1982). A border zone study employing a modified MDO oxygen electrode (Walfridsson et al 1984), indicates that an ischemic border zone exists. The next step in this type of research would be to try to improve the viability of the border zone to save myocardial tissue.

In 1978 Brian Duling stated, with regard to oxygen delivery, that: "more data and knowledge are required on shunting, the nature of capillary flow, sites of control, existence or lack of existence of precapillary sphincters, and detailed geometrical considerations".

In 1984 we have more data, but much remains to be satisfactorily explained.

Acknowledgements

Studies included in this review were supported by the Swedish Medical Research Council (05956), the Tore Nilson Foundation (83/94) and the Östergötland County Council (98/82, 14/83).

REFERENCES

Block, E. H., Iberall, A. S. 1982. Toward a concept of the functional unit of mammalian skeletal muscle. Am J Physiol., 242: R411.

Bourdeau-Martini, J., Honig, C. R. 1973. Control of coronary intercapillary distance: effect of arterial pCO_2 and pH. Microvasc Res., 6:286.

Damon, D. H., Duling B. R. 1984. Distribution of capillary blood flow in the microcirculation of the hamster: an in vivo study using epifluorescence microscopy. Microvasc Res., 27: 81.

Duling, B. R. 1978. Oxygen, metabolism, and microcirculatory control. In: Microcirculation, Vol. II, pp. 401-29. Eds: Kaley, G, Altura, B. M. University Park Press, Baltimore.

Duling, B. R. 1981. Coordination of microcirculatory function with oxygen demand in skeletal muscle. Adv Physiol Sci., 7:1.

Eriksson, E., Myrhage, R. 1972. Microvascular dimensions and blood flow in skeletal muscle. Acta physiol scand., 86:211.

Faber, J. E., Harris, P. D., Wiegman, D. L. 1982. Anesthetic depression of microcirculation, hemodynamics and respiration in decerebrated rats. Am J Physiol., 243:H837.

Grunewald, W. A., Sowa, W. 1977. Capillary structures and O_2 supply to tissue. In: Reviews of Physiology, Biochemistry and Pharmacology, Vol. 77, pp 149-209. Springer-Verlag, Berlin, Heidelberg, New York.

Hammersen, F. 1968. The pattern of the terminal vascular bed and the ultrastructure of capillaries in skeletal muscle. In: Oxygen Transport in Blood and Tissue, pp 184-97. Ed: Lübbers, D. W. et al, Georg Thieme Verlag, Stuttgart.

Honig, C. R., Bourdeau-Martini, J. 1974. Extravascular component of oxygen transport in normal and hypertrophied hearts with special reference to oxygen therapy. Circ Res., 34-35, suppl. II: 97.

Hearse, D. J., Yellon, D. M. 1982. The three-dimensional geometry
     of regional myocardial ischemia: the role of the coronary
     microcirculation in determining patterns of injury. In:
     Microcirculation of the heart, pp 149-63. Eds., Tillmanns,
     H., Kübler, W., Zebe, H. Springer-Verlag, Berlin, Heidel-
     berg, New York.
Jackson, W. F., Duling, B. R. 1983. The oxygen sensitivity of
     hamster cheek pouch arterioles. Circ Res., 53:515.
Kanabus, E. W., Feldstein, C., Crawford, D. W. 1980. Excursion of
     vibrating microelectrodes in tissue. J Appl Physiol., 48:737.
Kirk, E. S., Honig, C. R. 1964. Non-uniform distribution of blood
     flow and gradients of oxygen tension within the heart. Am
     J Physiol., 207:661.
Kunze, K. 1969. Das Sauerstoffdruckfeld im normalen and pathologisch
     veränderten Muskel. Schriftenreihe Neurologie, Band 3.
     Springer-Verlag, Berlin, Heidelberg, New York.
van der Laarse, A. 1978. On the multiple polarographic measurement
     of myocardial oxygen tension. Ph.D.-dissertation, University
     of Amsterdam.
Lindbom, L., Tuma, R. F., Arfors, K-E. 1980. Influence of oxygen
     on perfused capillary density and capillary red cell velocity
     in rabbit skeletal muscle. Microvasc Res., 19:197.
Longmuir, I. S. 1981. Channels of oxygen transport from blood to
     mitochondria. Adv Physiol Sci., 25:19.
Longnecker, D. E., Harris, P. D. 1980. Microcirculatory actions of
     general anesthetics. Fed Proc., 39:1580.
Lund, N., Ödman, S., Lewis, D. H. 1980. Skeletal muscle oxygen
     pressure fields in rats. Acta anaesth scand., 24:155.
Lund, N., Jorfeldt, L., Lewis, D. H. 1980. Skeletal muscle oxygen
     pressure fields in healthy human volunteers. Acta anaesth
     scand., 24:272.
Moss, A. J. 1968. Intramyocardial oxygen tension. Cardiovasc Res.,
     3:314.
Nylander, E., Lund, N., Wranne, B. 1983. Effect of increased blood
     oxygen affinity on skeletal muscle surface oxygen pressure
     fields. J Appl Physiol., 54:99.
Plyley, M. J., Sutherland, G. J., Groom, A. C. 1976. Geometry of
     the capillary network in skeletal muscle. Microvasc Res.,
     11:161.
Potter, R. F., Groom, A. C. 1983. Capillary diameter and geometry
     in cardiac and skeletal muscle studied by means of corro-
     sion casts. Microvasc Res., 25:68.
Saborowski, F., Kessler, M., Höper, J., Greitschus, F., Rath, K.,
     Dickmans, H. A., Thiele, K. G. 1983. Skeletal muscle oxygen
     pressure in patients with chronic renal insufficiency. In:
     Determination of Tissue Oxygen Pressure in Patients, pp 79-
     84. Ed.; Ehrly, A. M. Pergamon Press, Oxford.

Seyde, W. C., McGowan, L., Lund, N., Duling, B. R., Longnecker, D.E.
Influences of pharmacological anesthesia or decerebration on
central and regional hemodynamics in normovolemic and hemor-
rhaged rats. Submitted for publication.

Silver, I. A., 1981. Heterogeneity in tissue oxygenation; systemic
and local factors. Adv Physiol Sci., 25:67.

Skolasinska, K., Harbig, K., Lübbers, D.W., Wodick, R., 1978, pO_2
and microflow histograms of the beating heart in response
to changes in arterial pO_2. Basic Res Cardiol., 73:307.

Steinhausen, M., Tillmanns, H., Thederan, H., 1978. Microcirculation
of the epimyocardial layer of the heart. Pflügers Arch.,
378:9.

Thorborg, P., Malmqvist, L-Å, Lund, N. Surface oxygen pressure
fields in skeletal muscle: dependence on arterial pO_2.
Submitted for publication.

Turek, Z., Kreuzer, F., Hoofd, L. J. C., 1973, Advantage or disadvantage of a decrease of blood oxygen affinity for tissue
oxygen supply at hypoxia. Pflügers Arch., 342:185.

Vetterlein, F., dal Ri, H., Schmidt, G. 1982. Capillary density in
rat myocardium during timed plasma staining. Am J Physiol.,
242:H133.

Walfridsson, H., Lewis, D. H., Lund, N., Acute coronary occlusion:
oxygen pressure in the border zone studied in the pig.
Accepted for publication.

Wiener, L., Santamore, W. P., Venkataswamy, A., Plzak, L.,
Templeton, J. 1982. Postoperative monitoring of myocardial
oxygen tension: experience in 51 coronary artery bypass
patients. Clin Cardiol., 5:431.

Wieringa, P. A., Spaan, J. A. E., Stassen, H. G., Laird, J. D.,
1982. Heterogeneous flow distribution in a three dimensional network simulation of the myocardial microcirculation
- a hypothesis. Microcirculation. 2(2):195.

Wilson, G. J., Mac Gregor, D. C., Holness, D. E., Lixfeld, W.,
Yasni, H., 1973, Mass spectrometry for measuring changes in
intramyocardial pO_2 and pCO_2. Adv Exp Med Biol., 37A:547.

Wranne, B., Berlin, G., Jorfeldt, C., Lund, N., 1983, Tissue oxygenation and muscular substrate turnover in two subjects
with high hemoglobin oxygen affinity. J Clin Invest., 72:
1376.

DIFFUSION WITH CHEMICAL REACTION IN BIOLOGICAL SYSTEMS

Pieter Stroeve

Chemical Engineering Department
University of California
Davis, CA

INTRODUCTION

The interplay between diffusion and chemical transformation takes place in practically an infinite number of systems, either in nature or in the chemical industry. A variety of academic disciplines have actively studied the phenomena of diffusion with chemical reaction in order to understand the basic laws and to utilize them in predicting the behavior of systems or to design chemical processes which produce desirable species. Obviously, the study of mass transport and chemical transformation in biological systems is of great importance in the biological sciences. Likewise, the chemical reactions of molecules in industrial systems often involve significant diffusion effects and the interplay of the two effects needs to be understood to design efficient chemical systems. The laws that describe diffusion with chemical reaction are very general and apply to very disparate systems. As was pointed out by Weisz (1973) in an informative review article, discoveries made in various disciplines often were made independently of each other. The emergence of the interdisciplinary field of bioengineering has helped in bringing together knowledge developed in engineering, the pure and the biological sciences.

In this paper, I will review some of the important developments during this century in the phenomena of diffusion with chemical reaction and their applications to oxygen and carbon dioxide transport in biological systems. The discussion in this paper will be general and have a personal flavor since the subject is too extensive to cover in a single paper. Further, I would like to point out the similarities in development both in Physiology and Chemical Engineering.

45

For those readers who would like to further explore the subject, there are a number of important books and reviews available in the literature. In the chemical engineering literature, the texts by Astarita (1967), Danckwerts (1970), Aris (1975) and Astarita et al. (1983) are excellent sources of the theoretical developments in diffusion with chemical reaction. Useful review articles are those by Schultz et al. (1974), Goddard et al. (1974), Goddard (1977), and Meldon et al. (1982). In the field of physiology the articles of Wittenberg (1970), Kreuzer (1970) and Kreuzer and Hoofd (1984) focus on the specific problem of oxygen utilization and carbon elimination in physiological systems. The review by Weisz (1973) discusses the interdisciplinary nature of the phenomena. A recent symposium on diffusion and chemical transformation, conducted by the American Institute of Chemical Engineers, contains papers dealing with a spectrum of problems (Stroeve and Ward, 1981).

COMPLEXITY

The transport of mass is described by conservation equations for all species in each phase of the system. In the case that i) the phases' densities are constant, ii) the diffusion coefficients are independent of concentration, iii) the species are uncharged and iv) their concentrations are small, the conservation equations for all species i in phase j are of the form

$$\frac{\partial c^{i,j}}{\partial t} + \underline{v}^j \cdot \underline{\nabla} \, c^{i,j} = D^{i,j} \nabla^2 \, c^{i,j} + R^{i,j} \qquad (1)$$

The integer i is the index for all the chemical species involved in the chemical reaction of interest while j is the index for all phases existing in the system, e.g. cellular and extracellular phases. If the velocity vectors $\underline{v}^j$ are known in each phase, the formal statement of the problem requires initial conditions, coupling boundary conditions between the phases and system boundary conditions. In the case that the velocity vector is not known it can be obtained for Newtonian liquids in laminar flow from the Navier-Stokes Equations

$$\rho^j \left(\frac{\partial \underline{v}^j}{\partial t} + \underline{v}^j \cdot \underline{\nabla} \, \underline{v}^j \right) = - \underline{\nabla} \, p^j + \rho^j \underline{g} + \mu^j \nabla^2 \underline{v}^j \qquad (2)$$

subject to the appropriate initial, boundary and coupling conditions for fluid flow in the system. Solutions for equations (1) and (2) can be exceedingly complex and simplifying assumptions, which are physically satisfied, are necessary to obtain a solution. Examples of assumptions are steady state and zero flow for stagnant media. In addition, the biological system often has to be modelled as a simpler geometric system to further reduce the complexity of the problem.

46

THE IMPORTANCE OF MODELLING

Biological media such as tissues, cell suspensions or single cells are so complex that exact solutions of the conservation equations are often impossible. The complexity of a biological system must be reduced to a simpler model which is easier to solve but maintains the essential elements of the original problem. In the field of chemical engineering very complex systems are also encountered such as emulsions, dispersions, packed bed reactors, porous catalysts particles, etc., and one must devise models which are physically realistic but can be solved theoretically.

Some Examples

One of the early simple models which met with much success in modeling mass transfer across interfaces is the Whitman film model (1923). According to this model the physical absorption rate of a gas in an agitated liquid is controlled by two hypothetical stationary films of gas and liquid at the interface between the two phases. Mass transfer of the absorbed gas occurs by diffusion through these two films. This simple model is basically derived from the film model of Nernst (1904). The film model gives for the mass transfer rate of a species A into a liquid medium

$$N_A = \frac{D_A}{\delta} (C_i - C_B) \tag{3}$$

where δ is the thickness of the stationary liquid film, D_A is the diffusivity, C_i is the interfacial concentration and C_B is the bulk concentration of A in the liquid. In terms of a mass transfer coefficient, the flux is given by

$$N_A = k_A (C_i - C_B) \tag{4}$$

The film model predicts that for the physical absorption of a gas the liquid-side mass transfer coefficient is given by the diffusivity divided by the film thickness. The film model was later improved by other models such as the penetration theory and the surface renewal model (Danckwerts, 1970). These models have been useful in understanding gas absorption and desorption in industrial systems where the rigorous solutions of the mass conservation and Navier-Stokes equations are too difficult. For simple reactive systems with well-defined flow geometry, exact solutions are possible (Bird et al., 1960). It has been shown, in situations where there is fluid flow, that it is the boundary layers near interfaces which represent the resistance for mass transfer so that the concept of a stationary film in flow situations is an approximation. Concentration and velocity changes are most significant in the boundary layer compared to the bulk solution.

The problem of gas absorption accompanied by chemical reaction was considered by Hatta (1928) for CO_2 absorption into an agitated KOH solution and Hill (1928) who studied the diffusion of oxygen into a layer of fatigued muscle tissue. Although the systems described above are very different, there are certain similarities. The effect of the chemical reaction is to lower the concentration of the diffusion species leading to an increase in its concentration gradient and, consequently, an increase in the mass transfer rate. Both Hatta and Hill considered the case of instantaneous reaction and assumed the existence of a sharp reaction front defining a plane where all reaction was completed.

The construction of simple models by Hatta and Hill allowed for the derivation of accurate approximate solutions. In Hill's study which dealt with the study of oxygen diffusion into fatigued muscle, the oxygen reacts rapidly with the lactic acid so that the reaction occurs in an extremely thin layer called a front. The reaction front slowly moves into the tissue until recovery is complete. Hill assumed that the diffusion of lactic acid is much slower than the diffusion of oxygen. The mass conservation equation for oxygen (A) is

$$\frac{\partial C}{\partial t} = D_A \frac{\partial^2 C}{\partial x^2} \qquad 0 \leq x \leq \eta \tag{5}$$

with the initial conditions

1) $t = 0$, there is an oxygen debt λ moles/cc of tissue and $C = C_o = 0$ \hfill (6)

2) $x = 0$, $\quad C = C_i$, $t \geq 0$ \hfill (7)

3) $x = \eta$, $\quad -D_A \frac{dC}{dx} = \lambda \frac{d\eta}{dt}$, $\quad t > 0$ \hfill (8)

Hill further assumed that the reaction front advances so slowly into the tissue that a steady-state oxygen concentration profile is set up behind it.
Equation (5) becomes

$$D_A \frac{d^2 C}{dx^2} = 0 \tag{9}$$

for which the solution is

$$C = C_i (1 - x/\eta) \tag{10}$$

At the advancing front

$$\lambda \frac{d\eta}{dt} = \frac{D_A}{\eta} \frac{C_i}{} \tag{11}$$

48

which is an ordinary differential equation in η for which the solution is

$$\eta = \sqrt{\frac{2D_c C_i t}{\lambda}} \tag{12}$$

The advancing front moves with the square root of time. The instantaneous mass transfer rate into a stagnant reactive layer can be obtained from equations (11) and (12) and is

$$N_A = \sqrt{\frac{D_A \lambda}{2C_i t}} \quad (C_i - C_o) \tag{13}$$

where the initial gas concentration C_o in the muscle is zero. Clearly, an increase in λ causes an increase in the mass transport rate so that reaction enhances the mass transfer rate. A better theoretical expression is obtained with the application of the penetration theory to instantaneous irreversible reaction. In this case (Danckwerts, 1970)

$$N_A = \frac{1}{erf(\beta/\sqrt{D_A})} \sqrt{\frac{D_A}{\pi t}} \quad (C_i - C_o) \tag{14}$$

where C_o is again zero. Here β is obtained from

$$e^{\beta^2/D_B} erfc(\beta/\sqrt{D_B}) = \frac{B_o}{C_i} \sqrt{\frac{D_B}{D_A}} e^{\beta^2/D_A} erf(\beta/\sqrt{D_A}) \tag{15}$$

Equations (14) and (15) take into account the mobility of the reactant B. When there is no reactant B present, the penetration theory gives

$$N_A = k_A \quad (C_i - C_o) \tag{16}$$

where the mass transfer coefficient is given by

$$k_A = \sqrt{\frac{D_A}{\pi t}} \tag{17}$$

Since the term

$$\frac{1}{erf(\beta/\sqrt{D_A})} \geq 1 \tag{18}$$

the penetration theory also predicts enhancement of the mass transfer rate.

Hatta's model is a problem of gas absorption into a reactive agitated liquid containing a reactant at concentration B_o. Hatta modelled the reaction front to occur inside the hypothetical stagnant film of Whitman (1923). At the reaction front (for a bimolecular reaction), the film model yields (in terms of the mass transfer coefficient given by the film theory)

$$N_A = k_A \left(1 + \frac{D_B B_o}{D_A C_i} \right) (C_i - C_o) \qquad (19)$$

Comparison of these theories with the absorption of a nonreactive gas (Eq.4) shows that the chemical reaction: 1) enhances the mass transfer rate compared to purely physical absorption, 2) decreases the rate of the depth of penetration of the species A. Solutions for the local species concentration predict very different concentration profiles for the reactive case compared to the inert case. In addition we can state that chemical reaction: 3) changes concentration levels, 4) increases solution capacity for the species in case of reversible reactions. Other effects such as oscillatory phenomena due to chemical reactions will not be considered here.

Although the models of Hill and Hatta have deficiencies, they were very important in that they yielded approximate analytical solutions and gave a physical insight into the mass transfer process. The papers were the stimulus for further developments in this area. For example, the advancing front theory of Hill has been extensively used in more complex systems such as the design and modelling of oxygen transport in artificial membrane oxygenators (Lightfoot, 1968; Oomens et al., 1977; Dorson and Voorhees, 1976). Comparisons of predictions with results from numerical techniques have shown that Hill's advancing front theory gives accurate results for a wide range of parameters (Spaan, 1973).

ENHANCED AND FACILITATED TRANSPORT

For mass transfer with irreversible reaction, it can be shown that the mass transfer rate for species A can always be presented by

$$N_A = k_A E (C_i - C_o) \qquad (20)$$

as is apparent from the equations in the previous section. The dimensionless parameter E is known as the enhancement factor. If the mass transfer coefficient k_A^* for reaction is defined as

$$N_A = k_A^* (C_i - C_o) \qquad (21)$$

then it follows that the enhancement factor is the ratio of the mass transfer coefficient with reaction to the mass transfer coefficient without reaction. The enhancement factor is always greater or equal to one. In the case of reversible reaction where the species A complexes with a carrier species, the term facilitation factor has become common. In this case the transport is given by

$$N_A = k_A \ (1 + F) \ (C_i - C_o) \tag{22}$$

where the facilitation factor is defined as the ratio of carrier-facilitated transport to transport solely by Fickian diffusion of species A. The relationship between enhancement factors and facilitation factors is from the above equations

$$E = 1 + F \tag{23}$$

The facilitation factor is always greater than or equal to zero.

THE IMPORTANCE OF TIME SCALES

In any transport problem it is important to consider the competition of various rate processes. In diffusion with chemical reaction in stagnant media, the rate processes are diffusion and chemical reaction. The intrinsic rate of chemical reaction can be expressed in terms of a chemical reaction time scale t_R while diffusion rates can be characterized in terms of a diffusion time t_D. For first order reaction the reaction time can be defined as the time required to change the concentration of the reactive species, C^i, when the reaction takes place at the reaction rate at that concentration, i.e.,

$$t_R = \frac{C^i}{R^i} \tag{24}$$

The diffusion time can be defined as the diffusion coefficient divided by the square of the mass transfer coefficient

$$t_D = \frac{D}{k_A{}^2} \tag{25}$$

For the film model the diffusion time therefore becomes

$$t_D = \frac{\delta^2}{D} \tag{26}$$

which is the square of the film thickness divided by the diffusion coefficient.

The dimensionless ratio of the time scales is a measure of the relative rates of reaction and diffusion. We define the parameter

$$\gamma = \frac{t_D}{t_R} \tag{27}$$

When γ is much smaller than one, t_R is very large relative to t_D so chemical reaction rates are small relative to diffusion rates, so that diffusion predominates over reaction. As a consequence, one does not expect a significant lowering of the concentration of the reactive species in absorption and no enhancement of transport takes place. This is known as the slow reaction regime or near-diffusion regime. If γ is much greater than one, the chemical reaction rate prevails over diffusion. This case is called the instantaneous reaction equilibrium regime and the chemical reaction approaches equilibrium so that the term near-equilibrium regime is also common.

The use of a dimensionless parameter to characterize problems of diffusion with chemical reaction was independently developed by Damköhler (1937), Thiele (1939) and Zeldovitch (1939). The parameter γ is often called the Damköhler number and for a single reaction it can be expressed as

$$\gamma = \frac{R^i l^2}{C^i D^i} = \left(\frac{1}{\lambda}\right) = \phi^2 \qquad (28)$$

where l is the typical length scale of the phase of interest where the reaction is occurring. The parameter λ is called the characteristic reaction-diffusion length scale and is a measure of the thickness of a region where deviations from chemical reaction equilibrium are significant (Friedlander and Keller, 1965). The Thiele modulus ϕ is the square root of the Damköhler number. The Damköhler number or Thiele modulus is not highly sensitive to the exact geometry of the system so that the size of the particle, l, can be considered to be a typical length parameter (Aris, 1957; Roughton, 1952).

In solutions of the mass conservation equations, the Damköhler number will always arise when reaction exists in the system. The utility of γ is obvious in the asymptotic regimes. When $\gamma \to 0$, the assumption of Fickian diffusion of the reactive species is a good approximation, and when $\gamma \to \infty$ the assumption of chemical reaction equilibrium is valid. Such assumptions can lead to considerable simplification in the mass conservation equations. In the intermediate regime where γ is neither very small nor large, approximate analytical solution for some problems have been devised. The dependency of the enhancement factor E, and the facilitation factor F as a function of the Thiele modulus or the Damköhler number has been calculated for a large number of diffusion-reaction type problems (Danckwerts, 1970; Kreuzer and Hoofd, 1984; Astarita et al., 1983). In all cases when $\gamma \to 0$, then $F \to 0$ and $E \to 1$, while for $\gamma \to \infty$, F and E reach the maximum allowable value obtained for instantaneous chemical reaction.

Thiele introduced the concept of effectiveness for the transformation of molecules in catalyst particles. For diffusion into reactive particles where the diffusion species is consumed at a concentration-dependent intrinsic rate inside the particles, depletion of the species will lead to low conversion rates. The maximum reaction will occur at the highest possible concentration of the diffusing species inside the particle. This situation will only arise when the characteristic dimension of the particle, l, is made sufficiently small, or since the Thiele modulus depends on l as shown in equation (28), when ϕ is sufficiently small. Maximum reaction is obtained when the concentration gradient of the species A is negligible throughout the particle. The effectiveness factor can be defined as the actual reaction rate in the particle divided by the maximum attainable reaction rate. The Thiele effectiveness factor varies from $\eta = 1$ when $\phi \to 0$ to $\eta = 0$ when $\phi \to \infty$. The Thiele effectiveness factor is relatively insensitive to system geometry or reaction order (Weisz, 1973).

For any system of reactive particles to operate near maximum efficiency ($\eta = 1$) for chemical conversion, Weisz and Prater (1954) formulated the criterion

$$\phi \leq 1 \tag{29}$$

It appears that some biological systems are optimized for chemical transformation: calculation of representative Damköhler numbers indicates that they satisfy the criterion expressed by equation (29). In other words, the Thiele effectiveness factor is near one for sufficiently small Damköhler numbers. On the other hand, for the case of oxygen transport through red blood cells, the reaction inside the red blood cells appears to be at equilibrium leading to a maximum facilitation factor for oxygen, as determined for in vitro experiments and accompanying theoretical calculations at 37ºC (Stroeve et al., 1976 a). A plausible hypothesis is that biological systems, such as the red blood cell where one of the major functions is carrier-facilitated species transport, are optimized for maximum facilitation factors under normal physiological conditions. Unfortunately, insufficient data are available to test this hypothesis.

For some complex biological systems, such as bacterial cells, the Damköhler number for oxygen transport is sufficiently large for certain oxygen concentrations that the cells may become anoxic (Bailey and Ollis, 1977). In such cases, the Thiele effectiveness factor is below one and enhanced oxygen transport may take place. However, the enhancement of oxygen may not be sufficient to deliver oxygen into the interior of the cell or ensembles of cells because the relatively high reaction rate may consume all oxygen supplied. For complex systems where a multitude of chemical transformations and species transport occurs, the various Damköhler numbers for each species may not all be optimized.

OXYGEN AND CARBON DIOXIDE TRANSPORT IN BIOLOGICAL SYSTEMS

The theoretical and experimental study of the interaction of diffusion and chemical reaction in biological systems has been extensive (Wittenberg, 1970; Wittenberg and Wittenberg, 1981; Kreuzer, 1970; Kreuzer and Hoofd, 1984; Meldon et al., 1982; Bauer et al., 1980). Oxygen transport in hemoglobin solutions and red blood cell suspensions has been especially of interest since the papers by Klug et al. (1956a, 1956b), Wittenberg (1959) and Scholander (1960) showed that oxygen transport is facilitated in hemoglobin and myoglobin solutions. These papers were the stimulus for many theoretical papers which modeled the oxygen-hemoglobin and oxygen-myoglobin systems. A variety of approximate analytical solutions have appeared which have attempted to predict the facilitation factor for hemoglobin- or myoglobin-facilitated oxygen transport. The accuracy of the solutions has been ascertained by comparing theoretical predictions to solutions of the conservation equations as obtained by numerical analysis (Kutchai et al., 1970; Smith et al., 1973). The most accurate and versatile of these analytical solutions was devised by Hoofd and Kreuzer (1981) which allows the calculation of facilitation factors, oxygen transport rates and local concentrations of all species over the full range of Damköhler numbers. In essence, the Hoofd-Kreuzer technique is the sum of two solutions: the small and large Damköhler number approximations, i.e. the solutions for the near-diffusion regime and the near-equilibrium regime. The use of an accurate theory which can predict facilitated transport in the non-equilibrium regime is also useful in extracting kinetic data from the oxygen-hemoglobin system from accurate oxygen transport data through thin films of hemoglobin solutions (Bouwer et al., 1984).

Transport of oxygen in red blood cell suspensions and tissues has also been investigated. In vitro experiments have shown facilitated transport to exist in red blood cells (Kutchai and Staub, 1969; Stroeve et al., 1976b) and muscle tissue (Wittenberg et al., 1975; De Koning et al., 1981) although the importance for in vivo systems has not yet been established. Theoretical solutions for facilitated transport in heterogeneous media are available (Stroeve et al., 1976c; Goddard, 1981b).

Diffusion and chemical reaction of carbon dioxide in biological systems became of great interest after Longmuir et al. (1966) experimentally verified the suggestion by Hill (1928) that bicarbonate could facilitate carbon dioxide transport in aqueous systems. Accurate experiments on CO_2 transport in protein solutions were reported by Gros and Moll (1974) and Stroeve and Ziegler (1980) while Kawashiro and Scheid (1976) found facilitated CO_2 transport in muscle tissue. In the CO_2-water diffusion-reaction system in biological media charged species are produced and diffusion potentials, induced by the mobility difference of the various ionic species, especially charged protein species, lead to a significant reduction of the facilitated CO_2 transport due to bicarbonate (Meldon et al., 1978). Obviously the transport relationships given by equations 1 and 2 are modified to contain terms which take into account the electrical field and charge effects. The importance of electrical fields in diffusion-reaction systems involving ionic systems has been shown in biological transport and in possible separation schemes (Goddard, 1981a; Sasidhar and Ruckenstein, 1983; Meldon and Kang, 1983; Ivory, 1982; Gallagher et al., 1984). The problem of nonequilibrium CO_2 facilitated transport in biological solutions has not yet been addressed. Similar to oxygen transport, well-defined in vivo transport experiments are needed to determine the importance of chemical reaction in carbon dioxide transport. Improved theoretical models for in vivo oxygen and carbon dioxide transport will be necessary to interpret the experimental results and to make predictions.

VOLUME AVERAGING TECHNIQUES

Biological media are often heterogeneous in nature. For systems where the characteristic cell size is much smaller than the size of the system, transport phenomena are often described by homogenized equations. These conservation equations are similar to the conservation equations for single-phase media. The homogenized equations yield effective or bulk parameters for the physical properties such as diffusion coefficients and reaction rates (Stroeve, 1984). The dependence of the effective physical properties of all phases and the geometry of the interphase in the system are desired. A possible approach would be to conduct a variety of experiments to extract the desired information. However, biological media are so complex and changes in physical properties may damage the media that it is often impossible to carry out the experiments for the variety of conditions that can be encountered. The development of a theory that can rigorously predict the dependency of the effective parameters on the properties of the system is required.

One successful approach to modelling transport phenomena in multi-phase systems is the volume averaging technique introduced by Slattery (1981) and Whitaker (1973). The standard approach is to volume average the conservation equations and boundary conditions for the phases present in the system to obtain homogenized equations. For a two-phase system, containing phase β and σ, the volume-average for a property is defined for the β phase by

$$\langle \psi_\beta \rangle = \frac{1}{V} \int_{V_\beta} \psi_\beta \, dV \tag{30}$$

where V_β is the volume of the β-phase contained in the averaging volume V which is

$$V = V_\beta + V_\sigma \tag{31}$$

The averaging volume V is much smaller than the system volume. Use is also made of the spatial averaging theorem for the gradient in a property

$$<\underline{\nabla}\psi_\beta> = \underline{\nabla} <\psi_\beta> + \frac{1}{V} \int_{A_{\beta\sigma}} \underline{n}_{\beta\sigma}\, \psi_\beta \; dA \qquad (32)$$

The homogenized equations are then solved by analytical or numerical techniques. Often the homogenized equations need to be simplified by making order of magnitude analysis on the terms appearing in the equations. Obviously, order of magnitude analysis can impose important constraints on the model.

Ryan et al. (1981) considered the diffusion into reactive porous catalysts. They used a spatially periodic porous medium as the model of the porous catalyst. The advantage of this model is that one can divide the system into identical unit cells. If the array is very large, each unit cell sees virtually the same surroundings so that solutions for one unit cell are applicable to other cells. In this case, the problem can be solved for only one cell where the boundary conditions are replaced by periodicity conditions which consider symmetry and skew-symmetry conditions.

FUTURE CONSIDERATIONS

The theoretical formalism of volume averaging is now being applied to complex multi-phase transport problems in reactive, heterogeneous media in the presence of flow (Whitaker, 1983). Examples of problems are heat transfer with reaction in packed beds, and the catalysis of reactions in a reactor filled with catalyst particles. In these problems convection of fluid has a significant effect on the overall transport rate. Figure 1 shows a situation of flow and chemical reaction in a heterogeneous medium. This is the type of problem that chemical engineers are now attempting to solve. One can observe that the problems encountered in chemical engineering are strikingly similar to transport processes in cellular media. The cells are surrounded by extracellular fluid in which convection may exist. The diffusing species may react at different rates inside the cells, the cell membranes and the extracellular fluid. The present and future knowledge on reactive multiphase transport phenomena obtained from techniques such as volume averaging may be effectively applied to transport problems in tissues as long as the cells' characteristic size is much smaller than the system dimension. Volume averaging is a technique which allows for exact analysis of the homogenized equations applied to geometric models which mimic complex heterogeneous media.

The state of the art of theoretical and numerical analysis of diffusion with reactions in simple stagnant geometrical systems is reasonably developed. In vitro, measurements on systems with slab geometry have been conducted extensively, and comparisons of data

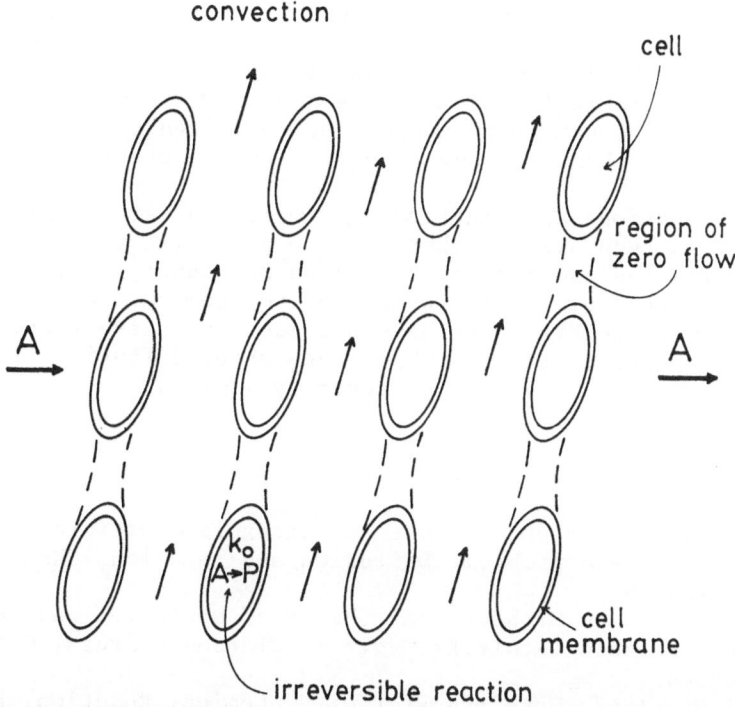

Fig. 1. Example of a problem with transport of A across a two-phase heterogeneous medium in the presence of chemical reaction and convection.

to theory have been favorable. It is difficult to determine enhancement and facilitation factors or effectiveness factors in vivo for many biological systems due to their geometric complexity and the difficulty to make measurements within the system.

For many transport problems, knowledge of the microcirculatory flow in tissues is necessary. The presence of convective flow in extracellular fluid must be considered to fully assess the importance of chemical reactions in affecting the total transport. Our present knowledge of flow in biological systems is limited. In addition, in many biological systems the typical cell size may be of the same order of magnitude as the characteristic system size so that homogenizing techniques such as volume averaging may not be applicable. An example is a system of cells that forms a lining such as the epithelia. Perhaps an area-averaging technique combined with an analysis which takes into account the presence of just one or two layers of cells may be an appropriate approach. Flow across epithelia must also be considered. We do not know if convective transport overwhelms enhanced or facilitated transport in those systems. In biological systems where many functions take place, will the values of the Damköhler numbers be optimized such that there will be maximum chemical conversion and transportation?

Many reactions are kinetically complex and are coupled to other reactions. In such systems there is the possibility of multiple steady states and oscillatory phenomena may take place. Oscillatory phenomena in physiological systems due to chemical reaction in oxygen and carbon dioxide transport have not been extensively studied. At best we can conclude that our knowledge about diffusion with chemical reaction for in vivo systems is severely limited.

REFERENCES

Aris, R., 1957, On shape factors for irregular particles - I. the steady state problem. Diffusion and reaction, Chem. Eng. Sci., 6, 262-268.

Aris, R., 1975, The Mathematical Theory of Diffusion and Reaction in Permeable Catalysts, Vol. 1. Clarendon Press, Oxford, England.

Astarita, G., 1967, Mass Transfer with Chemical Reaction, Elsevier, Amsterdam, The Netherlands.

Astarita, G., Savage, D.W., and Bisio, A., 1983, Gas Treating with Chemical Solvents. Wiley-Interscience, New York, U.S.A.

Bailey, J.E., and Ollis, D.F., 1977, Biochemical Engineering Fundamentals, McGraw-Hill, New York, U.S.A.,

Bauer, C., Gros, H., and Bartels, H., eds., 1980, Biophysics and Physiology of Carbon Dioxide, Springer, Berlin, West Germany.

Bird, R.B., Stewart, W.E., and Lightfoot, E.N., 1960, Transport Phenomena. Wiley, New York, U.S.A.

Bouwer, S., Hoofd, L., and Kreuzer, F., 1984, Private communications, University of Nijmegen, The Netherlands.

Damköhler, G., 1937, Einfluss von Diffusion, Stromung und Warmtetransport auf die Ausbeute bei chemisch-technischen Reaktionen, in: Der Chemieingenieur., A. Eucken, M. Jacob, eds. Bd. 3, Teil, p. 359., Leipzig, Germany.

Danckwerts, P.V., 1970, Gas-Liquid Reactions. McGraw-Hill, New York, U.S.A..

De Koning, J., Hoofd, L.J.C., and Kreuzer, F., 1981, Oxygen Transport and the function of myoglobin. Theoretical model and experiments in chicken gizzard smooth muscle, Pflügers Arch., 389, 211-217.

Dorson, W.J., and Voorhees, M.E., 1976, Analysis of oxygen and carbon dioxide transfer in membrane lungs. in: Artificial Lungs for Acute Respiratory Failure. Theory and Practice. W.M. Zapol and J. Qvist, eds., p. 43, Academic Press, New York, U.S.A.

Friedlander, S.K., and Keller, K.H., 1965, Mass transfer in reacting systems near equilibrium, Use of the affinity function. Chem. Eng. Sci., 20, 121-129.

Gallagher, P.M., Athayde, A.L., and Ivory, C.F., 1984, The facilitated transport of carbon dioxide through aqueous bicarbonate membranes. I. Formulation and solution. Unpublished manuscript, Notre Dame University, U.S.A..

Goddard, J.D., 1977, Further applications of carrier-mediated transport theory, A survey. Chem. Eng. Sci., 32, 795-809.

Goddard, J.D., 1981a, Electric field effects in carrier-mediated ion transport, AIChE Symp. Ser., 77(202), 114-122.

Goddard, J.D., 1981b, A model of facilitated transport in concentrated two-phase dispersions, Chem. Engr. Commun., 9, 345-361.

Goddard, J.D., Schultz, J.S., and Suchdeo, S.R., 1974, Facilitated transport via carrier-mediated diffusion in membranes: Part II. Mathematical aspects and analysis, AIChE Journ., 20, 625-645.

Gros, G., and Moll, W., 1974, Facilitated diffusion of CO_2 across albumin solutions, J. Gen. Physiol., 64, 356-371.

Hatta, S., 1928, On the absorption velocity of gases by liquids. I. Absorption of carbon dioxide by potassium hydroxide solution, Technol. Report Tohoku Imperial University (Japan), 8, 1-25.

Hill, A.V., 1928, The diffusion of oxygen and lactic acid through tissues, Proc. Roy. Soc., B104, 39-96.

Hoofd, L., and Kreuzer, F., 1981, The mathematical treatment of steady state diffusion of reacting species, AIChE Symp. Ser., 77(202), 123-129.

Ivory, C.F., 1982, Forced facilitation in carrier-mediated transport. Paper 51f. AIChE Meeting, November 14-19, Los Angeles, California, U.S.A..

Kawashiro, T., and Scheid, P., 1976, Measurement of Krogh's diffusion constant of CO_2 in respiring muscle at various CO_2 levels: Evidence for facilitated diffusion, Pflügers Arch. 362, 127-133.

Klug, A., Kreuzer, F., and Roughton, F.J.W., 1956a, Simultaneous diffusion and chemical reaction in thin layers of haemoglobin solution, Proc. Roy. Soc. B., 145, 452-472.

Klug, A., Kreuzer, F., and Roughton, F.J.W., 1956b, The diffusion of oxygen in concentrated haemoglobin solutions, Helv. Physiol. Pharm. Acta., 14, 121-128.

Kreuzer, F., 1970, Facilitated diffusion of oxygen and its possible significance: a review, Respir. Physiol., 9, 1-30.

Kreuzer, F., and Hoofd, L., 1984, Facilitated diffusion of O_2 and CO_2, in: Handbook of Physiology, Am. Physiol. Soc. Washington, D.C., U.S.A., in press.

Kutchai, H., Jacquez, J.A., and Mather, F.J., 1970, Nonequilibrium facilitated oxygen transport in hemoglobin solution,

<u>Biophys J.</u>, 10, 38-54.

Kutchai, H., and Staub, N.C., 1969, Steady-state, hemoglobin-facil-
itated O_2 transport in human erythrocytes, <u>J. Gen. Physiol.</u>,
53, 576-589.

Lightfoot, E.N., 1968, Low-order approximations for membrane blood
oxygenators, <u>AIChE J.</u>, 14, 669-670.

Longmuir, I.S., Forster, R.E., and Woo, C.-Y., 1966, Diffusion of
carbon dioxide through·thin layers of solution, <u>Nature</u>,
209, 393-394.

Meldon, J.H., De Koning, J., and Stroeve, P., 1978, Electrical
potentials induced by CO_2 gradients in protein solutions
and their role in CO_2 transport, <u>Bioelectrochem. Bioenerg.</u>,
5, 77-87.

Meldon, J.H., and Kang, Y.-S., 1983, The transport of carbon dioxide in purified protein solutions, <u>AIChE Symp. Ser.</u>, 79
(227), 36-42.

Meldon, J.H., Stroeve, P., and Gregoire, C.E., 1982, Facilitated
transport of carbon dioxide: A review, <u>Chem. Eng. Commun.</u>,
16, 263-300.

Nernst, W., 1904, Theorie der Reaktionsgeschwindigkeit in hetero-
genen Systemen, <u>Z. Phys. Chem.</u>, 47, 52-79.

Oomens, J.M.M., De Koning, J., and Stroeve, P., 1977, A comparison
of oxygen transfer into hemoglobin solutions and whole
blood flowing in rectangular channels, <u>AIChE J.</u>, 23, 390-
393.

Roughton, F.J.W., 1952, Diffusion and chemical reaction velocity in
cylindrical and spherical systems of physiological interest,
<u>Proc. Roy. Soc. London B</u>, 140, 203-229.

Ryan, D., Carbonell, R.G., and Whitaker, S., 1981, A theory of diffusion and reaction in porous media, <u>AIChE Symp. Ser.</u>, 77
(202), 46-62.

Sasidhar, V., Ruckenstein, E., 1983, Relaxation method for facilitated transport, <u>J. Membr. Sci.</u>, 13, 67-84.

Scholander, P.F., 1960, Oxygen transport through hemoglobin solutions, <u>Science</u>, 131, 85-90.

Schultz, J.S., Goddard, J.D., Suchdeo, S.R., 1974, Facilitated transport via carrier-mediated diffusion in membranes. Part I.
Mechanistic aspects, experimental systems and characteristic
regimes, <u>AIChE J.</u>, 20, 417-445.

Slattery, J.C., 1981, Momentum, Energy and Mass Transfer in Continua,
<u>Krieger</u>, Huntington, N.Y., U.S.A..

Smith, K.A., Meldon, J.H. and Colton, C.K., 1973, An analysis of
carrier-facilitated transport, <u>AIChE J.</u>, 19, 102-111.

Spaan, J.A.E., 1973, Transfer of oxygen into haemoglobin solution,
<u>Pflügers Arch. ges. Physiol.</u>, 342, 289-306.

Stroeve, P., 1984, Diffusion with Chemical Reaction in Two-Phase
Heterogeneous Media, <u>in</u>: Advances in Transport Processes,
Vol. III, p. 361-386, A.S. Mujumdar, R.A. Mashelkar, eds.,
Wiley Eastern, New Delhi, India.

Stroeve, P., Smith, K.A., and Colton, C.K., 1976a, Facilitated diffusion of oxygen in red blood cell suspensions, Adv. Exptl. Med. and Biol., 75, 191-198.

Stroeve, P., Smith, K.A., and Colton, C.K., 1976b, An analysis of carrier facilitated transport in heterogeneous media, AIChE J., 22, 1125-1132.

Stroeve, P., Colton, C.K., and Smith, K.A., 1976c, Steady state diffusion of oxygen in red blood cell and model suspensions, AIChE J., 22, 1133-1142.

Stroeve, P., and Ziegler, E.M., 1980, The transport of carbon dioxide in high molecular weight buffer solutions, Chem. Eng. Commun., 6, 81-103.

Stroeve, P., Ward, W.J., 1981, Transport with chemical reactions, AIChE Symp. Ser., 202, Vol. 77.

Thiele, E.W., 1939, Relation between catalytic activity and size of particle. Industrial Engr. Chem., 31, 916-920.

Weisz, P.B., 1973, Diffusion and chemical transformation. An interdisciplinary excursion, Science, 179, 433-440.

Weisz, P.B., and Prater, C.D., 1954, Interpretation of measurements in experimental catalysis. Adv. Catalysis, 6, 143-207.

Whitaker, S., 1973, The transport equations for multi-phase systems, Chem. Engr. Sci., 28, 139-147.

Whitaker, S., 1983, Transport processes with heterogeneous reaction, 25th Conicet Anniversary Reactor Design Conference, Santa Fe, Argentina, August.

Whitman, W.G., 1923, The two-film theory of absorption, Chem. and Met. Engr. 29, 147-153.

Wittenberg, J.B., 1959, Oxygen transport - a new function proposed for myoglobin, Biol. Bull., 117, 402-403.

Wittenberg, J.B., 1970, Myoglobin in oxygen entry into muscle, Physiol. Rev., 50, 559-636.

Wittenberg, B.A., Wittenberg, J.B., and Caldwell, P.R.B., 1975, Role of myoglobin in the oxygen supply to red skeletal muscle, J. Biol. Chem., 250, 9038-9043.

Wittenberg, J.B. and Wittenberg, B.A., 1981, Facilitated oxygen diffusion by oxygen carriers, in: Oxygen and Living Processes, D.L. Gilbert, ed., Springer-Verlag, New York, U.S.A..

Zeldovitch, J.B., 1939, On the theory of reactions on powders and porous substances, Acta Phys.-chim. URSS, 10, 583-594.

BLOOD GAS TRANSPORT AND 2,3-DPG

Jerry H. Meldon

Chemical Engineering Department
Tufts University
Medford, Mass. 02155

INTRODUCTION

Since the discovery of the sensitivity of oxygen-hemoglobin interaction to the concentration of red cell 2,3-diphosphoglycerate (Benesch and Benesch, 1967; Chanutin and Curnish, 1967), a great number of investigators have explored its biochemical, physiological and clinical ramifications. The following is a brief overview of this work, with particular emphasis upon the role of DPG in blood oxygen transport in health and disease.

The significance of DPG in gas transport is generally assessed in terms of its contribution to the satisfaction of tissue oxygen demand. Thus, pertinent discussions often begin with the following mathematical accounting for the difference between the oxygen contents of the blood leaving the left ventricle and entering the right auricle of the heart in the steady-state (i.e., when the body's O_2 stores - e.g., myoglobin - function at a capacity level essentially invariant with time):

$$\dot{V}_{O_2} = \dot{Q} \ [Hb] \ (S^A - S^V) \tag{1}$$

where $\dot{V}_{O_2}$ is tissue oxygen consumption rate (e.g., in mMol O_2/min), $\dot{Q}$ is cardiac output (in liters blood/min), $[Hb]$ is hemoglobin concentration (in mMol heme/liter blood), S is fractional saturation of hemoglobin with oxygen (in mMol O_2/mMol heme), and the superscripts A and V denote the respective conditions in mixed arterial and venous blood.

Immediately apparent from equation (1) is the implication that an increase in at least one of the three factors - cardiac output, hemoglobin concentration or arterio-venous saturation difference - is a necessary response to a decrease in one or more of the remaining factors, if O_2 consumption is to be maintained. It is often reasoned, moreover, that arterial blood pO_2 is fixed by ambient and pulmonary conditions, while venous pO_2 is regulated to provide the driving force for diffusion from peripheral capillary to metabolizing tissue. It follows, then, that blood whose oxyhemoglobin dissociation curve (ODC - see figure 1) is shifted to the right without reducing S^A appreciably, provides enhanced $S^A - S^V$, and may therefore compensate for impaired cardiac output.

This conclusion is unaltered by evidence that invalidates the theoretician's typical assumptions of regular "Krogh cylinder" capillary/tissue geometry (Ellis et al., 1983) and negligible intracapillary pO_2 gradients radially, as opposed to between the arterial and venous ends (Honig et al., 1984). Blood with a right-shifted ODC, as just described, is inherently advantageous as long as: a) passive (including facilitated) diffusion is the process by which oxygen transfers from erythrocytes to mitochondria, b) hemoglobin affinity for oxygen reflects association/dissociation kinetics that do not limit O_2 transport, and c) what leads to the shift in the ODC does not also have counter-acting side effects.

Thus, the discovery that an increase in red cell DPG concentration is, by itself, responsible for a rightward shift in blood's ODC has prompted research into a) its effect upon the ODC under widely ranging conditions and its additional effects upon blood pH and carbon dioxide transport, b) the biochemical mechanisms by which red cell DPG level is regulated, c) the correlation of DPG level with anemia, hypoxia and many other pathophysiological conditions, and d) the significance of hemoglobin oxygen affinity in transfusion.

DPG AND BLOOD-GAS CHEMISTRY

Hydrogen ions and DPG each reduce hemoglobin's oxygen affinity "allosterically" - i.e., their binding to specific "oxygen-linked" sites in the protein induces conformational changes, and hence alterations in the chemical and electrostatic environment of heme O_2 sites, such that the "deoxy" conformation is energetically stabilized (Baldwin, 1975). Carbon dioxide acts in analogous fashion. However, the ODC shift due to changing pCO_2 is largely an indirect one caused by the associated change in pH. Figure 1 illustrates the effect of changes in either plasma pH or red cell DPG concentration, in whole human blood at 37°C.

Recent experimental studies have greatly extended the range of conditions over which oxygen-hemoglobin equilibrium may be calculated. Samaja, Winslow and coworkers have published a series of papers

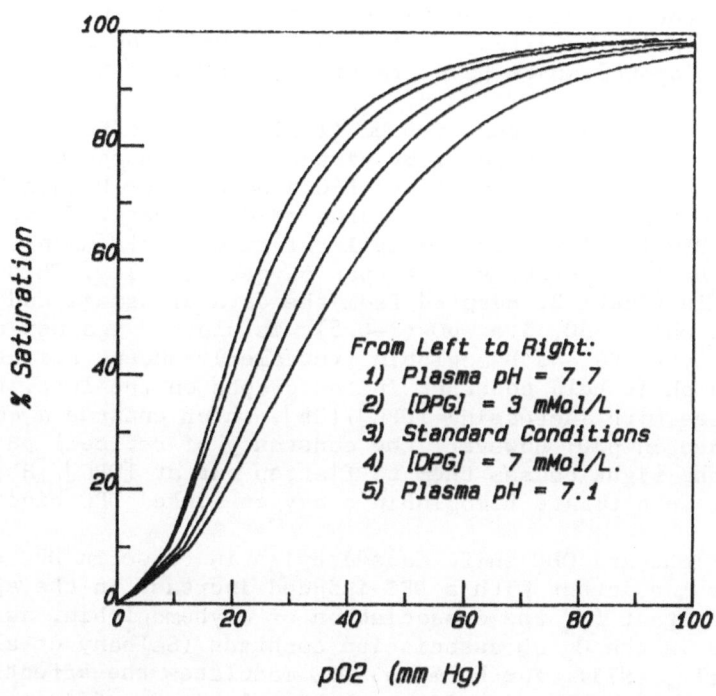

Figure 1.   Oxyhemoglobin dissociation curve (ODC) for whole human
             blood under standard conditions of pCO_2 = 40 mm Hg, T =
             37°C, plasma pH = 7.4 and red cell DPG concentration =
             5 mMol/liter; and under conditions altered as indicated.
             Based on the data of Arturson et al., (1974).

that allow accurate estimation of $S(pO_2)$ with plasma pH 7.2-7.8, pCO_2 7-70 mm Hg and [DPG]/[Hb] 0.2-2.7 mol/mol. Their results are conveniently presented both as a nomogram (Samaja et al., 1981) and as values for the four constants in the Adair equation:

$$S = \frac{a_1 p + 2a_2 p^2 + 3a_3 p^3 + 4a_4 p^4}{4(1 + a_1 p + a_2 p^2 + a_3 p^3 + a_4 p^4)} \tag{2}$$

Values for the a_i are expressed as empirically determined functions of pH, pCO_2 and [DPG]/[Hb], all at 37° (Winslow et al., 1983). O_2 tension is denoted above by p, rather than pO_2.

As first demonstrated by Duhm (1971), DPG's effect on hemoglobin O_2 affinity is multifold. By virtue of its charge of ca. −4 and negligible membrane permeability, DPG enhances the Donnan-type potential and hence the red cell/plasma pH difference. Thus, an increase in DPG level lowers red cell relative to plasma pH, which magnifies DPG's apparent effect upon oxygen affinity. This is illustrated in figure 2, adapted from the data of Samaja and Winslow (1979), in which p50, i.e. $pO_2(S=0.5)$, is plotted against the ratio of erythrocyte DPG and hemoglobin (tetramer) concentrations. Since the plasma pH is held constant in the graphs on the left, red cell pH decreases with increasing [DPG]/[Hb], which ensures a continuous increase in p50. However, the constancy of red cell pH in the plots on the right causes them to flatten out at [DPG]/[Hb] values sufficient to saturate hemoglobin's oxygen-linked DPG binding site.

The rightward ODC shift caused by an increase in DPG concentration is consistent with a DPG-induced increase in the apparent kinetic constant for the dissociation of oxyhemoglobin, as well as a decrease in the O_2-Hb association constant (Salhany et al., 1970; Bauer et al., 1973). Furthermore, DPG modulates the effects of hydrogen ions and carbon dioxide upon hemoglobin O_2 affinity. The hydrogen effect, expressed as the "Bohr factor" - the ratio of the change in $\log_{10} pO_2$ to the change in plasma pH, at constant S and DPG level, is sensitive to a change in DPG concentration, because of the pH-dependence of hemoglobin DPG binding. The CO_2 effect is DPG-sensitive because DPG and CO_2 competitively bind at the same hemoglobin amino groups. Thus, DPG decreases the magnitude of the "CO_2 Bohr factor" - i.e., that measured when the pH change is brought about by a change in pCO_2, and increases the magnitude of the "fixed acid Bohr factor" - that measured when the pH change is caused by the addition of non-volatile acid or base (Hlastala and Woodson, 1983). For an early, but highly authoritative review of this chemistry, see Kilmartin and Rossi-Bernardi (1973).

Finally, because DPG contains two phosphate groups which are titrated in the physiological pH range, it makes a contribution to the blood's buffer capacity, albeit a small one compared to that of

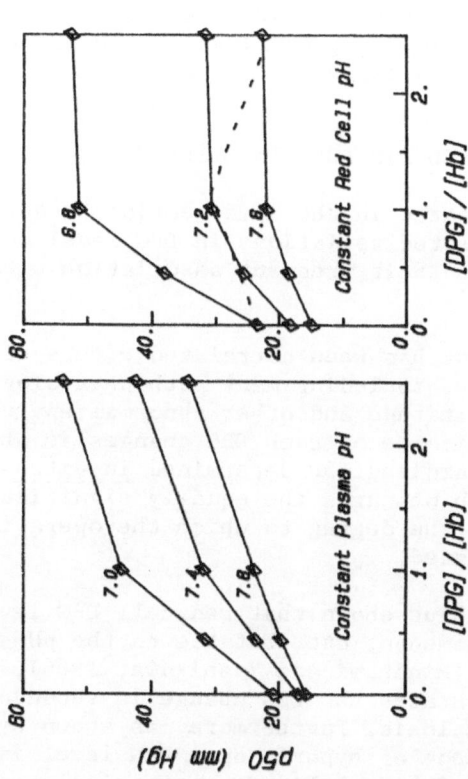

Figure 2. Dependence of p50 of human blood at 37°C and pCO_2 40 mm Hg, upon the ratio of red cell DPG and Hb (tetramer) concentrations, at constant values of plasma pH (left) and red cell pH (right). Symbols denote data of Samaja and Winslow (1979). Broken lines (right) adapted from correlation of DPG level and red cell pH reported by Astrup et al. (1970).

hemoglobin (Siggaard-Andersen, 1974). Duhm (1976) has demonstrated
that under certain conditions DPG magnification of the red cell/
plasma pH differential, together with the greater pH change under-
gone by plasma than cells during titration of high-DPG blood, make
it appear that DPG decreases blood buffer capacity.

Any buffer influences blood CO_2 transport, since the extent of
carbon dioxide transformation to bicarbonate ion is limited by the
capacity to buffer the hydrogen ions formed from carbonic acid. In
addition, DPG competition for hemoglobin's CO_2 binding sites restricts the contribution of carbamino formation to CO_2 transfer between peripheral and pulmonary capillaries (Bauer, 1970). However,
the influences of DPG upon blood CO_2 carriage and pH are each small
by comparison with its role in oxygen transport.

REGULATION OF DPG IN VIVO AND ITS ROLE IN DISEASE

These subjects are treated in the same section because the significance of disease-correlated variations in DPG level must be interpreted in the context of their frequent association with and apparent cause by pH changes.

Erythrocyte DPG content has been correlated with a wide variety
of physiological conditions, including many pathophysiological
states and adaptation to altitude and other abnormal environments
(Harken, 1977). The significance of such DPG changes is often measured in terms of the standardized p50 determined in vitro at a plasma pH of 7.4. This approach obscures the equally significant effect
of in vivo pH. In general, the degree to which the operating ODC has
been shifted is over-estimated.

Astrup et al. (1970) have shown that red cell DPG level increases with pH. This phenomenon, attributable to the pH-sensitivity
of erythrocyte glycolysis (Minakami and Yoshikawa, 1966), indicates
that in many pathological states the DPG change is secondary to a
prevailing acidosis or alkalosis. Furthermore, as shown by Duhm and
Gerlach (1971), the influence of hypoxia upon DPG level is itself
mediated by the influence of hemoglobin O_2 saturation upon pH.

The broken lines in figure 2 indicate combinations of erythrocyte pH and DPG consistent with the data of Astrup et al. (1970).
They suggest that, when sustained for the ca. 24-hr period for DPG
response (Valeri and Hirsch, 1969), an in vivo pH change will normally effect a DPG change that largely compensates for the pH-induced perturbation in p50. For example, Lichtman et al. (1974) found
that increased DPG offset the alkalosis of hypoproliferative anemia,
but not the decrease in blood hemoglobin content.

The rule has many exceptions; e.g., DPG and pH no longer correlate simply in the presence of disorders of glycolytic enzymes or of the availability of inorganic phosphate. Nonetheless, the role of pH in DPG regulation is of primary importance in the understanding of disease-induced O_2 affinity changes.

THE SIGNIFICANCE OF BLOOD OXYGEN AFFINITY IN TRANSFUSION

Although long-term p50 adjustment via DPG is not feasible, evidence is accumulating that transfusion of blood with normal or elevated p50 is vital for the recovery from acute cardio-respiratory disturbances (Valeri, 1984). The switch to citrate-phosphate-dextrose (CPD) from acid-citrate-dextrose (ACD) solution for storage of red cells in blood banks has been prompted by the need to avoid DPG depletion. Furthermore, incubation with inosine, pyruvate and phosphate (Deuticke et al., 1971) yields supranormal DPG levels, which may become increasingly important in light of recent studies indicating that blood O_2 affinity is a key to sustaining tissue oxygen consumption when a second factor - e.g., the heart - is compromised.

Table 1 lists the results of such studies, which may be assessed after first returning to equation (1) of the introductory section. This states that metabolism requires the release of a certain fraction of the oxygen supplied to tissue by the flowing blood. When the supply rate is compromised, the fraction released must rise. This can be realized by operating at a lower venous pO_2 - which is tolerable in the event of capillary recruitment and thus a decrease in oxygen diffusion distance. Alternatively, with venous pO_2 fixed, greater extraction can be accomplished with a right-shifted ODC - unless arterial pO_2 is so low as to substantially diminish S^A.

Ross and Hlastala (1981) found that, when blood flow was maintained constant, isolated canine muscle sustained its O_2 consumption in response to a decrease in p50, with a decrease in venous pO_2 - except in the case of DPG-depleted, stored blood. This is difficult to explain without entertaining the possibility that some factor in stored blood interferes with capillary recruitment or the kinetics of erythrocyte O_2 release (the latter being less likely). While muscle may generally be able to cope with compromised O_2 supply, the results of Woodson and Auerbach (1982) indicate that heart and brain tissue require from two to four times normal blood flow when perfused with low p50 blood, the results being more extreme in the case of anemic rats. The sensitivity of brain O_2 consumption to increased blood O_2 affinity and constant blood flow was further emphasized by Woodson et al. (1982) who observed substantial decreases in metabolic rate and EEG signal with perfusion of canine brain with low p50 blood.

While Nylander et al. (1983) again demonstrated the resilience of muscle tissue to alterations in p50, Soulard et al. (1983) demon-

Table 1. Results of Recent Studies of the Effects of Altered Blood O_2 Affinity

Investigators	Organs	Blood flow	p50 Range*	Results
Ross and Hlastala (1981)	Isolated canine muscle	Controlled	Normal(30) Metabisulfite(24) Storage(22) Cyanate(14)	O_2 consumption maintained with decrease in venous pO_2, except with stored blood, in which case venous pO_2 was unchanged
Woodson and Auerbach (1982)	Normal and anemic rats	Measured in various organs	Lowered by cyanate and metabisulfite	Unchanged cardiac output which was, however, redistributed to brain and heart
Woodson et al. (1982)	Isolated canine brain	Controlled	Normal(30) Cyanate(18) Alkalosis(17)	O_2 consumption and EEG signal lower with left-shifted oxyhemoglobin dissociation curve
Nylander et al. (1983)	Rats, normal and exposed to 12% oxygen	----------	Normal(35) Cyanate(17)	Skeletal muscle pO_2 histograms unaffected by affinity changes
Soulard et al. (1983)	Guinea pig	Measured	Normal(25) Transfused rat blood(37)	Reduced flow of rat blood due to increase in peripheral resistance
Apstein et al. (1983)	Isolated rabbit heart	Controlled	Stored blood(16) DPG-rejuvenated blood(33)	Greater myocardial O_2 consumption with low affinity blood

*Numbers in parentheses denote the p50 in mm Hg, under standard conditions.

strated low affinity blood reduces the number of active capillaries in guinea pigs, thereby increasing peripheral resistance and decreasing cardiac output. Finally, Apstein et al. (1983), working with isolated rabbit hearts, have demonstrated compromised myocardial oxygen consumption in the controlled flow of high-affinity, stored blood, and substantially greater O_2 consumption in corresponding experiments with DPG-restored, low affinity blood.

These studies underline the need to experiment under carefully controlled conditions, as well as the importance of capillary recruitment viz-a-viz both oxygen diffusion distance and peripheral resistance. Furthermore, they demonstrate the particular sensitivity of brain and cardiac tissue to affinity changes, especially in conjunction with compromised blood flow or hemoglobin content. Since transfusion is called upon particularly in cases involving such compromises, the importance of ensuring proper blood oxygen affinity is clear.

CONCLUSIONS

a) DPG has the effect of stabilizing the position of the oxyhemoglobin dissociation curve in the face of chronic changes in pH.

b) Manipulation of hemoglobin oxygen afinity via DPG may be vital during acute disturbances in arterial blood O_2 delivery, particularly in heart and brain tissue.

ACKNOWLEDGMENT

This work was supported by NIH funds made available by the Tufts Faculty Research Awards Committee.

REFERENCES

Apstein, C. S., Dennis, R. C., Briggs, L., Vogel, W. M., Frazer, J., and Valeri, C. R., 1984, Effect of red blood cell storage on cardiac performance: Improved myocardial oxygen delivery and function during constant flow coronary perfusion with low oxy-hemoglobin affinity human red blood cells in normothermic and hypothermic rabbit hearts, Office of Naval Research, Contract N0014-79-C-0168, Technical Report No. 83-01.
Arturson, G., Garby, L., Robert, M. and Zaar, B., 1974, The O_2 dissociation curve of normal human blood with special reference to the influence of physiological effector ligands, Scand. J. clin. Lab. Invest., 34:9.
Astrup, P., Rørth, M., and Thorshauge, C., 1970, Dependency on acid-base status of oxyhemoglobin dissociation and 2,3-diphospho-

glycerate level in human erythrocytes. II. In vivo studies, Scand. J. clin. Lab. Invest., 26:47.

Baldwin, J. M., 1975, Structure and function of hemoglobin, Prog. Biophys. Molec. Biol., 29:225.

Bauer, C., 1970, Reduction of the carbon dioxide affinity of human hemoglobin solutions by 2,3-diphosphoglycerate, Resp. Physiol., 10:10.

Bauer, C., Klocke, R. A., Kamp, D., and Forster, R. E., 1973, Effect of 2,3-diphosphoglycerate and H^+ on the reaction of O_2 and hemoglobin, Am. J. Physiol., 224:838.

Benesch, R. and Benesch, R. E., 1967, The effect of organic phosphates from the human erythrocyte on the allosteric properties of hemoglobin, Biochem. Biophys. Res. Commun., 26:162.

Chanutin, A. and Curnish, P., 1967, Effect of organic and inorganic phosphate on the oxygen equilibrium of human erythrocytes, Arch. Biochem. Biophys., 121:96.

Deuticke, B., Duhm, J., and Dierkesmann,R.,1971, Maximal elevation of 2,3-diphosphoglycerate concentrations in human erythrocytes: Influence on glycolytic metabolism and intracellular pH, Pflugers Arch., 326:15.

Duhm, J., 1971, Effects of 2,3-diphosphoglycerate and other organic phosphate compounds on oxygen affinity and intracellular pH of human erythrocytes, Pflugers Arch., 326:341.

Duhm, J., 1976, Influence of 2,3-diphosphoglycerate on the buffering properties of human blood. Role of the red cell membrane, Pflugers Arch., 363:61.

Duhm, J. and Gerlach,E.,1971, On the mechanism of the hypoxia-induced increase of 2,3-diphosphoglycerate in erythrocytes, Pflugers Arch., 326:254.

Ellis, C. G., Potter, R. F., and Groom, A.C.,1983, The Krogh cylinder is not appropriate for modelling O_2 transport in contracted skeletal muscle, Adv. Exper. Med. Biol., 159:253.

Harken, A. H., 1977, The surgical significance of the oxyhemoglobin dissociation curve, Surg. Gynec. Obstet., 144:935.

Hlastala, M. P. and Woodson, R. C., 1983, Bohr effect data for blood gas calculations, J. Appl. Physiol., 55:1002.

Honig, C. R., Gayeski, R. E. J.. Federspiel, W., Clark, A. Jr., and Clark, P., 1984, Muscle O_2 gradients from hemoglobin to cytochrome: new concepts, new complexities, Adv. Exper. Med. Biol., 169:23.

Kilmartin, J.V. and Rossi-Bernardi, L., 1973, Interaction of hemoglobin with hydrogen ions, carbon dioxide and organic phosphates, Physiol. Rev., 53:836.

Lichtman, M. A., Murphy, M. S., Whitbeck, A. A., and Kearney, E. A., 1974, Oxygen binding to haemoglobin in subjects with hypoproliferative anaemia, with and without chronic renal disease: Role of pH, Brit. J. Haemat., 27:439.

Minakami, S. and Yoshikawa, H., 1966, Studies on erythrocyte glycolysis. III. The effects of active cation transport, pH and inorganic phosphate concentration on erythrocyte glycolysis, J. Biochem. (Tokyo), 59:145.

72

Nylander, E., Lund, N. and Wranne, B., 1983, Effect of increased blood oxygen affinity on skeletal muscle surface oxygen pressure fields, J. Appl. Physiol., 54:99.

Ross, B. K. and Hlastala, M. P., 1981, Increased hemoglobin-oxygen affinity does not decrease skeletal muscle oxygen consumption, J. Appl. Physiol., 51:864.

Salhany, J. M., Eliot, R. S., and Mizukami, H., 1970, The effect of 2,3-diphosphoglycerate on the kinetics of deoxygenation of human hemoglobin, Biochem. Biophys. Res. Commun., 39:1052.

Samaja, M., Mosca, A., Luzzana, M., Rossi-Bernardi, L., and Winslow, R., 1981, Equations and nomogram for the relationship of human blood p50 to 2,3-diphosphoglycerate, CO_2 and H^+, Clin. Chem., 27:1856.

Samaja, M. and Winslow, R., 1979, The separate effects of H^+ and 2,3-DPG on the oxygen equilibrium curve of human blood, Brit. J. Haemat., 41:373.

Siggaard-Andersen, O., 1974, "The Acid-Base Status of the Blood," Munskgaard, Copenhagen.

Soulard, C. D., Teisseire, B. P., Teisseire, L. J., and Herigault, R. A., 1983, Consequences of an acute increase in p50 in anaesthetized guinea pigs, Respir. Physiol., 51:21.

Valeri, C. R., 1984, Clinical importance of the oxygen transport function of preserved red blood cells, in: "Proc. 12th Katzir-Katchalsky meeting on oxygen transport by red blood cells", Pergamon, Oxford, in press.

Valeri, C. R. and Hirsch, N. M., 1969, Restoration in vivo of erythrocyte adenosine triphosphate, 2,3-diphosphoglycerate, potassium ion and sodium ion concentration following transfusion of acid-citrate-dextrose-stored human red blood cells, J. Lab. Clin. Med., 73:722.

Winslow, R. M., Samaja, M., Winslow, N. J., Rossi-Bernardi, L., and Shrager, R. I., 1983, Simulation of continuous blood O_2 equilibrium curve over physiological pH, DPG and pCO_2 range, J. Appl. Physiol., 54:524.

Woodson, R. D. and Auerbach, S., 1982, Effect of increased oxygen affinity and anemia on cardiac output and its distribution, J. Appl. Physiol., 53:1299.

Woodson, R. D., Fitzpatrick, J. H. Jr., Costello, D. J., and Gilboe, D. D., 1982, Increased brain oxygen affinity decreases canine brain oxygen consumption, J. Lab. Clin. Med., 100:411.

CENTRAL NERVOUS SYSTEM

OXYGEN SUPPLY OF THE BLOOD-FREE PERFUSED GUINEA PIG BRAIN

AT THREE DIFFERENT TEMPERATURES

U. Heinrich, J. Hoffmann, H. Baumgärtl, B. Yu,
D.W. Lübbers

Max-Planck-Institut für Systemphysiologie
Rheinlanddamm 201, 4600 Dortmund 1, FRG

INTRODUCTION

Spectrophotometric measurements were used to study the redox-state of the cytochromes of the respiratory chain in the blood-free perfused brain. An evaluation method was investigated which allows to obtain information about the true absorption spectra and the influence of scattering.

The analysis of local tissue oxygen supply was performed by measuring Po_2 histograms. To have a better insight in the oxygen supply, we combined measurements of the Po_2 distribution on the brain surface with measurements of the Po_2 in deeper layers of the brain, using a Pt-needle electrode.

Tissue respiration was varied by changing the temperature of the perfusion medium.

METHODS

Since hemoglobin has a very strong absorption spectrum in the same wavelength range as the cytochromes, it was necessary to perfuse the brain with a clear, colourless solution. The brain perfusion was performed according to Heinrich et al. (1984). As perfusion medium we used a Macrodex 6% solution with addition of glucose (5.5 mmol·1^{-1}), KCl (4.7 mmol·1^{-1}), $CaCl_2$ (1.25 mmol·1^{-1}), KH_2PO_4 (1.2 mmol·1^{-1}), $NaHCO_3$ (24.9 mmol·1^{-1}), $MgSO_4$ (0.3 mmol·1^{-1}) and papaverine (4.0 mg/100 ml perfusion solution).

The perfusion medium was equilibrated with carbogen and heated up to three different temperatures (18°C, 24°C and 37°C). The perfusion rate was 30 ml/min.

All recordings of reflection spectra of the perfused brain were performed by the rapid spectrometer T 13/3 according to Lübbers and Niesel (1957) in the wavelength range of 510 - 630 nm. The depth of the penetration of the light beam was about 1 to 1.5 mm.

Local cortical tissue Po_2 was measured polarographically with a multiwire Pt surface electrode according to Kessler and Lübbers (1966) and modified by Yu et al. (1984).

To obtain additional information about the deeper layers of the brain, experiments were performed with the Po_2 needle electrode according to Baumgärtl and Lübbers (1983), beginning from the brain surface up to 3 mm depth.

RESULTS AND DISCUSSION

The evaluation method for the reflection spectra of biological material considers absorption and scattering using the two-flux-theory of Kubelka and Munk (1931). For the analysis of reflection spectra we used a non-linear multicomponent analysis according to Hoffmann et al. (1984).

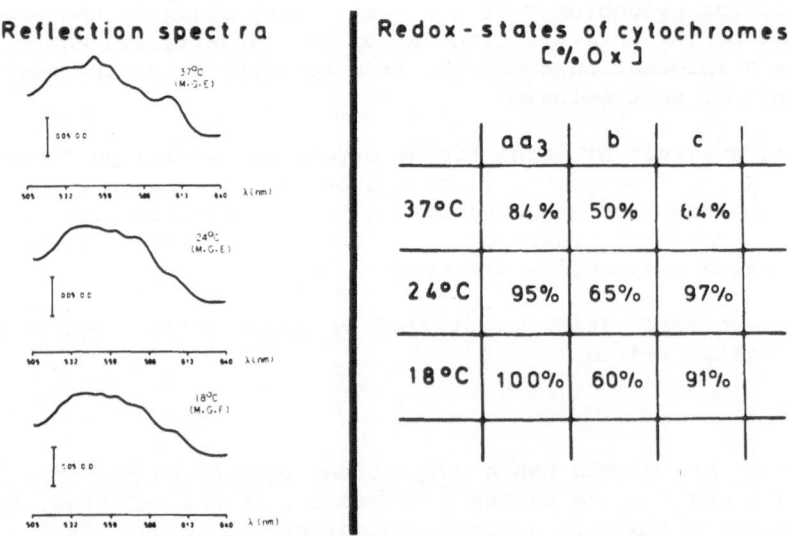

Fig. 1. Reflection spectra and redox-states of the blood-free per-fused guinea-pig brain at 18°C (lower trace), 24°C (middle trace), and 37°C (upper trace). The perpendicular bar corresponds to an absorption change of 0.05 OD. The wavelengths (x-axis) ran from ≈ 505 to 640 nm

To change the oxygen consumption and the oxygen supply, we perfused the guinea pig brain with solutions of different temperatures. The left side of Fig. 1 shows the reflection spectra at the perfusion temperatures 18°C, 24°C and 37°C. The right side of Fig. 1 gives information about the redox state of the cytochromes aa_3, b and c during our perfusion conditions.

Calculations of the redox-states during a perfusion stop has the result that the cytochromes follow different kinetics. Whereas cytochrome aa_3 behaves similarly to cytochrome c, cytochrome b behaves differently in the redox state during normoxia and in the kinetics during hypoxia (Heinrich et al., 1983).

To compare the absolute values of the redox-states during the experiments with the oxygen supply of the brain surface, we combined the measurements of the redox-states of cytochromes with measurements of Po_2 histograms on the brain surface (Fig. 2).

The redox-state of cytochrome aa_3 serves as an indicator of the intracellular mitochondrial oxygen supply, whereas the measured surface Po_2 histogram characterizes only the O_2 supply of the surface layer.

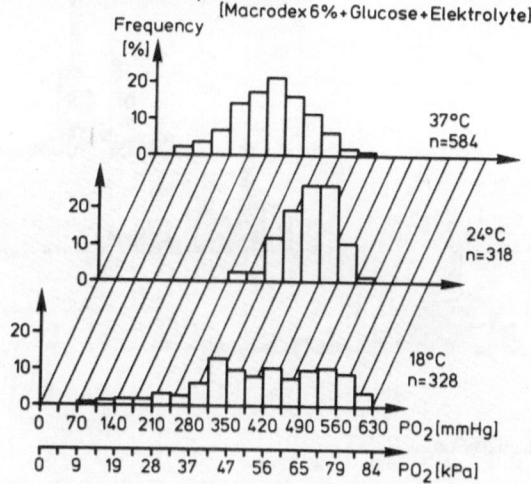

Fig. 2. Po_2 surface histograms of the blood-free perfused guinea pig brain at 18°C, 24°C and 37°C

In the perfused brain, the mean surface Po_2 amounts to about 450 torr at 18°C, to about 350 torr at 24°C and to about 200 torr at 37°C. These very high Po_2 values correspond to the high Po_2 of the inflowing medium, which is about 600 torr.

To obtain additional information about the oxygen supply in deeper layers of the brain, we performed experiments with the Po_2 needle electrode, beginning from the brain surface up to 3 mm depth.

These experiments were of special interest, because our photo-metric measurements are made up to a depth of about 1 to 1.5 mm.

The following figures show the oxygen supply, measured with the Po_2 needle electrode according to Baumgärtl and Lübbers (1983) at the temperature 18°C, 24°C and 37°C.

The Po_2 histograms for each temperature are divided into different parts (Figs. 3-5).

The lowest one shows the complete Po_2 distribution from the brain surface up to 3 mm depth. The second from the surface to 0.5 mm. The third histogram shows the scope from 0.5 mm to 2 mm, which corresponds to the grey matter of the brain and to the re-flection measurements. The fourth and uppermost histogram shows the white matter Po_2 distribution from 2 mm to 3 mm depth.

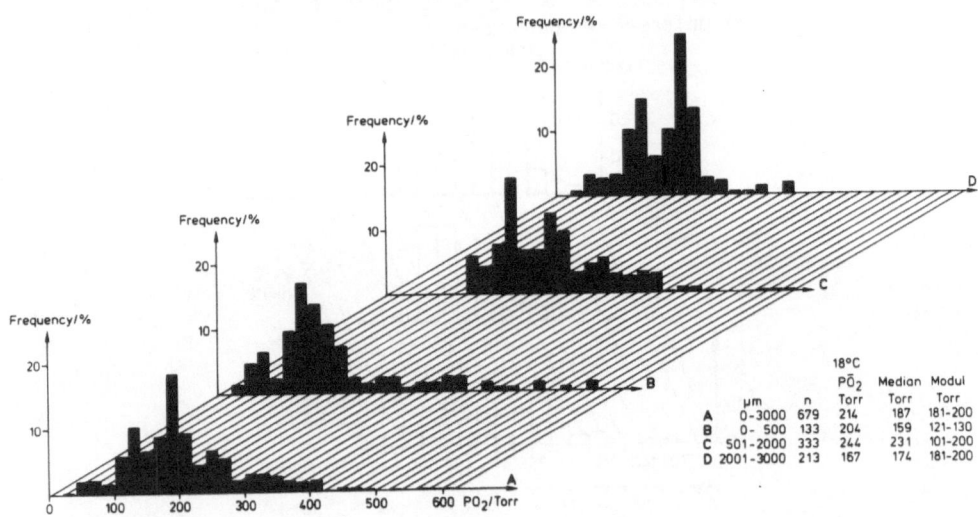

Fig. 3. Po_2 needle-electrode histogram of the blood-free perfused guinea-pig brain at 18°C (measured from the brain surface up to 3 mm depth)

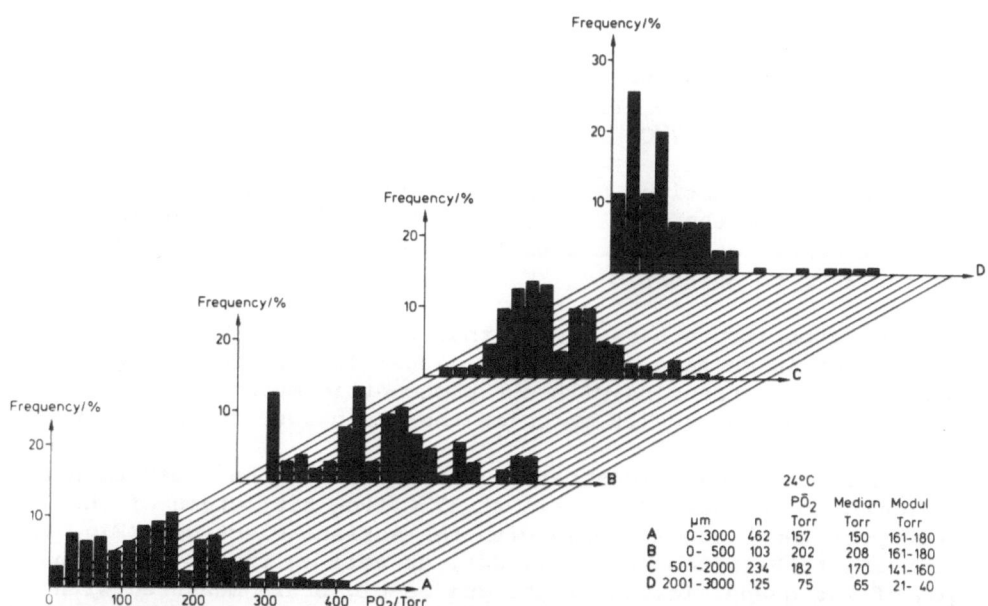

Fig. 4. Po₂ needle electrode histogram of the blood-free perfused
guinea-pig brain at 24°C (measured from the brain surface
up to 3 mm depth)

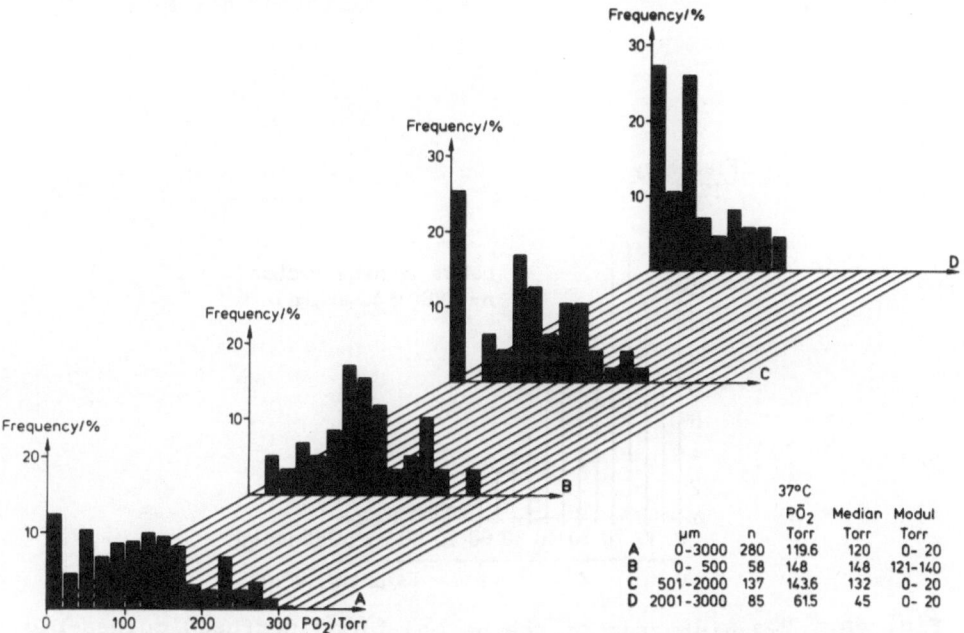

Fig. 5. Po₂ needle electrode histogram of the blood-free perfused
guinea-pig brain at 37°C (measured from the brain surface
up to 3 mm depth).

The mean values of the Po_2 distribution from the brain surface up to 3 mm depth, including the grey matter and the white matter of the brain, amounted to 214 torr at 18°C, to 157 torr at 24°C and to 120 torr at 37°C.

There is a distinct difference between the surface Po_2 on the brain cortex and the mean Po_2 distribution of the deeper layers. The difference for 18°C amounts to 236 torr, for 24°C to 193 torr and for 37°C to 80 torr.

The experiments have shown, that the Po_2 values are decreasing from the brain surface towards the deeper layers of the brain. These results correspond with our photometric measurements, in which tissue up to 1.5 mm below the brain surface is involved.

These findings demonstrate a difference to the measurements of the normal blood perfused brain at 37°C. Po_2 histograms of the blood perfused brain measured with the surface electrode (Fig. 6a) according to Heinrich et al. (1984), as well as the Po_2 distribution of the deeper layers of the guinea-pig brain measured with pO_2 needle electrode (Fig. 6b) according to Lübbers (1981) did not show a significant difference between both histograms.

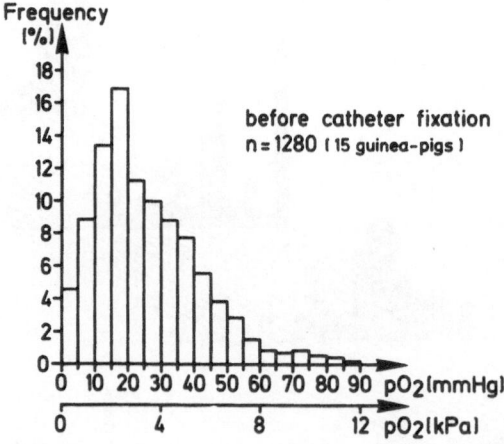

Fig. 6a. Po_2 histogram of the normal blood perfused guinea-pig brain at 37°C, measured with the Po_2 surface electrode

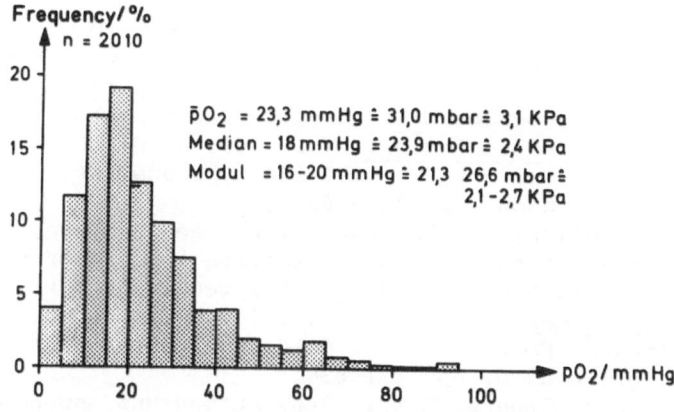

Fig. 6b.   PO$_2$ histogram of the normal blood perfused guinea-pig
brain at 37°C, measured with the Po$_2$ needle
electrode

The differences between the blood perfused brain and the
blood-free perfused brain can be explained by the particular
vascular pattern of the brain and the diffusion conditions (shunt
diffusion).

Our investigations show that only at the lowest temperature
(18°C) the oxygen consumption became so small, that it is
possible to provide sufficient oxygen supply of the brain. Whereas
at 24°C and at 37°C the lower Po$_2$ values measured with the
needle electrode and the decreased redox-state of the cytochromes
point to a beginning hypoxia.

REFERENCES

Baumgärtl, H., Lübbers, D. W., 1983, Microcoaxial needle sensor
    for polarographic measurement of local O$_2$ pressure in the
    cellular range of living tissue – its construction and
    properties, in: "Polarographic Oxygen Sensors", E. Gnaiger,
    H. Forstner, eds., Springer-Verlag, Berlin-Heidelberg,
    pp. 37-65
Heinrich, U., Hoffmann, J., and Lübbers, D. W., 1983, Quantitative
    analysis of reflection spectra on the perfused brain in
    different states of oxygen supply, in: "Oxygen Transport to
    Tissue IV," Adv. Exp. Med. and Biol., Vol. 159, H. I.
    Bicher, D. F. Bruley, eds., Plenum Press, New York-London,
    pp.119-127.

Heinrich, U., Yu, B., Hoffmann, J., and Lübbers, D. W., 1984,
The effect of glucose on the oxygen supply of the blood-free
perfused guinea pig brain as measured by reflection spectra
and pO_2 histograms, in: "Oxygen Transport to Tissue V,"
Adv. Exp. Med. and Biol., Vol. 169, D. W. Lübbers, H. Acker,
E. Leniger-Follert, T. K. Goldstick, eds., Plenum Press,
New York-London, pp. 261-269.

Hoffmann, J., Wodick, R., Hannebauer, F., and Lübbers, D. W., 1984,
Quantitative analysis of reflection spectra of the surface
of the guinea pig brain, in: "Oxygen Transport to Tissue V,"
Adv. Exp. Med. and Biol., Vol. 169, D. W. Lübbers, H. Acker,
E. Leniger-Follert, T. K. Goldstick, eds., Plenum Press,
New York-London, pp. 831-839.

Kessler, M., and Lübbers, D.W., 1966, Aufbau und Anwendungsmöglichkeiten verschiedener Po_2-Elektroden, Pflügers Arch. ges.
Physiol., 291:R82.

Kubelka, P., and Munk, F., 1931, Ein Beitrag zur Optik der
Farbanstriche, Techn. Physik, 12:593-603.

Lübbers, D. W., 1981, Grundlagen und Bedeutung der lokalen Sauer-
stoffdruckmessung und des pO_2-Histogramms für die Beurtei-
lung der Sauerstoffversorgung der Organe und des Organismus,
in: "Messung des Gewebesauerstoffdruckes bei Patienten,"
A. M. Ehrly, ed., Gerhard Witzstrock, Baden-Baden-Köln-New
York, pp. 11-21.

Lübbers, D. W., and Niesel, W., 1957, Ein Kurzzeit-Spektralanaly-
sator zur Registrierung rasch verlaufender Änderungen der
Absorption, Naturwissenschaften, 4:59-60.

Yu, B., Baumgärtl, H., and Lübbers, D. W., 1984, An improved
polarographic multiwire surface Po_2 electrode, particularly for measurement of high Po_2 values, in: "Oxygen Transport to Tissue V," Adv. Exp. Med. and Biol., Vol. 169,
D. W. Lübbers, H. Acker, E. Leniger-Follert, T. K. Goldstick, eds., Plenum Press, New York-London, pp. 877-886.

QUANTITATIVE ANALYSIS OF REFLECTION SPECTRA AND TISSUE METABOLITES

OF THE BLOOD-FREE PERFUSED GUINEA PIG BRAIN

U. Heinrich, J. Hoffmann, and D.W. Lübbers

Max-Planck-Institut für Systemphysiologie
Rheinlanddamm 201, 4600 Dortmund 1, FRG

INTRODUCTION

Absorption spectra of the blood-free perfused guinea-pig brain were determined by cytochrome aa_3, b, and c at three different temperatures (18° C, 24° C, 37° C) with the rapid spectrometer according to Lübbers and Niesel (1957). ECoG recordings were used to define the brain function throughout the experiments. Tissue metabolism was investigated by measuring the labile metabolites ATP, ADP, AMP and P_i as well as Lactate and Pyruvate in the guinea-pig brain.

METHODS

Guinea-pigs weighing about 300 g were pretreated with 0.5 ml Liquemin 30 min before starting the experiment. For the anaesthesia we used Nembutal (60 mg/ml) in a concentration of 0.1 ml/100 b.w. with an addition of 0.1 ml Atropine (1mg/ml). The brain perfusion was performed according to Heinrich et al. (1984a). As perfusion medium we used a Macrodex 6% solution with an addition of glucose and different electrolytes (Heinrich et al., 1984b). The perfusates were heated up to temperatures of 18° C, 24° C, and 37° C and aerated with carbogen (95% O_2 + 5% CO_2) by a disk oxygenator. The pH value of perfusates amounted to 7.3 and the perfusion rate was 30 ml/min.

All measurements of reflection spectra were performed with the rapid spectrometer according to Lübbers and Niesel (1957) in the wavelength range of 510 - 630 nm. The penetration of the light beam in tissue was about 1 to 1.5 mm. Reflection spectra were evaluated by applying the two-flux-theory of Kubelka and Munk (1931) and Hoffmann et al. (1984).

ECoG-measurements during the brain perfusions were recorded monopolarly with a silver wire.

Labile tissue metabolites were determined by the following freezing technique: The brain was removed from the skull with a pre-cooled spoon and pressed between two frozen metal disks. The pressed tissue was immersed immediately in liquid nitrogen. The frozen tissue was pulverized under further addition of liquid nitrogen and prepared for biochemical analysis.

For the quantitative analysis of the tissue metabolites we used the Boehringer-Test-Combinations.

ATP was determined according to Bücher (1947), ADP/AMP according to Jaworek (1974), Lactate according to Noll (1974), and Pyruvate according to Czok and Lambrecht (1974). Inorganic phosphorus was determined by Sigma Test-Box No. 670.

RESULTS AND DISCUSSION

Exact analysis of the redox-states of the cytochromes aa_3, b, and c was determined by using a non-linear multicomponent analysis according to Hoffmann et al. (1984). Table 1 shows the redox-states of the measured cytochromes during the brain perfusion at different temperatures in percent of oxidation.

The measurements show that only at the lowest temperature (18°C) the oxygen consumption became so small, that cytochrome aa_3, as a direct reaction partner of molecular oxygen is 100 % oxidized. By increasing the temperature all cytochromes become more reduced.

Table 1. Redox-states of the cytochromes (% ox) during brain perfusion at different temperatures

	Cyt.aa3	Cyt.b	Cyt.c
37° C	84 %	50 %	64 %
24° C	95 %	65 %	97 %
18° C	100 %	60 %	91 %

The error of the values in Table 1 amounts to ca. 3% (least square sum).

The results correspond to our polarographic measurements of the oxygen supply in different layers of the perfused guinea-pig brain (Heinrich et al., 1984b). There exists a great diffusion shunt of the oxygen from the brain surface up to a depth of about 3 mm. The measurements of the reflection spectra are made in a depth up to 1.5 mm.

Another parameter of the brain function throughout the experiments were ECoG measurements, recorded with a silver wire at three different temperatures.

The comparison of ECoG power analysis of the brain perfusion experiments with EcoG power analysis of the blood perfused brain does not show significant differences, as demonstrated in Figs. 1 and 2.

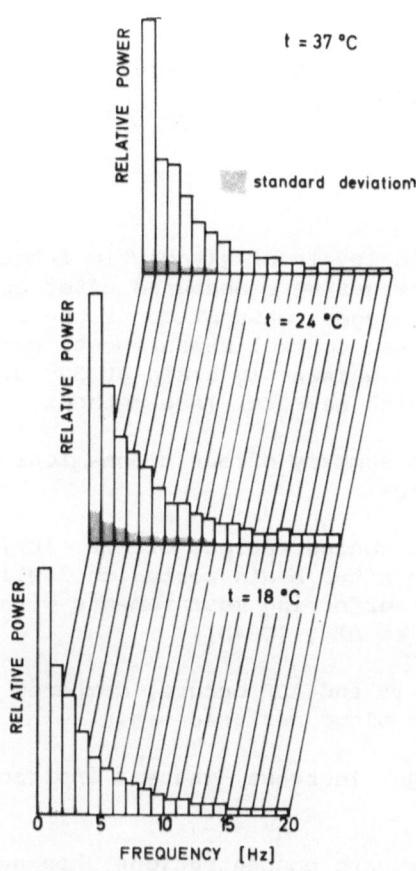

Fig. 1. ECoG-measurements of the perfused guinea-pig brain at the temperatures 18° C, 24° C, and 37° C

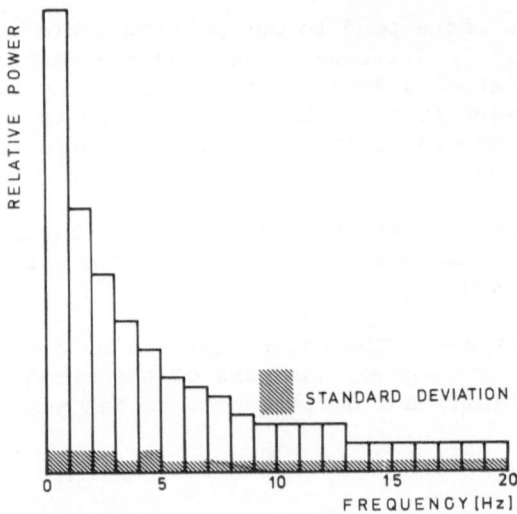

Fig. 2.   ECoG-measurements of the normal blood perfused guinea-pig
          brain at 37° C

Guinea-pig brain levels of glycolytic intermediates and high-
energy phosphate reserves were measured after brain perfusion and
correlated with the oxygen consumption of the brain at three
different temperatures. Control measurements were made of the
normal blood perfused guinea-pig brain at 37° C. All animals
were aneasthesized with Nembutal (see methods).

Table 2 shows a summary of our biochemical investigations of
the tissue metabolites.

We obtained the concentrations of ATP, ADP, AMP, P_i,
Lactate and Pyruvate after brain perfusion lasting about 1 to
1.5 hours and after performing measurements with the Po_2-needle
electrode (Heinrich et al., 1984b).

A decrease of ATP and ADP occurs, compared to the control
values of the normal blood perfused brain.

AMP shows a light increase, whereas inorganic phosphorus is
clearly higher.

Lactate and Pyruvate concentrations show no distinct
difference.

Table 2. Concentrations of ATP, ADP, AMP, P_i, Lactate and
Pyruvate of the blood-free perfused guinea-pig brain at
37° C and control values of the blood perfused
guinea-pig brain at 37° C

Tissue metabolites

Tissue metabolites during brain perfusion

[µmol/g]	ATP	ADP	AMP	Pi	Lac	Pyr	n
37°C	0.747 ± 0.259	0.372 ± 0.121	0.448 ± 0.139	10.11 ± 1.75	6.98 ± 1.04	0.281 ± 0.118	26

Controls : Blood perfused brain (37°C)

[µmol/g]	ATP	ADP	AMP	Pi	Lac	Pyr	n
37°C	3.55 ± 0.35	0.782 ± 0.023	0.409 ± 0.081	6.95 ± 0.84	5.10 ± 1.63	0.128 ± 0.033	10

   The comparison of the control values of the normal blood
perfused brain at 37° C with experiments of other authors
(Siesjö, 1978; Bergmeyer, 1974) shows a similar distribution of the
concentrations. However our measured tissue metabolite concentrations are generally higher than those of the other authors.

   The reason might be that Siesjö and the other investigators,
summarized by Bergmeyer, usually worked with rats and sometimes
with mice, but there is very few information about metabolism
changes in the guinea-pig brain.

   It has been shown that the photometric measurements as well
as the tissue metabolites react in the same way to changed
conditions of the oxygen supply in tissue. The redox-states of the
cytochromes as well as the metabolite concentrations point to a
beginning hypoxia, whereas the ECoG-measurements did not show a
significant difference. Additional measurements of tissue metabolites at 18°C and 24°C will be completed in the future.

REFERENCES

Bergmeyer, H. U., 1974, "Methoden der enzymatischen Analyse,"
    Verlag Chemie, Weinheim.
Bücher, Th., 1947, Biochim. biophys. Acta 1:292.
Czok, R., Lambrecht, W., 1974, Methoden der enzymatischen Analyse,
    Verlag Chemie, Weinheim, pp. 1491.
Heinrich, U., Yu, B., Hoffmann, J., Lübbers, D.W., 1984a, The
    effect of glucose on the oxygen supply of the blood-free
    perfused guinea-pig brain as measured by reflection spectra
    and Po_2-histograms, in: "Oxygen Transport to Tissue V,"
    Adv. Exp. Med. and Biol., Vol. 169, D. W. Lübbers, H.
    Acker, T. K. Goldstick, E. Leniger-Follert, eds., Plenum
    Press, New York, pp. 261-269.
Heinrich, U., Hoffmann, J., Baumgärtl, H., Yu, B., Lübbers, D.W.,
    1984b, in: "Oxygen Transport to Tissue VII," Kreuzer et
    al., eds, in print.
Hoffmann, J., Wodick, R., Hannebauer, F., and Lübbers, D. W., 1984,
    Quantitative analysis of reflection spectra of the surface
    of the guinea pig brain, in: "Oxygen Transport to Tissue V,"
    Adv. Exp. Med. and Biol., Vol. 169, D. W. Lübbers, H. Acker,
    E. Leniger-Follert, T. K. Goldstick, eds., Plenum Press,
    New York-London, pp. 831-839.
Jaworek, D. et al., 1974, in: H. U. Bergmeyer, "Methoden der en-
    zymatischen Analyse," Verlag Chemie, Weinheim, pp. 2178.
Kubelka, P., and Munk, F., 1931, Ein Beitrag zur Optik der
    Farbanstriche, Techn. Physik, 12:593-603.
Lübbers, D. W., and Niesel, W., 1957, Ein Kurzzeit-Spektralanalysa-
    tor zur Registrierng rasch verlaufender Änderungen der
    Absorption, Naturwissenschaften, 4:59-60.
Noll, F., 1974, in: H. U. Bergmeyer, "Methoden der enzymatischen
    Analyse," Verlag Chemie, Weinheim, pp. 1521.
Siesjö, B. K., 1978, "Brain Energy Metabolism," John Wiley & Sons,
    Chichester, New York, Brisbane, Toronto.

REGULATION OF CEREBRAL BLOOD FLOW (CBF) DURING HYPOXIA AND

EPILEPTIC SEIZURES

Eörs Dóra and Arisztid G.B. Kovách

Experimental Research Department and 2nd Institute
of Physiology, Semmelweis University Medical School
1082 Budapest, Hungary

INTRODUCTION

The exact mechanism as how cerebral vessels are dilated and
CBF increases during arterial hypoxia and epileptic seizures is
still poorly understood (Kuschinsky and Wahl, 1978; Winn et al.,
1981a; Dóra, 1984a). Because recently it was suggested that
adenosine may fulfill a critical role in the regulation of CBF
(Winn et al., 1981a), and Jöbsis (1977) postulated cytochrome
oxidase as being responsible for the dilatation of cerebral vessels during hypoxia, the present study was devoted to get further
data on these issues.

METHODS

The experiments were carried out on cats anaesthetized with
50-60 mg/kg alpha-D-glucochloralose, immobilized with flaxedil, and
artificially ventilated. Arterial blood gases and pH determined in
the normoxic animals during the control period were in the physiological range. The heads of the animals were mounted in stereotaxic stands and a cranial window was made into the right parietal
bone. The cranial window, described previously (Dóra, 1984a), was
used to superfuse the brain cortex with various drugs, and for optical monitoring of cerebrocortical microcirculation and NADH fluorescence. Electrical activity of the exposed cortex and the other
brain hemisphere was measured by silver electrodes built in the
plastic ring of the cranial window and by copper screws fixed into
the left parietal bone. Intracranial pressure was measured by metal
tubes sealed also into the plastic ring of the cranial window. Intracranial pressure and arterial blood pressure were measured by
Statham P23/d electromanometers.

Cerebrocortical reflectance (sum of scattered and reflected light) and NADH fluorescence were measured at 366 nm and 450 nm, respectively, through the cranial window with a microscope fluoro-reflectometer (Kovách et al., 1983; Dóra, 1984a). Cereborcortical vascular volume (CVV) and mean transit time of cortical blood flow (t_m) were measured, CBF calculated, with the modified (Dóra, 1984b) method of Eke et al. (1979). The reference values of these parameters were regarded as 100%.

For superfusion of the brain cortex, the artificial cerebro-spinal fluid (mock CSF) of Wahl and Kuschinsky (1976) was used. The various drugs were dissolved in mock CSF, bubbled with 5% CO_2 balanced in air and thermostated at 38° C. For perfusion a 2-chan-nel Harvard infusion pump with a perfusion rate of 1 ml/min was used. The pH of the CSF containing various drugs, except the CSF containing cyanide, was the same as the pH of the mock CSF (pH 7.20-7.25).

Experimental Procedures and Analysis of the Data

In the first series of experiments, the vasodilative potencies of the mitochondrial electron transport inhibitor amytal (inhibits at site I) and cyanide (inhibits at site III) were compared. Both drugs were applied by superfusion into the brain cortex.

In the second series of experiments, the vasodilative potency of topically applied adenosine and 2-chloroadenosine was tested. 2-chloroadenosine is a stable analogue of adenosine. It is not deaminated by adenosine deaminase and is taken up less rapidly by the brain as compared to adenosine (Winn et al., 1981b).

In the third series of experiments, it was tested how topically applied adenosine deaminase (5 U/ml) affects the hypoxic and functional hyperemic responses of cerebrocortical vessels. 5 U/ml adenosine deaminase deaminates 5×10^{-6} mol/ml/min adenosine into the nonvasoactive inosine. This enzyme activity is more than necessary to deaminate the extracellularly released adenosine, because during profound arterial hypoxia and epileptic seizures extracellular adenosine concentration in the brain does not increase to a higher value than approximately 10^{-8} mol/ml (Winn et al., 1981a).

In the fourth series of experiments, in order to get further insight into the significance of adenosine in the regulation of CBF, the brain cortices were topically treated with the vascular adenosine receptor antagonist theophylline (10^{-7} mol/ml). In the third and fourth series of experiments, arterial hypoxia, lasting some 3-4 min, was evoked by ventilating the animals with a gas mixture containing 6% oxygen. Epileptic seizures, lasting some

92

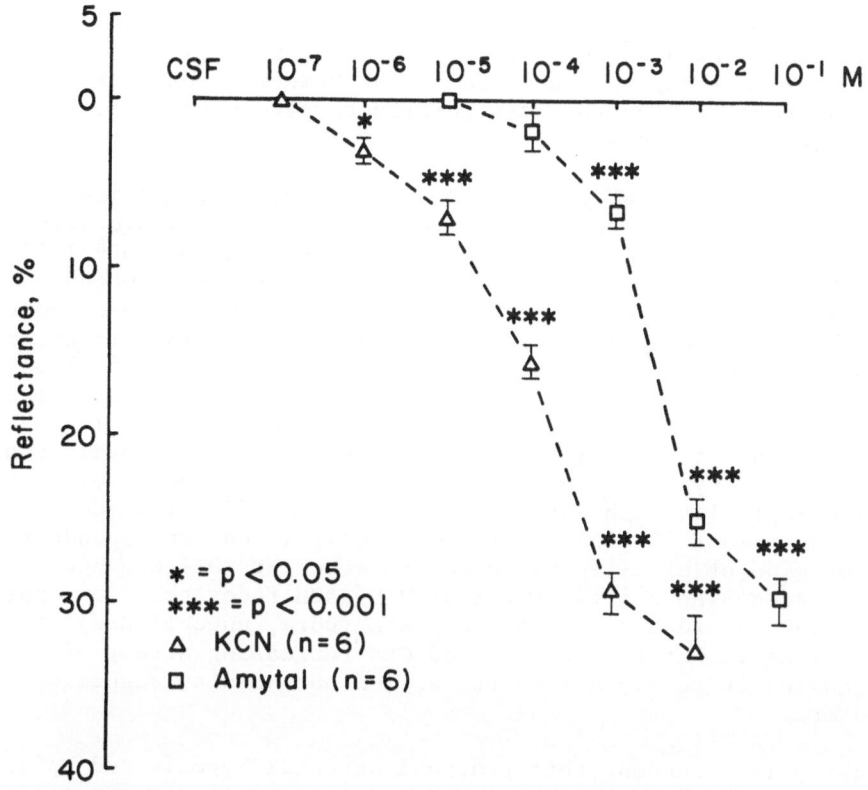

Fig. 1. Effect of cyanide and amytal superfusion of the brain cortex on cortical cascular volume (reflectance). The tested concentrations of amytal and cyanide are shown on the abscissa. Bars represent SEM; n is the number of experiments averaged; asterisks indicate the significant changes as compared with the values in mock CSF-superfused brain cortex. Decrease in reflectance means increase in cerebrocortical vascular volume.

60-120 s, were produced by injecting 3-6 mg/kg of metrasol into the lingual artery. Transient arterial hypoxia and epileptic seizures were used as test reactions.

The results are expressed as means $\pm$ SE. Statistical analysis of the data was performed by analysis of variance and a modified t test.

(amytal) oxidizes, at site III (cyanide) reduces cytochrome oxidase, though inhibition at both sites leads to maximum vasodilatation, it is very unlikely that changes in the reduction-oxidation state of cytochrome oxidase have a significant role in the hypoxic dilatation of cerebral vessels.

In Fig. 2, the effects of topically applied adenosine and its stable analogue 2-chloroadenosine on cerebrocortical microcirculation are demonstrated. In the concentration range of 10^{-6}-10^{-3} M, adenosine and 2-chloroadenosine led to concentration-dependent vasodilatation (increase in CVV), increase in the speed of cortical blood flow (decrease in t_m), and increase in CBF. Since 2-chloroadenosine is not deaminated by adenosine deaminase and is less rapidly taken up by the brain than adenosine, 2-chloroadenosine led to more marked increase in CBF than adenosine. At physiologically relevant concentration (10^{-5} M), adenosine and 2-chloroadenosine increased CBF by 49.6 $\pm$ 5.6% and 80.4 $\pm$ 10,3%, respectively. At pharmacologically high concentration (10^{-3} M), 2-chloroadenosine led to an almost fivefold increase in CBF, which corresponds to the data of Winn et al. (1981b). However, since at 10^{-3} M concentration, 2-chloroadenosine shifted cortical NAD/NADH redox state by approximately 15% toward a more reduced state (Dóra, unpublished), it is very unlikely that the very marked CBF increasing effect of 2-chloroadenosine is solely due to its action on vascular adenosine receptors.

Taking into account that profound arterial hypoxia and epileptic seizures increase CBF in the cat by approximately 2.5 and 4 times, respectively, but 10^{-5} M 2-chloroadenosine increases CBF only by 80.4 $\pm$ 10.3%, it seems unlikely that adenosine plays a critical role in the regulation of CBF during hypoxia and epileptic seizures. This assumption is strongly supported by our findings, which show that topically applied adenosine deaminase did not attenuate the vasodilative and NAD reducing potency of arterial hypoxia (Fig. 3), and attenuated slightly the vasodilative effect of transient epileptic seizures (Dóra et a., 1984). Similarly to this, superfusion of the brain cortices with CSF containing 10^{-7} mol/ml theophylline failed to diminish the CBF increasing effect of profound arterial hypoxia (Fig. 4) and of transient epileptic seizures (Fig. 5).

Concerning the significance of extracellularly released adenosine in the regulation of CBF, our results disagree with some of the data from literature (Emerson and Raymond, 1981; Winn et al., 1981a; Morii et al., 1983), but correspond to others (Nilsson et al., 1978; Rehncrona et al., 1978). For the explanation of our disparate finding, it is assumed that perivascular adenosine concentration in the brain cortex is either not increased to 10^{-5} M during profound arterial hypoxia and epileptic seizures, as suggested by Winn et al. (1981a), or some other vasoregulatory

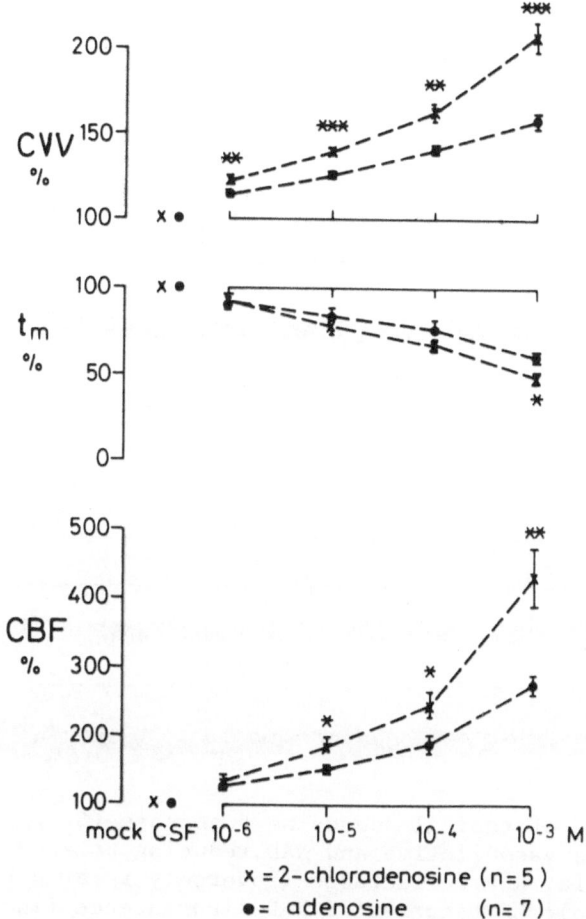

Fig. 2. Effect of topically applied adenosine and 2-chloroadenosine on cerebrocortical vascular volume (CVV), mean transit time of cortical blood flow (t_m), and cortical blood flow (CBF). Vertical bars represent SEM; n shows the number of experiments averaged. The reference values of CVV, t_m, and CBF, measured in artificial cerebrospinal fluid (mock CSF) superfused brain cortices during the control period, were regarded as 100%. Significant differences between the adenosine group and the 2-chloroadenosine group are marked by asterisks, as shown in Fig. 1.

RESULTS AND DISCUSSION

As Fig. 1 shows, the mitochondrial electron transport inhibitors amytal and cyanide resulted in concentration-dependent increase in cortical vascular volume, cyanide being more potent than amytal. Because inhibition of mitochondrial electron transport at site I

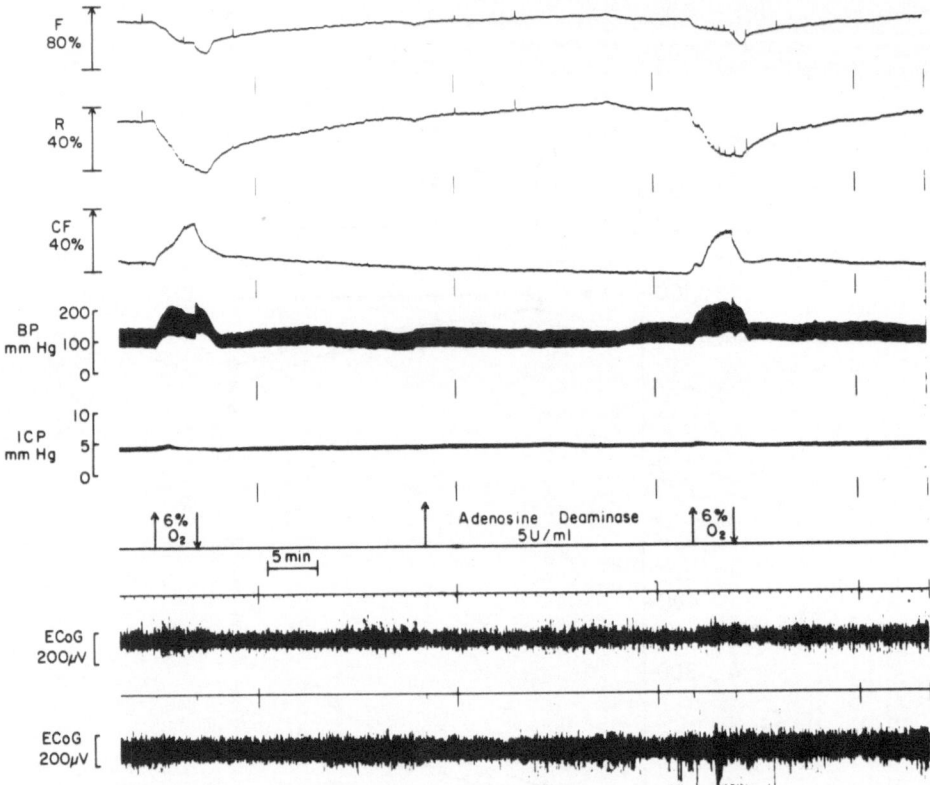

Fig. 3. Effect of topical adenosine deaminase (5 U/ml) treatment
on the vasodilative and NAD reducing potency of arterial
hypoxia. R = reflectance (inversely related to vascular
volume); CF = corrected NAD fluorescence (increase in CF
implies NAD reduction); BP = arterial blood pressure;
ICP = intracranial pressure.

mechanisms may oppose or entirely replace the vasoregulatory effect
of adenosine. The former assumption is supported by the experimental data of Nilsson et al. (1978) and Rehncrona et al. (1978), who
failed to reveal a significant increase in cerebral AMP and adenosine content during arterial hypoxia and epileptic seizures. The
second assumption is supported by those data from literature
(Astrup et al., 1978; Leniger-Follert, 1984), which show that extracellular H^+ and K^+ activities are increased to that high level
during arterial hypoxia and epileptic seizures, which according to

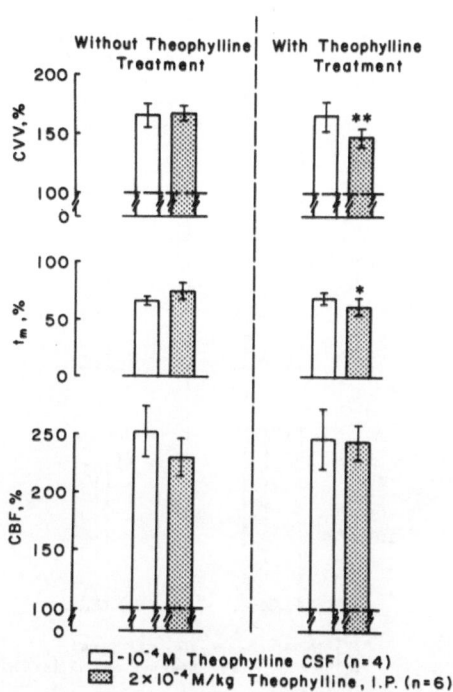

Fig. 4. Effect of topical theophylline treatment (10^{-7} mol/ml in CSF) (open columns) on the changes of cerebrocortical vascular volume (CVV), mean transit time of cortical blood flow (t_m), and cerebrocortical blood flow (CBF) evoked by profound arterial hypoxia. Vertical bars represent SEM; n shows the number of experiments averaged. The normoxic reference values of CVV, t_m, and CBF were regarded as 100%. Dotted columns show the effect of systemic (i.p. = intraperitoneal) theophylline treatment.

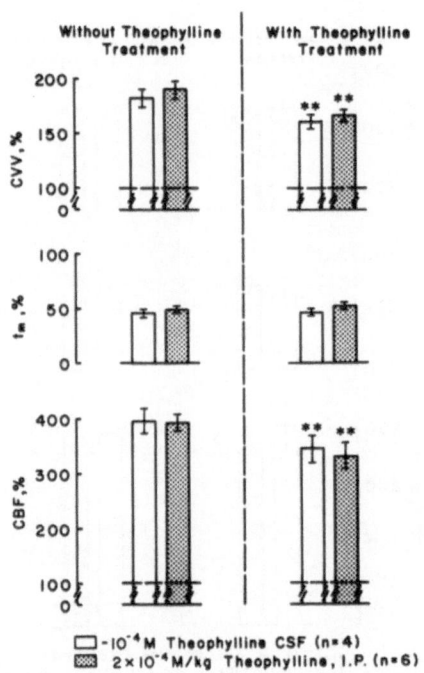

Fig. 5. Effect of topical theophylline treatment (10^{-7} mol/ml in
CSF) (open columns) on the changes of cerebrocortical vascular volume (CVV), mean transit time of cortical blood flow
(t_m), and cerebrocortical blood flow (CBF) evoked by transient epileptic seizures. Vertical bars represent SEM;
n shows the number of experiments averaged. Asterisks
($xx = p < 0.01$) show the significant differences between
the treated and untreated groups. Other marks are the same
as in Fig. 4.

Wahl and Kuschinsky (1977) can practically abolish the vasodilative effect of adenosine.

SYMMARY

In conclusion, our results suggest that neither the redox state of cytochrome oxidase nor adenosine are critical factors in the regulation of cerebral blood flow during arterial hypoxia and epileptic seizures.

REFERENCES

Astrup, J., Heuser, D.J., Lassen, N.A., Nilsson, B., Norberg, K., Siesjö, B.K., 1978, Evidence against H^+ and K^+ as main factors for the control of cerebral blood flow, in: Cerebral Vascular Smooth Muscle and its Control, Ciba Foundation Symposium 56, new series pp. 313-332, Elsevier, Amsterdam.

Dóra, E., 1984a, A simple cranial window technique for optical monitoring of cerebrocortical microcirculation and NAD/NADH redox state. Effect of mitochondrial electron transport inhibitors and anoxic anoxia. J. Neurochem. 42:101-108.

Dóra, E., 1984b, Further studies on the reflectometric method used for monitoring of cerebrocortical microcirculation. Importance of lactate anions, per se, in the coupling between cerebral blood flow and metabolism. Acta Physiol. Hung. in press.

Dóra, E., Koller, A., Kovách, A.G.B., 1984, Effect of topical adenosine deaminase treatment on the functional hyperemic and hypoxic responses of cerebrocortical microcirculation. J. Cereb. Blood Flow Metabol., 4:447-457.

Eke, A., Hutiray, Gy., Kovách, A.G.B., 1979, Induced hemodilution detected by reflectometry for measuring microregional blood flow and blood volume in cat brain cortex. Am. J. Physiol., 236:H759-768.

Emerson, T.E., Raymond, R.M., 1981, Involvement of adenosine in cerebral hypoxic hyperemia in dog. Am.J. Physiol. 241:H134-138.

Jöbsis, F.F., 1977, What is a molecular oxygen sensor? What is a transduction process?, in: Tissue Hypoxia and Ischmia, M. Reivich, R. Coburn, S. Lahiri, B. Chance, eds., pp. 3-17, Plenum Press, New York.

Kovách, A.G.B., Dóra, E., Szedlacsek, S., Koller,A., 1983, Effect of the organic calcium antagonist D-600 on cerebrocortical vascular and redox responses evoked by adenosine, anoxia, and epilepsy. J. Cereb. Blood Flow Metabol., 3-51-61.

Kuschinsky, W., Wahl, M., 1978, Local chemical and neurogenic regulation of cerebral vascular resistance. Physiol. Rev.,58:656-689.

Leniger-Follert, E., 1984, Mechanisms of regulation of cerebral microflow during bicuculline-induced seizures in anaesthetized cats. J. Cereb. Blood Flow Metabol., 4:150-165.

Morii, S., Winn, H.R., Berne, R.M., 1983, Effect of theophylline, an adenosine receptor blocker, on cerebral blood flow (CBF) during rest and transient hypoxia. J. Cereb. Blood Flow Metabol., 3, suppl. 1:S480.

Nilsson, B., Rehncrona, S., Siesjö, B.K., 1978, Coupling of cerebral metabolism and blood flow in epileptic seizures, hypoxia, and hypoglycemia, in: Cerebral Vascular Smooth Muscle and its Control, Ciba Foundation Symposium 56, new series, pp 199-214, Elsevier, Amsterdam.

Rehncrona, S., Siesjö, B.K., Westerberg, E., 1978, Adenosine and cyclic AMP in cerebral cortex of rats in hypoxia, status epilepticus and hypercapnia. Acta Physiol. Scand., 104:453-463.

Wahl, M., Kuschinsky, W., 1976, The dilatatory action of adenosine on pial arteries of cats and its inhibition by theophylline. Pflügers Arch., 362:55-59.

Wahl, M., Kuschinsky, W., 1977, Influence of H^+ and K^+ on adenosine induced dilatation at pial arteries of cats. Blood Vess., 14: 285-293.

Winn, H.R., Rubio, G.R., Berne, R.M., 1981a, The role of adenosine in the regulation of cerebral blood flow. J. Cereb. Blood Flow Metabol., 1:239-244.

Winn, H.R., Rubio, R., Curnish, R.R., Berne, R.M., 1981b, Changes in regional cerebral blood flow (rCBF) caused by increases in CSF concentrations of adenosine and 2-chloroadenosine (CHL-ADO). J. Cereb. Blood Flow Metabol., 1, suppl. 1:S401.

REDISTRIBUTION OF CEREBROCORTICAL MICROFLOW DURING INCREASED

NEURONAL ACTIVITY

Andras Eke

Experimental Research Department and 2nd Department of
Physiology, Semmelweis Medical University, Budapest
H-1082, Hungary, and
Department of Neurology, The University of Alabama in
Birmingham, Birmingham AL 35294

INTRODUCTION

It is well established[1], that among a wide range of circumstances the cerebral blood flow is tightly coupled via different
mechanisms to the metabolic activity of the neuronal tissue in
volumes down to several cubic millimeters. Many of these adjusting
mechanisms (O_2, CO_2, H^+, K^+, metabolites, neurotransmitters, etc.)
coexist in the brain and can be equally influenced in their
effectiveness by the distribution pattern of the cerebral
intraparenchymal circulation in tissue microareas, which along with
these factors will ultimately determine the distribution of blood
flow among the smallest groups of neurones in functional integrity
at any given functional state of the tissue. Experimental data on
high resolution distribution pattern of cerebrocortical microflow
in resting conditions and during increased metabolic demand in
focal tissue areas, therefore, seems to be important to acquire. A
recently accomplished television densitometric method[2,3] imaging
microflow over the brain cortex has provided the means to study the
question outlined above at adequate spatial and temporal resolution
in the cat in control conditions and during cold paw stimulation.

METHODS

Distribution pattern of cerebrocortical red cell flow has been
determined by a television densitometric method[2,3] in cats
anesthetized by Chloralose among an array of cylindrical volumes of

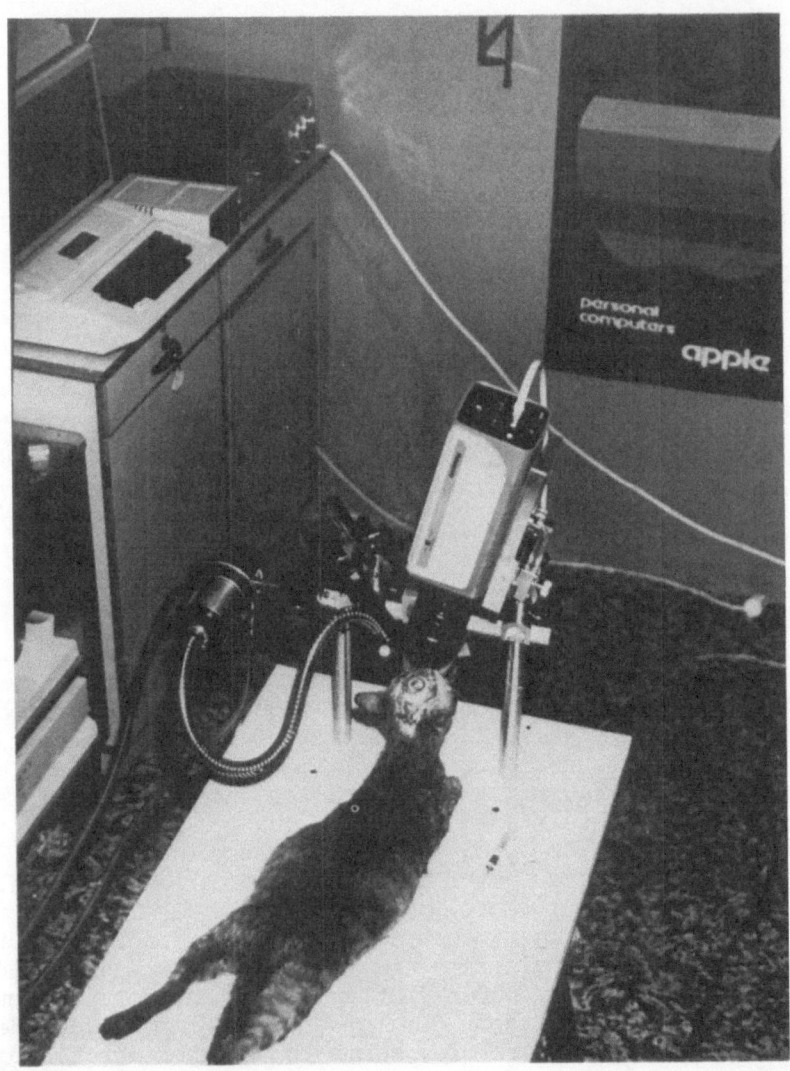

Fig. 1. Experimental setup for imaging cerebrocortical microflow in
the laboratory. The cerebrocortical transit of the
hemodilution pulse – introduced by a bolus injection of
isotonic mannitol solution into the common carotid artery –
is monitored by a TV camera through a cranial window under
epiillumination and recorded on tape for storage and
off-line frame-by-frame densitometric analysis by an Apple
II computer system for a map of microflow within the
window's area.

neuronal tissue each of which measured 0.01 cubic mm (See Fig. 1).
The spatial resolution of this microflow imaging technique is 10000
elements/image at data acquisition, 625 elements/image at the
calculation stage and being increased to 2500 elements/image by
extrapolation when the images are displayed. It permits repetitive
imaging of microflow at a maximal rate of 5 images/minute.

Microregional distribution pattern and degree of heterogeneity
was determined from the microflow images by averaging their
parenchymal pixel data (pixel data corresponding to visible pial
vessels were defined as non-parenchymal and have been excluded from
the calculations) by the sum of these pixel data (that is the total
regional parenchymal flow) and displaying them in a frequency
distribution histogram, called fractionation histogram[4]. A
heterogeneity factor was calculated for each histogram as the ratio
of the half-peak-width over the peak of the histograms.

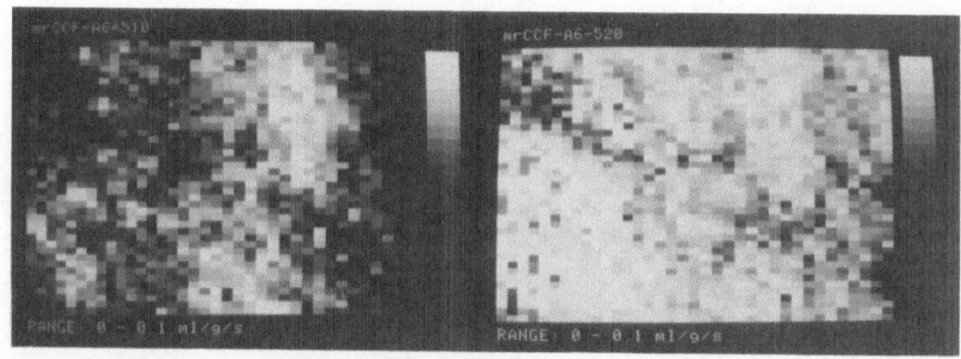

Fig. 2. Representative cerebrocortical microflow images of an
        anesthetized cat in control condition (left) and at the 1st
        minute of contralateral cold paw stimulation (right). The
        mapped area is 9 mm^2. The intensity code of the display
        covers a range of microflow from 0 ml/g/s (black) to 0.1
        ml/g/s (white).

Activation of neurones within the scope of our measurement was
made by stimulating the contralateral paw of the animal by
immersing it into a mixture of ice and water maintained at a
temperature of 0 $^{\circ}$C.

103

RESULTS

In response to cold paw stimulation the cerebrocortical blood
flow rose quickly to a higher, often oscillating level (Fig. 2). In
the groups of those experiments where cortical response in blood
flow to cold stimulation of the contralateral paw could be readily
evoked, the heterogeneity factor doubled during stimulation and
returned to the control level afterwards. Microflow images
representative to these cases along with their absolute and
normalized histograms are shown in Fig. 3.

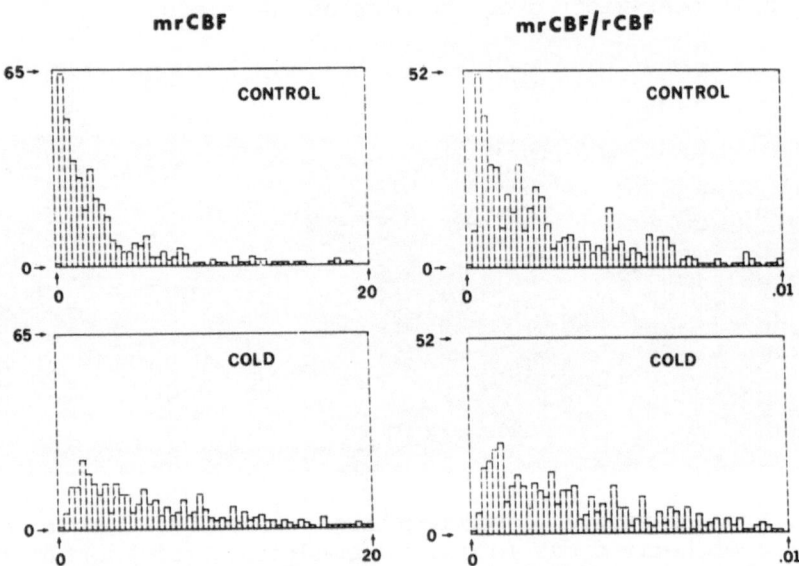

Fig. 3. Absolute and normalized (fractionation) histograms of
cerebrocortical microflow images shown in Fig. 2. Note the
markedly increased heterogeneity during cold paw
stimulation as defined by the half-peak-width over peak
ratio of the histograms. Range of microflow is indicated by
relative units on the absolute histograms (0-20). This
range corresponds to 0-0.02 ml/g/sec in absolute units.

CONCLUSION

These experiments have shown that the distribution of cerebro-cortical microflow becomes more heterogeneous during increased neuronal activity. The presented results are in agreement with our findings in Metrazol induced epileptic seizure[2].

It remains to be seen if the increase in heterogeneity during neuronal activity occurs within an intraparenchymal vascular network of unchanged complexity or within one that responded to the increased neuronal activity by rearranging its microcirculatory routes to enhance supply. A most recently proposed[5] mathematical treatment of our cerebrocortical dilution arrays[5] or similar methods can yield an image of a complexity factor and corresponding histogram that can possibly provide valuable data about the nature of the heterogeneity of intraparenchymal blood flow and its change during increased neuronal activity.

REFERENCES

1. R.M. Berne, H.R. Winn, and R. Rubio, Metabolic regulation of cerebral blood flow, in:"Vasodilatation," P.M. Vanhoutte and I. Leusen, eds., Raven Press, New York (1981).
2. A. Eke, Heterogeneity of cerebrocortical microflow in epileptic seizure, in:"Current Problems in Epilepsy," M. Baldy-Moulinier, D. H. Ingvar, B. S. Meldrum, eds., John Libbey, London, Paris (1983).
3. A. Eke, Reflectometric mapping of microregional blood flow and blood volume in the brain cortex, J. Cereb. Blood Flow Metabol. 2:41-53 (1981).
4. A. Eke, Distribution of cerebrocortical microflow in normo- and hypertensive rats, in:"Oxygen Transport to Tissue VI", Plenum Press, New York (1984).
5. M. Tomita, F. Gotoh, T. Amano, N. Tanahashi, M. Kobari, T. Shinohara, and B. Mihara, Transfer function through regional cerebral cortex evaluated by a photoelectric method, Am. J. Physiol. 245:H385-H398 (1983).

ACKNOWLEDGEMENTS

This work was supported by NIH Grant NS-08802.

DISTRIBUTION OF CEREBROCORTICAL MICROFLOW IN NORMO- AND HYPERTENSIVE RATS: STUDIES IN ISCHEMIA

Andras Eke* and James H. Halsey, Jr.

Department of Neurology, The University of Alabama in Birmingham, Birmingham AL 35294, USA
* Experimental Research Department and 2nd Department of Physiology, Semmelweis Medical University, Budapest H-1082, Hungary

INTRODUCTION

A television version of the densitometric method of Eke (1981)[1] for imaging cerebrocortical microflow[2] has revealed a distinctly different distribution of cerebrocortical microflow in groups of normo- and spontaneously hypertensive rats (NTR, SHR respectively) in control condition, when the distribution of microflows within one map´s area was normalized by the map´s mean and averaged for each group[3]. These, so called, fractionation histograms of microflow showed a partial decrease of the intraparenchymal vascular resistance in the SHR group as likely being a secondary response to an excessively increased extraparenchymal resistance.

In our present series of experiments, fractionation histograms of cerebrocortical microflow have been collected and compared to those of control conditions in NTR and SHR groups during transient ischemia induced by temporary ligation of both carotid arteries.

METHODS

Distribution pattern of cerebrocortical red cell flow has been determined by a television densitometric method[1,2] in rats among an array of cylindrical volumes of neuronal tissue each of which measured 0.01 cubic mm. The spatial resolution of this microflow imaging technique is 10000 elements/image at data acquisition, 625 elements/image at the calculation stage and being increased to 2500 elements/image by extrapolation when the images are displayed. It permits repetitive imaging of microflow at a maximal rate of 5 images/minute.

Male white rats of 200-250 gr body weight have been used for the experiments. Animals from the WKY strain were used as controls (n=5) and the ones from the SHR strain as a hypertensive group (n=5). General anesthesia was performed by the inhalation of an appropriate mixture of Fluothane and 100 % oxygen, that ensured painless conditions for the surgical procedure and the experiment. Catheters were introduced into a small branch of the carotid artery toward the common carotid through which bolus injections of isotonic mannitol solution in an amount of 0.02-0.04 ml were made at the time of the blood flow measurements. In the final phase of surgery, a window of 4x3 mm was cut into the skull with a scapel adjacent to the midline over the parietal region in a very delicate procedure. When the dura looked thick and vascularized, it was cut and removed from within the windows area. A tiny pool of saline was then formed over the window by a ring of semicured dental acrylic and covered leak-tight by a cover slip. Detection of the transit of the hemodiluted bolus from the brain cortex was done through this window under epiillumination by a television densitometer and sequential reflectance images of the brain cortex were stored on tape for off-line digitazation and calculation of microflow images according to Eke (1981).

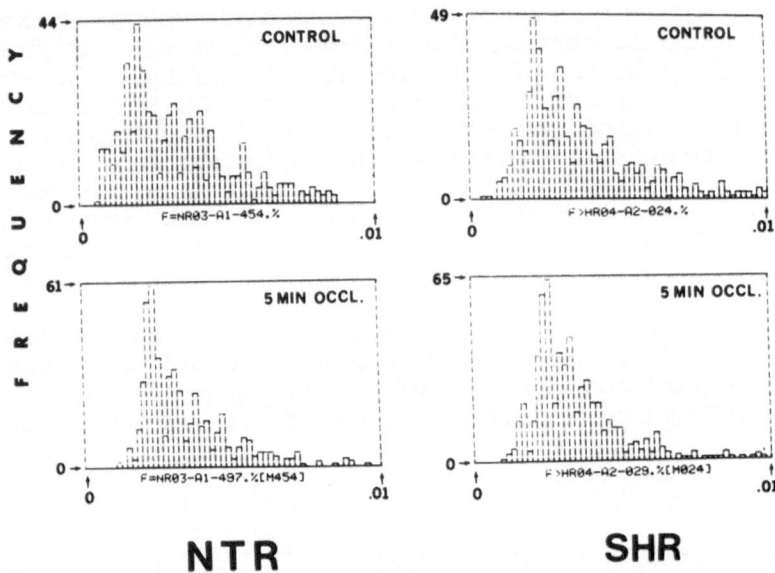

Fig. 1. Representative microflow fractionation histograms of a normotensive and a hypertensive animal in control and at 5 minutes in ischemia.

108

RESULTS

Figure 1 shows two sets of microflow fractionation histograms, one for a normotensive (left), the other for a hypertensive animal (right), that represents typical changes we observed in the studied cases. According to these, the numbers of microareas found in low-fraction classes of the histograms were greater in the NTR than in the SHR group in control condition whereas they showed no significant difference by the fifth minute of cerebral ischemia induced by bilateral carotid occlusion.

CONCLUSION

Although our results are of preliminary nature, they seem to support our hypothesis about the importance of a narrowed range of circulatory adaptation of the SHR brain in the explanation of the smaller survival rate of the SHR animals in ischemia[4,5]. This explanation relies on the fact that a fewer number of microareas per region with the greatest capacity for dilatation is available in the SHR animal for circulatory adaptation in ischemia. This role of these low-fraction microareas can be appreciated by the fact that the fractionation microflow histograms show no significant difference by the fifth minute of the ischemia in the two groups.

REFERENCES

1. A. Eke, Reflectometric mapping of microregional blood flow and blood volume in the brain cortex, J. Cereb. Blood Flow Metabol. 2:41-53 (1981).
2. A. Eke, Heterogeneity of cerebrocortical microflow in epileptic seizure, in:"Current Problems in Epilepsy," M. Baldy-Moulinier, D. H. Ingvar, B. S. Meldrum, eds., John Libbey, London, Paris (1983).
3. A. Eke, Distribution of cerebrocortical microflow in normo- and hypertensive rats, in:"Oxygen Transport to Tissue VI", Plenum Press, New York (1984).
4. J. Choki, T. Jamaguchi, Y. Takeya, Y. Morotomi, T. Omae, Effect of carotid artery ligation on the regional cerebral blood flow in normotensive and spontaneously hypertensive rats, Stroke, 8:374-379 (1977).
5. J. H. Halsey, M. O'Brien, E. Strong, Amelioration of cerebral ischemia by prior treatment of hypertension, Stroke, 11(3):235-239 (1980).

ACKNOWLEDGEMENTS

This work was supported by NIH Grant NS-08802.

CHANGES IN REGIONAL CEREBROVASCULAR RESISTANCE

DURING PARTIAL CEREBRAL ISCHEMIA IN RATS

Antal G. Hudetz*, Karl A. Conger, James H. Halsey,
John McCormick, Tom A. Wilson, and James F. Roesel

Departments of Neurology and Neuropathology, The
University of Alabama in Birmingham, Birmingham
Alabama 35294

INTRODUCTION

Secondary changes in regional cerebral blood flow (rCBF) have
been observed to occur within hours to days in acute focal
cerebral ischemia. Following experimental occlusion of the middle
cerebral artery (MCA) the secondary decline in rCBF during the
first 4 hours of ischemia appeared to correlate with progressive
brain swelling (Hossmann and Schuier, 1980). In subsequent studies
the delayed rise in intracortical vascular resistance as the cause
of the decrease in rCBF was noted (Shima et al, 1983). It is
assumed that the continuing failure of cerebral hemodynamics
associated with the delayed rise in regional cerebral vascular
resistance (rCVR) can aggravate the ischemia and in this way can
contribute to the extension of cerebral infarction.

Ischemic brain edema develop as a function of postocclusion
rCBF (Symon et al, 1979) and the changes in rheological properties
of blood in ischemia are also flow dependent (Fischer, 1973).
Since the rate of changes in rCVR as a function of flow during
ischemia have not yet been determined, the present study was
devoted to the evaluation of the time course of rCVR changes in
partial cerebral ischemia.

---

*Dr. Hudetz is a visiting scientist from the Experimental Research
 Department, Semmelweis Medical University, Budapest 1082,
 Hungary.
This work was supported by the NIH research grant NS-08802.

METHODS

The method of Pulsinelli and Brierley (1979) was employed for producing experimental cerebral ischemia in 7 Sprague-Dawley rats. Three days prior to the experiments 8 platinum electrodes (diameter: 0.01 inch, bare tip length: 1 mm) were implanted in 4 locations of each cerebral hemisphere of the animals under halothane anesthesia. In the first 4 animals the electrodes were placed stereotaxically in the cerebral cortex, habenular nucleus, posterior commissura and superior colliculus. In further 3 animals the electrodes were placed in the hippocampus, thalamus, substantia nigra and the cortex (Figure 1). Disregarding the microheterogeneities in rCBF, these areas were previously found to have relatively uniform blood flow in the ischemic model used here. In addition to electrode implantation both vertebral arteries were excised and coagulated at this time.

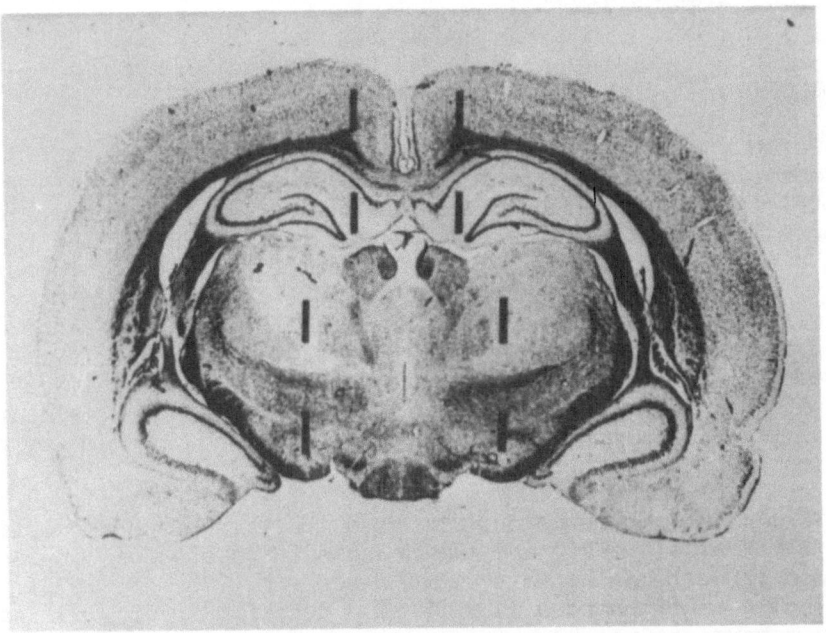

Figure 1. Approximate location of the 8 hydrogen electrodes in the brains of the animals of the second group. The distances of the electrodes from the saggital suture were 1 mm and 3 mm, and from the bregma 2 mm and 3.6 mm, respectively. the electrodes were introduced 1, 4, 6 and 9 mm deep into the brain.

112

During the experiment EEG, systemic arterial pressure (SAP), carotid back pressure (CBP) and, in the last 3 animals, cerebral venous pressure (CVP) were monitored continuously. The external carotid artery was tied off at the side of pressure measurement in the last 3 animals. The rCBF was measured intermittently, at every 5-10 minutes before ischemia and 10-15 minutes during ischemia by hydrogen clearance (Aukland, 1964; Haining et al, 1968). Initiation and timing of hydrogen inhalation and washout, data storage and analysis were performed by a TRS-80 microcomputer.

After 4-7 control flow measurements the animals were heparinized, the other common carotid artery was occluded and the SAP was lowered by withdrawing blood by a controlled roller pump connected to the line in the femoral artery. The SAP was adjusted continuously by computer control (TRS-80) to maintain the CBP at 15 ± 1 mmHg throughout the ischemic period of the experiment. With the 4 major cerebral arteries occluded, this level of CBP was found to produce critical rCBF leading to regional cerebral infarction. The ratio of extracerebral (and collateral) and intracerebral vascular resistance was approximated by (SAP-CBP)/(CBP-CVP). When CVP was not measured its value was taken as zero. In the second group of animals an approximate mean hemispheric flow (MHF) was also calculated by summing the rCBF values weighted by appropriate tissue volumes. The approximate volumes of cerebral structures were determined planimetrically, using a stereotactic atlas (König and Klippel, 1963). Having MHF calculated the extracerebral resistance was estimated as (SAP-CBP)/MHF.

The values of rCVR were calculated from each rCBF measurement as (CBP-CVP)/rCBF. The rate of change in local resistance was defined as the slope of rCVR in the function of time as obtained from the linear regression of rCBF at each electrode.

RESULTS

Global Observations

Prior to ischemia the mean SAP for the 7 animals was 71 ± 6 (SD) mmHg and the mean CBP was 42 ± 11 (SD) mmHg. Average CVP, when measured, was 3.3 ± 0.5 (SD) mmHg. The mean resistance ratio was 0.77 ± 0.10 (SD) and the MHF was 54 ± 17 (SD) ml/min/100g. Spontaneous electrical activity as indicated by the EEG was undisturbed during the control period.

Following the occlusion of the other common carotid artery CBP fell and the EEG was reduced significantly by the time the CBP was decreased near to 15 mmHg by lowering the SAP. The MHF fell to

18 + 8 ml/min/100g (p<0.005). During several hours postocclusion
the SAP had to be decreased in order to maintain constant CBP.
Within the first hour SAP was in the range of 38-66 mmHg, the
average being 48 + 10 (SD) mmHg. The resistance ratio also decreased with time in all animals except one (R254) of the first group
(Figure 2). This animal showed recovery of cerebral blood flow
after 2 hours postocclusion. In two experiments (R401 and R402)

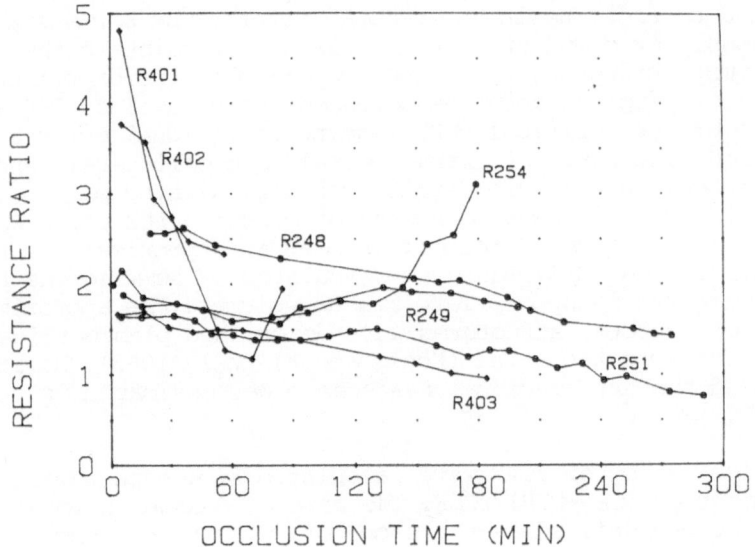

Figure 2. Time course of the ratio of extracerebral and
intracerebral resistances from the time of occlusion of
the carotid artery. R248 - R254 and R401 - R403 indicate
rats of the first and second groups, respectively.

the resistance ratio was initially higher but decreased more rapidly
than in the others. These animals belonged to the second group in
which the external carotid artery was tied off at the side of CBP
measurement resulting in an increased collateral resistance. Extracerebral resistances of the animals R401, R402 and R403 were 0.31,
0.48 and 0.22 Hgmm.min/ml, respectively.

Table 1.   Regional cerebral blod flow before and during early
           cerebral ischemia (mean ± SE).

Location of electrode	Preocclusion (ml/min/100g)	5 minute postocclusion (ml/min/100g)	(%)
Cerebral Cortex	78.1 ± 8.2	24.9 ± 4.6	33 ± 6
Habenular Nucleus	82.7 ± 6.6	29.9 ± 3.9	36 ± 7
Posterior Commissure	91.6 ± 8.3	43.1 ± 2.9	52 ± 7
Superior Colliculus	90.5 ± 6.2	34.3 ± 3.6	41 ± 7
Hippocampus	48.4 ± 6.2	18.6 ± 4.6 *	37 ± 8 *
Thalamus	53.9 ± 10.3	23.5 ± 3.6 ⌐	48 ± 9 ⌐
Substantia Nigra	68.8 ± 8.0	43.0 ± 4.2 ⌐	66 ± 7 ⌐
Cerebral Cortex	51.3 ± 7.7	9.6 ± 4.5 ⌐	16 ± 7 ⌐

Brackets indicate significant differences between the means at the
p<0.05 level from unpaired T-test. For the first group of
structures N = 8, for the second group N = 6, except where the *
indicates N = 5.

Regional Observations

        Control and ischemic mean rCBF values in various cerebral
structures are given in Table 1. The preocclusive flows shown
there are average values of those collected at 5-10 minute
intervals during the last 40-70 minutes prior to occlusion. The
ischemic flows are average values of those measured at about 5
(4-6) minutes following occlusion and lowering the SAP, and they
are expressed in both absolute units and in percent of the mean
preocclusive rCBF at the same electrode. Due to the relatively
large variance there was no statistically significant difference
among the mean rCBF's of any cerebral structures in the first
group of animals. The 5-min rCBF was the lowest in the cerebral
cortex in 5 of the 8 hemispheres and it was the highest in the
posterior commissure in all but one hemispheres of the first group.
In the second group, the mean postocclusive rCBF was significantly
(p<0.05) higher in the substantia nigra while it was significantly
lower in the cerebral cortex than in any other structures.
Cortical rCBF fell to zero immediately following occlusion in 2
animals of the second group. The relative changes in rCBF showed
similar significant differences (see Table 1). No correlation was

found between the mean preocclusive and 5-min postocclusive rCBF (r=0.38, N=54).

Changes in rCBF during the ischemic period had a decreasing tendency except in one animal (R254) with relatively high initial rCBF which continued to rise until the experiment was terminated at 3 hours postocclusion.

Table 2. Regional cerebral vascular resistance before and during early cerebral ischemia (mean ± SE).

Position of electrode	Preocclusion (mmHg.min/ml)	5 minute postocclusion (mmHg.min/ml)	(%)
Cerebral cortex	0.64 ± 0.10	0.80 ± 0.10⌉	143 ± 12 +
Habenular Nucleus	0.56 ± 0.06	0.72 ± 0.15⎥	133 ± 23
Posteror Commissure	0.53 ± 0.07	0.43 ± 0.04⌋	83 ± 8
Superior Colliculus	0.48 ± 0.05	0.53 ± 0.08	113 ± 14
Hippocampus	0.68 ± 0.05	0.94 ± 0.20⌉	136 ± 26
Thalamus	0:68 ± 0.10	0.76 ± 0.15⎥	118 ± 19
Substantia Nigra	0.49 ± 0.07	0.37 ± 0.04⌋	79 ± 11
Cerebral Cortex	0.74 ± 0.17	1.51 ± 0.47 *	274 ± 71 *

Brackets indicate significant differences between the means at the p<0.05 level from unpaired T-test. Sign + denotes significant (p<0.05) change based on paired T-test. For the first group N = 8, for the second one N = 6, except where the * indicates N = 4.

Table 2 presents the mean values of control and 5-min postocclusive rCVR in both absolute and relative units. The rCVR rose significantly (p<0.05) by 5 minute postocclusion in the cerebral cortex in the first group. At 5-min ischemia rCVR was significantly lower in the posterior commissure than in the cerebral cortex. A similar difference in rCVR between the substantia nigra and the hippocampus was seen in the second group. No structure independent correlation was found between postocclusive rCVR and preocclusive rCBF (r=0.38, N=54).

Further changes in resistance were determined by the initial postocclusion flow. The dependence of the rate of change in rCVR on the 5-min postocclusive rCBF at the same electrode is displayed in Figure 3. From this we can see that rCVR rose rapidly when 5-min rCBF was below 15-20 ml/min/100g. A similar relationship between the rate of rCVR and the 5-min relative rCBF was obtained with a corresponding flow threshold of 30-35 % of the control rCBF. The mean rate of rCVR of the 6 cases with distinctly high rates was 0.080 + 0.021 mmHg/ml. These high resistance rates occurred at the electrodes, 3 of which were in the cortex, two were in the hippocampus and one was in the thalamus.

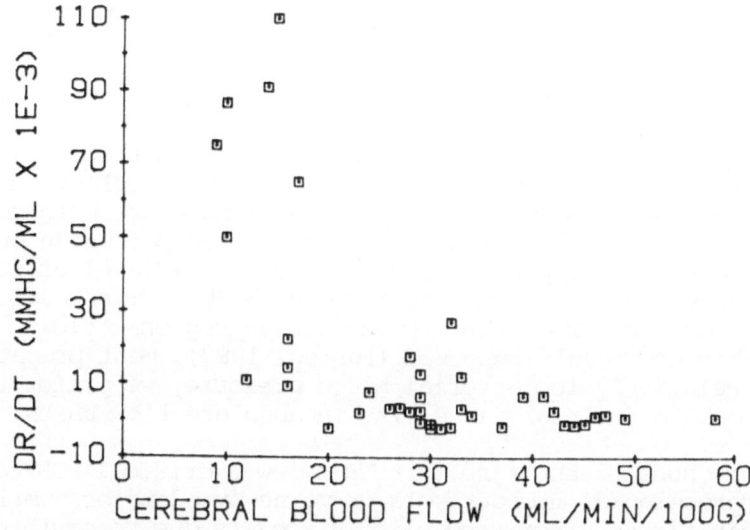

Figure 3. Dependence of the rate of change in regional cerebral vascular resistance on the initial (5-minute) ischemic regional cerebral blood flow. Each point represents the average rate of resistance at one electrode for the postocclusion period of the experiment.

DISCUSSION

The primary objective of this study was to determine the rate and dependence of regional cerebral vascular resistance on regional cerebral blood flow in partial ischemia. rCVR was calculated from the local blood flow and from the carotid back pressure which was maintained at 15 mmHg during ischemia. The advantage of controlling CBP was the resulting ability to (1)

control the depth of ischemia and (2) eliminate the possible occurrence of arterial steal. Steal did not occur at the venous
side either since CVP was constant within ± l mmHg throughout the
experiments. For the calculation of rCVR the CBP is an appropriate
index for cerebral perfusion pressure for all cerebral regions
both in control and in ischemia if the ischemia is produced by the
occlusion of cerebral arteries proximal from the Circle of Willis.
In addition, the CBP could be used for the estimation of the ratio
of extracortical and intracortical vascular resistance (Fujishima
and Omae, 1976).

The major finding of this study was the threshold type
dependence of the rate of change in vascular resistance on local
blood flow. The resistance rise, on the other hand, seemed to be
independent of the cerebral structure in which it occurred.
Although such a relationship based on the measurement of the time
course of cerebrocortical blood flow (Hossmann and Schuier, 1980)
and on the semiquantitative determination of intracortical
vascular resistance (Shima et al, 1983) in MCA occlusion has been
suggested, until now the resistance rates have not been calculated
for various cerebral regions under controlled perfusion pressure
condiditons. In the present study the critical level of rCBF for
the progressive rise in resistance was 15-20 ml/min/100g or 30-35
% of the control rCBF. Since preocclusive regional flows were
lower than previously reported (Furlow, 1982), most probably due
to the relatively low arterial blood pressure, we prefer to define
the threshold for resistance rise in absolute flow units.

The cause of the rise in rCVR below a critical rCBF could be
the compression of microvessels or veins by edema or swelling of
the brain tissue, increased blood viscosity due to erythrocyte
aggregation, or capillary obstruction by leukocytes (Yamakawa et
al, 1984). All these phenomena occur at low flow states. Hossmann
and Schuier (1980) have reported about the secondary changes of
cerebrocortical blood flow as associated with the development of
cerebral edema between 1 to 4 hours following MCA occlusion, when
the blood flow was below 10-15 ml/min/100g. A higher threshold of
20ml/min/100g was found for ischemic water increase in the same
experimental model by Symon et al (1979). They observed secondary
flow decreases of about 5 ml/min/100g at 1-2 hours postocclusion.
Whether edema does, in fact, compress capillaries during the first
few hours of ischemia remains a matter of debate. Microcirculatory
obstruction, as indicated by impaired microvascular filling by
carbon perfusion, becomes evident three hours following MCA
occlusion, partly as a result of perivascular glial swelling and
developing edema (Little et al, 1976). At 1-2 hours postocclusion
no evidence of no reflow as measured by hydrogen clearance was
found (Morawetz et al., 1978), while unperfused cortical regions
were clearly demonstrated by single dye passage of carbon black or
Evans blue (Hossmann and Schuier, 1980) after 1 hour of MCA

118

occlusion. Since in our experiments significant increases in the vascular resistance were seen at comparable flow rates within 30-60 minutes of ischemia, the observed increase in microvascular resistance must be at least in part reversible by reperfusion during the first few hours of ischemia. Rheological changes of blood resulting in increased microvascular resistance in ischemia may also be reversible. We have recent theoretical evidence (unpublished) that partial obstruction of capillaries in networks, although it increases local microvascular resistance, does not impair regional blood flow significantly before more than 50 % of the capillaries with low flow velocity are obstructed.

The threshold of 15-20 ml/min/100g for the rise in resistance found in the present study coincides with the flow range where the EEG and evoked potentials decrease and disappear (Branston et al, 1974) but it is higher than the threshold of 9-11 ml/min/100g reported for membrane failure as indicated by the depletion of ATP and the increased extracellular potassium concentration (Branston et al, 1977). The highest resistance rates in our experiments occurred in the range of the ischemic penumbra (10-15 ml/min/100g), that is in the flow gap between reversible functional and irreversible structural cell damage. Why the infinite time threshold of 18 ml/min/100g (Heiss, 1983) for morphological damage can be nearly 2 times higher than that for the energy failure, may perhaps be explained by the rising cerebovascular resistance. At the initial flow rates of 10-15 ml/min/100g the rapid rise in rCVR could easily convert the functionally inactive but still viable tissue into an infarcted mass.

REFERENCES

Ames, A.III., Wright, R.L., Kowada, M., Thurston, J.M., and Majno, G., 1968, Cerebral ischemia. II. The no-reflow phenomenon, Am. J. Phath. , 52:437.

Astrup, J., Siesjo, B.K., and Symon, L., 1981, Thresholds in cerebral ischemia - the ischemic penumbra, Stroke , 12:723.

Aukland, K., Bower, B.F., and Berliner, R.W., 1964, Measurement of local blood flow with hydrogen gas, Circ. Res. , 14:164.

Branston, N.M., Strong, A.J., and Symon, L., 1977, Extracellular potassium activity, evoked potential and tissue blood flow: relationship during progressive ischemia in baboon cerebral cortex, J. Neurol. Sci. , 32:305.

Branston, N.M., Symon, L., Crockard, H.A., and Pasztor, E., 1974, Relationship between the cortical evoked potential and local cortical blood flow following acute middle cerebral artery occlusion in the baboon, Exp. Neurology , 45:195.

Fischer, E.G., 1973, Impaired perfusion following cerebrovascular stasis, Arch. Neurol. , 29:361.

Fujishima, M., and Omae, T., 1976, Lower limit of cerebral

autoregulation in normotensive and spontaneously hypertensive rats, *Experientia*, 32:1021.

Furlow, T.W., Jr., 1982, Cerebral ischemia produced by four-vessel occlusion in the rat: A quantitative evaluation of cerebral blood flow, *Stroke* ., 13:852.

Haining, J.L., Turner, D., and Pantall, R.M., 1968, Measurement of local cerebral blood flow in the unanesthetized rat using a hydrogen clearance method, *Circ. Res.* , 23:313.

Halsey, J.H., Jr., and Clark, L.C., Jr., 1970, Some regional circulatory abnormalities following experimental cerebral infarction, *Neurology* , 20:238.

Heiss, W.D., 1983, Flow thresholds of functional and morphological damage of brain tissue, *Stroke* , 14:329.

Hossmann, K.A., and Schuier, F.J., 1980, Experimental brain infarcts in cats, *Stroke* , 11:583.

König, J.F.R., and Klippel, R.A., 1963, "The Rat Brain," Robert E. Krieger, Huntington.

Little, J.R., Kerr, F.W.L., and Sundt, T.M., 1976, Microcirculatory obstruction in focal cerebral ischemia: An electron microscopic investigation in monkeys, *Stroke* , 7:25.

Morawetz., R.B., DeGirolami, U., Ojemann, R.G., Marcoux, F.W., and Crowell, R.M., 1978, Cerebral blood flow determined by hydrogen clearance during middle cerebral artery occlusion in unanesthetized monkeys, *Stroke* , 9:143.

Pulsinelli, W.A., and Brierley, J.B., 1979, A new model of bilateral hemispheric ischemia in the anesthetized rat, *Stroke* , 10:267.

Shima, T., Hossman, K.A., and Date, H., 1983, Pial arterial pressure in cats following middle cerebral artery occlusion, *Stroke* , 14:713.

Symon, L., Branston, N.M., and Chikovani, O., 1979, Ischemic brain edema following middle cerebral artery occlusion in baboons: Relationship between regional cerebral water content and blood flow at 1 to 2 hours, *Stroke* , 10:184.

Yamakawa, T., Sugiayama, I., and Niimi, H., 1984, Behaviours of white blood cells in microcirculatory of the cat brain cortex during hemorrhagic shock: intravital microscopic study, *Int. J. Microcirc.* , 3:588.

THE EFFECT OF PEPTIDES ON CEREBROVASCULAR RESISTANCE IN CATS

M. Wahl

Department of Physiology, University
of Munich, Pettenkoferstr. 12
8000 Munich 2, FRG

INTRODUCTION

It was the aim of the present study to investigate the effect of several naturally occurring peptides and synthetic analogues on cerebral resistance vessels. These peptides appear to be generated and released in the brain from vascular nerve endings or parenchymal cells. Neurotensin, a tridecapeptide, was first isolated from extracts of hypothalamus by Carraway and Leeman (1973) and later also detected in other brain regions such as cortex, thalamus, and pituitary (Bisette et al., 1978; Brown and Miller, 1982). In addition, neurotensin immunoreactive fibres have been detected in cerebral vessels by Chan-Palay (1977).

After the discovery of endogenous opioid peptides by Hughes et al. (1975) and Terenius and Wahlström (1975) enkephalin-immunoreactive neurones and enkephalinergic pathways in the central nervous system have been found in various studies (Del Fiacco et al., 1982; Gramsch et al., 1979; Uhl et al., 1979). Recently, a close relationship between enkephalin-like immunoreactive profiles and the basement membranes of capillaries and small veins was observed by Kapadia and de Lanerolle (1984). In addition, a small population of opiate receptors has been demonstrated in microvessels using radioactive ligands (Peroutka et al., 1980).

Bradykinin has been discovered some 55 years ago but its presence in the brain has only been detected during the last 15 years. Although there is no evidence for bradykinin-containing fibres innervating cerebral vessels it appears to be generated and released from neuronal cells in various regions of the brain since all components of an intracerebral kinin system have been found (for re-

ferences see Wahl et al., 1983 a and b). Furthermore, under pathological conditions with disruption of the blood-brain barrier, blood
borne kininogen has been shown to penetrate into the brain and after conversion to bradykinin to act as a mediator in vasogenic brain
edema (Maier-Hauff et al., 1984; Unterberg and Baethmann, 1984).
One factor involved in the determination of the intensity and duration of the effects induced by bradykinin is its enzymatic degradation. Several enzymes with kininase-like activity have been found
in the brain (for references see Wahl et al., 1983 b). A part of
the cerebral kininase activity is due to kininase II. This enzyme
can be blocked by in vivo applicable inhibitors. Using such compounds the role of kininase II in the degradation of bradykinin can
be quantified in vivo.

The above mentioned peptides have been found to affect smooth
muscle cells in various parts of the body by different mechanisms.
Direct effects mediated by receptors of smooth muscle cells have
been reported for neurotensin (Kitabgi and Freychet, 1978), enkephalins (Hanko and Hardebo, 1978), and bradykinin (Regoli and Barabe, 1980). However, in several cases these peptides appear to act
indirectly on the smooth muscle by influencing the release of neurotransmitters (Kitabgi and Freychet, 1978; Knoll, 1976; Starke et
al., 1977) or of divergent mediator compounds (Chand and Altura, 1981;
Cherry et al., 1982; Marceau et al., 1981; Rioux et al., 1980; Yau
et al., 1983). Therefore, the effects of these peptides on segments
of pial arteries were tested in situ using microapplication into the
perivascular space thus mimicking the normal route of penetration
of a compound released and acting from the extravascular side.

METHODS

Experiments were performed on anaesthetized (α-chloralose)
and immobilized (gallamine) cats. End-tidal CO_2, arterial blood
pressure, and body temperature of the artificially ventilated animals were recorded continuously. The acid base status of the arterial blood was measured intermittently. Craniectomy was performed
with a cooled dental drill. After covering the brain and the dura
with a 1 - 2 cm thick layer of paraffin oil heated to between 37
and 38° C the dura was slit. The diameter of arteries and arterioles
of the parietal lobe was measured using an image-splitting method
(Wahl and Kuschinsky, 1979 a). The following compounds were used:
neurotensin (Serva), leu-enkephalin (Serva), D-ala^2-leu-enkephalin-
amide (Serva), D-ala^2-met-enkephalinamide (Serva), morphine (Merck),
naloxone (gift of Endo Labs.), bradykinin (Serva), met-lys-bradykinin (Serva), des-arg^9-bradykinin (Serva), des-arg^9-leu^8-bradykinin
(Serva), bradykinin potentiator C (Peninsula), and captopril (gift
of Squibb). The substances were dissolved in an inert artificial
cerebrospinal fluid (CSF) of the following composition (mM): Na$^+$,
159.5; K$^+$, 2.5; Ca^{2+}, 1.5; Cl$^-$, 150.5; HCO$_3^-$, 14.5. The pH was 7.25

(38°C), and osmolarity 308 mosmol/l. The values of pH and K^+ of the artificial CSF are the same as those found in the natural CSF of the cortical subarachnoid space under corresponding experimental conditions (Wahl and Kuschinsky, 1979 b; Kuschinsky and Wahl, 1979). Fresh solutions were prepared daily, bubbled with a mixture of 5% CO_2 and 95% N_2 (equilibrated with water), and stored at 0°C in a refrigerator. Immediately before application, test solutions were filled into siliconized glass capillaries with sharpened tips. Using micropuncture technique 5 µl were applied into the perivascular space of individual extraparenchymal arteries. Methodological details are described in a previous paper (Wahl et al., 1983 a). After testing the vascular reactivity to alteration in pH (Wahl et al., 1970; Kuschinsky et al., 1972), the effect of the inert artificial CSF was measured. Thereafter, data were obtained by application of ascending concentrations or random injections of single concentrations of the compounds under investigation. The statistical analysis of the data was performed by analysis of variance and multiple comparisons according to the method of Scheffé(1953). In addition, a paired t-test with the sequentially rejective Bonferroni procedure was used to assure the multiple level of significance, according to the method of Holm (1979). The 99% level was taken as significant.

RESULTS

The compounds were tested on pial arteries with a resting diameter of 55 to 310 µ. Perivascular application of artificial CSF did not significantly change the diameter of the arteries (mean dilatation of 0.52 ± 0.25%). The effects of the various compounds tested were calculated after subtraction of the effect of the solvent on the individual vessels.

1. Neurotensin

The effect of neurotensin was tested in concentrations ranging from 10^{-12} to 10^{-5}M. Neurotensin did not induce a significant change of vascular diameter which varied between a constriction of 0.08% and a dilatation of 1.09% independent of concentration.

2. Opiate receptor agonists and antagonists

Table 1 summarizes the effects of four opiate receptor agonists: leu-enkephalin, D-ala^2-leu-enkephalinamide, D-ala^2-met-enkephalinamide, and morphine. No change of vascular diameter was observed at concentrations between 10^{-11} and 10^{-5}M. At 10^{-4}M only the dilatation (4.3%) elicited by D-ala^2-leu-enkephalinamide was statistically significant (p<0.01). All four agonists elicited

Table 1. Vascular Effects of Opiate Receptor Agonists (Means $\pm$ SEM)

Substance	Concentration (M)								
	10^{-11}	10^{-10}	10^{-9}	10^{-8}	10^{-7}	10^{-6}	10^{-5}	10^{-4}	10^{-3}
Leu-enkephalin	0.02 $\pm$0.38		-0.43 $\pm$0.45		-0.46 $\pm$0.36		-0.07 $\pm$0.32	3.70 $\pm$1.73	7.58 $\pm$2.02
D-ala^2-leu-enkephalinamide	0.98 $\pm$0.76		-0.50 $\pm$0.60		0.53 $\pm$0.97		-1.01 $\pm$2.17	4.30 $\pm$0.87	13.63 $\pm$2.47
D-ala^2-met-enkephalinamide	-0.12 $\pm$0.63		0.82 $\pm$0.68		0.05 $\pm$0.40		2.48 $\pm$1.68		6.02 $\pm$1.59
Morphine		-0.52 $\pm$0.33		0.55 $\pm$1.01		0.03 $\pm$0.43		1.87 $\pm$1.24	5.45 $\pm$1.28

Table 2. Vascular Effects of Bradykinin Receptor Agonists (Means $\pm$ SEM)

Substance	Concentration (M)							
	10^{-13}	10^{-11}	10^{-8}	10^{-7}	10^{-6}	10^{-5}	10^{-4}	10^{-3}
Bradykinin	0.15 $\pm$0.51	1.40 $\pm$1.19	3.31 $\pm$0.98	11.22 $\pm$1.46	29.10 $\pm$2.57	44.75 $\pm$2.62	35.96 $\pm$2.82	
Met-lys-bradykinin			1.94 $\pm$1.42	9.54 $\pm$1.81	20.60 $\pm$4.95	46.93 $\pm$9.42	31.70 $\pm$3.44	
Des-arg^9-bradykinin			0.06 $\pm$0.57	0.22 $\pm$0.89	0.61 $\pm$1.09	0.23 $\pm$0.59	0.99 $\pm$1.15	5.92 $\pm$2.31

Table 3. Vascular Effects of Kininase II Inhibitors on the Bradykinin Response (Means $\pm$ SEM, Paired Data)

Substance	Bradykinin (M)			
	10^{-8}	10^{-7}	10^{-6}	10^{-5}
Bradykinin (BK)	4.03 $\pm$2.30	17.40 $\pm$4.40	34.60 $\pm$5.60	58.10 $\pm$6.60
BK + Captopril (10^{-5}M)	3.10 $\pm$1.92	12.40 $\pm$3.20	35.60 $\pm$4.20	53.40 $\pm$7.40
Bradykinin (BK)	0.07 $\pm$1.74	2.64 $\pm$1.73	33.52 $\pm$7.26	41.52 $\pm$6.84
BK + Potentiator C (10^{-5}M)	0.22 $\pm$1.32	5.35 $\pm$2.37	31.30 $\pm$5.46	42.86 $\pm$4.79

125

significant (p $<$ 0.01) dilatations at 10^{-3}M varying between 5.4% (morphine) and 13.6% (D-ala^2-leu-enkephalinamide). The maximal dilatations induced by leu-enkephalin and D-ala^2-met-enkephalinamide were 7.6% and 6%, respectively. To test whether these dilatations were mediated by specific opiate receptors the opiate receptor antagonist naloxone was used. At the same vessels D-ala^2-leu-enkephalinamide (10^{-4} and 10^{-3}M) was tested first, then the agonist was administered simultaneously with 10^{-4}M naloxone. Naloxone (10^{-4}M) induced per se an insignificant dilatation of 0.56 $\pm$ 0.64%. During the simultaneous perivascular administration naloxone reduced the dilatations induced by 10^{-4} and 10^{-3}M D-ala^2-leu-enkephalinamide completely and by 85%, respectively.

3. Bradykinin receptor agonists and antagonists

Table 2 shows the effects of three bradykinin receptor agonists: bradykinin, met-lys-bradykinin (both acting on B$_1$ and B$_2$ receptors), and des-arg^9-bradykinin (acting on B$_1$ receptors). Bradykinin and met-lys-bradykinin induced similar dose dependent dilatations with maximal effects of 45.5% and 46.8% at 10^{-5}M, respectively. However, the relative potency of met-lys-bradykinin was less than that of bradykinin as found under in vivo and in vitro conditions by Whalley and Wahl (1983 a). Des-arg^9-bradykinin did not change arterial diameter when concentrations of 10^{-8} to 10^{-4}M were administered. An insignificant dilatation of 5.9% was measured at 10^{-3}M. That this bradykinin-induced dilatation is mediated by B$_2$ receptors could be confirmed by application of the B$_1$ receptor antagonist des-arg^9-leu^8-bradykinin which did not reduce the dilating effect of bradykinin (Whalley and Wahl, 1983 a).

4. Kininase II inhibitors

The effect of kininase II inhibitors, potentiator C or captopril, on the action of bradykinin was investigated on the same artery: first, bradykinin (10^{-8} to 10^{-3}M), then 10^{-5}M potentiator C or captopril, and finally kininase II inhibitor simultaneously with bradykinin were tested. The paired data obtained are shown in table 3. At 10^{-5}M, potentiator C and captopril induced per se insignificant dilatations of 0.21% and 1.07%, respectively (Wahl et al., 1983 b). Both compounds did not change significantly the effect of bradykinin.

DISCUSSION

Neurotensin had no effect on the diameter of feline pial arteries in situ. That this finding was not caused by a loss of its biological activity was shown in parallel experiments using the guinea pig ileum (Wagner and Wahl, 1984). In addition, Hanko et al. (1981) could not detect any effect of neurotensin on feline cerebral arteries in vitro.

Enkephalins and morphine did not significantly change pial arterial diameter at concentrations up to 10^{-5} or 10^{-4} M/l. The concentrations of enkephalins found in natural CSF are in the range of 10^{-11} to 10^{-9}M (Terenius and Wahlström, 1978; Nyberg and Terenius, 1982). Although the concentrations will be increased in the immediate vicinity of enkephalinergic synapses it is improbable that enkephalins are important for the adjustment of pial arterial resistance. The dilatations measured at high concentrations are mediated by opiate receptors since they can be blocked by naloxone. It appears likely that the dilatation-inducing μ- and δ- opiate receptors are located on vascular smooth muscles since the resting tone of the vessels is obviously not influenced by nerves. Therefore, the effects of the opioids appear not to be mediated by prejunctional receptors modulating the release of neurotransmitters. The present results are not in contradiction to findings of Hanko and Hardebo (1978) on isolated feline cerebral arteries, since these authors later (Hardebo, 1983) found that they had overestimated the relaxing effect of opioid agonists previously.

Bradykinin has been shown to be a potent dilator of feline pial arteries in situ not only during perivascular microapplication, but also during cortical superfusion (Wahl et al., 1983 c and 1984; Unterberg et al., 1984). Corresponding results have been obtained in isolated human pial (Toda, 1977; Wahl et al., 1983 a), feline pial and middle cerebral (Wahl et al., 1983 a and b; Whalley and Wahl, 1983 a and b), and rabbit basilar artery (Whalley et al., 1983 a and b). Using various bradykinin receptor agonists and antagonists the dilating effect of bradykinin on feline pial arteries in situ has been shown to be mediated by B_2-receptors. The same has been reported for cat middle cerebral (Whalley and Wahl, 1983 a), and rabbit basilar (Whalley et al., 1983 a) artery in vitro. The effect of bradykinin was not influenced by inhibitors of kininase II under in situ and in vitro conditions (Wahl et al., 1983 b, Whalley and Wahl, 1983 b; Whalley et al., 1983 a and b). From this it can be concluded that kininases other than kininase II are involved in the degradation of bradykinin in the cerebral arteries tested. Considering the vasomotor response of bradykinin and its effect on the blood-brain barrier (Wahl et al., 1983 c and 1984; Unterberg et al., 1984) bradykinin appears to be an important factor in the regulation of cerebral microcirculation and oxygen supply.

REFERENCES

Bisette, G., Manberg, P., Nemeroff, C.B., and Prange, A.J., 1978, Neurotensin, a biologically active peptide, Life Sci., 23: 2173-2182.

Brown, D.R., and Miller, R.J., 1982, Neurotensin, Brit.Med.Bull.,
    38: 239-245.
Carraway, R., and Leeman, S.E., 1973, The isolation of a new hypo-
    tensive peptide, neurotensin, from bovine hypothalami, J.Biol.
    Chem., 248: 6854-6861.
Chand, N., and Altura, B.M., 1981, Inhibition of endothelial cell-
    dependent relaxations to acetylcholine and bradykinin by lip-
    oxygenase inhibitors in canine isolated renal arteries, Micro-
    circulation, 1: 211-223.
Chan-Palay, V., 1977, Innervation of cerebral blood vessels by nor-
    epinephrine, indoleamine, substance P and neurotensin fibres
    and the leptomeningeal indoleamine axons: their roles in vaso-
    motor activity and local alterations of brain blood composition,
    in: "Neurogenic control of the brain circulation," Owman, Ch.,
    Edvinsson, L., eds., Pergamon Press, Oxford, pp. 39-54.
Cherry, P.D., Furchgott, R.F., Zawadzki, J.V., and Jothianandan, D.,
    1982, Role of endothelial cells in relaxation of isolated arter-
    ies by bradykinin, Proc.Nat.Acad.Sci., 79: 2106-2110.
Del Fiacco, M., Paxinos, G., and Cuello, A.C., 1982, Neostriatal en-
    kephalin-immunoreactive neurones project to the globus palli-
    dus, Brain Res., 231: 1-17.
Gramsch, C., Höllt, V., Mehraein, P., Pasi, A., and Herz, A., 1979,
    Regional distribution of methionine-enkephalin- and beta-endor-
    phine-like immunoreactivity in human brain and pituitary, Brain
    Res., 171: 261-270.
Hanko, J.H., and Hardebo, J.E., 1978, Enkephalin-induced dilatation
    of pial arteries in vitro probably mediated by opiate receptors,
    Eur.J.Pharmacol., 51: 295-297.
Hanko, J.H., Hardebo, J.E., and Owman, Ch., 1981, Effects of various
    neuropeptides on cerebral blood vessels, J.Cereb.Blood Flow
    Metab., 1, Suppl.1: S346-S347.
Hardebo, J.E., 1983, Personal communication.
Holm, S., 1979, A simple sequentially rejective multiple test pro-
    cedure, Scand.J.Statist., 6: 65-70.
Hughes, J., Smith, T.W., Kosterlitz, H.W., Fothergill, L.A., Morgan,
    B.A., and Morris, H.R., 1975, Identification of two related
    pentapeptides from the brain with potent opiate agonist acti-
    vity, Nature, 258: 577-579.
Kapadia, S.E., and de Lanerolle, N.C., 1984, Immunohistochemical and
    electron microscopic demonstration of vascular innervation in
    the mammalian brain stem, Brain Res., 292: 33-40.
Kitabgi, P., and Freychet, P., 1978, Effects of neurotensin on iso-
    lated intestinal smooth muscles, Eur.J.Pharmacol., 50: 349-357.
Knoll, J., 1976, Neuronal peptide (enkephalin) receptors in the ear
    artery of the rabbit, Eur.J.Pharmacol., 39: 403-407.
Kuschinsky, W., and Wahl, M., 1979, Perivascular pH and pial arter-
    ial diameter during bicuculline seizures in cats, Pflügers
    Arch., 382: 81-85.
Kuschinsky, W., Wahl, M., Bosse, O., and Thurau, K., 1972, Perivas-

cular potassium and pH as determinants of local pial arterial diameter in cats. A microapplication study, Circ.Res., 31: 240-247.

Marceau, F., Knap, M., and Regoli, D., 1981, Pharmacological characterization of the vascular permeability-enhancing effects of kinins in the rabbit skin, Can.J.Physiol.Pharmacol., 59: 921-926.

Maier-Hauff, K., Baethmann, A.J., Lange, M., Schürer, L., and Unterberg, A., 1984, The kallikrein-kinin system as mediator in vasogenic brain edema. Part 2: Studies on kinin formation in focal and perifocal brain tissue, J.Neurosurg., 61: 97-106.

Nyberg, F., and Terenius, L., 1982, Endorphins in human cerebrospinal fluid, Life Sci., 31: 1737-1740.

Peroutka, S.J., Moskowitz, M.A., Reinhard, J.F., and Snyder, S.H., 1980, Neurotransmitter receptor binding in bovine cerebral microvessels, Science, 208: 610-613.

Regoli, D., and Barabe, J., 1980, Pharmacology of bradykinin and related kinins, Pharmacol.Rev., 32: 1-46.

Rioux, F., Quirion, R., Leblanc, M.A., Regoli, D., and St-Pierre, S., 1980, Possible interactions between neurotensin and prostaglandins in the isolated rat portal vein, Life Sci., 27: 259-267.

Scheffé, H., 1953, A method for judging all contrasts in the analysis of variance, Biometrica, 40: 87-104.

Starke, K., Peskar, B.A., Schumacher, K.A., and Taube, H.D., 1977, Bradykinin and postganglionic sympathetic transmission, Naunyn-Schmiedeberg's Arch.Pharmacol., 299: 23-32.

Terenius, L., and Wahlström, A., 1975, Search for an endogenous ligand for the opiate receptor, Acta Physiol.Scand., 94: 74-81.

Terenius, L., and Wahlström, A., 1978, Physiological and clinical relevance of endorphins, in: "Centrally acting peptides," Hughes, J., ed., MacMillan, London, pp. 161-178.

Toda, N., 1977, Actions of bradykinin on isolated cerebral and peripheral arteries, Amer.J.Physiol., 232: H267-H274.

Uhl, G.R., Goodman, R.R., Kuhar, M.J., Childers, S.R., and Snyder, S.H., 1979, Immunohistochemical mapping of enkephalin containing cell bodies, fibres and nerve terminals in the brain stem of the rat, Brain Res., 166: 75-94.

Unterberg, A., and Baethmann, A.J., 1984, The kallikrein-kinin system as mediator in vasogenic brain edema. Part 1: Cerebral exposure to bradykinin and plasma, J.Neurosurg., 61: 87-96.

Unterberg, A., Wahl, M., and Baethmann, A., 1984, Effects of bradykinin on permeability and diameter of pial vessels in vivo, J.Cereb.Blood Flow Metab., (in press).

Wagner, F., and Wahl, M., 1984, The effect of neurotensin on vascular and intestinal smooth muscle, Pflügers Arch., (in press).

Wahl, M., Deetjen, P., Thurau, K., Ingvar, D.H., and Lassen, N.A., 1970, Micropuncture evaluation of the importance of perivascular pH for the arteriolar diameter on the brain surface, Pflügers Arch., 316: 152-163.

Wahl, M., and Kuschinsky, W., 1979 a, The dilating effect of histamine on pial arteries of cats and its mediation by H_2 receptors, Circ.Res., 44: 161-165.

Wahl, M., and Kuschinsky, W., 1979 b, Unimportance of perivascular
  H^+ and K^+ activities for the adjustment of pial arterial diameter during changes of arterial blood pressure in cats, Pflügers Arch., 382: 203-208.
Wahl, M., Young, A.R., Edvinsson, L., and Wagner, F., 1983 a, Effects
  of bradykinin on pial arteries and arterioles in vitro and in
  situ, J.Cereb.Blood Flow Metab., 3: 231-237.
Wahl, M., Young, A.R., Edvinsson, L., and Wagner, F., 1983 b, Effects
  of kininase II inhibitors on the vasomotor response to bradykinin of feline intracranial and extracranial arteries in vitro
  and in situ, J.Cereb.Blood Flow Metab., 3: 339-345.
Wahl, M., Unterberg, A., and Baethmann, A., 1983 c, Effects of bradykinin on permeability and diameter of cerebral vessels, in:
  "The cerebral veins, an experimental and clinical update," Auer
  L.M., Loew, F., eds., Springer, Wien, pp. 119-122.
Wahl, M., Unterberg, A., and Baethmann, A., 1984, Intravital fluorescence microscopy for the study of blood-brain barrier function, Int.J.Microcirc.Clin.Exp., (in press).
Whalley, E.T., and Wahl, M., 1983 a, Analysis of bradykinin receptor
  mediating relaxation of cat cerebral arteries in vivo and in
  vitro, Naunyn-Schmiedeberg's Arch.Pharmacol., 323: 66-71.
Whalley, E.T., and Wahl, M., 1983 b, The effect of kininase II inhibitors on the response of feline cerebral arteries to bradykinin and angiotensin, Pflügers Arch., 398: 175-177.
Whalley, E.T., Fritz, H., and Geiger, R., 1983 a, Kinin receptors
  and angiotensin converting enzyme in rabbits basilar arteries,
  Naunyn Schmiedeberg's Arch.Pharmacol., 324: 296-301.
Whalley, E.T., Wahl, M., and Sampaio, C.A.M., 1983 b, Angiotensin-
  converting enzyme, bradykinin, angiotensin and cerebral vessel
  reactivity, Hypertension, 5, Suppl. V: V34-V37.
Yau, W.M., Verdun, P.R., and Youther, M.L., 1983, Neurotensin: a mo-
  dulator of enteric cholinergic neurons in the guinea pig small
  intestine, Eur.J.Pharmacol., 95: 253-258.

ACKNOWLEDGEMENTS

The assistance of Miss Eveline Karoline Dolischan and Dr.
Lothar Schilling is gratefully appreciated. I wish to thank especially Franz Friedrich Waldemar Wagner for the statistical analysis
of the results.
Supported by Deutsche Forschungsgemeinschaft Wa 441/2-3.

EFFECTS OF INCREASES IN THE INSPIRED OXYGEN FRACTION ON BRAIN
SURFACE OXYGEN PRESSURE FIELDS AND REGIONAL CEREBRAL BLOOD FLOW

Christina Eintrei, Svante Ödman and Niels Lund

Departments of Anesthesiology and Biomedical Engineering
University Hospital
S-581 85 Linköping, Sweden

It has been shown that hyperoxemia causes abnormal tissue oxygenation in, e.g., skeletal muscle (Lund 1979). An inspired oxygen fraction (FIO_2) of approx. 0.6-0.7 caused signs of abnormal muscle tissue oxygenation (p_tO_2) (Lund et al 1980).

Kety and Schmidt (1948) and Lambertsen et al (1953) studied the effect of oxygen breathing on cerebral blood flow (CBF). Their results showed a relationship between arterial pO_2 (P_aO_2) and CBF in man. CBF decreased when p_aO_2 was increased. However, no specific p_aO_2-levels were given. Johansson and Siesjö (1975) and Borgström et al (1975) obtained the same results in studies on rats.

The present study was done in order to evaluate the effects of changes in FIO_2 on brain p_tO_2 and regional CBF (rCBF).

MATERIAL AND METHODS

The experiments were performed on five minipigs (approx. 20 kg b.w.). Induction of anesthesia was carried out with 80 mg of azaperon and 0.5 mg atropine i.m. followed by 150-300 mg of metomidate i.v.. Anesthesia was maintained with a continuous infusion of ketamine 0.25-0.35 mg $\cdot$ kg-1 $\cdot$ min-1. The animals were paralyzed with pancuronium 0.20-0.30 mg $\cdot$ kg-1 $\cdot$ min-1. The pigs were tracheotomized and mechanically ventilated to a normal arterial carbon dioxide pressure (p_aCO_2) and maintained at this p_aCO_2 level throughout the experiment. Temperature of the brain surface and the heart rate were monitored continuously. The femoral artery and femoral vein or one jugular vein were cannulated for blood sampling, continuous blood pressure monitoring, infusions and injections. Arterial blood samples were drawn for blood gas analysis.

Measurements of brain surface oxygen pressure fields were performed with the MDO oxygen electrode (Kessler & Lübbers 1966). The
skull and dura were opened with the utmost care to avoid trauma
to the cortical surface. A small plastic holder for the electrode
was placed on the cortex, and the rest of the exposed brain surface
was moistened with saline and covered with a soft membrane imper-
meable to oxygen. In order to avoid pressure on the cortex the
electrode was suspended in an arm counterbalanced with an adjustable weight.

In order to obtain a sufficient number of observations (n>80)
for statistical evaluation and to enable construction of tissue
oxygen pressure histograms (Lübbers 1977), eight oxygen pressure
values were collected every 15 sec. The observed values were fed
into a computer (Luxor ABC 800, Luxor AB, Sweden) and corrected
for electrode drift, temperature and air pressure changes.

To measure rCBF a modification of the Kety and Schmidt (1945,
1948) method was used. Directly on the brain cortex a 1 cm^2 polyester film (Mylar®) was placed. Then 0.6-1.3 mCi of ^{133}Xenon in
saline was applied under the polyester film. The wash-out curve of
the isotope from the brain was registered with an external CdTL-
detector at a distance of 5 cm from the brain. The clearance curve
was monitored for 10 min. From the obtained curve blood flow was
calculated (Eintrei et al 1985).

In varying sequences the pigs were ventilated with different
FIO_2's: 0.21, 0.35, 0.7, and 1.0. To obtain baseline measurements
and for control purposes the pigs were always ventilated with air
between each change of FIO_2. The rCBF measurements with ^{133}Xenon
were done immediately after the p_tO_2 measurements. The blood flow
measurements were not done during the control measurements with a
FIO_2 of 0.21.

Statistical methods: comparisons between group means were made
using paired t-test (Lindgren 1976). Statistically significant
differences were determined at the levels indicated in the text.
Mean values are given ±SD. Changes in histogram distribution types
were tested with the two-sample Kolmogorov-Smirnov test (Lindgren
1976) as modified by Ödman and Lund (1980).

RESULTS

Blood pressure, hematocrit, pH and p_aCO_2, which all influence
cerebral blood flow, were almost constant throughout the experiments (Table 1) and should thus not influence the p_tO_2-measurements.

TABLE 1. Basic physiological parameters at the corresponding FIO_2-levels. Values in the table are mean ±SD. Blood gases are in kPa.

FIO_2	Blood pressure	Hemato-crit	paO_2	P_aCO_2	pH	Brain sur-face temp
0.21	98 ±9 / 66 ±16	29 ±3.4	15.0 ±1.3	4.4±0.6	7.43±0.05	37.2 ±0.4
0.35	119±20 / 80±20	28 ±1.8	26.6±4.2	4.5±0.4	7.41±0.08	37.0±0.3
0.70	109±13 / 70±15	28±2.4	50.0±7.3	4.2±0.5	7.44±0.04	37.3±0.2
1.0	125±28 / 74±17	35±1.3	71.6±4.1	4.5±0.5	7.40±0.09	37.4±0.6

The influence of increased pressure on tissue when applying the electrode was negligible. The weight of the MDO electrode used was 1.4 g and the touching area 0.6 cm^2 causing a pressure of 0.23 kPa when applied directly on brain tissue. By a counterweight lever this pressure was balanced out. Pressure measurements on a balanced scale (Mettler P.E. 360) showed that it was possible to achieve a pressure force of only 0 ±0.001 N in the best case (limits due to digital reading of the scale). In the worst case when the counter-balance lever was maximally out of balance a force of 0.039 ±0.001 N was measured, corresponding to a pressure of 6.5 Pa. Even if we did not manage to apply the electrode with the lowest surface pressure possible in all cases, a lower pressure than 0.14 Pa used by Ödman and Lund (1980) or recommended by Kessler (1968) should have been exerted on the brain surface in this study. Movements of the brain mainly caused by breathing (frequency 0.2 Hz and ampli-tude 5 mm) caused at most an acceleration of $(2\pi \cdot 0.2)^2 \cdot 5 = 7.9 \cdot 10^{-3}$ m/s^2. Together with the mass of the MDO electrode this gave a periodical momentum of force with a peak value of 108 N and a pressure of 0.18 Pa.

In Table 2 the p_tO_2 results are presented. During baseline measurements the SD was small indicating normal tissue oxygen pressure fields. Table 3 shows rCBF at different FIO_2's. There was a decrease in rCBF when FIO_2 was increased. Paired t-tests between the four p_tO_2 group means were statistically significant with $p<0.01$.

TABLE 2. Mean tissue pO$_2$'s (in kPa) at the different FIO$_2$-levels.

	FIO$_2$			
Pig no	0.21	0.35	0.70	1.0
1	4.1±1.0	11.2±2.0	16.9±6.4	25.6±10.4
2	2.4±2.6	6.1±3.7	8.5±10.3	6.6±6.0
3	3.4±2.1	4.4±2.1	8.6±4.0	18.1±9.3
4	3.7±1.2	12.5±3.7	14.8±6.1	6.0±2.4
5	5.4±1.2	12.1±1.5	19.0±1.6	22.5±1.8
MEAN ± SD	3.8±1.1	9.5±1.5	13.6±1.6	15.8±9.0

TABLE 3. Regional cerebral blood flow (rCBF) measured with ^{133}Xenon locally applied at different FIO$_2$'s. Values in ml·100 g^{-1} ·min^{-1} in grey matter.

Pig no	1	2	3	4	5	Mean
0.21	134	95	84	81	148	108
0.35	86	88	73	75	62	77
0.70	107	74	50	74	61	73
1.0	82	59	70	46	63	64

DISCUSSION

In this study the baseline measurements (FIO$_2$ 0.21) had a ptO$_2$ between 2.4 and 5.4 kPa. Leniger-Follert et al (1975) found a ptO$_2$ between 0-90 mm Hg (0-12 kPa) in the superficial layers of the cat cortex at normoventilation. Metzger et al (1971) reported a pt O$_2$ of 4 mm Hg (0.6 kPa) at normoxia measured in the rat cortex with a needle electrode. Their low ptO$_2$ may have been caused by the electrode compressing the tissue and thus influencing the microcirculation (Lund 1984). Nair et al (1975) also used needle electrodes for measuring pO$_2$ in the cortex of cats. During air breathing they found a range in p_tO_2 from 0 to 99 mm Hg (0-13 kPa) with a mean of 38 mm Hg (5 kPa). The p_tO_2 values from the present study thus correspond well with the results of other studies at normoxia.

Increasing the FIO_2 to 0.35 increased p_aO_2 and p_tO_2 to a total average of 9.5 kPa (range 4.4-12.5 kPa). However, the histogram distribution type changed significantly ($p<0.05$) in all cases compared to baseline results. All histograms were now of the scattered type (Fig. 1). Nair et al (1975) reported an increase in p_tO_2 in 22 of 29 locations at a FIO_2 of 1.0, however, they gave no p_tO_2 values. At a FIO_2 of 0.4 Leniger-Follert et al (1975) registered p_tO_2's from 15 to 85 mm Hg (2 to 11 kPa). When they increased FIO_2 to 0.6 they found an increase in p_tO_2 in three different locations to 40, 85 and 110 mm Hg (5, 11 and 15 kPa). Metzger et al (1971) found that p_tO_2 increased with increasing FIO_2, but the increase in p_tO_2 depended on initial pO_2 in different tissue areas, i.e. scattering increased with increasing FIO_2. However, our study does not allow direct comparisons with the studies discussed as they either used other techniques or presented their results in other ways than histograms.

The rCBF decreased with increasing FIO_2 (Table 3). At FIO_2 1.0 the decrease in rCBF was from 20% to 55% when compared to initial flow. However, on two occasions we noted a slight increase in rCBF when FIO_2 was increased. Kety and Schmidt (1948) and Lambertsen et al (1953) also found a decrease in rCBF in man breathing 100% oxygen. These results were confirmed by Jóhansson and Siesjö in 1975 and Borgström et al (1975) in studies on rats.

Thus, our study and those of others have shown that a relationship exists between brain surface oxygen pressure and regional cerebral blood flow. However, we did not find a correlation between mean tissue oxygen pressure and rCBF. This was not surprising since mean p_tO_2 is not the decisive parameter in describing p_tO_2 (Lübbers 1977).

Our conclusion is that a FIO_2 of 0.35 or higher affects brain p_tO_2. Also, increasing FIO_2's lead to a decrease in rCBF.

ACKNOWLEDGEMENTS

This study was supported by the Swedish Medical Research Council (05956), The Östergötland County Council (96/82, 98/82, 14/83) and the Tore Nilson Foundation (83/94). We are greatly indebted to Lars-Åke Malmqvist and Anita Forsman for skilful technical assistance.

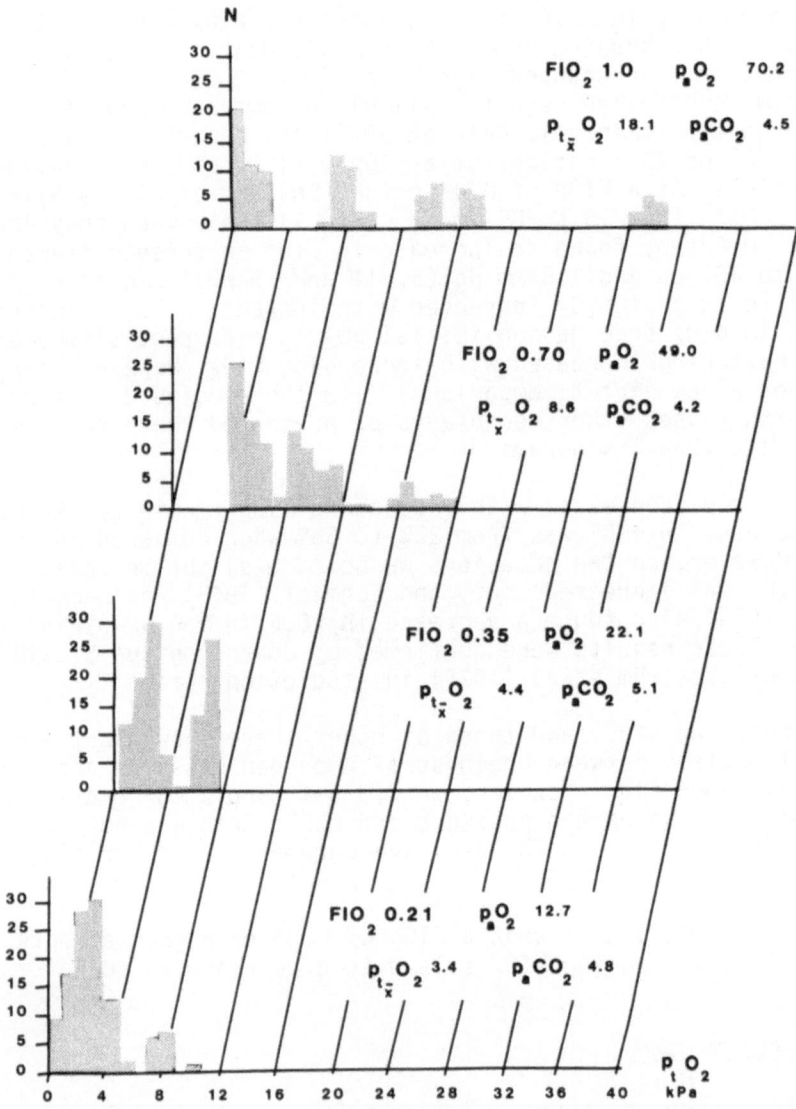

FIGURE 1. Histograms from pig brain at different FIO_2's. Note the increasing scattering at increasing FIO_2.

REFERENCES

Borgström, L., Jóhansson, H., Siesjö, B.K. 1975. The relationship
    between arterial pO2 and cerebral blood flow in hypoxic
    hypoxia. Acta Physiol Scand., 93:423.
Eintrei, C., Leszniewski, W.,Ödman, S., Lewis, D.H. 1985. Locally
    applied ^{133}Xenon for the measurement of regional cerebral
    blood flow rCBF - An experimental study in the pig. Accep-
    ted for publication in Acta Physiol Scand.
Jóhansson, H., Siesjö, B.K. 1975. Cerebral blood flow and
    oxygen consumption in the rat in hypoxic hypoxia. Acta
    Physiol Scand., 93:296.
Kessler, M. 1968. Normal and critical O -supply of the liver.
    In: Oxygen transport in blood and tissue. Eds: Lübbers,
    D.W., Luft, U. C., Thews, G., Witzleb, E. Georg Thieme
    Verlag, Stuttgart.
Kessler, M., Lübbers, D. W. 1966. Aufbau und Anwendungsmöglich-
    keiten verschiedener PO2-Elektroden. Pflügers Arch., 291:
    R82.
Kety, S. S., Schmidt, C. F. 1945. The determination of cerebral
    blood flow in man by the use of nitrous oxide in low
    concentrations. Am J Physiol., 143:53.
Kety, S. S., Schmidt, C. F. 1948. The effects of altered arterial
    tensions of carbon dioxide and oxygen on cerebral blood
    flow and cerebral oxygen consumption of normal young men.
    J Clin Invest., 27:484.
Lambertsen, C. J., Krough, R. H., Cooper, D. Y., Emmel, G. L.,
    Loeschcke, C. F., Schmidt, 1953. Oxygen toxicity. Effects
    in man of oxygen inhalation at 1 and 3.5 atmospheres upon
    blood gas transport, cerebral circulation and cerebral
    metabolism. J Appl Physiol., 5:471.
Leniger-Follert, E., Lübbers, D., and Wrabetz, W. 1975. Regulation
    of local tissue pO2 of the brain cortex at different arterial
    O2 pressures. Pflügers Arch., 359:81.
Lindgren, B.W. 1976. Statistical theory. The Macmillan Company,
    New York.
Lübbers, D. W. 1977. Quantitative measurement and description of
    oxygen supply to the tissue. In: Oxygen & Physiological
    Function, pp 254-276. Ed., Jöbsis, F. F.. Professional In-
    formation Library, Dallas, TX, USA.
Lund, N. 1979. Studies on skeletal muscle surface oxygen pressure
    fields. Linköping University, Medical Dissertations No 71.
Lund, N. 1984. Skeletal and cardiac muscle oxygenation. Adv Exp
    Med Biol., this volume.
Lund, N., Jorfeldt, L., Lewis, D. H. 1980. Skeletal muscle oxygen
    pressure fields in healthy human volunteers. Acta anaesth
    scand., 24:161.

Metzger, H., Erdmann, W., Thews, G. 1971. Effect of short periods of hypoxia, hyperoxia and hypercapnia on brain O_2 supply. J Appl Physiol., 31(5):751.

Nair, P., Whalen, W. J., Buerk, D. 1975. pO_2 of cat cerebral cortex: response to breathing N_2 and 100% O_2. Microvasc Res., 9:158.

Ödman, S., Lund, N. 1980. Data acquisition and information processing in MDO oxygen electrode measurement of tissue oxygen pressure. Acta anaesth scand., 24:161.

ASSESSMENT OF THE IN VIVO RECORDING OF LOCAL CEREBRAL BLOOD FLOW

USING A THERMISTOR DEVICE

J. Coremans, H. Vermariën, F. Vereecke and R.H. Bourgain

Laboratory for Physiology and Physiopathology, V.U.B.
Laarbeeklaan 103, B-1090 Brussels, Belgium

ABSTRACT

In order to obtain a continuous measurement of local blood flow in the cerebral cortex of a laboratory animal using chronically implanted sensors, we have developed a device based on the heat clearance principle. Flow information is obtained from temperature measurement by means of two thermistors one of them being heated at a defined level above ambient tissue temperature; as such, cooling of the heated thermistor caused by convection phenomena in its vicinity, can be related to local perfusion rate. In a first step "in vitro" measurements were performed in order to study the behaviour, sensitivity and reliability of the device; a physical model was established explaining the results. In this paper we describe "in vivo" tests in the rabbit's brain cortex with the miniature thermistors (0.5 mm diameter) chronically implanted (at the cortical surface). Results are correlated with oxygen tension measurements using (smaller) pO_2 electrodes inserted into the cortical tissue. We have observed that all sensors are well tolerated by the animals who remain symptom free. Test experiments, inducing a well known physiological effect on local blood flow, such as arterial clamping, inhalation of CO_2 gas mixtures, etc., are performed. The phenomena during induced anoxic anoxia are also shown. These preliminary investigations are essential in order to attempt by future experiments the establishment of a correlation between "in vivo" recorded flow signals and the "in vitro" measured characteristics.

INTRODUCTION

In a previous report (Vermariën et al., 1984) we described a thermistor device developed for the continuous recording of local blood flow applying chronical sensor implantation. Our method is based on the heat clearance principle and makes use of accurate temperature measurement. As sensors thermistors are used, one of them being heated by a high frequency wave; temperature measurement is performed at DC level. The convective cooling of the heated thermistor with as a reference the non-heated one is thus a measure for the surrounding fluid flow velocity. Additionally we realized a method for the "in vitro" calibration of the device and we developed a mathematical model explaining the measured results, i.e. the relation between the cooling of the heated thermistor and the (uniform) velocity in the test fluid. As test fluids water and glycerin were used, having thermal characteristics approximating the ones of brain tissue.

With the experiments reported in this paper we intend to evaluate the "in vivo" applicability of the device, with the thermistors chronically implanted on the brain cortical tissue. For this purpose we have chosen some experiments of which the physiological effect on flow is well known (CO_2 inhalation causing vasodilation (Betz, 1972; Mamo and Seylaz, 1974) and arterial clamping). As the flow measuring method is intended to be used during anoxic anoxia experiments (Van Waeyenberge et al., in this issue), we also describe the results from a similar procedure.

MATERIALS AND METHODS

The thermistors used are miniature types having an external diameter of 0.5 mm. The thermistor property is used for temperature measurement (DC) as well as for heating (high frequency). Technical details are described in our previous paper (Vermariën et al., 1984). Two application modes can be defined: the non-heated mode with both thermistors measuring local temperature in tissue and a heated mode with one of the thermistors (Th) heated to a certain level above the surrounding (measured by the reference thermistor Tref). Before implantation on the cerebral cortex of the rabbit, the thermistors used are calibrated in a thermostatic bath with as a reference a precision Pt100 digital thermometer. Additionally local pO_2 is measured with the aid of polarographic electrodes inserted into the cortical tissue (0.1 mm diameter). The thermistors, having a larger diameter, are positioned at the surface of the cortex and fixed by tissue glue. Generally we use 3 pO_2 electrodes (parietal, occipital and frontal zone), the thermistors being located at both sides of the parietal electrode (at a 5 mm distance). More details about the preparation of the animal are given by Van Waeyenberge et al. (in this issue). After

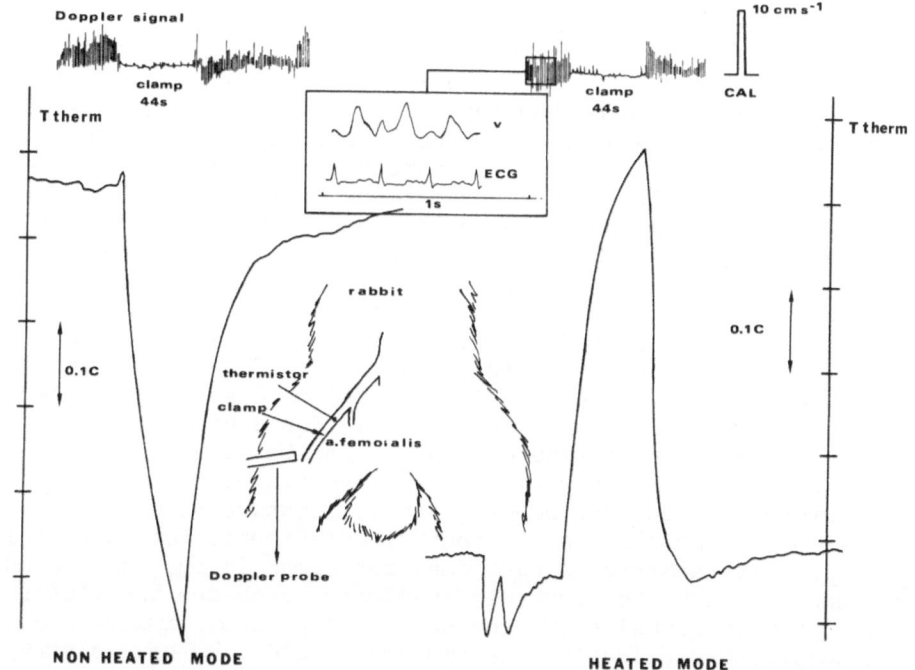

Fig. 1. Clamping of the a. femoralis under Doppler control. One thermistor is glued to the surface of the artery and temperature is measured in the non-heated mode and in the heated mode.

two weeks the animal has recovered from anaesthesia and surgical procedure. It appears that electrodes and thermistors are very well tolerated, as no pathological symptoms can be observed. ECoG and somatosensory evoked potentials also remain unaffected.

EXPERIMENTS AND RESULTS

All experiments were performed on animals prepared according to the procedure described above. Additional surgery and specific tests have been performed using adequate anaesthesia.

The applicability of our heat clearance device can firstly be illustrated by the following preliminary test. We perform clamping of the a. femoralis and observe the results of temperature measurement using only one thermistor applied either in the non-heated mode or, thereupon, in the heated mode. The a. femoralis is exposed over a distance of about 30 mm and a thermistor is fixed on the surface of the artery. The total preparate is covered with cotton wool imbued with paraffin oil in order to prevent disturbances due to convective air cooling. The blood velocity in the artery is measured about 20 mm distally from the thermistor site with a Doppler apparatus (continuous mode). Figure 1 shows the results. Clamping reduces the velocity to zero (only artefacts are visible). In the non-heated mode clamping causes a temperature decrease as can be explained by the loss of heat supply due to discontinued blood flow. In extremis temperature would drop towards environmental level. In the heated mode during clamping temperature increases because the convective heat loss measured by the thermistor and caused by flowing blood is reduced to zero.

Further we focus our attention on the results obtained with the thermistors implanted on the cortical surface. From our "in vitro" results we could conclude that the surface temperature of the heated thermistor is much lower than the one of its nucleus as the electrical insulation is responsible for a high, constant (i.e. flow independent) temperature drop (Vermariën et al., 1984). As such, from our tests in water and in glycerin we estimated this temperature gradient and adapted the temperature values, referring to the thermistor's surface. Control experiments for observation of variability and trends have been performed in the non-heated mode and in the heated mode; in the latter case one thermistor is heated 10°C (nucleus) above the surrounding level, implying a surface temperature elevation (estimated) of 2°C. We have observed that the heating thermistor slightly influences the non-heated one (about 0.1 °C increase). Furthermore we assume that the heating

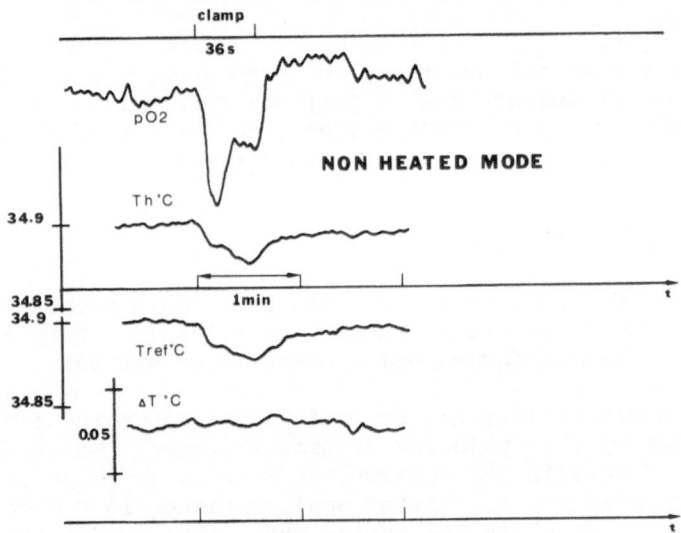

Fig. 2a. Clamping of both carotid arteries in the non-heated mode. pO_2 shows a marked decrease followed by a slight overshoot; both thermistors demonstrate a temperature decrease, whereas temperature difference ($\Delta T = Th - Tref$) is not affected.

did not influence the physiology of the surrounding tissue, as no specific alteration was observed on the pO_2 measured in the vicinity.

Figures 2a and 2b show the effect of clamping of both carotid arteries during about 30 s. The effect on pO_2 is characterized by an initial large decrease (about 15 s) followed by a partial increase towards an intermediary level. After discontinuing the clamp pO_2 increases, goes into a slight overshoot and thereupon regains its normal level. This evolution is observed in the non-heated as well as in the heated mode. In the non-heated mode (figure 2a) a decrease in temperature of both thermistors is observed, temperature difference ($\Delta T = T_h - T_{ref}$) remaining practically constant, which indicates a correct temperature compensation. In the heated mode (figure 2b) temperature T_h increases and, similarly, ΔT during clamping. Interpretation of the data is corresponding with the one developed for clamping of the a. femoralis: increase of ΔT is related to reduced flow in the cortical tissue (not zero flow as the aa. vertebrales remain unaffected).

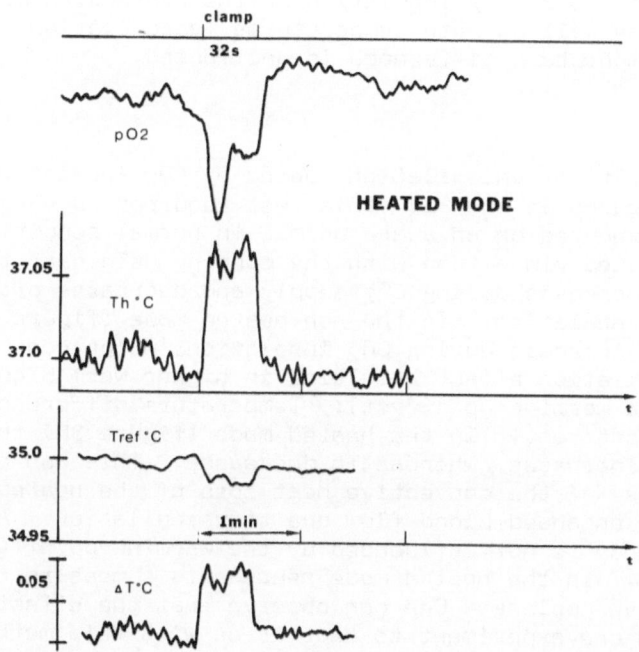

Fig. 2b. Clamping of both carotid arteries in the heated mode. pO_2 evolves similarly as in the non-heated mode, temperature difference demonstrates a clear increase corresponding with flow diminution (reduced scale!).

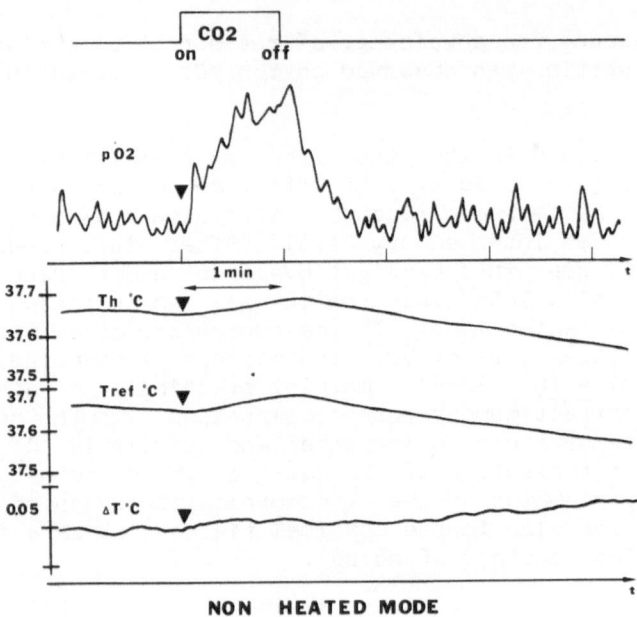

Fig. 3a. Effect of CO_2 inhalation in the non-heated mode.   pO2
increases, as well as both temperatures (vasodilation, warming-up
effect), temperature difference is unaffected.

    The results of vasodilation caused by CO_2 inhalation are pre-
sented in figures 3a and 3b. This test requires no surgery at all
and can be executed on an awake animal in normal condition. CO_2
is then supplied via a tube with the opening held near the animal's
nose. pO2 increases during CO_2 supply and decreases after discontinuing CO_2 inhalation. In the non-heated mode (figure 3a) both
temperatures increase during CO_2 inhalation, which can be explained
by the vasodilation effect resulting in higher warm blood supply to
the tissue (a warming-up effect). Temperature difference is approximately constant. In the heated mode (figure 3b) the reference
temperature increases, whereas Th decreases. This can be explained
as an increase of the convective heat loss of the heated thermistor
caused by an enhanced blood flow due to vasodilation. As ΔT in the
non-heated mode is not influenced by the warming-up effect of CO_2
inhalation, ΔT in the heated mode represents a measure exclusively
for convective cooling. One can observe that the effect of CO_2
differs from one experiment to another as with this method the
exact composition of the gas mixture inhaled by the rabbit is unknown. Nevertheless, this method allows quick and easy testing of
the well functioning of the implanted sensors.

    Similar effects have been observed on the rabbit in exper-
iments where artificial ventilation was used: enhanced pO2 during
CO_2 administration, the warming-up effect on both thermistors;

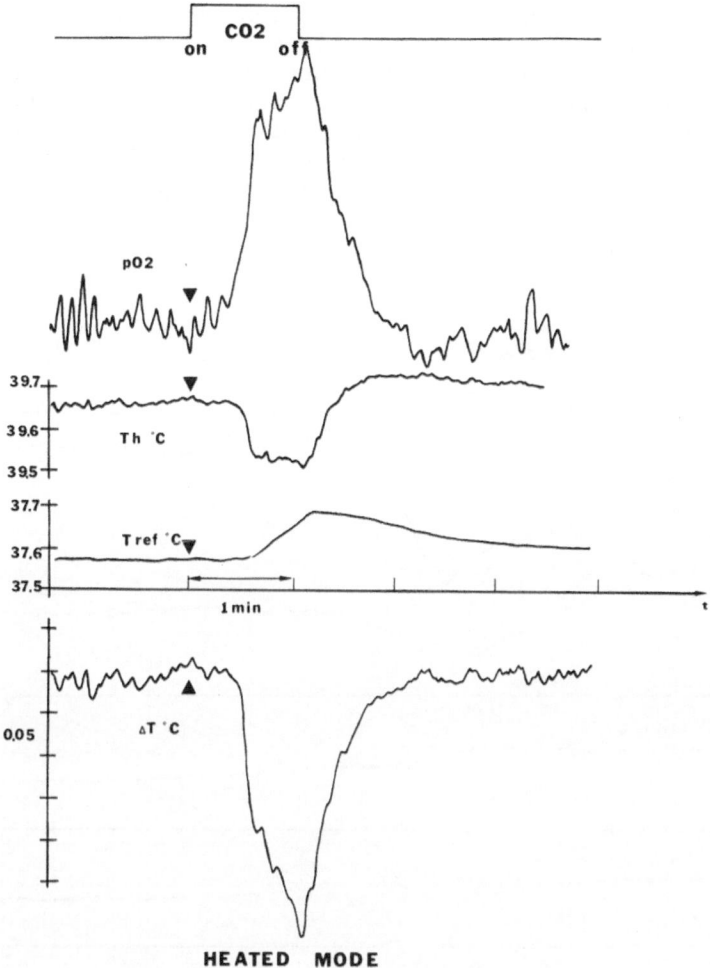

Fig. 3b. Effect of CO_2 inhalation in the heated mode. pO_2 evolves similarly as in the non-heated mode, temperature difference shows a clear decrease corresponding with flow increase.

negligible variation on ΔT in the non-heated mode, large cooling on ΔT in the heated mode.

Figure 4 displays results during anoxic anoxia induced by pure nitrogen breathing (a 100 s period) (according to Van Waeyenberge et al., in this issue). pO_2 diminishes during the anoxia time. T_{ref} slightly increases, whereas T_h decreases; as such, ΔT decreases remarkably, which is in accordance with the increase of blood flow during anoxia (Siesjö, 1978).

Finally we present results (figure 5) obtained when the animal was sacrificed by an overdose of Nembutal which induces an immediate heart arrest. As a consequence of blood flow interruption (following cardiac standstill), temperature (Tref, Trec (rectal temperature)) decreases, whereas Th initially increases. As such, ΔT, having the shape of a smoothed step function, displays two levels: 1) normal flow and 2) zero flow. By using these levels all preceding responses (increase or diminution of flow) can be standardized.

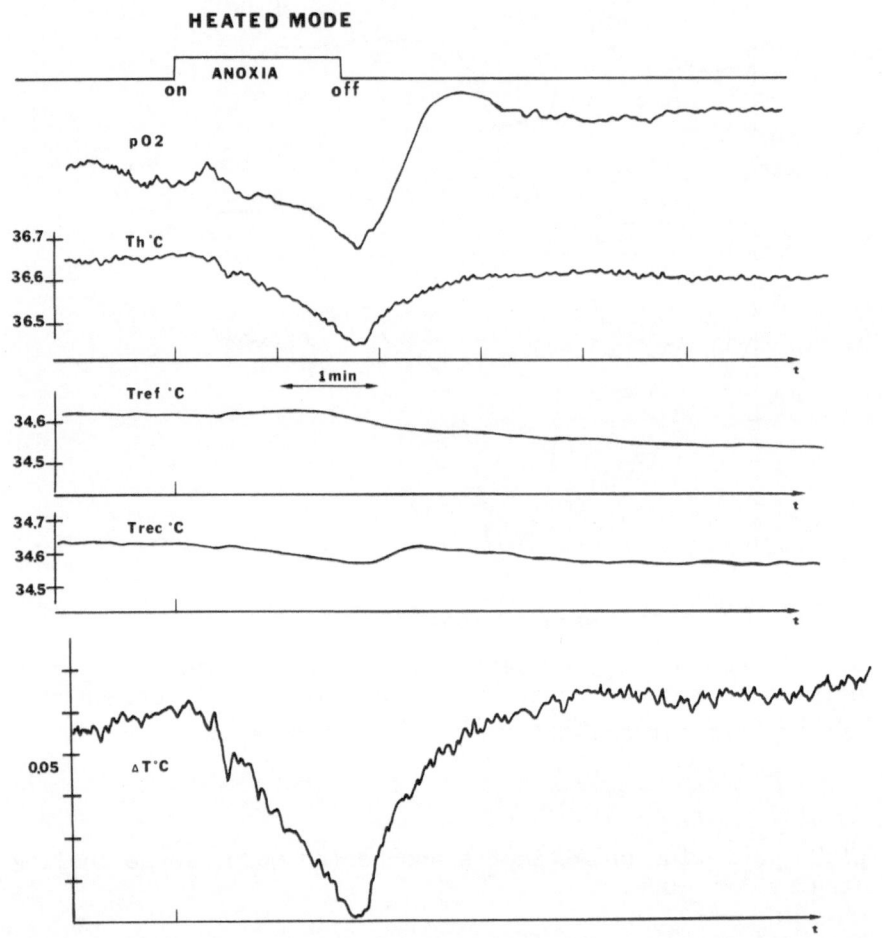

Fig. 4. Results during anoxic anoxia (heated mode). Whereas Tref slightly increases, Th decreases remarkably and, similarly, ΔT, demonstrating an enhancement in local blood flow during the anoxia period. A small variation is visible on the rectal temperature (Trec).

146

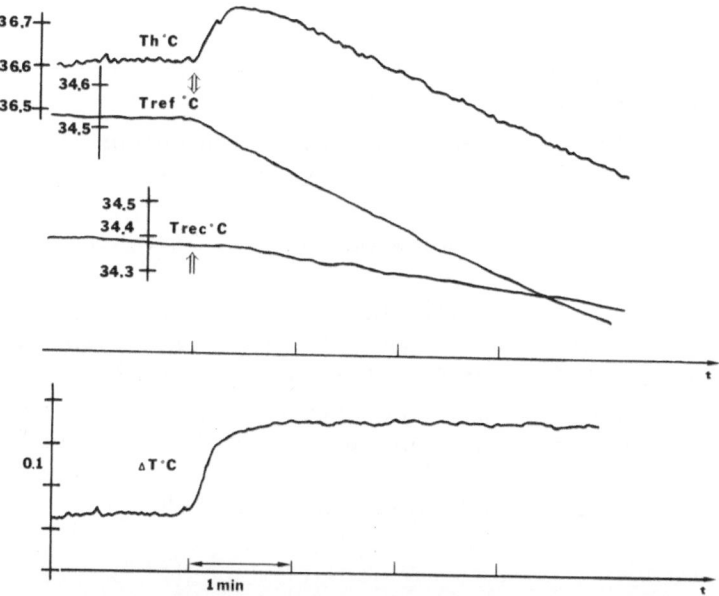

Fig. 5. Recordings before and following cardiac standstill (indicated by the arrow). Whereas Tref and Trec (rectal temperature) decrease, Th is initially enhanced. The latter phenomenon corresponds with the interruption of blood flow: ΔT shows a typical step function characterized by two levels: 1) normal flow, 2) zero flow.

CONCLUSIONS

From these experiments we can conclude that variation in local blood flow is accompanied by two different important effects. Firstly, flow alteration introduces temperature variation: increased warm blood supply to the superficial cortical tissue introduces a temperature elevation. Therefore the use of two thermistors is unavoidable. We observed that the influence on temperature difference between both of them is negligible. The second effect, i.e. the influence of flow alteration on the temperature of the heated thermistor referred to the non-heated one is thus a measure exclusively for flow variation (temperature difference). Zero flow can be determined after the animal's death. All experiments implying increased flow (CO_2, anoxia) or decreased flow (clamping) gave consistent results in the measured temperature difference. However, in order to obtain quantitative data in relation to localization of the thermistors, dimension of the thermistors (how "local" are the measured results) and finally the accordance with the "in vitro" calibration and linearization, still large research efforts will be necessary.

REFERENCES

Betz, E., 1972, Cerebral blood flow: its measurement and regulation, Physiological Reviews, 52: 595-630.

Mamo, H. and Seylaz, J., 1974, La circulation cérébrale. Données méthodologiques et physiologiques, Rev. d'E.E.G. Neurophysiol., 4: 194-209.

Siesjö, B.K., 1978, Brain Energy Metabolism, Wiley and Sons, New York.

Van Waeyenberge, M., Vermariën, H., De Backer, H., Manil, J. and Bourgain, R.H., 1984, Discriminant parameters representing cerebral function during anoxic anoxia investigations (in this issue).

Vermariën, H., Coremans, J., Vereecke, F. and Bourgain, R.H., 1984, A thermistor device for the continuous recording of mass transport velocity in tissue based on the heat clearance principle, to be published in Oxygen Transport to Tissue VI, Plenum Press, New York.

DISCRIMINANT PARAMETERS REPRESENTING CEREBRAL CORTICAL FUNCTION

DURING ANOXIC ANOXIA INVESTIGATIONS

M. Van Waeyenberge, H. Vermariën, H. De Backer,
J. Manil and R.H. Bourgain

Laboratory for Physiology and Physiopathology
Laarbeeklaan 103, B-1090 Brussels, Belgium

ABSTRACT

In order to quantify the effect of specific drugs on the cerebral cortex an "in vivo" model has been developed for the induction and the observation of anoxic anoxia. Rabbits are used as test animals. Sensors for the assessment of local parameters are chronically implanted: ECoG electrodes are applied; pO_2 electrodes are inserted into the cortical tissue. The derived somatosensory evoked potentials are used for evaluating the cerebral cortical function. Animals are cannulated with a tracheal tube, curarized and artificially ventilated. Anoxic anoxia, controlled by a special purpose microprocessor system, may then be induced and repeated in a reproducible way. During the experiments local (pO_2, ECoG, SEP) as well as general parameters (ECG, heart rate, systemic blood pressure, rectal temperature) are recorded and stored on analog magnetic tape as well as digitized with the microprocessor system. The cortical pO_2 is measured with a polarographic method, the SEP's are obtained on-line by time coherent averaging and the ECoG states (e.g. epilepsy during anoxia) are derived by using band-pass filters and rms detectors. Off-line the signals (pO_2, heart rate, mean systemic blood pressure, temperature) are standardized and represented together with parameters derived from ECoG and SEP. SEP-waveform parameters indicating intensity (norm) and similarity with a reference SEP signal (correlation value) are used.

The measuring and processing method is still being optimized; special attention is being paid towards the quality of the calculated SEP's which are to be used for the quantification of the cortical function during reference, anoxia and recovery period. As such, in order to improve the signal-to-noise ratio of the SEP's and, consequently, of the derived parameters, ECoG signals are digitized off-line and subjected to a preprocessing, implying filtering and spectral analysis procedures.

INTRODUCTION

In previous investigations the specific modifications of the evoked cortical somatosensory potentials in anoxic anoxia were described in detail (Manil et al., 1978; Colin et al., 1980); studies on the control mechanisms involved in the regulation of cortical tissue pressure in oxygen were performed (Bourgain et al., 1981). It was then deemed essential to correlate these findings with the parameters of local blood flow in the cortex, the electrocorticogram and the systemic blood pressure.

More detailed correlative studies have been made possible by the development of a special purpose microprocessor controlled apparatus allowing flexible experimental organizing and data acquisition. Simultaneously recorded parameters are subjected to off-line processing with a PDP-11/70 computer, resulting eventually in convenient data representation and reporting. In these conditions the mechanisms regulating cortical tissue pressure in oxygen and local blood flow correlated with the electrogenesis can be investigated in specific physiopathological and pharmacological conditions by a standardized reproducible procedure.

INDUCTION AND RECORDING OF ANOXIC ANOXIA: SURVEY OF THE METHOD

The test procedure implies "in vivo" induction of anoxic anoxia and recording of the effects, specially in the brain cortex, using chronically implanted sensors. The method is standardized and can be repeated several times provided a limited anoxia duration is applied. Figure 1 shows a block diagram of the apparatus.

A specially designed microprocessor system controls the test procedure. The microprocessor times the anoxia sequence and drives stepping motors which control the valves of the gasmixture supplies used for artificial ventilation of the test animal; furthermore it generates trigger pulses for the stimulating device, thus controlling the sequence and the recording of the somatosensory evoked potentials (SEP's). The system digitizes measured signals, performs on-line a part of the preprocessing, i.e. the calculation of the SEP's out of the recorded electrocorticogram (ECoG) and stores resulting data on tape. Off-line data are sent to a PDP-11/70 computer for further processing and storage.

Local and systemic parameters are recorded, monitored and processed afterwards. Local oxygen pressure is recorded using miniature electrodes inserted into the cortical tissue of the test animal. ECoG and derived parameters obtained through band-pass filters and

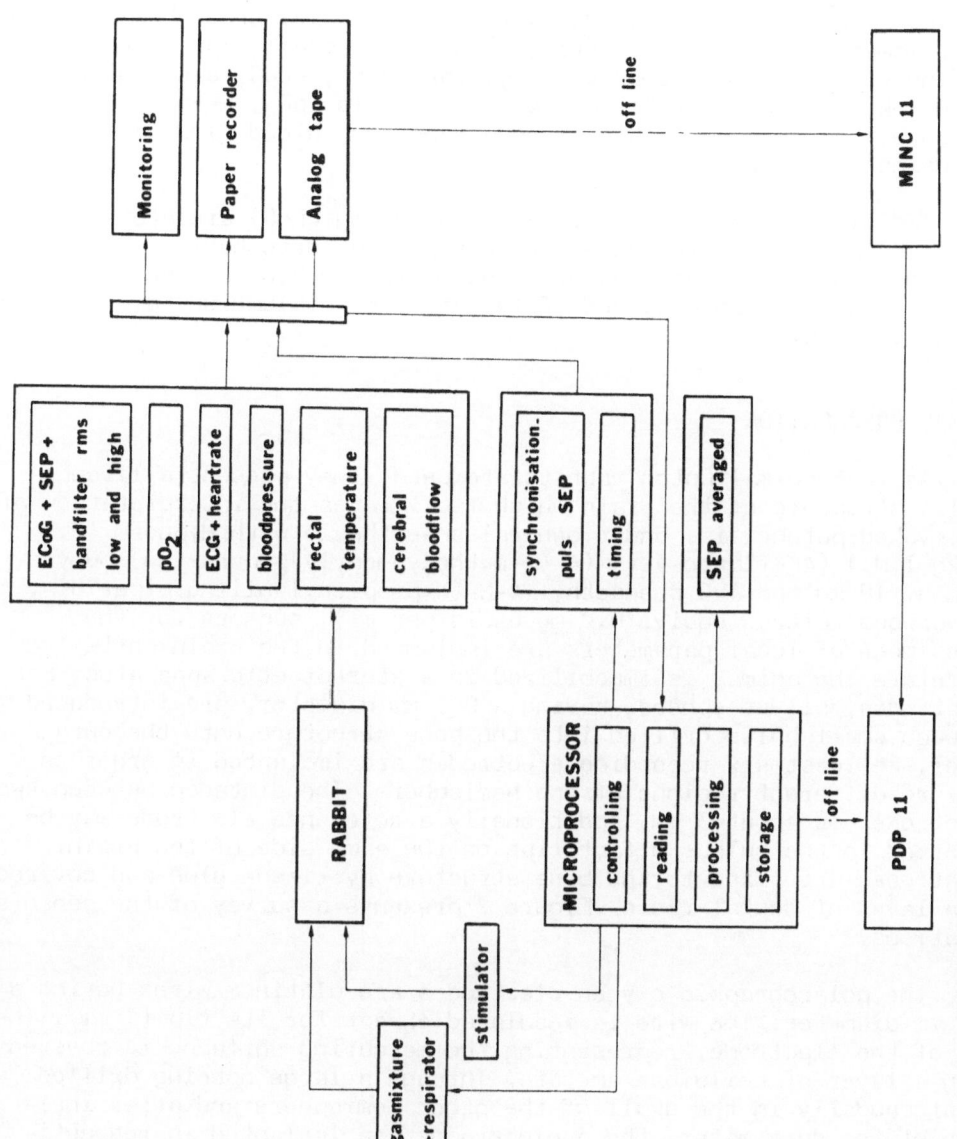

Fig. 1. Block diagram of the experimental apparatus for the induction and recording of anoxic anoxia.

151

"root mean square" (rms) detectors, represent spontaneous cortical activity. In order to have a direct indication of the functional state of the brain cortical tissue the SEP's are obtained by time coherent averaging of the ECoG and the result is continuously visualized on a scope. Assessment of local cerebral blood flow by using a thermistor method based on the heat clearance principle is being developed. Furthermore, general parameters are measured: ECG and heart rate, momentary and mean arterial pressure, rectal temperature. "Fast" varying signals (ECG, momentary blood pressure, ECoG) are registered on an ink jet recorder; "slow" varying signals (pO_2, mean arterial pressure, heart rate, ECoG derived parameters, blood flow) are recorded using a pen writer.

Additionally all original data (including ECoG) are stored on two 8-channel analog instrumentation tape recorders having larger storage capacity as compared with the microprocessor system. As such original data can be disposed of for off-line evaluation, digitization and processing.

ANIMAL PREPARATION

As test animal Dutch rabbits are used. They present a lisence-phalic structure of the brain which facilitates the interpretation of the evoked potentials. Under general anaesthesia with Hypnorm (0.5 mg/kg I.M.) (4'-fluoro-4-(1-(4-(2-methoxyphenyl))piperazino)-butyro-phenon, 10 mg and 1-2 phenaethyl-4-N-(N-propionylanilino)piperidin, dihydrogen, citras equiv; 0.2 mg basis per ml), sensors for the assessment of local parameters are implanted in the brain cortex. Therefore the animal is immobilized in a stereotactic apparatus. EcoG electrodes, silver spheres having a 0.5 mm diameter, are introduced through small holes drilled into the bone structure onto the dura mater. At least six recording electrodes are implanted in order to explore different regions of one hemisphere. The distance between two electrodes is about 3 mm. Additionally a reference electrode may be inserted in the bulbus olfactorius on the same side of the brain. Electrodes are fixed to the bone structure by tissue glue and covered by a layer of dental resin. Figure 2 presents a survey of the sensors' locations.

The polarographic oxygen electrodes are platinum wires having a 100 μm diameter. The wire is insulated except for its tip (1 mm). The tip of the electrode, representing the measuring surface, is covered with a layer of cellulose acetate. Through a large opening drilled rostrocaudally in the skull of the other hemisphere and after incision of the dura mater, the 3 electrodes are implanted in respectively the frontal, parietal and occipital regions. Figure 3 shows a sketch of the electrode as it is inserted into the cortical tissue. Recently we also apply a couple of miniature thermistors (spheres with a 0.5 mm diameter), placed onto the cerebral cortical surface for the purpose of evaluating local blood flow (Vermariën et al., 1984; Coremans et al., in this issue). The area of the rabbit's head surgically treated is covered with a thick layer of dental resin.

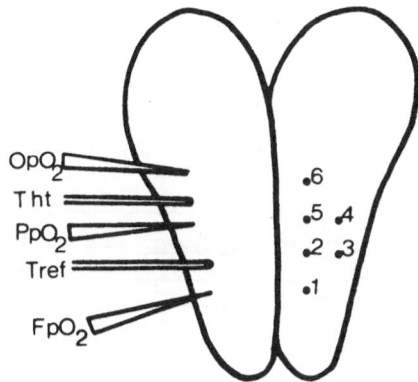

Fig. 2. Survey of electrode implants. Points 1 to 6 indicate the
location of ECoG electrodes. The electrodes 1, 2, 5 and 6, about
equally spaced (3 mm), are located rostrocaudally at a distance of
3 mm from the sagittal midline, electrodes 3 and 4 another 3 mm
farther. Electrodes 1, 2 and 3 are placed rostrally of the sutura
coronalis, electrodes 4, 5 and 6 caudally. OpO_2 (occipital), PpO_2
(parietal) and FpO_2 (frontal) indicate the sites of the pO_2 electrodes. Two thermistors, T_{ref} (reference) and T_{ht} (heated), are
used for local blood flow measurement (heat clearance method).

All connecting wires are soldered to a plug attached to the skull
by stainless steel screws embedded in the resin.

Antibiotic therapy is performed for five days with Chloromycetin
(Chloramphenicoli natrium succinum, Parke-Davis, 100 mg/kg I.M.
daily). The animals were allowed to recover for at least two weeks.

On the day of the experiment the rabbit is cannulated with a
tracheal tube under fluothane anaesthesia. Positive pressure ventilation with a gas mixture containing 80% N_2 and 20% O_2 is performed;
gas flow is controlled with the aid of rotameters. The animal is curarized by intravenous administration of Flaxédil (Gallamine triethio-
didum, 20 mg/ml). A polyethylene catheter (1.3 mm external diameter)
is inserted into the femoral artery and the blood pressure is
obtained by a Beckmann transducer. An Ag/AgCl reference electrode is
attached to the animal's ear for the purpose of pO_2 measurement
(polarographic method). This point is connected to the ground. ECG is
obtained by using two needle electrodes and a heart rate signal is·
derived. Rectal temperature is obtained with the aid of a thermistor
sensor. The stimuli for evoking somatosensory potentials are rectangular pulses, having a duration of 1 ms and about 10 V amplitude
(supramaximal stimulation), and are delivered through a pair of ring
electrodes attached to the animal's contralateral forepaw, coupled
to the skin with a conductive paste. ECoG derivations are unipolar
with the reference Ag-electrode in the bulbus olfactorius or alternatively with an Ag/AgCl electrode glued on the ear. Test procedures
may then be started as soon as the animal has regained its normal
state, as can be checked on the ECoG pattern.

153

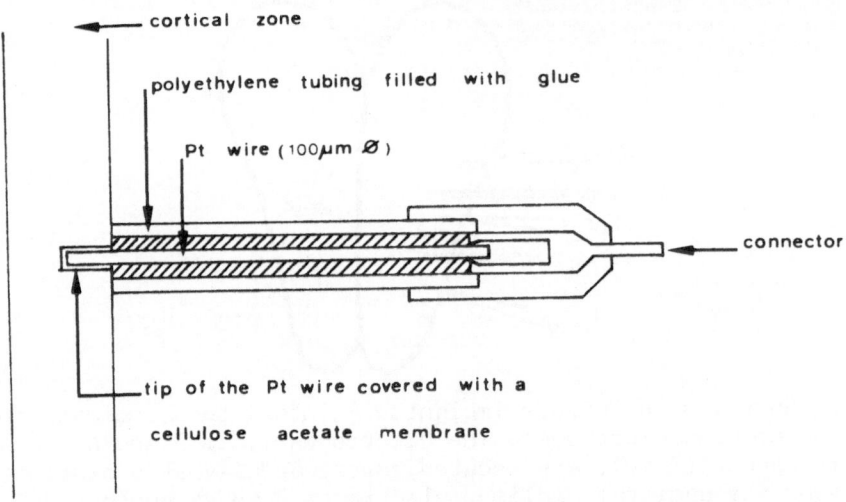

cortical zone

polyethylene tubing filled with glue

Pt wire (100μm Ø)

connector

tip of the Pt wire covered with a

cellulose acetate membrane

Fig. 3. A polarographic miniature disposable oxygen electrode, inserted into the cortical tissue (constructed and applied according to Silver (1965), Bicher (1973), Leniger-Follert and Hossman (1977)). The electrode is fixed by gluing the protective polyethylene tubing to the cortical surface.

ANOXIC ANOXIA TEST PROCEDURE

The use of a microprocessor system allows a relatively flexible control of the experimental protocol. Additional information concerning drugs, treatment, etc., can easily be introduced and added to the data set via the keyboard. Protocol parameters can be adapted; in the following description we will present typical values. A test procedure is essentially composed of three parts: a reference interval, a period with induced anoxia and, following, a recovery period; duration and hypoxia depth can be chosen. Measuring functions and derived parameters have been selected on the basis of their alterations during anoxia as compared with the reference period.

The derived SEP, used as a quantitative index for cerebral cortical function, is obtained on one of the six electrodes (i.e. the one with the largest response) (figure 4). This is performed on-line by time coherent averaging of an adaptable number of responses. The stimulation frequency is set at 0.5 Hz, to prevent adaptation phenomena. The number of averaged responses (10) is thus a compromise between, on the one hand, the signal (evoked response)-to-noise (spontaneous activity) ratio, requiring a larger number, and, on the other hand, time resolution of waveform alteration during the anoxia experiment (requiring a lower number). The duration of the SEP being about 200 ms, sampling time is set at 480 ms with a 48 ms period preceding the stimulus. Sampling rate is 500 samples per second. We have observed that the signal's spectrum is limited to 150 Hz: with a 1st order low-pass filter cutting at 150 Hz no distortion is introduced to the P-wave (the one with the highest frequency content). The microprocessor stores the derived SEP's (1 for every 20 s period), together with the "slow" varying signals digitized at a rate equal to the stimulation frequency (pO_2, mean arterial pressure, rectal temperature, ECoG parameters, cerebral blood flow, heart rate). Different states of the cortical spontaneous activity are detected with two band-pass filters (1st order, centre frequency at respectively 0.5 and 16 Hz), followed by rms detectors delivering a measure for the intensity of the electrical activity around the mentioned frequencies (figure 5). These frequencies are typically observed during the "on" (anoxia) and "off" (reoxygenation) epilepsy period.

Before starting anoxia test procedures a control period is recorded, allowing evaluation of variability and trend in the measured and calculated parameters. Provided no permanent damage is caused to the cortical tissue anoxia test procedures can be executed and repeated several times. Typically we use a reference interval of 180 s, an anoxia period of 120 s. Total reading and processing period including

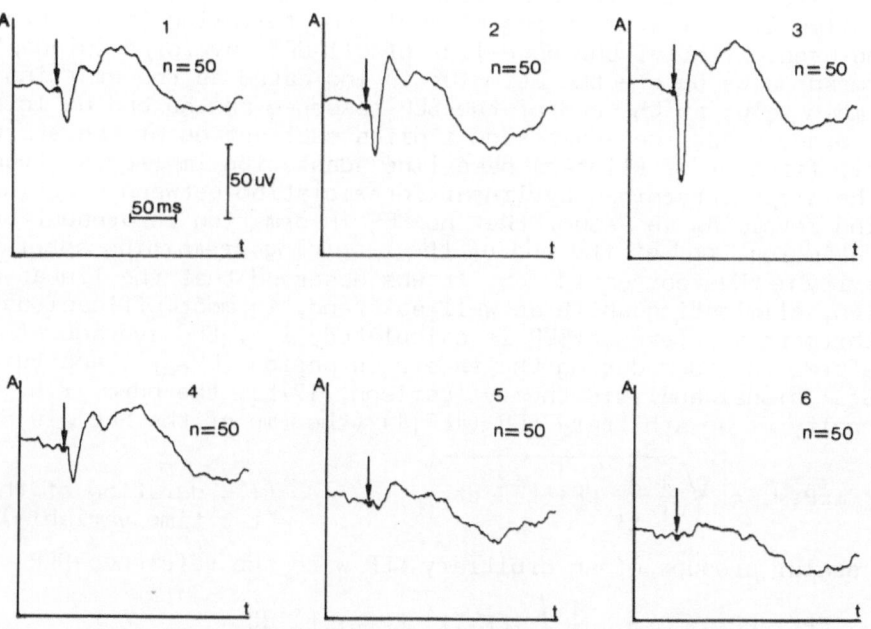

Fig. 4. Off-line calculated SEP's derived from 6 adjacent electrodes (figure 2) (average of 50 responses) illustrating spatial distribution. The arrow indicates the stimulation moment. Location 3 presents the best response, having the largest P-wave (sharply downwards) and N-wave (upwards).

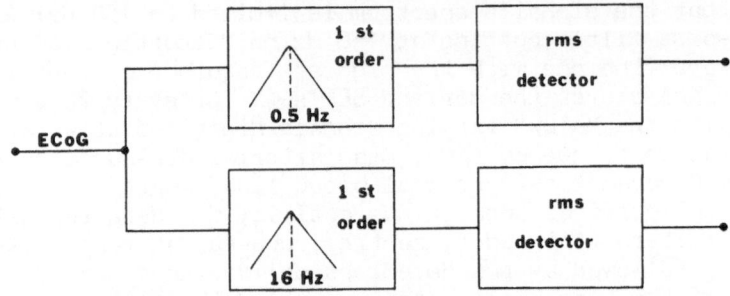

Fig. 5. Block diagram for ECoG parameters derivation: 1st order band-pass filters (0.5 Hz and 16 Hz) and rms detectors.

reference, anoxia and recovery is 840 s. Between two procedures usually a waiting time of minimally 20 min is applied.

Off-line digitized data are sent to a PDP-11/70 computer. Here data are standardized and all signals are presented at an identical time scale together with calculated data from SEP signals. For the quantification of alterations of SEP's the following parameters are being used. Firstly, the base-line of all SEP waveforms is adapted. The mean value before the stimulus is indicated as the starting level, the mean value at the end of the SEP response as the ending level. Zero order base-line adaptation implies subtraction of the starting level, first order (linear) base-line adaptation implies subtraction of the slope determined by linear interpolation between starting and ending level. As we assume that no SEP information is present before the stimulus, nor at the end of the recording, remaining spontaneous activity is thus corrected for. It was observed that the linear adaptation, eliminating shift as well as trend, is most efficacious. Furthermore a reference SEP is calculated, i.e. the average of the waveforms recorded during the reference period (EP_{ref}). According to general signal analysis theory (Carlson, 1975), the norm, i.e. the intensity of an arbitrary SEP ($\|EP_i\|$) (the rms of the SEP), is defined as

$$\|EP_i\| = \sqrt{\frac{1}{T} \int_T EP_i(t)^2 \, dt} \qquad \begin{array}{l} (T = \text{duration of the SEP}) \\ (t = \text{time variable}), \end{array}$$

the scalar product of an arbitrary SEP with the reference SEP

$$\langle EP_i, EP_{ref} \rangle = \frac{1}{T} \int_T EP_i(t) \, EP_{ref}(t) \, dt$$

and the correlation value, representing the similarity between two waveforms

$$c_i = \langle EP_i, EP_{ref} \rangle / (\|EP_i\| \, \|EP_{ref}\|) \qquad \text{with} \quad -1 \leqslant c_i \leqslant 1$$

In order to standardize our parameters with respect to the reference
period we have calculated
  1. the relative norm $rn_i = \|EP_i\|/\|EP_{ref}\|$
  2. the correlation value c_i
  3. the relative scalar product $rsp_i = <EP_i, EP_{ref}>/\|EP_{ref}\|^2$

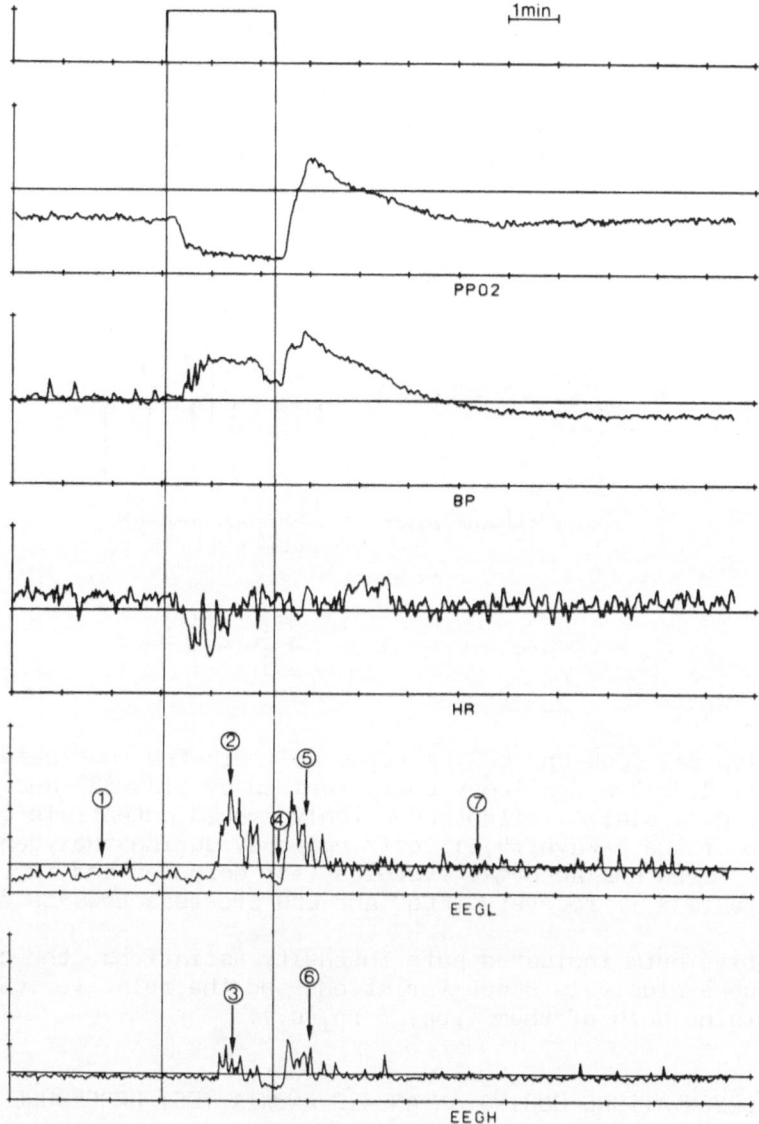

Fig. 6. Parietal oxygen tension (PpO_2), blood pressure (BP), heart
rate (HR), ECoG derived parameters (EEGL (0.5 Hz) and EEGH (16 Hz)).
Numberings in the latter signals refer to intervals characterized by
typical waveform patterns (presented in figure 7).

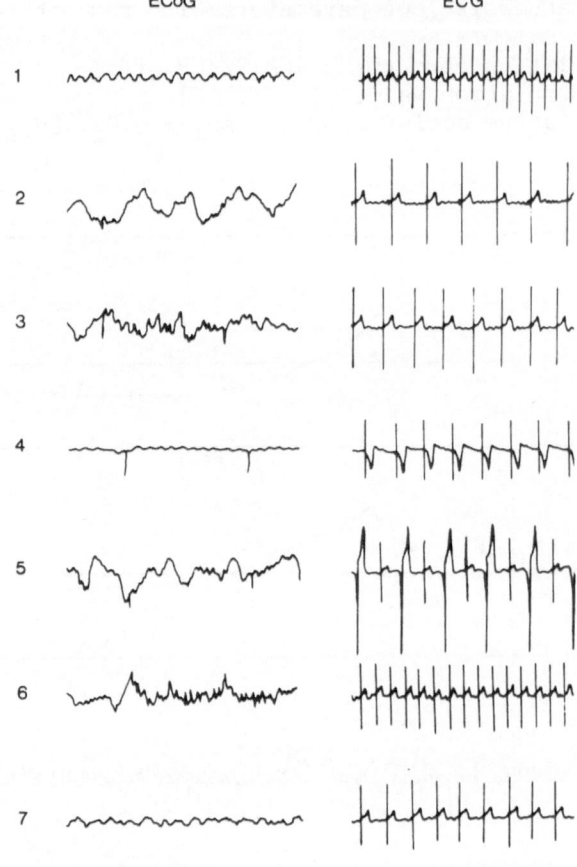

ECoG   ECG

Fig. 7. Typical ECoG and ECG patterns as indicated in figure 6;
1: normal; 2,3: "on" epilepsy characterized by slow (2) and fast (3)
waves; bradycardia; 4: silent ECoG (only evoked potentials visible);
inversion of the T-wave; 5,6: "off" epilepsy during reoxygenation:
slow ECoG waves and abnormal systoles (5); spindles and increased
heart rate (6); 7: recovery (ECoG and ECG progress towards normal).

The relative norm indicates pure intensity variations, the correlation value exclusively shape variations and the relative scalar product contains both of them ($rsp_i = rn_i \, c_i$).

TYPICAL OBSERVATIONS DURING AN ANOXIC ANOXIA TEST PROCEDURE

Figure 6 shows the evolution of the parameters during an anoxia
test procedure. The first signs of anoxia are an abrupt decrease of
the oxygen tension in the cortex and a bradycardia, whereas the blood
pressure increases. At this time ECoG and SEP are still normal.

158

Changes in the ECoG begin with slow large waves (low frequency) and spindles (high frequency), typical for an epileptical pattern (figure 7). At the same time altering of the SEP occurs: the P-wave enlarges and the N-wave decreases, disappears and becomes negative, the latter being clearly visible in the decrease and sign inversion of the correlation value (figure 8). These phenomena persist when the spontaneous electrocortical activity has completely disappeared (only the evoked activity remains) (figure 7). Bradycardia with arrhythmia occurs and there are obvious signs of myocardial impairment such as indicated by inversion of the T-wave.

Oxygen is readministered after 2 min. The intracortical pO_2 demonstrates a typical overshoot and blood pressure, decreased during the ECoG silent period, once more increases to a maximal level corresponding with the pO_2 overshoot (figure 6). In this period a similar epileptic pattern occurs in the ECoG with slow waves and spindles. Thereupon pO_2 decreases slowly to its normal value, as well as blood pressure, whereas the heart rate regains its normal level; SEP-waveforms also recover (figure 8).

The occurrence of a distorted SEP during the period of silent ECoG demonstrates that the functional state of the cortex during anoxic anoxia can be more accurately monitored by the somatosensory evoked cortical potentials than by the electrocorticogram (Manil et al., 1978; Colin et al., 1980).

OPTIMIZATION OF THE METHOD

As one can observe in figure 8b, the noise level at the SEP parameters is rather high, which implies that too much of the spontaneous activity is still present in the waveforms. As it is most important for the quantification of the cortex functioning, we intend to improve the signal-to-noise ratio of these signals. Therefore the data stored on analog tape (2×8 channels) are digitized on a MINC-11 multichannel satellite processor and transferred to the PDP-11/70 computer. A preprocessing procedure of the raw ECoG data is being developed, applying filtering techniques, selection criteria, artifact removal, etc.

CONCLUSION

Although our method is described for anoxic anoxia procedures, it may be used for any experiment during which the animal is ventilated with a special gas mixture (e.g. hypercapnia). The presentation of the parameters, measured as well as calculated, gives a satisfactory survey of the data which are (compared with the original) extremely reduced. The apparatus and the processing software are flexible, the experiment driven by the microprocessor is largely controllable.

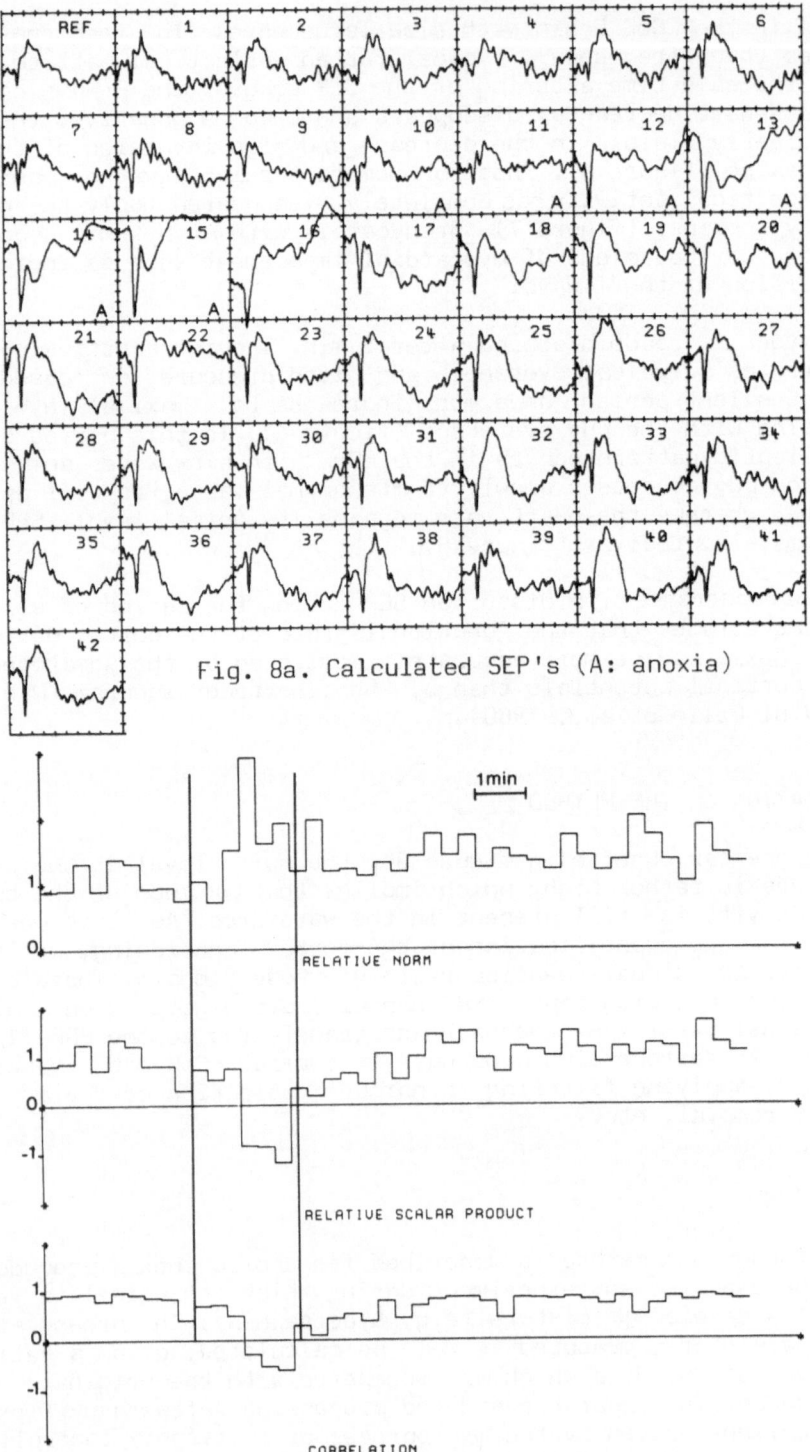

Fig. 8a. Calculated SEP's (A: anoxia)

Fig. 8b. Waveform parameters derived from SEP's (time scale according to figure 6).

REFERENCES

Bicher, H.I., 1973, Autoregulation of oxygen supply to brain tissue, in: Oxygen Transport to Tissue (eds H.I. Bicher and D.F. Bruley), Plenum Press, New York, 215-222.

Bourgain, R.H., Colin, F., Vermariën, H., Maes, L. and Manil, J., 1981, Control mechanisms involved in the regulation of cerebral tissue pressure in oxygen, in: Adv. Physiol. Sci., vol. 25, Oxygen Transport to Tissue, A.G.B. Kovach, E. Dóra, M. Kessler, I.A. Silver (eds), 207-213.

Carlson, A.B., 1975, Communication systems, McGraw-Hill Kogakusha, Tokyo.

Colin, F., Manil, J. and Bourgain, R.H., 1980, Properties of cortical somatosensory evoked potentials in the awake rabbit, Neurol. Res., 1: 247-264.

Coremans, J., Vermariën, H., Vereecke, F. and Bourgain, R.H., 1984, Assessment of the in vivo recording of local cerebral blood flow using a thermistor method (in this issue).
Leniger-Follert, E. and Hossmann, K.A., 1977, Microflow and cortical oxygen pressure during and after prolonged cerebral ischemia, Brain Res., 124: 158-161.

Manil, J., Colin, F. and Bourgain, R.H., 1978, Modifications of somatosensory evoked cortical potentials during hypoxia in the awake rabbit, in: Oxygen Transport to Tissue III (eds I.A. Silver, M. Erecinska and H.I. Bicher), Plenum Press, New York, 509-516.

Silver, I.A., 1965, Some observations on the cerebral cortex with an ultramicro, membrane-covered, oxygen electrode, Med. Electron. Biol. Engng., 3: 377-387.

Vermariën, H., Coremans, J., Vereecke, F. and Bourgain, R.H., 1984, A thermistor device for the continuous recording of mass transport velocity in tissue based on the heat clearance principle, to be published in Oxygen Transport to Tissue VI, Plenum Press, New York.

FUNCTION AND ELECTRONMICROSCOPIC STRUCTURE OF ANTERIOR HORN CELLS

DURING GRADUATED TEMPORARY ISCHEMIA (MOVIE FILM)

W. Blasius and G. Merker

Department of Physiology, University of Giessen
Aulweg 129, D-6300 Giessen, Federal Republic of Germany

INTRODUCTION

In this paper we will summarize the main features of a movie film that was shown at the ISOTT Meeting in Nijmegen. This film was originally produced in German and was provided with an English synchronization of its text for this Meeting, both in cooperation with the "Institute for the Production of Scientific Films" in Göttingen (Blasius and Merker, 1974), whose support is greatly appreciated. Copies of both the German and English version are available from this Institute.

We produced this film for three reasons. First, we wanted to demonstrate the theoretical and experimental results of our investigations of neuronal function during and after ischemia as examined simultaneously by physiological and electronmicroscopic methods, this combination providing a correlation between structure and function. The second reason for the production of this film was to document these relationships without the need for new animal experiments during courses and student laboratory exercises in physiology. Third, the didactic message of the film was enhanced by handing out a questionnaire with 16 questions to the students to check their comprehension of the film's results and conclusions.

CONTENT OF THE FILM

In a rabbit anesthetized with urethane a laparotomy is performed and the aorta is prepared. A temporary clamping of the aorta can be achieved by a light metal clamp loosely fixed at the aorta (Fig. 1). A thread is placed under the aorta with a modified ligation needle and fixed at the clamp. This clamp permits the occlu-

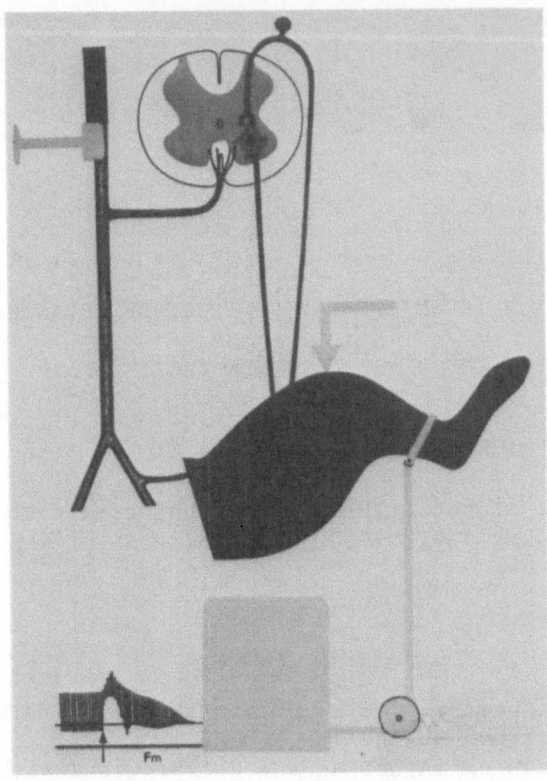

Fig. 1. Diagram of ligature of the aorta with reduction of blood
supply to specific parts of the reflex arc and method of
eliciting and recording the reflex.

sion of the aorta after the abdominal cavity has been closed. In
this way the blood supply to the lumbar spinal cord, the site of
the reflex center of the monosynaptic quadriceps reflex, can be
interrupted at will (Blasius, 1950).

The reflex excursions of the quadriceps reflex, showing the
functional condition of the spinal cord motoneurons, are elicited
by a motor-driven hammer. The excursions of the lower part of the
leg are recorded by electronic equipment. From this record the characteristic time intervals giving information on the efficiency of
function and the ability for recovery of the spinal cord anterior
horn cells can be derived.

Fig. 1 also shows the structural elements of this reflex: the
muscle spindle, the afferent sensory fiber with its spinal ganglion
cell, the anterior horn cell with its efferent motor nerve fiber,
and the muscle. Ligation of the aorta results in an ischemic para-

lysis of, in sequence, the anterior horn cell (after about 1 min), the spinal ganglion cell (after about 3 min), the sensory and motor nerve fibers (after about 60 min), and the muscle (after about 2 h) (Blasius, 1950).

Information on the function of the motor anterior horn cells is also obtained from summary potentials recorded with electrodes. For this purpose the lumbar spinal cord is prepared and an electrode holder is inserted and fixed. The intramedullary symmary potentials are recorded on an oscilloscope (Blasius et al., 1966).

During and after ischemia of the spinal cord due to temporary ligation of the aorta, the reflex excursions of the quadriceps reflex and the heigt of the reflex potential of the ganglion cells follow a course shown in Figs. 2 and 3 (Blasius et al., 1966) respectively. After occlusion the amplitude first is maintained and then declines exponentially toward zero. This time (F_m in Fig. 2) is called the "maximal function time" or "function maintenance time" during which reflex excitability of the neurons is maintained. When the occlusion is continued, reflex excitability is abolished reversibly while structural integrity is maintained ("structure maintenance time") (Fig. 4). If ischemia lasts even longer, irreversible abolition of reflex excitability ensues. When the occlusion is relieved with the fall of the amplitudes to zero, the following silent period is characterized as "disappearence time" (SF_m in Fig. 2, T_3 in Fig. 3). The subsequent "recovery time" (E in Fig. 2, T_4 in Fig. 3) includes the exponential return of the amplitude to the original level (after some overshoot in Fig. 2).

The decrease of the metabolic rate of the spinal cord during occlusion of blood supply is shown in Fig. 4 (Opitz and Schneider, 1950; Blasius, 1962). During the "function maintenance time" (ca. 50 sec) the metabolic rate is reduced to 50 %. After lapse of the

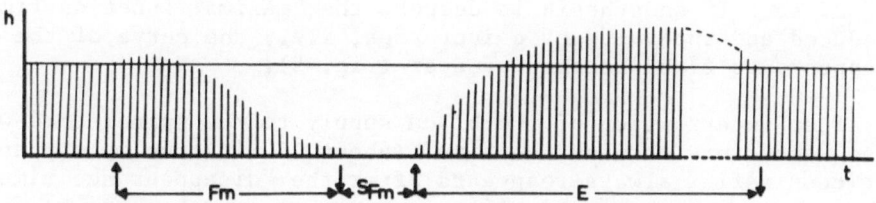

Fig. 2. Reflex excursions of quadriceps after ligature of the abdominal aorta with determination of the following standards: Fm:"maximal function time"; S_{F_m}: "disappearance time" after removal of the aortic clamp; E: "recovery time"; h: height of reflex excursions; t: time.

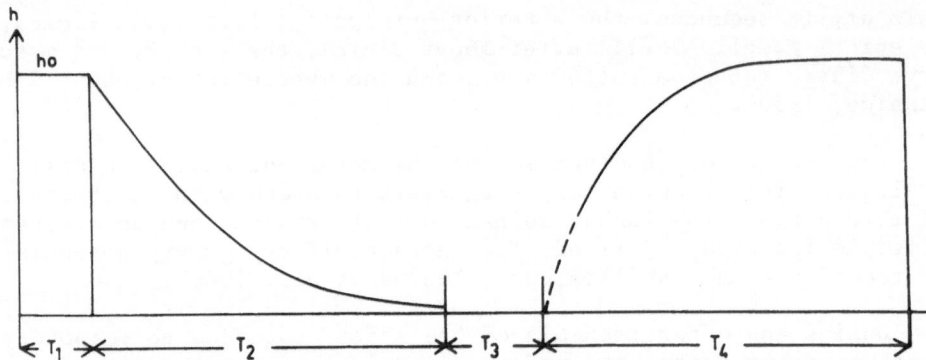

Fig. 3. Time course of the height of the reflex potential h during
and after clamping the aorta. T_1=phase of the same height
of the potential (h_o). T_2=phase of the exponential decrease
of the potential. T_3=phase of the disappearance of the potential. T_4=phase of the exponential return of the potential.
T_1 + T_2 = "maximal function time".

"structure maintenance time" (ca. 17 min), when metabolic rate is
reduced to 10 %, the limit of structural turnover necessary for
preservation of cellular structure is reached. If turnover is reduced below this value of 10 %, the changes become irreversible and
cell death ensues (Fig. 4).

Assuming reversibility, the "function time" F is directly
proportional to the time of ligation A until the "maximal function
time" F_m is reached: F = A for A < F_m (Fig. 5). The "disappearance
time" S, however, rises exponentially with increasing ligation time
A, i.e.: $S = e^{q \cdot A} + c$ (Blasius, 1950, 1962). In a typical case the
"maximal function time" is 70 sec, the corresponding "disappearance
time" 27 sec. If anesthesia is deeper, the "maximal function time"
is reduced and the value of q increases, i.e., the curve of the
"disappearance time" becomes steeper (Fig. 5).

After interruption of the blood supply to the spinal cord within the "structure maintenance time" (about 17 min) the monosynaptic
quadriceps reflex always reappears after the "disappearance time"
S. When, however, the aortic ligation is prolonged beyond the
"structure maintenance time", the reflex cannot be elicited again.
In this case the hind limbs of the animal remain paralyzed (Blasius,
1950).

Cellular respiration is dependent on the integrity of mito-
condrial structure. In order to understand possible structural
alterations of the mitochondria due to ischemia, it is important to

166

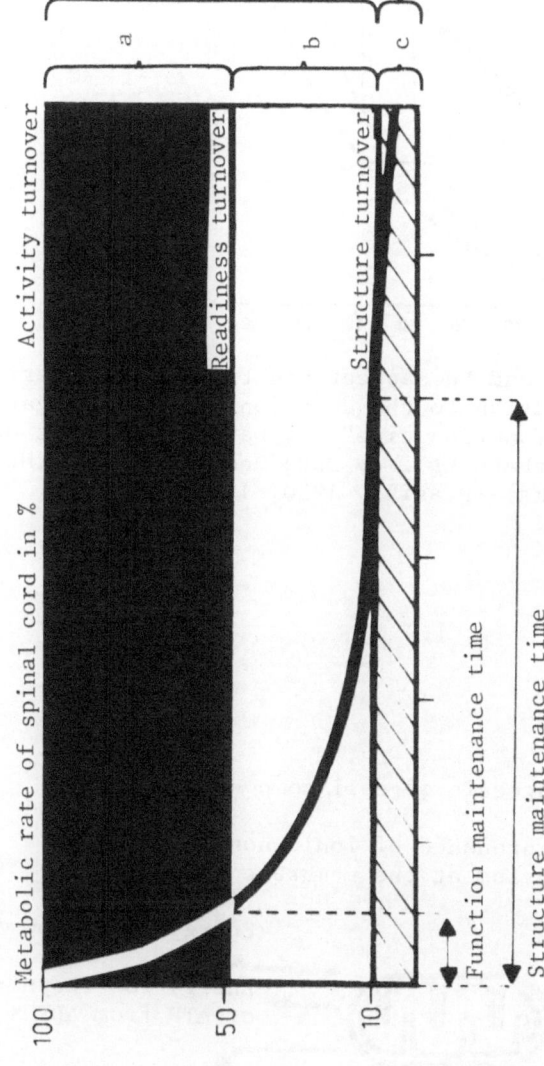

Fig. 4. Decrease of metabolic rate of the spinal cord during gradual reduction of blood supply. Normal or activity turnover equals 100 %; "Function maintenance time" (ca. 50 sec) with reduction of metabolic rate to 50 %; "Structure maintenance time" (ca. 17 min) with reduction of metabolic rate to 10 % (Blasius, 1962).
a = Excitation maintained;
b = Excitation paralyzed; excitability and structure maintained;
c = Cell death;
d = Range of reversible effects;
e = Range of irreversible effects.

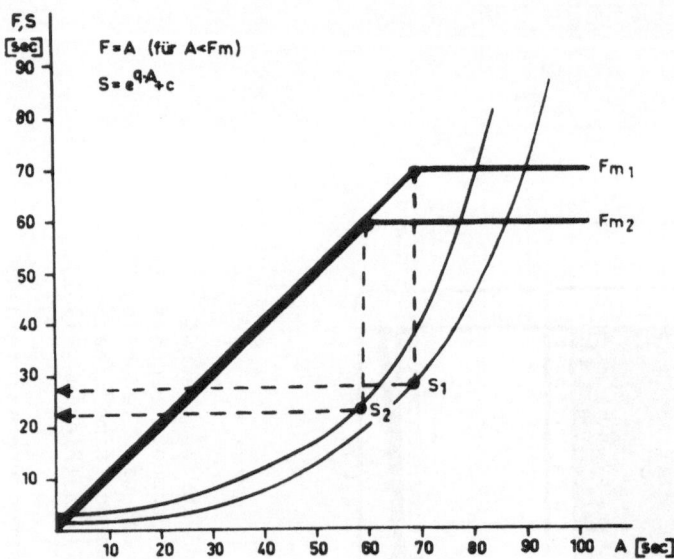

Fig. 5. "Function time" F and "disappearance time" S of anterior horn cells in relation to the duration of aortic ligature A. Fm = "maximal function time". 1: Data under light anesthesia (0.5 urethane/kg). 2: Data under deep anesthesia (0.75 g urethane/kg) (Blasius, 1950, 1962).

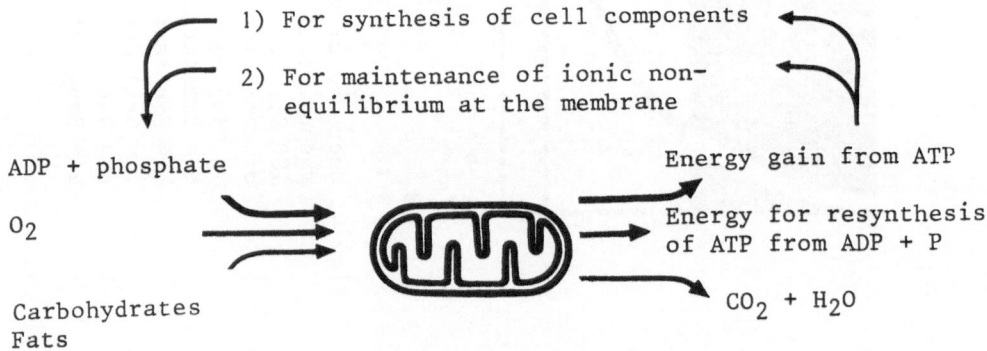

Fig. 6. The mitochondrion providing the cell with energy for synthesis of cell components and maintenance of ionic non-equilibrium at the membrane.

168

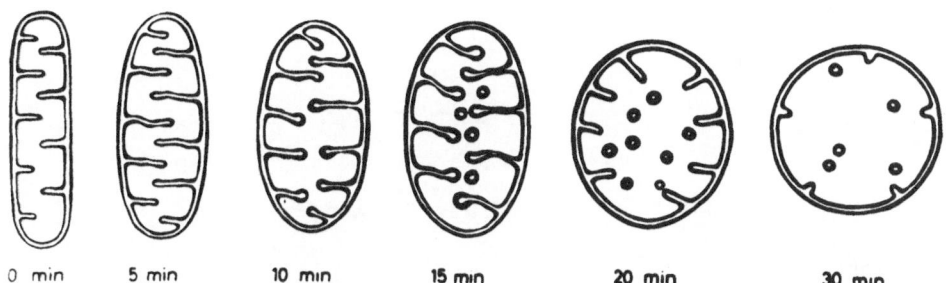

0 min   5 min   10 min   15 min   20 min   30 min

Fig. 7. Effects of temporary ischemia from 5 to 30 min on mitochondria of the anterior horn cells. After ischemia of less
than 17 min the structural alterations of the mitochondrial
membranes are reversible; occlusion of the blood supply for
more than 17 min, however, results in irreversible changes
of the mitochondrial structures (Merker 1969).

remember the detailed structure and function of the mitochondria
and their components (Merker, 1969). Mitochondria are long oval cytoplasmic organelles surrounded by a double membrane. The cristae,
foldings of the inner membrane, divide the internal space by incom-
plete septa. The basic substance or matrix is localized between these
septa. In the mitochondria the cellular oxidative metabolism takes
place. The enzymes for the citric acid cycle of the entire intermediary metabolism are located in the matrix whereas those of the
respiratory chain are arranged in the membrane in a mosaic-like repeating pattern and those for the information of ATP are also stored
separately in the membrane. Fig. 6 gives a summary of mitochondrial
energetic turnover (Blasius and Merker, 1974).

The structural alterations of the mitochondria are characteristic for the different times of ischemia. During increasing duration
of ischemia from 5 to 10 to 15 min a progressive increase in mitochondrial volume can be observed (Merker, 1969). The lamellar structure of the cristae becomes tubularly distended. The double-membrane
structure, however, is still preserved; during ischemia of up to 17
min therefore the structural alterations of the mitochondria are
reversible. Occlusion of blood supply from 20 to 30 min, however,
leads to further swelling and alteration of mitochondrial shape
accompanied by a progressive reduction of the cristae. Finally,
after ischemia of 30 min, most mitochondria are large empty vesicles
only (Figs. 7 and 8). The mitochondrial alterations have become
irreversible after 17 min of ischemia. The first structural changes
in the mitochondria are induced by the uncoupling of cellular respiration and oxidative phosphorylation after consumption of the
energy-rich phosphate compounds produced by the mitochondria
(Lehninger, 1962, 1970). The increased intracellular osmotic pres-

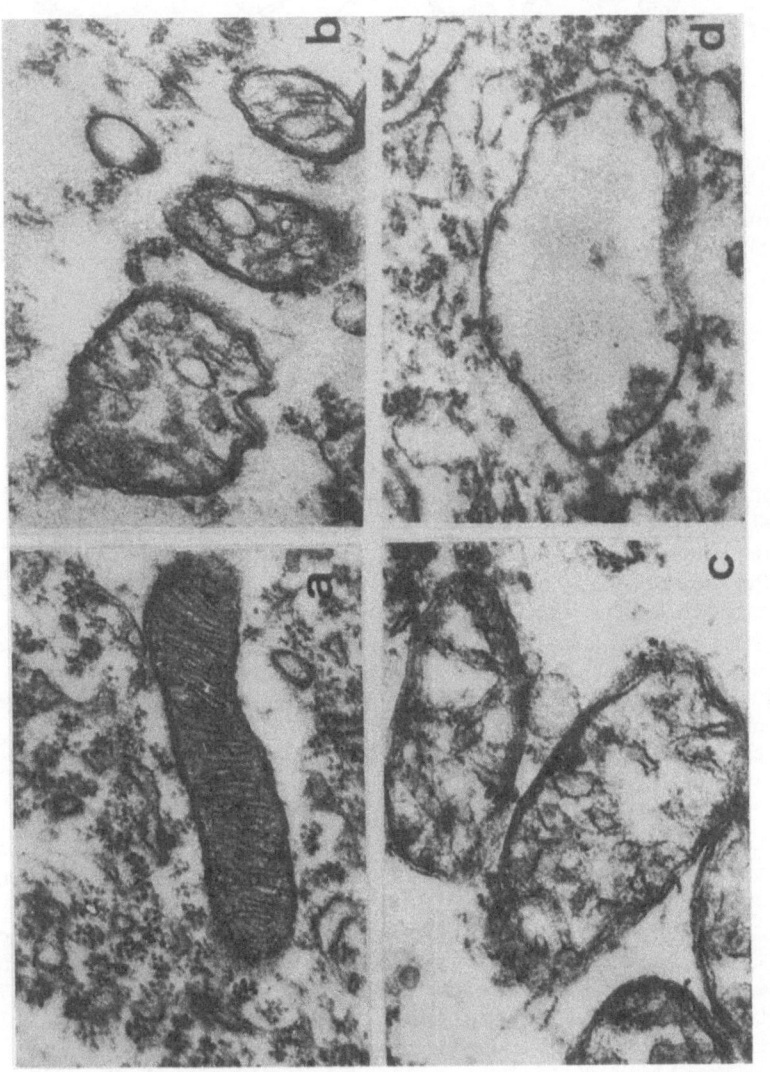

Fig. 8. Effect of temporary ischemia on the mitochondria of anterior horn motoneurons. Electronmicroscopical illustration. Scale: 1: 42000. a: Mitochondrion of an intact motoneuron; b-c: Reversible changes of mitochondrial structure after an ischemia of 5 min (b) and 10 min (c); d: Irreversible changes of mitochondrial structure after an ischemia of 30 min (Merker, 1969).

sure due to accumulation of low-molecular metabolic end-products results in increased water uptake and swelling. These derangements of cellular energy production and water balance due to ischemia are responsible for the observed structural changes in the spinal anterior horn motoneurons.

REFERENCES

Blasius, W., 1950, Das gesetzmässige Verhalten der Funktions- und Erholungsfähigkeit der Vorderhornganglienzelle bei zeitlich abgestufter Aortenabklemmung. Z. Biol., 103:209-252.

Blasius, W. 1962, Allgemeine Physiologie des Nervensystems. In: Landois-Rosemann "Lehrbuch der Physiologie des Menschen", 28. Aufl. Bd. II, p. 629-662. Urban & Schwarzenberg, München-Berlin.

Blasius, W., Repges, R., Schafé, M.K., 1966, Über Grösse und zeitlichen Verlauf von Reflexpotentialen der Vorderhornganglienzellen und des Muskels vor, während und nach Aortenabklemmung. Z. Biol., 115:248-264.

Blasius, W., Merker, G., 1974, Funktion und Ultrastruktur der Ganglienzellen des Vorderhorns unter zeitlich abgestufter Ischämie. Begleitveröffentlichung zum Wissenschaftlichen Film C 1130/1973 des Instituts für den Wissenschaftlichen Film, Göttingen 1974, mit 10 Abb. und einem Fragenkatalog zur Kontrolle des Lerneffektes des Films.

Lehninger, A.L., 1962, Water uptake and extrusion by mitochondria in relation to oxidative phosphorylation. Physiol. Rev., 42:467-517.

Lehninger, A.L., 1970, Bioenergetik. Stuttgart, 1970.

Merker, G., 1969, Ultrastrukturveränderungen motorischer Vorderhornzellen des Kaninchens unter abgestufter Ischämie. Z. Zellforsch., 95:568-593.

Opitz, E., Schneider, M., 1950, Über die Sauerstoffversorgung des Gehirns und den Mechanismus von Mangelwirkungen. Erg. Physiol. 46:126-260.

LUMBAR AND THORACIC SPINAL CORD OXYGEN TENSION

DURING AORTIC CROSS-CLAMPING

F. Wadouh, M. Hartmann, C. F. Arndt,
H. Metzger, and H. G. Borst

Div. Thoracic and Cardiovascular Surgery and
Dept. of Physiology, Medizinische Hochschule Hannover
3ooo Hannover 61, F.R.G.

INTRODUCTION

Cross-clamping of the descending thoracic aorta is followed by dramatic alterations in hemodynamics. The increase of the arterial blood pressure proximal to the occlusion (AP_{prox}) may cause cerebral hemorrage, pulmonary edema or cardiac dilation, whereas the marked distal pressure (AP_{dist}) decrease leads to impaired organ perfusion which can result in severe ischemic/anoxic organ dysfunction, especially in paraplegia. The reported postoperative incidence in the human ranges up to 24 % (Coles et al., 1983).

Cause and development of the spinal cord injury (SCI) are still being discussed (Wadouh et al., in press), particularly since the present theorues do not fully explain the disappointing results of intraoperative protections (e.g. shunt).

Certainly, the SCI depends on the duration and the position of the occlusion but also on the variations in arterial pressure distribution within the subsequent changes in blood supply, tissue oxygen and autoregulation. Furthermore, the morphological conditions of the collateral circulation must be taken into account.

In order to investigate the changes in tissue oxygen and the efficiency of the collateral circulation in the different regions of the spinal cord (SC) during aortic occlusion, surface PO_2 (sPO_2) was measured on the exposed SC in the pig in the lumbar and after a 45 minute occlusion. In addition, the pigs were examined neurologically 24 and 48 hours after operation.

MATERIALS AND METHODS

Basically, the experimental procedure has been described earlier. Note the differences between group IA and the older group I (Wadouh et al., in press).

Fourteen pigs (25-30 kg b.w.) were premedicated with azaperone (Stresnil, Janssen, Neuß, FRG) and atropine sulfate (Drobena, Berlin, FRG) and anesthetized with metomidate (Hypnodil, Janssen, Neuß, FRG) applied intravenously (ear vein). Following intubation the pigs were artificially ventilated with a 3:1 mixture of N_2O and O_2 using PEEP (6 mm Hg). Hypnodil and Stresnil were given as needed. $NaHCO_3$ was administered before and after release of blood flow into the aorta in order to counteract acidosis. The arterial blood pressure was measured in the aortic arch (AP_{prox}) and in the iliac artery (AP_{dist}), the central venous pressure was measured in the vena cava superior. The pigs were divided into two groups:

Group IA (n=7) - thoracotomy in the bed of the 4th left rib and cross-clamping of the descending thoracic aorta immediately below the left subclavian artery

Group II (n=7) - occlusion of the abdominal aorta by use of a Fogarty occlusion catheter (8-14 OC, Edwards Laboratories, Santa Ana, Cal., USA); the balloon was positioned (via the femoral artery) immediately above the origin of the arteria radicularis magna anterior (ARMA).

In both groups local surface PO_2 (sPO_2) was measured after laminectomy on the exposed SC in the lumbar (L_{3-5}) as well as in the thoracic regions (Th_{6-8}) before, during and after a 45 minute occlusion. The sPO_2 was registered using six gold cathodes ($\emptyset$ 15 μm) (resp. platinum cathodes according to Lübbers et al., 1969) arranged concentrically around an Ag/AgCl reference electrode ($\emptyset$ 200 μm). The gold (platinum) wires were embedded and isolated in Hysol (Dexter Corp., N. Y., USA). The electrode was wetted with 0.9 % saline solution and covered with a 25 μm thick polypropylene membrane (Radiometer Copenhagen, Krefeld, FRG). Calibration was performed in 0.9 % saline solution (36.5 ± 0.5 $^{\circ}$C), equilibrated with gas mixtures of known oxygen content (100 % N_2, 5 % O_2, 10 % O_2).

RESULTS

sPO_2: Before aortic cross-clamping, mean sPO_2 of the exposed SC in the lumbar regions was 42.3 mm Hg (group IA) and 28.0 mm Hg (group II), mean thoracic sPO_2 was 34.9 mm Hg resp. 32.2 mm Hg (Fig. 1 and Fig. 2).

In response to occlusion, the sPO_2 distal to the occlusion site always decreased drastically, reaching lowest levels in less than

5 (group IA) resp. 15 minutes (group II). Until the end of occlusion, the sPO_2 did not alter at all. The steady state values (group IA: thoracic sPO_2 = 3.9 mm Hg, lumbar sPO_2 = 3.2 mm Hg; group II: lumbar sPO_2 = 7.9 mm Hg) were significantly different from the initial values ($p < 0.001$). However, the differences concerning lumbar sPO_2 in both groups could not be established statistically. Thoracic sPO_2 in group II remained constant during the experiments. The rapidity of the sPO_2 decrease in the thoracic regions of group IA was only measured in additional experiments. It seems to be rather faster than in the lumbar parts.

Release of the aorta was followed by an sPO_2 overshoot (only measured in the lumbar regions) in both groups with a maximum increase above initial values of 30 % for group IA and 45 % for group II ($p < 0.002$). 20 minutes after release preocclusion values were restored in group II, whereas in group IA the overshoot lasted longer.

<u>Arterial pressure:</u> During occlusion, mean AP_{prox} increased in group IA from approx. 85 mm Hg to 110-130 mm Hg, in group II from approx. 70 mm Hg to 82-92 mm Hg, whereas mean AP_{dist} decreased to 19 mm Hg (group IA) resp. 15 mm Hg (group II).

<u>Postoperative observation:</u> 48 hours after operation, only two pigs of group II showed no neurological disorders, while all others experienced varying degrees of neurological lesions. The proportion of non-damage to paresis to paralysis was 0 : 4 : 3 in group IA and 2 : 2 : 3 in group II. The lumbar sPO_2 in the pigs without neurological disorders decreased only to approx. 55 % of the initial values, whereas in all other pigs the sPO_2 had fallen below 35 % (group IA) resp. 22 % (group II).

DISCUSSION

During aortic occlusion, the extraaortic collateral circulation can only induce a pressure of less than 20 mm Hg in the distal aorta. This is obviously not sufficient for an adequate supply of the SC (Wadouh et al.,in press). Blood flow direction in the distal vessels remains unexplained.

Adams and van Geertruyden (1956) suggested that the SCI following aortic occlusion is caused through an insufficient anterior longitudinal anastomotic chain (e.g. a. spinalis ant.), which is the most important part of the perimedullary circulation. Furthermore,they argued that within the anastomosis flow is directed from proximal to distal during occlusion, hence distal parts of the SC should carry the most pronounced flow reduction as well as degree of injury.

The results of our study show that the sPO_2 always distal to the occlusion decreased drastically, in response to high aortic

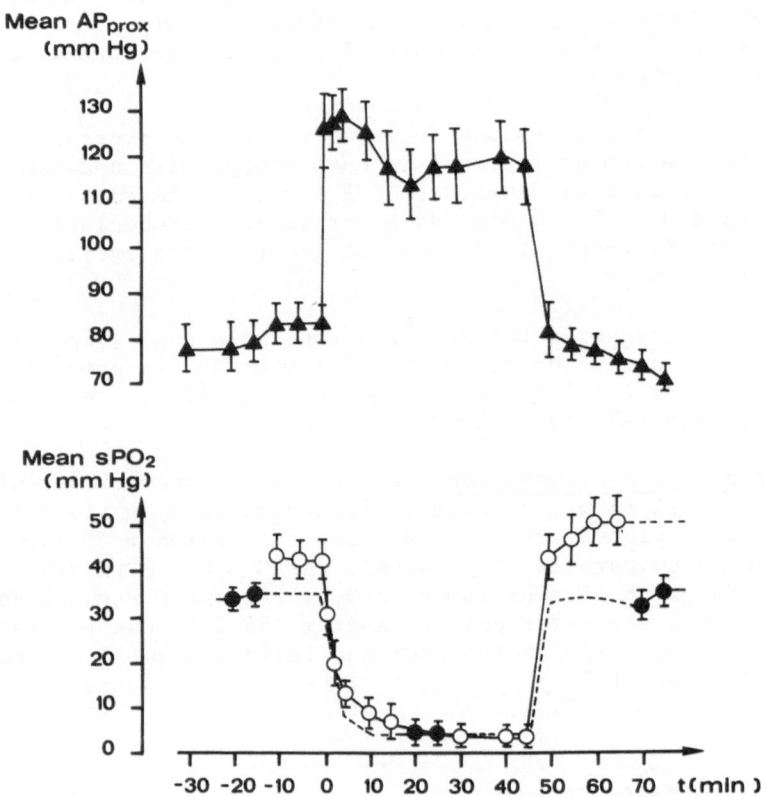

Fig. 1. Cross-clamping of the descending thoracic aorta immediately below the left subclavian artery (group IA). The curves show the mean lumbar (O) and mean thoracic (●) sPO_2 as well as mean AP_{prox} (▲) and the calculated SEM of group IA. Beginning of cross-clamping at t = 0 min., end of cross-clamping at t = 45 min.. The broken line shows extrapolated values. Concerning thoracic sPO_2, the rapidity of the decrease was only measured in additional experiments and seems to be faster than in lumbar regions. The sPO_2 measurement in this group was performed with gold wires.

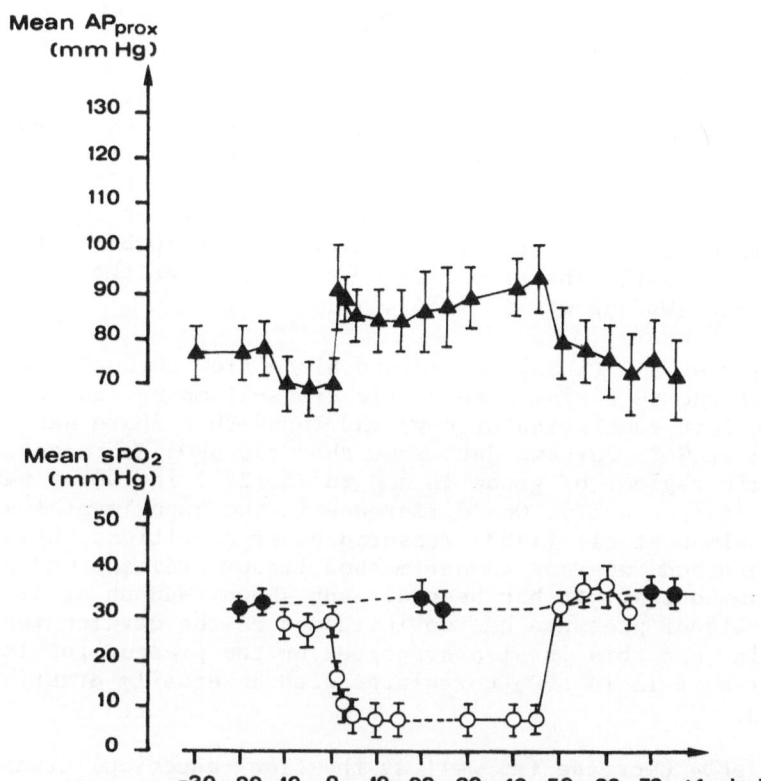

Fig. 2. Occlusion of the abdominal aorta immediately above the
origin pf the ARMA (group II). The curves show the mean
lumbar (O) and mean thoracic (●) sPO_2 as well as the
mean AP_{prox} (▲) and the calculated SEM of group II.
Beginning of occlusion at t = 0 min., end of occlusion
at t = 45 min.. The broken line shows extrapolated values.
The sPO_2 measurement in this group was performed with
platinum wires.

177

occlusion (group IA) already in the thoracic regions. No significant differences could be established between the lumbar parts of both groups and the thoracic region of group IA, neither in the first minutes after nor during occlusion.

Consequently it can be concluded that the spinal cord collateral vessels are insufficient at least during occlusion, in thoracic as well as in lumbar regions. Particularly, the marked sPO_2 decrease already in the thoracic parts of group IA can not be explained by the theory of Adams and van Geertruyden (1956). The sPO_2 decrease in lumbar parts of both groups demonstrates the importance of the ARMA for the lower regions.

Often, the extramedullary collateral pathways in thoracic (but not in lumbar) regions are sufficient. Blaisdell and Cooley (1962), Spencer and Zimmermann (1958), and Killen et al. (1965) have shown that ligature of all intercostal arteries only results in less than 20% SCI. Ligature, however, of the lumbar arteries (ARMA) gave rise to nearly the same rate of paraplegia as the occlusion of the aorta (Wadouh et al.,1984).

Gelman et al. (1983) determined blood flow through the distal regions of the SC during high aortic cross-clamping (immediately below the left subclavian artery) and found that there was a flow reduction of 94%. Our own data show that the sPO_2 decreases to 12% in thoracic regions of group IA and to 7% (25%) in lumbar parts of group IA (group II). One difference in the experimental setup is that Gelman et al. (1983) measured under conditions where liqour was not drained, whereas in our method liqour drainage was performed within laminectomy. It has been already shown (Wadouh et al., 1984) that the liquor pressure has no influence on the development of paraplegia, and this is also supported by the present results. Thus the observed fall in sPO_2 correlates with an equally drastic flow reduction.

The sPO_2 decrease (as well as the flow reduction) always distal to the occlusion can perhaps be explained by a steal syndrome: the blood flows from the collateral pathways into the aorta.

For applications of these results to clinical situation one has to consider the different vascular arrangement in human and in the investigated pigs. One of the most important differences is the position of the ARMA: in human it derives from the thoracic aorta (Th_{5-12}) in 75%, from the lumbar aorta in 25% (Jellinger, 1966; Piscol, 1972), whereas in the pig it always derives from the lumbar aorta (Wissdorf, 1970).

SUMMARY

In order to investigate the changes in tissue oxygen and the efficiency of the collateral circulation in the different regions of the spinal cord (SC) during aortic occlusion, surface PO_2 (sPO_2) was measured on the exposed SC in the pig in the lumbar (L_{3-5}) as well as in the thoracic (Th_{6-8}) parts before, during and after a 45 minute occlusion. The pigs were divided into two groups: group IA: cross-clamping of the aorta immediately below the left subclavian artery; group II: occlusion of the aorta immediately above the arteria radicularis magna anterior (ARMA).

In response to occlusion, the sPO_2 distal to the occlusion always decreased significantly (group IA: mean lumbar sPO_2 from 42.3 mm Hg to 3.2 mm Hg, mean thoracic sPO_2 from 34.9 mm Hg to 3.9 mm Hg; group II: mean lumbar sPO_2 from 28.0 mm Hg to 7.9 mm Hg). Mean thoracic sPO_2 in group II remained constant.

No statistically significant differences between the distal regions could be established. The collateral circulation in the thoracic as well as in the lumbar region was insufficient at least during occlusion.

REFERENCES

Adams, H. D., and van Geertruyden, H. H., 1956, Neurologic complications of aortic surgery, Ann. Surg. 144:574-609.

Blaisdell, F. W., and Cooley, D. A., 1962, The mechanism of paraplegia after temporary thoracic aortic occlusion and its relationship to spinal fluid pressure, Surgery 51:351-355.

Coles, J. G., Wilson, G. J., Sima, A. F., Klement, P., Tait, G. A., Williams, W. G., and Baird, R. J., 1983, Intraoperative management of thoracic aortic aneurysma, J. Thorac. Cardiovasc. Surg. 85:292-299.

Gelman, S., Reves, J. G., Fowler, K., Samuelson, P. N., Lell, W. A., and Smith, L. R., 1983, Regional blood flow during cross-clamping of the thoracic aorta and infusion of sodium nitroprusside, J. Thorac. Cardiovasc. Surg. 85:287-291.

Jellinger, K., 1966, Zur Orthologie und Pathologie der Rückenmarks-durchblutung, Springer Verlag, Wien-New York.

Killen, D. A., Edwards, R. H., Adkins, R. B., Jr, and Boehm, F. H., 1965, Spinal cord ischemia following mobilization of canine aorta from posterior parietes, Ann. Surg. 162:1063-1068.

Lübbers, D. W., Baumgärtl, H., Fabel, H., Huch, A., Kessler, M., Kunze, K., Riemann, H., Seiler, D., and Schuchhardt, S., 1969, Principle of construction and application of various

platinum electrodes, in: "Oxygen Pressure Recording in
Gases, Fluids, and Tissues", F. Kreuzer, ed., Progr. Resp.
Res. 3:136-146, S. Karger, Basel New York.

Piscol, K., 1972, Die Blutversorgung des Rückenmarkes und ihre
klinische Relevanz, Springer-Verlag, Berlin-Heidelberg-
New York.

Spencer, F. C., and Zimmermann, J. M., 1958, The influence of
ligation of intercostal arteries on paraplegia in dogs,
Surg. Forum 9:340-342.

Wadouh, F., Lindemann, E. M., Arndt, C. F., Hetzer, R., and Borst,
H. G., 1984, The arteria radicularis magna anterior as a
decisive factor influencing spinal cord damage during aortic
occlusion, J. Thorac. Cardiovasc. Surg. 88:1-10.

Wadouh, F., Metzger, H., Arndt, C. F., Hartmann, M., Schywalsky, M.,
and Hetzer, R., in press, Response of spinal cord oxygen
tension to aortic occlusion, to appear in:Adv. Exp. Med. Biol..

Wissdorf, H., 1970, Die Gefäßversorgung der Wirbelsäule und des
Rückenmarkes vom Hausschwein (Tierärztliche Hochschule
Hannover, Med. vet. Habilschrift), Parey-Verlag, Berlin.

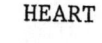HEART

HETEROGENEOUS pO_2 DISTRIBUTION AS A CONSEQUENCE OF THE CAPILLARY NETWORK

Peter A. Wieringa+, Henk G. Stassen*,
John D. Laird, and Jos A.E. Spaan+*

+Dept. of Physiology, Leiden University
2300 RC Leiden, and *Delft University of
Technology, Delft, The Netherlands

INTRODUCTION

The interconnectedness of the capillary network gives rise to a heterogeneous capillary fow distribution. Model studies have demonstrated that at normal overall perfusion some capillaries may receive no or little flow. However, capillary flow is an important factor in determining the degree of metabolic supply to adjacent tissue cells. Since the work of Krogh (1918), oxygen transport in capillary systems and tissue has been studied intensively. In the present model known non-linearities, such as the oxygen binding by the erythrocytes, the consumption rate in tissue cells and the resistance to diffusion of the capillary wall and cell membranes, are linearized. On the other hand the often oversimplified capillary network and capillary flow distribution have been added to the model allowing the study of convective mixing of confluent capillary blood flow. This is important for the description of tissue supply distal from a bifurcation. Moreover, the intercapillary distance in several organs is small, permitting diffusional shunting. The present three dimensional capillary and tissue network model has been based on observations of casts of the myocardial microcirculation (Bassingthwaighte et al., 1974; Tomanek et al., 1982). Heterogeneous capillary flow distribution in the myocardium has been observed experimentally. However, in order to calculate capillary and tissue $pO2$ distributions, a flow distribution has to be exactly defined as to satisfy the mass-balances. Therefore predictions on the heterogeneous capillary flow distribution (Wieringa et al. 1982) form the basis for the calculations on oxygen distribution in this study.

Compartmentation

The capillary network model consists of parallel capillaries being hexagonally stacked. Interconnecting capillaries were defined at a random fashion over the network such that the unbranched capillary segments satisfied an experimentally obtained distribution histogram (Bassingthwaighte et al., 1974). The unbranched capillary segments consist of one or more capillary elements (about 30 um long). A realistic number of arterioles and venules supplied and drained the network at random points. The flow distribution was calculated using a linear pressure-flow relationship for all capillaries. Fig. 1 depicts a diagram of a typical flow pattern in the network. The flow magnitudes and directions are marked by different line thicknesses and by arrows respectively. Highly perfused capillaries are present around arterioles and venules. Elsewhere in the network low perfused areas can be distinguished.

For each capillary element, i, the mass-balance requires that the amount of oxygen, J, which crosses the capillary wall is equal to the difference in oxygen content, ΔM, of the inlet and outlet blood, i.e.:

$$Q_i \cdot \Delta M_i = J_i, \qquad (1)$$

where Q_i is the capillary blood flow. We linearized the saturation curve (Altman and Dittmer, 1970) between 5 and 50 mmHg and assumed arteriolar pO_2 to be 50 mmHg (Duling et al., 1970). If the tangent of the linearized curve is α_b, the oxygen content difference can be written as:

$$M_i = \alpha_b \ (Pin_i - Pout_i). \qquad (2)$$

The tissue space between the capillaries was divided into units, such that each unit can be supplied by two capillary segments. This is illustrated in Fig. 2, showing a part from a slab perpendicular to the capillary orientation. Note the regular stacking of capillary and tissue units. The amount of oxygen diffusing from a capillary unit, i, into the six adjacent tissue units, ik=i1,i2,..,i6, is:

$$J_i = \sum_{k=1}^{6} J'_{ik}, \qquad (3)$$

where J'_{ik} equals the oxygen flow over the capillary wall between capillary, i, and tissue unit ik. From the two dimensional diffusion equation it can be shown that the oxygen flow into a tissue unit is proportional to the pO_2 difference between both adjacent capillaries plus the oxygen consumption of half a tissue unit m_{ik}:

$$J'_{ik} = a' \cdot (P_i - P_{ik}) + m_{ik}, \qquad (4)$$

where P_{ik} denotes the pressure in the capillary unit adjacent to

184

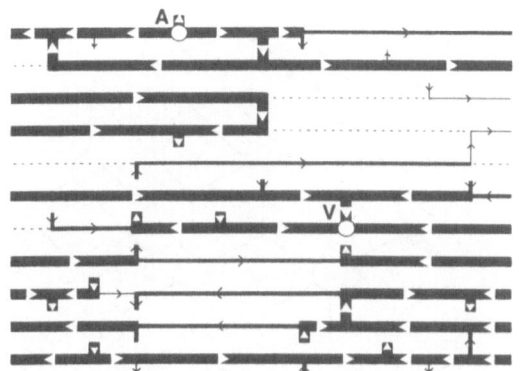

Fig. 1 Longitudinal section through the capillary network. Flow
       direction and magnitudes are indicated by arrows and line
       thicknesses respectively.High flow velocities are present
       around an arteriole (A) and venule (V). However, some
       capillaries receive very low flows (dotted lines).A flow
       velocity magnitude above 43% of the mean flow velocity
       (100 um/s) is indicated with a heavy line. Between 14 and
       43% with dark lines, from 7 to 14% with thin lines and
       below 7% with broken lines.

capillary, i, in the direction k. The coefficient of
proportionality, a', was caculated in the following way:

$$a' = a.D.\alpha_t.L.\frac{\pi}{3}.R_c/(Icd-R_c) \qquad (5)$$

The parameters D, α_t, R_c and Icd are defined in Table 1. L is the
length of a capillary unit and was equal to 30.1 um. Note that
Icd-R_c equals the distance between the walls of two adjacent
capillaries. With the aid of a finite element method (AFEP – Delft
University of Technology, The Netherlands) oxygen pressure
distributions, diffusional shunting between adjacent hexagonally
stacked capillaries and by the consumption in the tissue, were
calculated separately. The parameter a was estimated from the
pressure distributions to be 2,394. The results of the two
dimensional analysis will be published elsewhere.The driving
capillary oxygen pressure was assumed to equal the mean of inlet
and outlet capillary oxygen pressure:

$$P_i = (Pin_i + Pout_i)/2. \qquad (6)$$

Finally, the average pO_2 over the tissue unit was defined as the
pO_2 of the tissue unit.

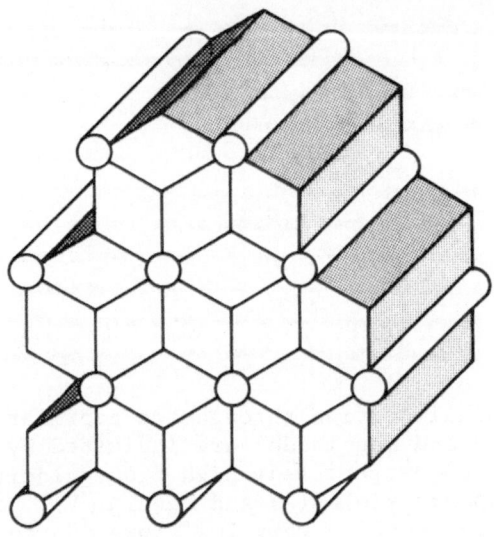

Fig. 2 Capillary and tissue units in a part from a slab of
simulated tissue.

The solution for the capillary and tissue pO_2's may be
expressed as a function of two variables. The first, so called
flow variable, F*, is proportional to several system parameters
(see Table 1) and the bulk flow, Q_b, which is an input variable
for the system:

$$F* = Q_b \cdot \frac{\alpha b^K}{D \cdot \alpha_t} , \qquad (7)$$

where K is a parameter determined by the geometry of the network.
The second variable, the consumption variable, C*, is proportional
to consumption rate, M:

$$C* = M \cdot \frac{K}{D \cdot \alpha_t \cdot pO_2\text{-art}} , \qquad (8)$$

where pO_2-art is the terminal arteriolar pO_2. The capillary and
tissue pO_2 are linear functions of C* but their dependency on F*
is more complex.

The geometry of the capillary network determines the relation
between Pin and Pout for different capillary units. Convective
mixing around confluent nodes of the interconnections was incorporated in the equations. To 2 out of 102 nodes of the network an
arteriole was connected. The position of 3 venules was randomly

distributed among the remaining 100 nodes of the network. The inlet pO_2's of each capillary element can now be described by a function of either one or more capillary outlet pO_2's and/or arteriolar pO_2's. From the Eqs.1, 2, 3 and the mass-balances around interconnections, three sets of lineair equations were defined. These equations were solved by matrix inversion. The software package used was developed by the United Kingdom Atomic Energy Authority HARWELL included in the NAG software library (Numerical Algorithms Group Mark 10). The FORTRAN subroutines make use of the sparsity of the matrices and apply pivoting to the elements.

RESULTS

Due to the amount of data which had to be stored and due to the restrictions by the virtual storage of the computer, the largest network which could be simulated contained 7x7 parallel capillaries. Seven capillary units were defined along the length of the network.

Fig. 3 shows the oxygen pressure histogram for the tissue elements.Venous pO_2, pO_2-ven, was higher than mean tissue pO_2. A test of accuracy of the matrix operation was performed by comparing the pO_2 in the venous effluent of the network with the pO_2 as determined by the overall mass-balance for the network

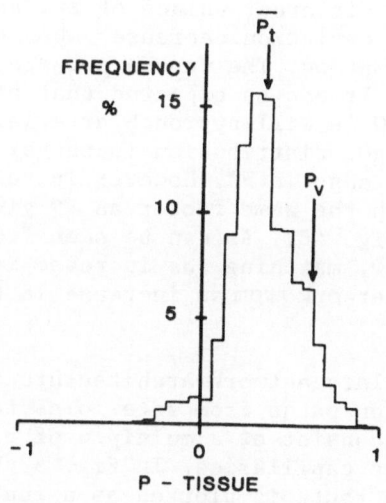

Fig. 3 Tissue pO_2 histogram. The pressures are normalized to pO_2-art.

Table 1

Symbols and values for parameters and variables (control).

Icd [2])	– Intercapillary distance	:	19 um
R_c	– Capillary radius	:	2.5 um
Q_b	– Bulk flow	:	1.0 min.$^{-1}$
α_b	– Tangent Dissociation curve	:	$4.2 \cdot 10^{-3}$ mmHg^{-1}
pO_2-art	– Artericolar pO_2	:	50 mmHg
α_t [1])	– O_2 Solubility of myocard	:	$27.6 \cdot 10^{-6}$ mmHg^{-1}
M	– O_2 Consumption rate	:	$8 \cdot 10^{-2}$ min.$^{-1}$
D [1])	– Diffusion coefficient	:	$9.0 \cdot 10^{-4}$ cm^2/min

[1]) – Altman and Dittmer, 1970, [2]) – Bassingthwaighte et al. 1974.

according to Eg. 9:

$$pO_{2\text{-ven}} = pO_{2\text{-art}} - M/\alpha_b/Q_b. \qquad (9)$$

Note that the value for pO_2-ven (31 mmHg) is independent of the capillary architecture and total capillary and tissue volume.

As can be seen from Fig. 3 the model predicts negative pO_2's. This of course is only possible mathematically and is related to the pO_2 independency of the consumption rate. At present an iteration procedure to correct for this irrealistic values is in development. The tissue units with negative pO_2's can be regarded as units with $pO_2 = 0$.

In Fig. 4 the influence of F* is depicted. The standard deviation and the values for mean and venous pO_2 are marked for each distribution at different values of F*. As can be seen from Fig. 4A the standard deviation decreases when blood flow increases at constant O_2 consumption. The venous pO_2 stays at the upper part of the distribution. It can be expected that at very high blood flow all capillary pO_2's will approach arterial pO_2. It is remarkable that the pO_2 distribution is rather sensitive to a two-fold increase or decrease in F*. However increasing the consumption rate with the same factor as F* gives a totally different picture (Fig. 4B). As can be seen from panel B an increase in bulk flow, matching the increase in O_2-consumption, cannot prevent the network from an increase in the number of units without oxygen.

Since the capillary network architecture of the model is well defined, all perfusion paths from arterioles to venules could be detected. The paths consist of a multiple of elementary capillaries and cross capillaries. In Fig. 5 the pO_2 of a capillary within the route is plotted as a function of the relative position of that capillary on the path. The bottom tracing shows a progressively decreasing capillary pO_2 similar to what is expected from a series of Krogh cylinders. However, the

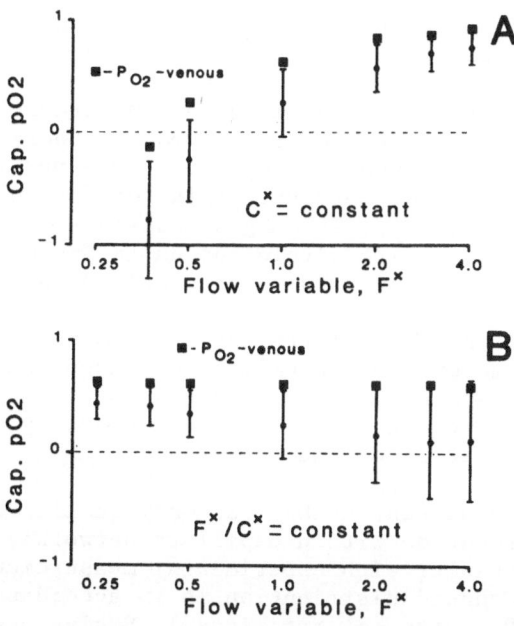

Fig. 4. Panel A: Effects of alteration of the flow variable on the tissue pO_2 distribution for a constant consumption variable. Mean, standard deviation and venous pO_2 are marked. Panel B: The distribution for constant ratio between flow and consumption variable.

other panels clearly show oxygen pressure patterns with hills and valleys. This can be explained by the convective mixing around confluent branching points in the network and by a diffusional shunting between adjacent capillaries. The paths shown in the second and third panels from the top are partly overlapping. From the arteriole up to the place marked with an asterix, the capillary pO_2 profiles are identical. Thereafter the routes divide and thus the pO_2 patterns become different. The pO_2 of the venous effluent of the different routes will be different. Summation of the oxygen content of blood drained from all the routes equals the supplied minus the consumed amount of oxygen.

DISCUSSION

A linear model was used to describe flow patterns through the capillary bed and, consequently, to calculate steady state solutions for the oxygen supply to tissue. Capillaries and tissue were divided into discrete units. Mass-balances for oxygen flow over the boundaries of the units were derived.

The linearization of the diffusion and transport processes is a prerequisite for the application of matrix operations. Besides blood rheology, the oxygen dissociation curve and the diffusion process were simplified. Moreover, axial diffusion and membrane influences were neglected. Inhomogeneously distributed physical and biochemical parameters within the units including pO_2 were assumed to be averaged over the entire unit volume.

The compartmentation of the capillaries and tissue was defined by capillary diameter, intercapillary distance and the assumption of a hexogonally stacking of capillaries. The length of each compartment was equal to the length of an elementary capillary as defined by the generation of the netword.

Although the present method can only qualitatively describe the oxygen distribution within capillary networks, it is tempting to compare the results with experimental measurements. At first glance the bell shaped distribution is in accordance with findings of Lübbers (1969, cortex of rat kidney), Skolasinska et al. (1978, cat heart), Schuchhardt (1971, guinea pig heart), Moss (1968, dog hearts). Calculations on various other types of three dimensional networks also show a heterogeneous pO_2 distribution (Grunewald and Sowa, 1977, 1978; Metzger, 1973; Kessler et al., 1973). Calculations of Metzger and our results clearly show a venous pO_2 which lay in the upper tail of the histograms. Venous pO_2 is therefore not representative for the worst condition of the tissue units as suggested by Grunewald and Sowa (1978).

As can be seen from Fig. 4, an alteration in bulk flow (or in the parameter associated with it) has a high influence on the pO_2 distribution histogram. At higher flow rates the range becomes smaller. For this case the diffusion process is less important and the oxygen supply to the tissue is completly determined by the flow distribution.

Our results clearly demonstrate that regardless of an adequate overall perfusion, small regions with low oxygen tension may appear. As is clear from Fig. 4 an increase in arteriolar flow will result in a higher pO_2 for all tissue units. However, if only one arteriole changes its blood flow delivery, the distribution over the network will be altered.

An important feature of interconnected capillary networks is that blood with different oxygen content will be mixed at

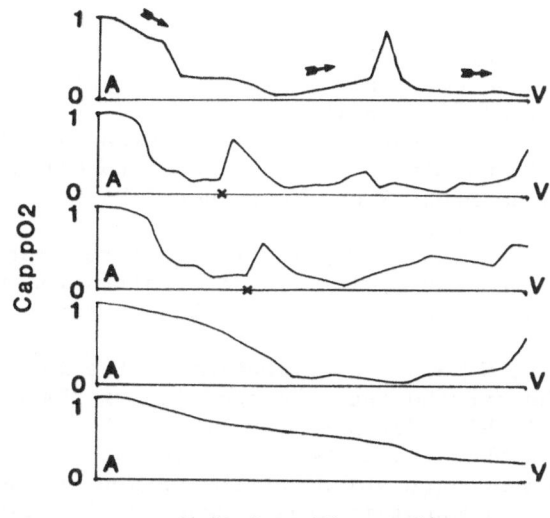

A-V Cap.Flowpaths

Fig.5. O_2 pressure along capillary arteriolar (A)-
        venular (V) paths. Path lengths are normalized.

confluent bifurcations. The implication will be that blood pO_2
along a capillary path can increase locally although overall
behaviour will show a decline.

    We conclude that the capillary flow pattern in the heart
plays an important role in the oxygen distribution among the
tissue cells. Furthermore, venous effluent pO_2 is not representative for the condition of the tissue cells.

ACKNOWLEDGEMENTS

    We are grateful to Ir. J.J.I.M. van Kan of the Delft Univer-
sity of Technology, Dept. of Mathematics for his support. We like
to thank Anette Waals and Heleen Bronsveld for typing this manuscript.

REFERENCES

Altman, P.L., Dittmer, D.S. (eds.). Respiration and
        Circulation, Federation of American Societies for
        Experimental Biology, Bethesda, Maryland, U.S.A.,1970.
Bassingthwaighte, J.B., T. Yipintsoi, R.B. Harvey.
        Microvasculature of the dog left ventricular myocardium.
        Micr. Vasc. Res. 7:229-249,1974.

Duling, B.R., R.M. Berne. Longitudinal gradients in peri-
    arteriolar oxygen   tension. A possible mechanism for the
    participation of oxygen in local regulation of blood flow.
    Circ. Res. 27:669-678,1970.

Grunewald, W.A., D.W. Lübbers. Die Bestimmung der intracapillären
    HbO_2-Sättigung mit einer kryo-mikrofotometrischen Methode
    angewandt am Myokard der Kaninchens. Pflügers Archiv.
    353:255-273,1975.

Grunewald, W.A., W. Sowa. Capillary structures and O_2 supply to
    tissue. An analysis with a digital diffusion model as
    applied to the skeletal muscle. Rev. Physiol. Biochem.
    Pharmacol. 77:149-209,1977.

Grunewald, W.A., W. Sowa. Distribution of the myocardial tissue
    pO_2 in the rat and the inhomogeneity of the coronary bed.
    Pflügers Archiv. 374:57-66,1978.

Krogh, A. The number and the distribution of capillaries in
    muscles with calculations of the oxygen pressure head
    necessary for supplying the tissue. J. Physiol., 52:409-415,
    1918.

Kessler, M., L. Görnandt, M. Lang. Correlation between oxygen
    tension in tissue and hemoglobin dissociation curve. Oxygen
    Supply Workshop, Dortmund, 1971

Lübbers, D.W. Exchange processes in the microcirculatory bed.
    Springer-Verlag,1977.

Metzger, H. Geometric considerations in modelling oxygen
    transport processes in tissue. Advances Exp. Med. Biol.
    37B,761-772,1973.

Moss, A.J. Intramyocardial oxygen tension. Cardiovasc. Res.
    3:314-318,1968.

Schuchhardt, S. Comparative physiology of the oxygen supply.
    Oxygen Supply Workshop, Dortmund 1971. Schuchhardt, S.
    Die Sauerstoffdruckverteilung im Hämoglobinfrei perfundierten
    Meerschweinchenherzen. Pflugers Archiv. 322:131-151, 1971.

Skolasinska, K., K. Harbig, D.W. Lübbers, R. Wodick. pO_2 and
    microflow histograms of the beating heart in response to
    changes in arterial pO_2. Basic Res. Cardiol.
    73:307-319,1978.

Tomanek, R.J., J.C. Searls, P.A. Lachenbruch. Quantitative changes
    in the capillary bed during developing,peak, and stabilized
    cardiac hypertrophy in the spontaneously hypertensive rat.
    Circ. Res. 51:295-304,1982.

Weiss, H.R., A.K. Sinha. Regional oxygen saturation of small
    arteries and veins in the canine myocardium. Circ. Res.
    42(1):119-126,1978.

Wieringa, P.A., J.A.E. Spaan, H.G. Stassen, J.D. Laird.
    Heterogeneous flow distribution in a three dimensional
    network simulation of the myocardial microcirculation.
    Microcirculation 2(2):195-216,1982.

MYOCARDIAL OXYGEN CONSUMPTION AND AUTOREGULATION OF THE CORONARY VASCULAR BED

Isabelle Vergroesen, Mark I.M. Noble*, Dirk L. Ypey
and Jos A.E. Spaan

Department of Physiology and Physiological Physics
State University, Leiden, The Netherlands
* King Edward VII Hospital, Midhurst, West Sussex

INTRODUCTION

The local control of vascular resistance is characterized by a relatively constant coronary flow during changes in perfusion pressure (autoregulation) and the ability of coronary flow to match increased metabolic requirements (metabolic regulation). Generally it is assumed that perfusion pressure does not affect heart metabolism (Feigl, 1983) although there is some evidence of the contrary (Gregg, 1963; Arnold et al., 1970). Under physiological conditions with aortic pressure as perfusion pressure of the coronary vascular bed, changes in mean aortic pressure (exercise, hypertension) cause significant changes in coronary blood flow via both myocardial oxygen consumption and perfusion pressure (Bugni et al., 1980). Relating coronary flow exclusively to oxygen consumption (Rubio & Berne, 1975; Eckenhoff et al., 1947) ignores the possible direct effect of perfusion pressure on flow. The oxygen hypothesis as formulated by Laird (Laird & Spaan, 1981; Drake-Holland et al., 1984) predicts a linear relation between coronary flow and both perfusion pressure and oxygen consumption. The aim of this study was to test this hypothesis applying multiple linear regression analysis to experimental data obtained from the in situ cannulated coronary bed of anaesthetised open chest dog and goat.

METHODS

Seven dogs and nine goats were used to study coronary autoregulation and metabolic regulation simultaneously.

Goat Experiments

Nine goats weighing 18-24 kg were anaesthetized after
sedation with 20 mg diazepam (Valium 10, La Roche) by injection
of ketamine hydrochloride (Ketaset, 15 mg/kg) into the right
jugular vein. Through the same needle atropine sulfate (0.1 mg/kg)
and 25 mg hydrocortisone (5 ml Hydroadreson, Organon) were
subsequently administered. The animal was ventilated with a Harvard
respirator using 2:1 nitrousoxide/oxygen mixture. Anaesthesia was
maintained by continuous infusion of ketamine hydrochloride.
Piritramide (Dipidolor, Janssen) was given intravenously as
analgetic in two doses of 3.2 mg at a four hours interval.

A left thoracotomy was done and both the 3rd and 4th rib were
removed, the pericardium was opened and a cradle formed. As with
the dogs the main stem of the left coronary artery was dissected
and a ligature placed around it. A stainless steel Gregg cannula
was inserted into the aorta via a purse string. The perfusion
system was activated and pumped continuously blood from the left
carotid artery via a pressure regulated reservoir through the
cannula. Pacing wires were sewn to the right auricle. The left
hemiazygos vein, which in the goat joins the great cardiac vein to
form the coronary sinus, was cannulated. From this cannula coronary
venous blood was pumped through the venous cuvette of the
Avox-system (Drake-Holland et al., 1984). With continuous perfusion
the Gregg-cannula, inserted in the aorta, was ligated into the left
main coronary artery (Spaan et al., 1981).

Dog Experiments

The preparation and the perfusion system used in the dog
experiments were quite similar to the ones used in the goat experiments and have been described elsewhere (Spaan et al., 1981;
Drake-Holland et al., 1984).

Protocols

The perfusion pressure was varied between 50 and 150 mmHg. The
oxygen consumption level was changed by either pacing at different
rates in dogs and goats or by the intravenous administration of
Hexamethoniumbromide (5 mg/kg), or adrenaline (.05 mg/kg/min – 5
mg/kg/min) in the goats. After a steady state was obtained the
following quantities were measured: mean perfusion pressure, mean
coronary flow, arteriovenous oxygen content difference (avox).
Oxygen consumption was calculated by coronary flow * avox. Where
possible perfusion pressure and oxygen consumption were varied
randomly.

Model

In fig. 1 the model (Laird & Spaan, 1981; Drake-Holland et
al., 1984) for the regulation of coronary vascular resistance by

194

extra-cellular PO2 is shown.The model equations yield under steady
state conditions (see appendix):

$$Q = A * (PP-P\emptyset) + B * \frac{M\dot{V}O2}{Hb*1.36}$$ 1)

where: A and B are parameters related to constants from the model
equations

Q   = coronary arterial flow
PP   = perfusion pressure
P∅   = perfusion pressure at zero Q
M V̇O2 = myocardial oxygen consumption
Hb   = the hemoglobin content of 100 ml blood in g%
       the factor of 1.36 equals the oxygen binding capacity
       of hemoglobin in ml O2/g.

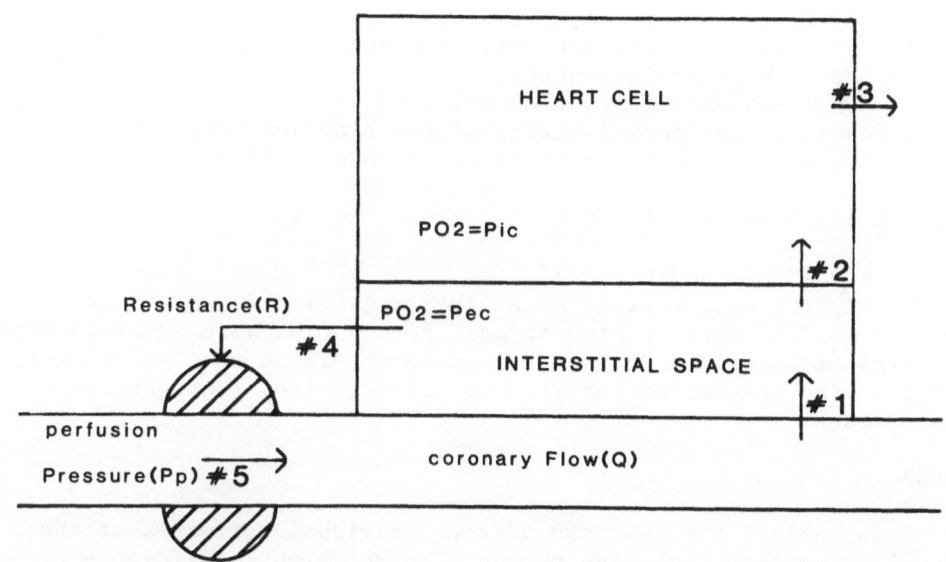

Fig. 1 Model of the regulation of coronary vascular resistance. The
       model equations applying to the processes indicated by
       numbered arrows in the figure are:
       #1: F1 = Q * Hb * 1.36 * (Sa-Sv) (Oxygen extraction)
       #2: F2 = K1 * (Pec-Pic) (diffusion of oxygen from
           extra-to intracellular space).
       #3: F3 = M V̇O2 (myocardial oxygen consumption)
       #4: R = R∅ + K2 * Pec (regulation law)
       #5: R = (PP-P∅)/Q (resistance to flow)

Normalization

The hemoglobin concentration of the blood was not the same for all animals. Moreover, due to infusion or transfusion the hemoglobin concentration could vary during an experiment. Hence the oxygen consumption data were normalized to an oxygen carrying capacity of 10 ml 02/100 ml blood. Differences due to the size of the coronary vasculature were corrected for as follows. The coronary arterial flow was divided by the peak reactive hyperemic flow (Qmax) at perfusion pressure of 100 mmHg due to an arterial occlusion of at least 10 sec and multiplied by a standard peak reactive flow arbitrarily defined as 1 ml/min/g at 100 mmHg perfusion pressure (see fig. 2).

$$\text{So: } Q_n = Q * \frac{1}{Q_{max}} \text{ ml/min/g}$$

$$\text{and } M\dot{V}O2_n = Q_n * avox * \frac{10}{Hb*1.36} \text{ ml02/min/g}$$

where: Q_n is normalized flow,
      Q is measured coronary arterial flow,
      $M\dot{V}O2_n$ is normalized oxygen consumption,
      avox is arterio-venous oxygen content difference
      Hb is hemoglobin content.
      Qmax has been defined above.
As a result of the normalization of the flow and oxygen consumption data the model equation 1) changes into

$$Q_n = a * (PP-P\emptyset) + b * M\dot{V}O2_n \qquad\qquad 2)$$

where $a = A/Q_{max}$ and $b = B/10$.
By multiple linear regression analysis equation 2) was fitted to the normalized data of each animal. $P\emptyset$ and Qmax were averaged from several measurements during an experiment. These mean values were used in the regression analysis of all data from that particular experiment.

RESULTS

In table 1 the mean ±SD of the individual estimates of the model parameters including the mean correlation coefficients of goats, dogs and dogs and goats combined are given. All correlation coefficients were significant at p .01. The estimates of the model parameters yielded no significant differences between dogs and goats as group. Individual animals however showed significant differences among each other; the intra-individual variance was significantly smaller than the inter-individual variance. The number of data points per animal varied between 12 and 45 with a mean of 28. The range of different oxygen consumption levels analysed showed significant variation between the animals.

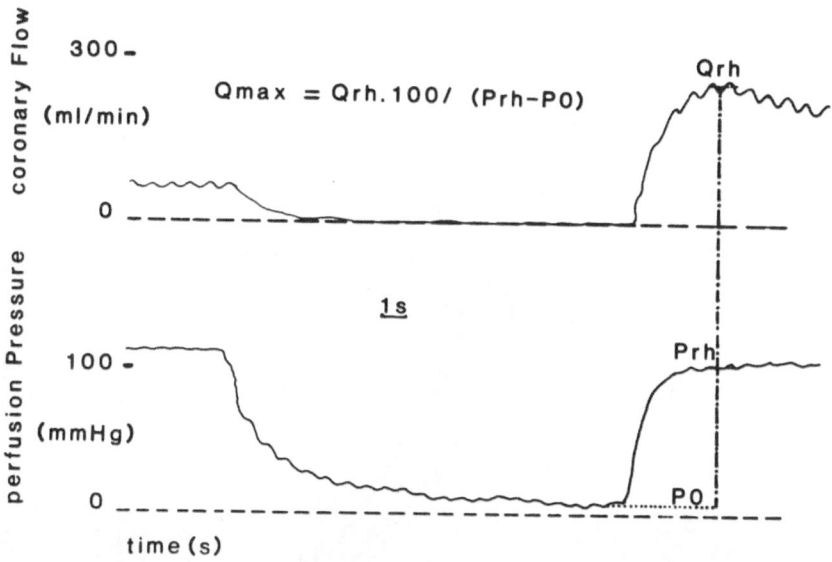

Fig. 2 Simultaneous recording of coronary arterial flow and
perfusion pressure showing an occlusion of the perfusion
line followed by Reactive Hyperaemia. Both signals were
filtered by a low pass filter (-3dB = .25Hz). The
principles of the measurement of Qmax are explained.

In fig. 3 the overal results of metabolic and autoregulation
of all experiments are shown using the model equation and
estimated parameters per animal. A fixed oxygen consumption level
(1.5 ml O2/min/g) was used for calculating the perfusion pressure –
flow relation for each animal depicted in the left panel. In the
right panel the oxygen consumption-flow relations are shown as
calculated for a perfusion pressure of 100 mmHg. The symbols
enclosing the individual lines in fig. 3 indicate the actual ranges
in which pressure and oxygen consumption were varied. The heavy
lines in both panels depict the relationships obtained with the
estimated parameters by fitting the model equation to all data from
all animals together (452 measurement points). From fig. 3 it is
obvious that none of the perfusion-pressure-flow relations are flat
after correction for oxygen consumption changes.

DISCUSSION

The normalization of the flow data do not affect the oxygen

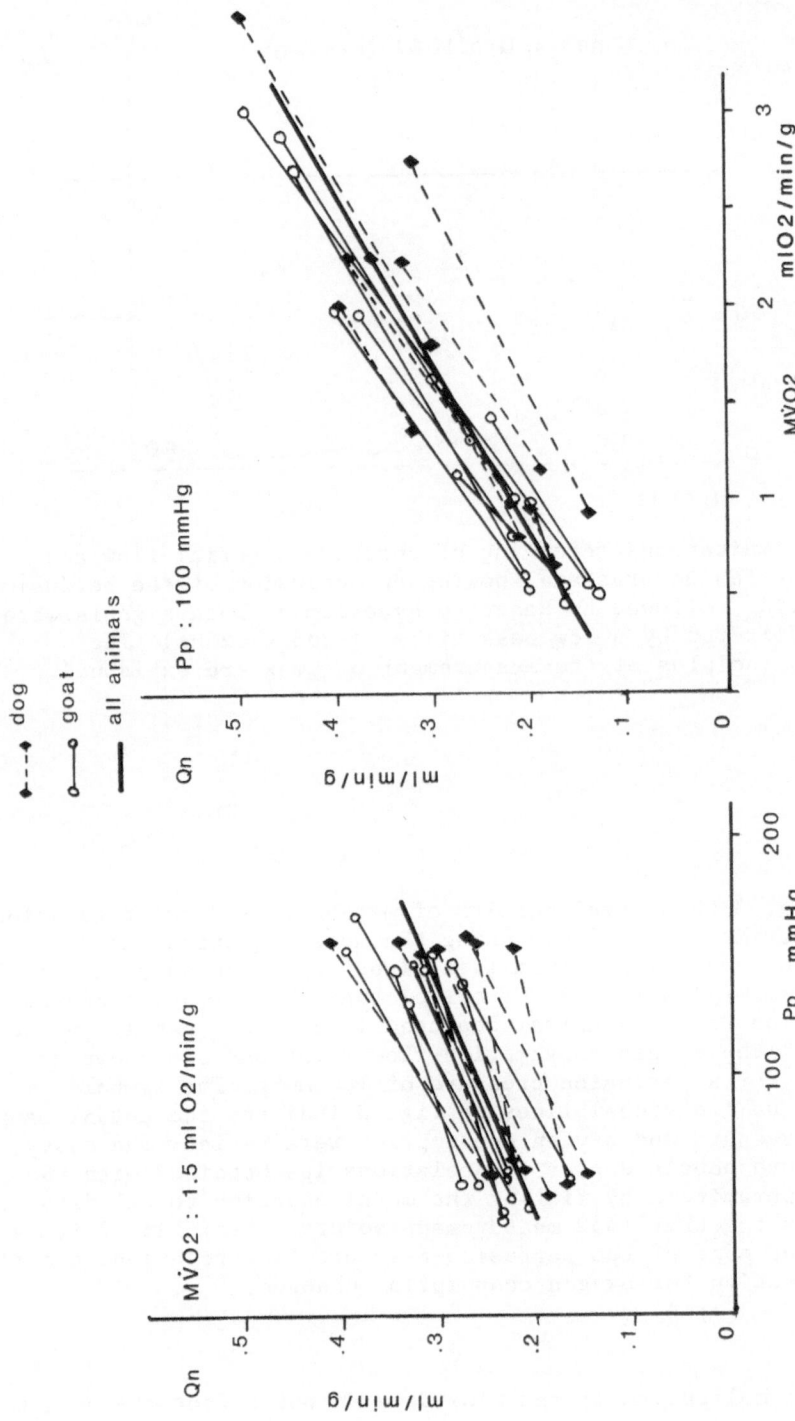

fig. 3: Left panel: The estimated flow-perfusion pressure lines for each individual animal at MVO2n = 1.5 ml O2/min/g. Right panel: The estimated flow-oxygen consumption relation at PP=100 mm Hg over the measured oxygen consumption range for each individual animal.

Table 1: Means and standard deviations of the individual best fitted parameters of the model: $Qn = a * (PP-P\emptyset) + b * M\dot{V}O2n$.

	$a * 10^3$	$b * 10$	r
goats (9)	1.02±0.29	1.25±0.26	0.86±0.11
dogs (7)	1.00±0.47	1.10±0.21	0.90±0.05
all animals (16)	1.10±0.37	1.19±0.24	0.88±0.09
all data (452) together	1.02±0.02	1.14±0.03	0.835

consumption-flow relation at a constant perfusion pressure. Only the flow-perfusion pressure relation was influenced by the normalization procedure. The inter-individual variation was reduced by 50% as a result of the normalization. Qmax was chosen as normalizing parameter because: 1) It was a well defined quantity, 2) It was measured a few times during each experiment under the same experimental conditions as the other experimental data, 3) The phenomenon of Reactive Hyperaemia is a quickly reversible process which does not affect the stability of the coronary circulation. An occlusion of 10 to 15 seconds is sufficient to reach the maximal coronary arterial flow (Fam & McGregor, 1969) and to estimate the perfusion pressure at zero flow. The pressure at zero flow has been introduced arbitrarily. However the physical basis of this quantity might be found in the Starling resistor behavior of the coronary venous circulation (Scharf et al., 1971). The choice for oxygen carrying capacity as normalizing factor was based on the model equation 1) and on the results of Jan & Chien (1977). They showed a linear relation between hematocrit and coronary flow over the ranges of hematocrits measured.

The oxygen hypothesis as formulated by Laird predicts a linear relationship between coronary arterial flow on the one hand and myocardial oxygen consumption and perfusion pressure on the other hand. As for all control systems, this linear relation exists only over a limited range of perfusion pressures. For example the linear relation between extracellular PO2 and resistance (the essential part of the model) obviously has only meaning at a positive resistance. Moreover the S-shaped relation between hemoglobin saturation and PO2 may only be linearized over a limited range of PO2. However, the model fits quite well to the data of individual animals despite these restrictions.

The model assumes independency of perfusion pressure and myocardial oxygen consumption with respect to their effects on the coronary arterial flow. In practice the measured perfusion pressure and oxygen consumption data were not always independent. In some

animals raising the perfusion pressure resulted in an increased
oxygen consumption level. This may be caused indirectly by a raised
aortic pressure (Arnold et al., 1970) or directly by decreasing
ventricular wall compliance (Gregg, 1963). The well known
oxygen-consumption-flow relation as published by Rubio & Berne
(1975) and Eckenhoff et al.(1947) has not been corrected for the
direct effects of perfusion pressure (= aortic pressure in their
experiments). However the autoregulation of the coronary vascular
bed is not so perfect that one can ignore the perfusion pressure
influence on flow.

CONCLUSION

     Coronary arterial flow can be predicted by from a linear
combination of perfusion pressure and myocardial oxygen
consumption. Under physiological conditions neither the perfusion
pressure nor myocardial oxygen consumption can be ignored in
studies concerning coronary arterial flow regulation.
Laird's oxygen hypothesis proved to be a useful framework for the
analysis of the regulation of the coronary arterial vascular bed.

APPENDIX

In steady state F1 = F2 = F3 (see fig. 1).
$$M\dot{V}O2 = Hb * 1.36 * (Sa-Sv) * Q \qquad\qquad 3)$$
where Sa = 0.97
We assume Pec = Pv (Pv = venous PO2)
and linearisation of O2 dissociaton curve of Hb in venous pO2
region yields:
$$Sv = S\emptyset + K3 * Pv \qquad\qquad 4)$$
where S$\emptyset$ = -0.1
       K3 = 0.024 (pH 7.4)

3) + 4): $M\dot{V}O2 = Hb * 1.36 * (1.07 - 0.024 \, Pec) * Q$ 5)
Combining #4 and #5 from fig 1 yields:

$$Pec = \frac{R-R\emptyset}{K2} \text{ and } R = \frac{PP-P\emptyset}{Q}$$

$$Pec = \frac{PP-P\emptyset}{Q*K2} - \frac{R\emptyset}{K2} \qquad\qquad 6)$$

5) + 6): $M\dot{V}O2 = Q * Hb * 1.36 * (1.07 - 0.024 * \frac{PP-P\emptyset}{Q*K2} - \frac{R\emptyset}{K2})$

rearranging yields:

$$Q = \frac{0.024}{1.07K2+0.024R\emptyset} * (PP-P\emptyset) + \frac{K2}{1.07K2+0.024R\emptyset} * \frac{M\dot{V}O2}{Hb*1.36} \qquad 7)$$

equation 7) is simplified to yield the model equation 1).

REFERENCES

Arnold, G., Morgenstern, O., Lochner, W., 1970. The
    autoregulation of the heart work by the coronary perfusion
    pressure. Pflügers Arch., 321:34.
Bugni, W.J., Kralios, A.C., Tsagaris, T.J., Kuida, H., 1980.
    Effect of arterial pressure on left ventricular O_2 consumption,
    coronary blood flow and reserve capacity following coronary
    occlusion. Am. Heart J., 100:657.
Drake-Holland, A.J., Laird, J.D., Noble, M.I.M.,
    Spaan, J.A.E., Vergroesen, I., 1984. Oxygen and coronary
    vascular resistance during autoregulation and metabolic
    vasodilation in the dog. J. Physiol., 348:285.
Eckenhoff, J.E., Hafkenschiel, J.H., Landmesser, C.M.,
    Harmel, M., 1947. Cardiac oxygen metabolism and control of the
    coronary circulation. Am. J. Physiol., 149:634.
Fam, W.M., McGregor, M., 1969. Pressure-flow relationships
    in the coronary circulation. Circ. Res., 25:293.
Feigl, E.O., 1983. Coronary Physiology. Physiol. Rev., 63:1.
Gregg, D.E., 1963. Effect of coronary perfusion pressure or
    coronary flow on oxygen usage of the myocardium. Circ. Res.,
    13:497.
Jan, K.M., Chien, S., 1977. Effect of hematocrit variations
    on coronary hemodynamics and oxygen utilization. Am. J.
    Physiol., 233:H106
Laird, J.D., Spaan, J.A.E., 1981. A simple computer model of
    coronary flow regulation based on interstitial oxygen tension.
    J. Physiol., 324:1P.
Rubio, R, Berne, R.M., 1975. Regulation of coronary blood
    flow. Prog. Cardiovasc. Dis., 18:105.
Scharf, S.M., Bromberger-Barnea, B., Permutt, S., 1971.
    Distribution of coronary venous flow. J. Appl. Physiol.,
    30:657-662.
Spaan, J.A.E., Breuls, N.P.W., Laird, J.D., 1981.
    Diastolic-systolic coronary flow differences are caused by
    intramyocardial pump action in the anesthetized dog. Circ.
    Res., 49:584.

MYOCARDIAL OXYGEN PRESSURE ACROSS THE LATERAL BORDER

ZONE AFTER ACUTE CORONARY OCCLUSION IN THE PIG HEART

H. Walfridsson, S. Ödman, and N. Lund

Departments of Internal Medicine, Biomedical Engineering
and Anesthesiology, University Hospital
S-581 85 Linköping, Sweden

INTRODUCTION

Since it was first understood[1] that it was possible to inter-
fere with the development of an acute myocardial infarction, that
it was indeed possible to reduce the amount of tissue damaged
because of ischemia[2,3], a lot of scientific interest has been
focused on this field. It became even more important when it was
shown that there was clinically a good correlation between myocardial infarct size and both morbidity and mortality[4,5,6]. Most of
this work was, and is, experimental using different animal models
where dog is the most commonly used species. Several clinical
studies have been made, some indicating infarct size reduction[7].
The major drawback of clinical studies is the difficulty concerning
infarct size estimation which is why the experimental approach is
still valid.

In the search for methods to preserve myocardium after acute
coronary occlusion much interest has been focused upon the tissue
between well perfused and ischemic myocardium. In the present study
this area will be referred to as the border zone. It was for a long
time regarded as a fact that there was a significant tissue volume
subjected to intermediate injury after coronary artery occlusion[8].
This tissue volume constituted the maximally salvageable tissue
with the appropriate intervention. More recent studies[9] have ques-
tioned earlier results concerning a border zone of only reversibly
damaged myocardium. This among other things because of lack of
sufficient resolution power of the techniques employed or because
of the time intervals used[9].

In a previous study we found that the lateral border zone

either had to be very narrow or that there was no intermediately damaged zone at all. On the other hand the results also supported the view that the border zone might be dynamic, i.e. the demarcation between normal and ischemic tissue could still be sharp but the demarcation line might move. In this earlier study we performed tissue surface oxygen pressure (p_tO_2) measurements with the standard MDO electrode which is a multichannel surface oxygen electrode of the Clark type[10,11]. It consists of eight randomly distributed platinum wires each 15 microns in diameter. To improve the possibility to register oxygen pressures across the border zone a modified MDO electrode was built. In this new electrode the eight measuring points are distributed along a straight line, 2.2 mm long.

The aim of the present study was to investigate the lateral border zone with the modified surface oxygen electrode and to follow the events immediately after an acute coronary occlusion as well as after reperfusion. In a longer perspective the aim of these investigations will be to try to reduce the amount of damaged myocardium inevitably caused by ischemia.

MATERIAL and METHODS

Technically successful experiments were carried out on 10 Swedish land race pigs with a weight of 28-36 kg. Anesthesia was induced with azaperon 4 mg/kg (Stresnil[R]) and atropine 0.05 mg/kg intramuscularly, followed by an initial dose of 15 mg/kg metomidate (Hypnodil[R]) intraperitoneally. Thereafter metomidate was given in continuous infusion in physiological saline. Muscle relaxation was achieved by pancuronium (Pavulon[R]) also given in continuous infusion. A tracheotomy was performed and the animals were ventilated with ambient air with an Engström ventilator. Positive end-expiratory pressure was kept at 5 cm of water in order to prevent pulmonary atelectasis. Arterial blood was drawn for gas analysis (ABL-3, Radiometer[R]) and the respiratory volume was adjusted in order to keep the arterial pO_2 and pCO_2 within normal ranges ($10 < pO_2 < 14$ kPa, $4.4 < pCO_2 < 5.5$ kPa)[12]. Catheters were placed in a superficial vein, in an external jugular vein and a red pigtail catheter (Cooks[R]) was placed in the left ventricle in a position inducing no persistent arrhythmias. Systolic and end-diastolic left ventricular pressures as well as surface ECG were registered with a Mingograf[R] recorder (Siemens-Elema).

A midsternal thoracotomy was performed and the heart suspended in a pericardial cradle to minimize movements due to respiration. A 2-0 silk ligature was placed around the left anterior descending coronary artery (LAD) after the third diagonal branch or in a corresponding position, i.e. approximately 2/3 of the distance from the base to the apex.

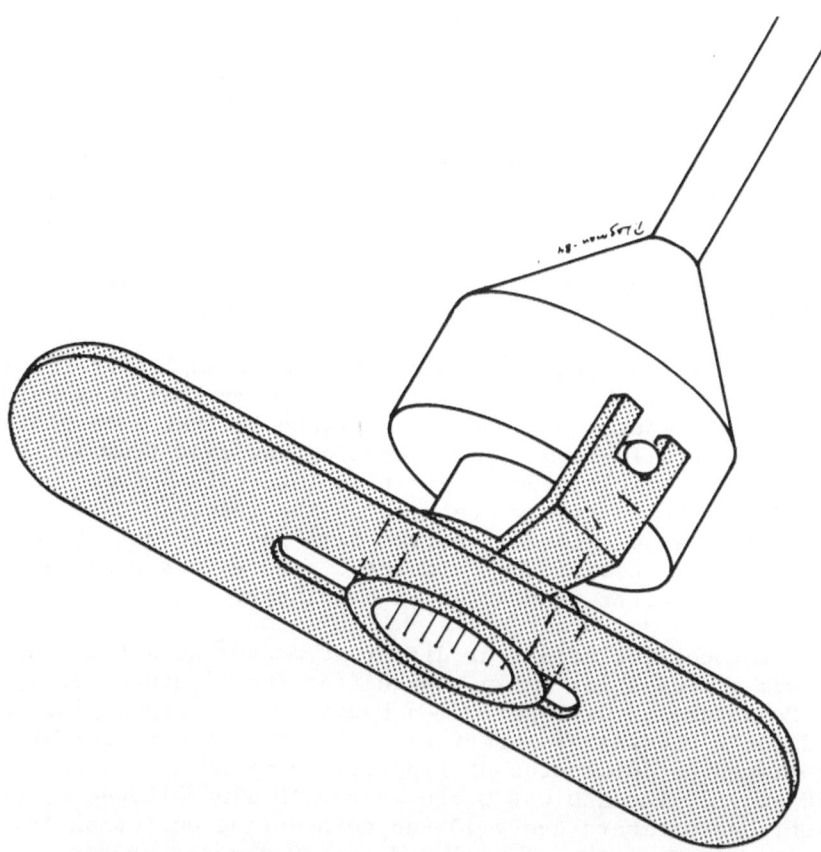

Fig. 1. The modified MDO electrode in its holder system. A plastic
film is sutured on to the left ventricular surface. The
electrode can be moved along the split in the plastic
while rotation is not possible.

The LAD was then obstructed temporarily for 30-90 sec to allow for
development of cyanosis in the area distal to the occlusion. The
area of cyanosis was clearly delineated from normal tissue. For the
tissue oxygen pressure measurements the modified MDO electrode
(Eschweiler & Co) was used. The electrode contains eight platinum
wires each 15 microns in diameter. In the conventional MDO electrode
these eight wires are distributed within a circle with 1.2 mm in
diameter. To improve the electrode for measurements across the
border zone the eight wires instead positioned in a straight line
2.2 mm long. This electrode has the same electrochemical characteristics as the conventional MDO electrode.

   To position the electrode on the left ventricular surface at
a precise point required a specially designed holder system
(Fig 1). This was sutured on to the left ventricle with 5-0 silk
sutures. The holder system allowed for controlled movements along

a line 15 mm long but all rotation was effectivly stopped. The electrode was positioned where the sharp demarcation between cyanotic and noncyanotic myocardium was seen after the first short occlusion of the LAD. The artery was again closed to ensure that both normal and ischemic tissue was found in the measuring area of the electrode. This required only a short lasting occlusion, 15-45 sec. The electrode was then left on the surface for 45 min of stabilization and during this time the LAD was left open.

The signals from the electrode were via an amplifier fed into an ABC 890 computer (Luxor, Sweden) where p_tO_2-values were calculated[13]. The computer program was designed so that each platinum wire was individually identified. Sampling was made from all eight measuring points simultaneously and time intervals between samplings could be chosen freely. Because of the response time of the electrode (approx. 6 seconds) shorter sampling intervals than 10 sec were never chosen. The calculated p_tO_2 values were plotted either on the computer display or on a printer.

The protocol included four different measuring situations: 1. The LAD was occluded for 2 min, thereafter the ligature was again opened. Measurements were performed every 10 sec both during occlusion and for 5 minutes of reperfusion. 2. The LAD was occluded for 5 min followed by 10 minutes of reperfusion with measurements every 10 sec. 3. The LAD was occluded for 10 min followed by reperfusion. Measurements every 10 sec both during occlusion and reperfusion. 4. The LAD was occluded for 30 minutes or for 60 minutes with at least 60 minutes of reperfusion. Measurements were done every 30 sec during both occlusion and reperfusion. During each period of p_tO_2 measurements we also measured systolic blood pressure, end-diastolic left ventricular pressure (LVEDP), an arterial blood sample was analysed and the ECG was continuously registered.

STATISTICAL METHODS

Mean values and S.D. were calculated. For analysis of differences Student´s t-test was used.

RESULTS

Ten pigs were used for these experiments. They were subjected to limited, repeated coronary artery occlusion with 45-60 minutes of reperfusion between each occlusion. Four pigs died during the experiments, all from ventricular fibrillation. Two of these occurred during ischemia while two occurred at reperfusion. In these 10 pigs 28 artery occlusions were studied: Eight occlusions of 2 min, 11 occlusions of 5 min, 4 occlusions of 10 min, 1 of 30 min and 4 of 60 min duration.

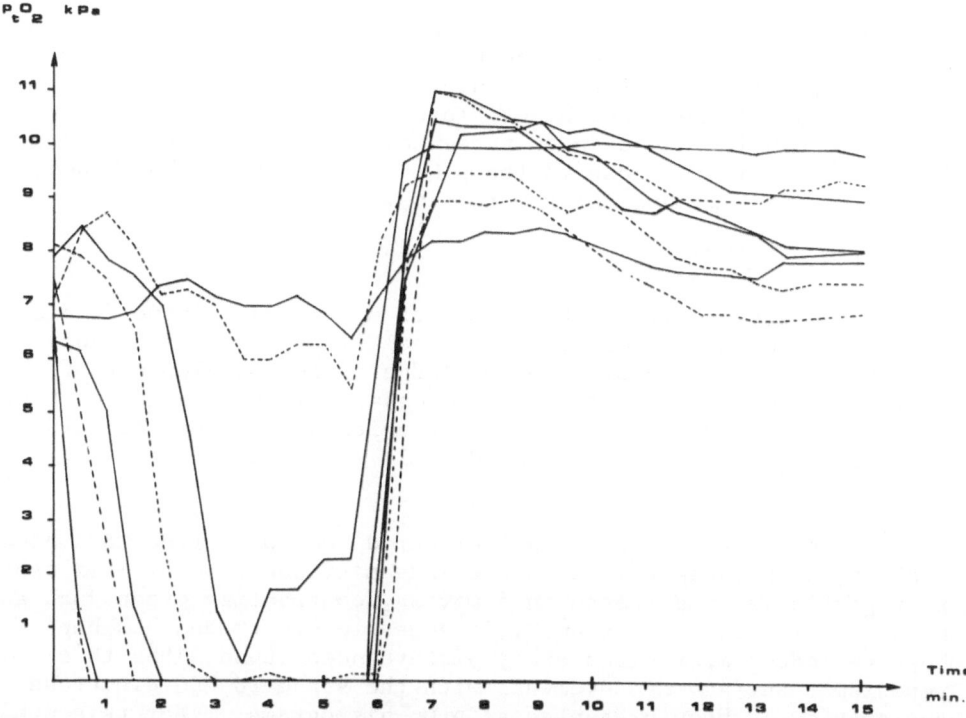

Fig. 2. P_tO_2 measurements from one experiment. The LAD is occluded at time 0 and kept occluded for five minutes
followed by reperfusion. Each one of the eight measuring
points can be individually followed.

The blood gas analyses showed a stable situation during each
experiment. Heart rate, systolic blood pressure and LVEDP showed
no significant changes before and after coronary occlusion.

The P_tO_2 values from one experiment are shown in Fig. 2. This
illustrates one of the two patterns seen after every artery occlusion. The P_tO_2 values measured at the point closest to the core of
ischemia dropped rapidly to zero. The next measuring point also
showed a fall to zero but not so fast. The third and fourth points
registered an even slower decrease of the P_tO_2. In this example
two measuring points registered normal values but in some other
experiments three or four remained normal. This pattern was seen
in seven animals, always the same pattern at repeated occlusions
in the same animal.

The other pattern seen after artery occlusion was initially

the same as for the seven animals described above but even without reperfusion there was a spontaneous rise in p_tO_2 from zero to values in the level 1-2 kPa. During reperfusion these values increased as in all the other cases. This spontaneous increase during arterial occlusion was seen in three animals. At reperfusion all 10 showed a rapid increase in the p_tO_2 values with an "overshoot" during the first minutes of reperfusion.

DISCUSSION

The ability to limit the extent of myocardial tissue damage because of ischemia is of great clinical importance. To be able to reach this goal a more precise knowledge of the development of irreversible myocardial damage is necessary. In this study we have used a surface oxygen electrode for studies across the lateral border zone in the pig heart immediately after coronary artery occlusion.

The use of a surface oxygen electrode was preferred to a needle electrode because this does not induce tissue trauma. This aspect is of particular importance in a moving, contracting organ such as the heart. The use of extremely fine needle electrodes has been shown to induce microcirculatory disturbances (Lund, 1984 this symposium). Surface measurements with the standard MDO electrode have previously been presented as p_tO_2-histograms[14]. For this study with the use of the modified MDO electrode an alternative form of presentation was chosen: Fig 2. With this form of presentation it is possible to follow the p_tO_2 values for the eight measuring points simultaneously. One major drawback of this technique is its limitation to the surface. The measurements only reflect the most superficial tissue down to approximately 25 microns.

The border zone and its precise shape has been disputed[9]. Some have found evidence for a diffuse "intermediate" zone between ischemic and well perfused myocardium[15] while others using other techniques have found evidence for a sharp border between ischemic and normoxic myocardium[16].

Our findings do not support the hypothesis of a cell to cell sharp demarcation between damaged and normoxic, well perfused myocardium. The finding of the stepwise slower decrease of the p_tO_2 values across the border could be explained by a residual blood flow that decreased over a distance of 550-1375 microns (corresponding to 2-5 measuring points of the electrode). This prevents, at least for some minutes, the development of ischemia in this area. We often observed that one measuring point registered intermediate p_tO_2 values which could be explained by diffusion. However when two points showed intermediate values diffusion alone probably does not explain this observation because of the distances involved being to long. This observation supports the hypothesis of a small, residual blood flow in the border zone. In some cases we observed a spontaneous increase in the p_tO_2 values during artery occlusion. This probably indicated opening of collaterals that in this situation seem to be able to support at least a small amount of myocardium.

Acknowledgements

This study was supported by the Swedisch Medical Research Council (05956), the Tore Nilsson Foundation (83/94) and the Östergötland County Council (15/82, 98,82, 14/83).

REFERENCES

1. P.R. Maroko, J. Kjekshus, B. Sobel, T. Watanabe, J. Ross, E. Braunwald, Factors influencing infarct size following experimental coronary artery occlusion. Circulation 18:67-82 (1971).
2. P.R. Maroko, E. Braunwald, Modification of myocardial infarct size after coronary occlusion. Ann Intern Med 79:720-733 (1973).
3. M. Rasmussen, K. Reimer, R. Kloner, R. Jennings, Infarct size reduction by propranolol before and after coronary ligation in the dogs. Circulation 56(5):794-798 (1977).
4. K.E. Hammermeister, T.A. DeRouen, H.T. Dodge, Variables predictive of survival in patients with coronary disease: selection by univariate and multivariate analyses from the clinical, electrocardiographic, exercise, arteriographic, and quantitative angiographic evaluations. Circulation 59(3):421-430 (1979).
5. H.T. Davis, J. DeCamilla, L.W. Bayer, A.J. Moss, Survivorship patterns in post-hospital phase of myocardial infarction. Circulation 60(6):1252-1258 (1979).
6. A. Vedin, L. Wilhelmsen, H. Wedel, B. Petterson, C. Wilhelmson, D. Elmfeldt, G. Tibblin, Prediction of cardiovascular deaths and non-fatal reinfarctions after myocardial infarction. Acta Med Scand 201:309-316 (1979).
7. T. Peter, R.M. Norris, E.D. Clarce, M.K. Heng, B.M. Singh, B. Williams, D.R. Howell, Reduction of enzyme levels by propranolol after acute myocardial infarction. Circulation 57(6):1091-1095 (1978).
8. M. Fishbein, C. Hare, S. Gissen, J. Spadara, D. Maclean, P. Maroko, Identification and quantification of histochemical zones during the evolution of myocardial infarction in the rat. Cardiovasc Res 14:41-49 (1980).
9. D.J. Hearse, D.M. Yellon, The "border zone" in evolving myocardial infarction: controversy or confusion? Am J Cardiol 47(6):321-324 (1981).

10. M. Kessler, W. Grunewald, Possibilities of measuring oxygen pressure fields in tissue by multiwire platinum electrodes. Prog Resp Res 3:147-152 (1969).

11. M. Kessler, D.W. Lübbers, Aufbau und Anwendungsmöglichkeiten verschiedener pO2-Electroden. Pflügers Arch ges Physiol R82:291 (1966).

12. W. v Engelhardt, Swine cardiovascular physiology - A review. In L.K. Bustad, R. McClellan, (eds),: Swine in biomedical research. Battelle North West, Richland, Washington (1965).

13. S. Ödman, N. Lund, Data acquisition and information processing in MDO oxygen electrode measurements of tissue oxygen pressure. Acta anaesth scand 24:161-165 (1980).

14. D.W. Lübbers, The meaning of the tissue oxygen distribution curve and its measurements by means of Pt electrodes. Prog Resp Res 3:112-123 (1969).

15. P.S. Vokonas, P.M. Malsky, S.J. Paul, S.L. Robbins, W.B. Hood, Radioautographic studies in experimental myocardial infarction: Profiles of ischemic blood flow and quantification of infarct size in relation to magnitude of ischemic zone. Am J Cardiol 42:67-75 (1978).

16. R.E. Patterson, E.S. Kirk, Analyses of coronary collateral structure, function, and ischemic border zone in the pigs. Am J Physiol 244:H23-31 (1983).

DISTRIBUTION OF MITOCHONDRIA RELATIVE TO CAPILLARIES IN GUINEA PIG MYOCARDIUM

Susan R. Kayar and N. Banchero

Department of Physiology
University of Colorado School of Medicine
Denver, Colorado 80262

INTRODUCTION

The distribution of mitochondria relative to capillaries is important in respiratory physiology because it reflects the distribution of distances over which oxygen diffuses from its source in capillaries to its site of utilization in mitochondria. Mitochondrial distribution also reflects the distribution of distances over which high-energy phosphates must be transferred from their site of formation in the mitochondria to their site of utilization in the myofibrils. In this study, we devised a simple method for measuring mitochondrial distributions. This method was then used to measure the distribution of mitochondria relative to capillaries in the right ventricles of four guinea pigs of differing capillary densities.

MATERIALS AND METHODS

The hearts of four guinea pigs (Cavia porcellus) ranging in age from approximately 3 weeks to 20 weeks were perfusion-fixed following the procedures described by Kayar and Banchero (1984). Blocks of tissue were cut from the right ventricles and embedded in Spurr medium. Four blocks were sectioned with an ultra-microtome (Sorvall II) perpendicularly to the primary axis of the fibers and capillaries, to a section thickness of approximately 0.5 um. These semithin sections were stained with Toluidine Blue and photographed under the light microscope (Zeiss) at 400x. The photographs were analyzed, using an x-y digitizer (GTCO Corp.) on line with a computer (Nova 4), to measure capillarity and fiber areas.

From previous analyses of heart tissue it was determined that myocardial capillaries are spaced in a uniform distribution for which the formulas for a hexagonal array fit well (Kayar and Banchero, 1983). In this case the intercapillary distance (L) can be approximated from the capillary density D as:

$$L = 0.88(D^{-1/2}).$$

The distance to the center of the hexagon, which is the point farthest from all capillaries, is also of length L. It is frequently more convenient mathematically and graphically, however, to consider the radial distance from capillaries in a hexagonal array within which 95% of the area of the hexagon has been included. This distance is:

$$R_{95} = 0.71(D^{-1/2}).$$

The radial distance from capillaries that represents the mean distance from a capillary within the hexagon is:

$$\bar{R} = 0.40(D^{-1/2}) \text{ (Kayar et al., 1982).}$$

Following the light-microscopic level of analysis of capillarity, two tissue blocks were cut again with the ultramicrotome to a section thickness of approximately 500 A and photographed under a transmission electron microscope (Zeiss Model EM 9 S-2). The distribution of mitochondria relative to capillaries was determined from these micrographs at a final magnification of approximately 11,000x. For the four animals in this study, 11 to 18 micrographs were analyzed per animal, depending on the number of micrographs representing good cross-sections of tissue.

Each photomicrograph contained one capillary near the center and 2 to 5 adjacent capillaries near its edges. These micrographs were then analyzed by a method of point-counting in concentric circles. A transparent template was made of a series of concentric circles in which the radius of the innermost circle was approximately equal to the radius roughly equal to one-half the mean intercapillary distance (1/2 L) as calculated from capillary density above. The space between the innermost and outermost circles was divided into 6 rings of equal area and therefore of ring widths that grew more narrow as radius increased. A regular grid of points was overlaid on this template, and because ring areas were equal, the number of grid points per ring (125) was also equal. A discussion of the rules for selection of grid point density is given by Weibel (1979). Briefly, the number of points per ring was selected to assure that every mitochondrial profile would be scored, and the number of micrographs was selected so that relative standard errors would be between 5 and 8% of means. This template of circles and points was superimposed on a photomicrograph with the center circle over the center capillary. The distance to each of the adjacent capillaries in the photomicrograph was measured and if any of the template rings extended closer to an adjacent capillary than one-half this distance, such portions of the photomicrograph were excluded from the analysis. Volume density of mitochondria per ring was calculated by standard stereological procedures (Weibel, 1979). This value is the ratio of the number of points per ring falling on the mitochondria to the total number of points overlying muscle fibers, excluding any points falling on interstitial space or fiber nuclei. There were usually one to three small areas in a photomicrograph that were farther from all capillaries than the radius of the outermost template circle (the so-called "dead spaces" of a tissue approaching distance L from a capillary); therefore, the volume density of mitochondria in these areas was calculated using the grid points in the innermost template circle centered over these areas. Thus only one average value for this region from 1/2 L to L was obtained.

RESULTS

As animals increased in body weight and heart weight, myocardial fibers increased in area and capillary density decreased (Table 1). However, mitochondrial volume densities were similar in these four hearts (Fig. 1). Volume density reached a peak of 30 to 33 volumes % near the capillary, with this peak appearing in the first template ring of the smallest animal with the highest capillary density, but in the second template ring in the other three animals. Volume density then declined to 24 to 27 volumes % in the regions farthest from capillaries in all animals, with a fairly stable volume density reached at or slightly before the distance corresponding to the $\bar{R}$ for each animal.

Table 1. Data from guinea pig right ventricle (RV). Mean fiber cross-sectional area (FCSA) and capillary density (CD) are expressed $\pm$ one standard error.

Body weight (g)	RV Weight (g)	FCSA (um^2)	CD (mm^{-2})
239	0.172	127 $\pm$ 19	3571 $\pm$ 130
341	0.255	140 $\pm$ 25	3210 $\pm$ 318
578	0.488	177 $\pm$ 4	2873 $\pm$ 150
940	0.600	241 $\pm$ 44	2661 $\pm$ 153

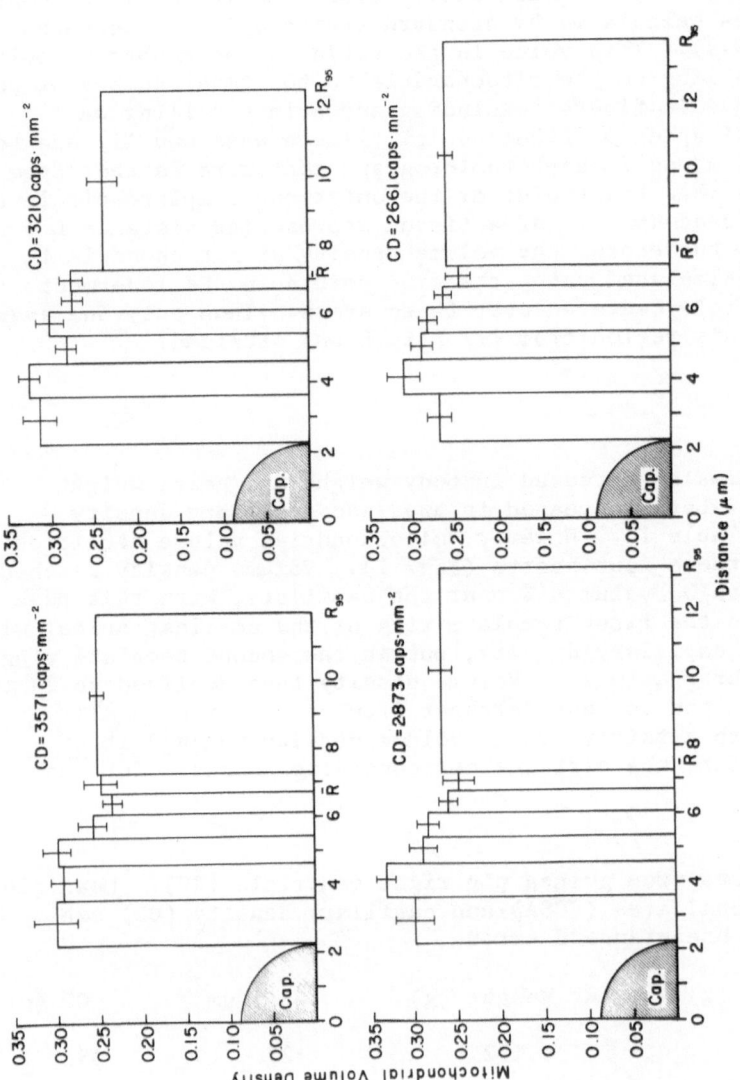

Fig. 1. Volume density of mitochondria relative to the distance from the center of a capillary in guinea pig right ventricle. Each panel represents data from 11 to 18 frames from one animal. Capillary density (CD) of each animal, and mean ($\bar{R}$) and maximal (R_{95}) oxygen diffusion distances calculated from capillary density are included. CAP indicates the capillary cross-section.

DISCUSSION

The total volume density of mitochondria in these four guinea pig right ventricles was similar, despite more than a three-fold difference in body weight and heart weight between the smallest and the largest animal. Thus there was an increase in the absolute volume of mitochondria in a ventricle that was in direct proportion to the total volume of tissue. There is a distinct region of higher mitochondrial volume density with its peak located at a distance well before the mean diffusion distance calculated for these hearts. Such a distribution has not previously been included in models of aerobic metabolism and oxygen diffusion in myocardia. The theoretical implications of a distribution of mitochondria clustered near capillaries has been considered by Mainwood and Rakusan (1982), who demonstrated that such a distribution would not only shorten oxygen diffusion distances, but would also greatly reduce PO_2 gradients across cells.

There is the additional problem of ATP delivery from inhomogeneously distributed mitochondria to working myofibrils throughout the fiber. Recent work with the "phosphocreatine shuttle" has suggested that theoretically, within the distances considered in these hearts, the diffusion of high-energy phosphates from inhomogeneously-distributed mitochondria should not be limiting to respiratory rate (Mainwood and Rakusan, 1982; Meyer et al., 1984). These and other implications of this distribution of mitochondria remain to be tested.

Supported by NIH grants HL-06527 and HL-28849. The authors wish to express their appreciation to Drs. Cynthea I. Blake and Catherine R. Jackson for their contribution to this project.

REFERENCES

Kayar, S.R., Archer, P.G., Lechner, A.J., and Banchero, N., 1982, The closest individual method in the analysis of the distribution of capillaries, Microvasc. Res., 24:326-341.

Kayar, S.R., and Banchero, N., 1983, Distribution of capillaries and diffusion distances in guinea pig myocardium, Pflugers Arch., 396:350-352.

Kayar, S.R., and Banchero, N., 1984, Myocardial capillarity in acclimation to hypoxia, Pflugers Arch., (in press).

Mainwood, G.W., and Rakusan, K., 1982, A model for intracellular energy transport, Can. J. Physiol. Pharmacol., 60:98-102.

Meyer, R.A., Sweeney, H.L., and Kushmerick, M.J., 1984, A simple
    analysis of the "phosphocreatine shuttle", *Am. J.
    Physiol.*, 246:(Cell Physiol. 15):C365-C377.
Weibel, E.R., 1979, "Stereological methods. Vol. 1. Practical
    methods for biological morphometry", Academic Press,
    London, 97-112.

OXYGEN SUPPLY TO HYPOTHERMIC ISOLATED WORKING HEART

DURING BLOOD ACID-BASE CHANGES

M. Sinet, M. Muffat-Joly, D. Henzel and J.J. Pocidalo

Institut National de la Santé et de la Recherche
Médicale, Unité 13
Hôpital Claude Bernard, 75019 Paris, France

INTRODUCTION

Alterations of thermal state induce changes in oxygen transport as a consequence of shifting metabolic demand, modifications
of acid-base parameters and changes in blood oxygen affinity. It is
now recognized that, when temperature is modified, variation in pH
of biological fluids parallels modifications in the neutral point
of water which is temperature dependent[1,2]. Therefore, pH adjustment, when organs from homeotherms are subjected to hypothermia
as presently practiced in cardiac surgery or organ preservation,
is justified.

Since little is known about the functional adaptation of an
organ to both temperature and acid-base changes, the present experiments were undertaken using blood perfused isolated working rat
hearts. The effects of blood pH variation on myocardial oxygenation
and mechanical function of working hearts during moderate hypothermia (26°C) were evaluated in conditions of normal and increased
workload and compared to results obtained at 37°C.

METHODS

Experiments were performed in a blood perfused working heart
apparatus[3,4].

Male Wistar rats, weighing 300-320g were anesthetized by ether
inhalation. The heart was rapidly excised, chilled in ice-cold
0.9% NaCl containing heparin and mounted by the aorta on a cannula.
Aortic cannula was fixed to the perfusion apparatus and the heart

was preperfused in a retrograde way until cannulation of the left atrium allowed working heart perfusion : perfusate entered the left atrium and was ejected from the left ventricle into a fluid column. The perfusion system reproduced an artificial systemic circulation and regulated afterload (fixed at 75 mmHg) and preload (adjustable to any chosen value under 25 mmHg). The left atrium could be perfused through one of two symmetrical circuits which contained different perfusates. The whole perfusion apparatus was enclosed in a thermostatic chamber.

Pig erythrocytes-enriched buffer at a final hematocrit of 30% was employed as perfusate. The P_{50} (P_{O2} necessary to half saturate hemoglobin) of this reconstituted blood was 32 torr at pH 7.4 and 37°C. Perfusate was filtered before use (pore size 10μm) and equilibration of blood with appropriate gas mixture was carried out using a membrane oxygenator (Hospal).

Blood was sampled from the perfusion tubing (arterial blood) and from the pulmonary arterial outflow (coronary venous blood). Blood was analyzed for P_{O2}, P_{CO2} and pH using blood gas electrodes calibrated and maintained at the temperature of experiment. Oxygen content of the blood was measured using a coulometric micromethod (Lex-O2-Con). Cardiac performance was assessed by measuring aortic pressure (Statham P23 Db pressure transducer), heart rate, aortic flow and coronary flow. Myocardial oxygen consumption ($M\dot{V}_{O2}$) was calculated as the product of coronary flow and arterial-coronary venous O_2 content difference. External work was calculated as the product of mean aortic pressure, cardiac output and a correction coefficient, and was expressed in $J.min^{-1}$. Aortic flow, coronary flow, $M\dot{V}_{O2}$ and external work were expressed per gram of the wet weight of both ventricles. Cardiac efficiency was computed as the ratio of external work to the product of $M\dot{V}_{O2}$ and the calorific value of oxygen ($20.3 J.1^{-1}$).

EXPERIMENTAL PROTOCOL

Group I : study of the effects of pH variation on mechanical function and myocardial oxygenation in hypothermia (26°C, 9 experiments) and comparison with control values at 37°C (8 experiments).

In hypothermia, blood normal pH was defined as that which, from pH 7.4 at 37°C, followed the pH-temperature relationship of neutral water and P_{CO2} was adjusted consequently. Variations in P_{CO2} used to generate acidosis or alkalosis were calculated at each temperature to provide a pH of ± 0.3 unit on both sides of normal pH. Composition of gas mixtures of the membrane oxygenator compartment was the following : at 37°C, 20% F_{O2} - 5, 15 or 1.5% F_{CO2} respectively for normal pH, acidosis or alkalosis ; at 26°C, 10% F_{O2} - 2.8, 7.6 or 0.9% F_{CO2}.

The experimental procedure was the same at both temperatures. After an equilibration period of 30 min at normal pH, the first measurement was taken. The perfusate was then changed every 50 min four times. First, alkaline or acid blood ; second, blood at normal pH ; third, acid or alkaline blood and last return to blood at normal pH. Two sets of measurements were performed during each 50 min period.

Group II : influence of pH on hemodynamic function and myocardial oxygenation in conditions of increased workload during hypothermia (26°C ; 6 experiments).

Ventricular performance was assessed at three levels of atrial filling pressure (7.7, 14.6 and 21.5 mmHg) and compared for normal pH perfusate (pH 7.6) and pH 7.4 perfusate as follows : after an equilibration period of 30 min at 7.7 mmHg atrial filling pressure with blood perfusate at pH 7.6, the different parameters were measured. Atrial filling pressure was then successively raised to 14.6 and 21.5 mmHg and then returned to 7.7 mmHg, for periods of 15 min. Each new state was maintained for 5 min before data were recorded. After return to the low atrial filling pressure, perfusate was changed to blood at pH 7.4. Atrial filling pressure was modified as above and finally the perfusate was changed back to blood at pH 7.6.

RESULTS

Group I : in these experiments the cardiac adaptation to temperature and acid-base changes was studied using a physiological perfusate where acid-base parameters were accurately controlled. It was first verified that experimental pH values for arterial and coronary venous blood at each level of acid-base equilibrium paralleled the temperature dependence of neutral water pH ($pN\ H_2O$). Between 37°C and 26°C, according to Weast et al.[5], $\Delta pN\ H_2O / \Delta T$ was - 0.0156 pH unit /°C. From blood experimental values, $\Delta pH / \Delta T$ was found to be in the range of - 0.0141 to - 0.0173 pH unit /°C. This parallelism of experimental values for blood $\Delta pH / \Delta T$ to the temperature relationship of neutral water attested that cardiac function was studied in the same acid-base conditions in normothermia and in hypothermia. Experimental values of acid-base parameters at the two temperatures are summarized in Table 1.

The effects of changes in arterial blood acid-base status on isolated heart were considered with respect to both myocardial oxygenation and mechanical function. The blood O_2 dissociation curve (ODC) was altered by varying both temperature and pH. P_{50} values, calculated from mean values of venous P_{O_2}, C_{O_2} and pH using Hill's equation are presented in Table 2 with the determinants

Table 1. Arterial (a) and coronary venous (v) acid-base parameters of hypothermic and normothermic working hearts.

		Acidosis		Normal pH		Alkalosis	
		a	v	a	v	a	v
pH	26°C	7.34 ± 0.01	7.32 ± 0.01	7.61 ± 0.01	7.58 ± 0.01	7.86 ± 0.02	7.80 ± 0.01
	37°C	7.15 ± 0.01	7.14 ± 0.01	7.45 ± 0.01	7.42 ± 0.01	7.68 ± 0.03	7.62 ± 0.02
P_{CO2}, Torr	26°C	43.6 ± 0.5	46.7 ± 0.4	19.9 ± 0.4	22.6 ± 0.4	9.7 ± 0.4	11.8 ± 0.4
	37°C	76.8 ± 0.8	81.6 ± 1.3	30.2 ± 0.4	35.4 + 0.5	14.2 ± 1.0	18.3 ± 1.2
$[HCO_3^-]$, $mmol.1^{-1}$	26°C	26.1 ± 0.5	27.0 ± 0.4	22.8 ± 0.5	24.1 ± 0.5	20.9 ± 0.8	21.9 ± 0.5
	37°C	25.7 ± 0.5	26.6 ± 0.5	20.6 ± 0.4	22.5 ± 0.4	16.9 ± 0.7	18.8 ± 0.4

Table 2. Calculated P_{50} values and determinants of oxygen supply and myocardial oxygen uptake.

		Acidosis	Normal pH	Alkalosis
P_{50}, Torr	26°C	21.6	15.6	11.0
	37°C	42.9	30.7	22.4
Ca_{O2}, $ml.100ml^{-1}$	26°C	12.6 ± 0.1	12.7 ± 0.2	12.9 ± 0.1
	37°C	11.0 ± 0.1	11.3 ± 0.1	11.5 ± 0.2
Pa_{O2}, Torr	26°C	82 ± 3	84 ± 6	87 ± 7
	37°C	120 ± 4	121 ± 3	111 ± 8
C.F., $ml.min^{-1}.g^{-1}$	26°C	4.7 ± 0.5	4.4 ± 0.5	3.9 ± 0.5
	37°C	5.7 ± 0.5	5.2 ± 0.6	4.9 ± 0.5
$Ca_{O2}-Cv_{O2}$, $ml.100ml^{-1}$	26°C	3.1 ± 0.2	3.4 ± 0.2	3.8 ± 0.3
	37°C	3.6 ± 0.1	4.1 ± 0.1	4.9 ± 0.2
Pv_{O2}, Torr	26°C	33 ± 1	24 ± 1	16 ± 1
	37°C	55 ± 2	38 ± 2	25 ± 2
$M\dot{V}O_2$, $ml.min^{-1}.g^{-1}$	26°C	0.143 ± 0.010	0.145 ± 0.010	0.143 ± 0.012
	37°C	0.200 ± 0.014	0.212 ± 0.026	0.232 ± 0.018

Values are mean ± SEM

of oxygen supply and oxygen consumption of isolated hearts. At both temperatures, a significant positive relationship was evidenced between pH and arterial-coronary venous O_2 difference ; coronary flow (C.F.) decreased with increasing pH. $\dot{M}V_{O2}$ was significantly related to pH at 37°C but no relationship was found at 26°C. Indices of cardiac function are reported on table 3 and assist comprehension of these apparent differences. Heart rate rose significantly with pH and the pH influence was greater at 37°C than at 26°C. However pH variations did not influence either stroke volume or $\dot{M}V_{O2}$ per beat. It therefore seems likely that the increase in $\dot{M}V_{O2}$ with pH observed at 37°C was only related to heart rate increase. These results indicate a satisfactory adaptation of the isolated working heart to hypothermia. At 26°C, external work and $\dot{M}V_{O2}$ decreased proportionately and therefore no difference in cardiac efficiency was found between normo and hypothermic hearts. When the ODC was left shifted by both decreased temperature and alkaline pH, Pv_{O2} mean value fell to 16 torr without any impairment of oxygen consumption and external work.

Group II : since no impairment in the O_2 supply-to-demand ratio was observed in the above experimental conditions, the study was extended to hypothermic working hearts in conditions of increased oxygen demand and hemodynamic performance was studied at different levels of atrial filling pressure. Hearts were perfused successively with blood at normal acid-base status (pH 7.590 ± 0.005 ; P_{CO2} 20.2 ± 0.5 torr) and with blood maintained at pH 7.4 (pH 7.394 ± 0.005 ; P_{CO_2} 36.5 ± 1.1 torr).

Table 3. Myocardial function of hypothermic and normothermic rat hearts.

		Acidosis	Normal pH	Alkalosis
Heart Rate, beat.min^{-1}	26°C	138 ± 3	148 ± 1	150 ± 1
	37°C	254 ± 9	285 ± 12	312 ± 9
Stroke Volume, µl.g^{-1}	26°C	172 ± 10	156 ± 11	165 ± 13
	37°C	123 ± 14	132 ± 7	120 ± 7
$\dot{M}V_{O2}$ per beat, µl.g^{-1}	26°C	1.03 ± 0.05	0.98 ± 0.06	0.95 ± 0.08
	37°C	0.79 ± 0.06	0.75 ± 0.09	0.75 ± 0.05
External Work, Joule.min^{-1}.g^{-1}	26°C	0.31 ± 0.02	0.30 ± 0.02	0.31 ± 0.02
	37°C	0.40 ± 0.05	0.44 ± 0.03	0.44 ± 0.03
Efficiency, per cent	26°C	10.7 ± 0.6	10.1 ± 0.4	11.1 ± 1.1
	37°C	9.9 ± 0.1	11.0 ± 1.0	9.9 ± 1.0

Values are mean ± SEM

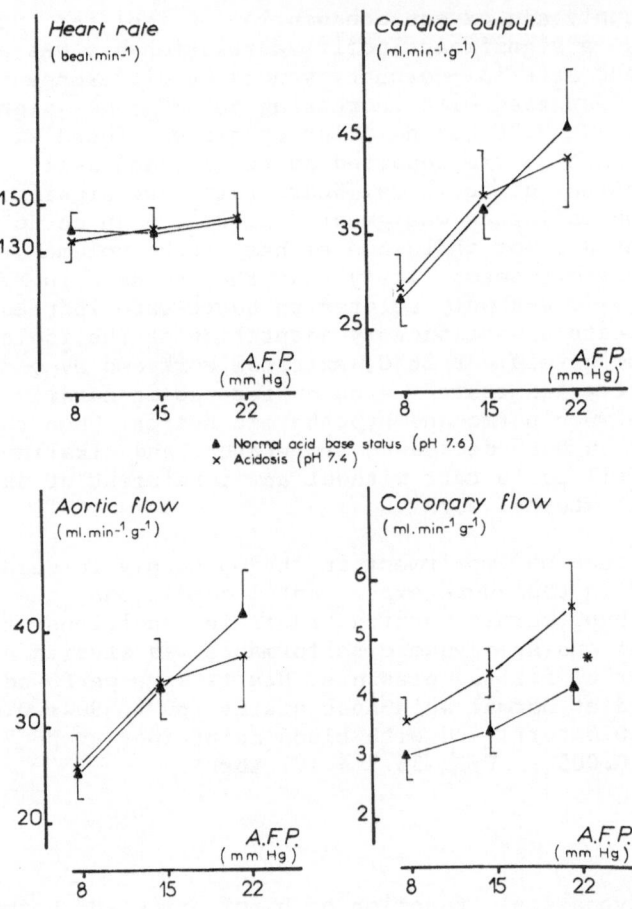

Fig 1.   Effect of pH on cardiac performance of the blood perfused
          isolated working heart. A.F.P.: atrial filling pressure.

    Figure 1 shows the effects of pH on cardiac performance at the
different levels of atrial filling pressure. Heart rate was not
significantly modified by the change in pH between the two perfusates. As expected, both aortic flow and coronary flow and consequently cardiac output increased with increasing workload. Even-
though cardiac output at the highest filling pressure tended to be
raised when heart were perfused with blood at normal pH, this
increase was not statistically significant. Therefore, pH change
did not significantly alter the cardiac response to increased
workload.

    Figure 2 describes the effects of pH on oxygen utilization and
external work at the different levels of workload. Arterio-venous
oxygen difference was increased at the highest workload at both

222

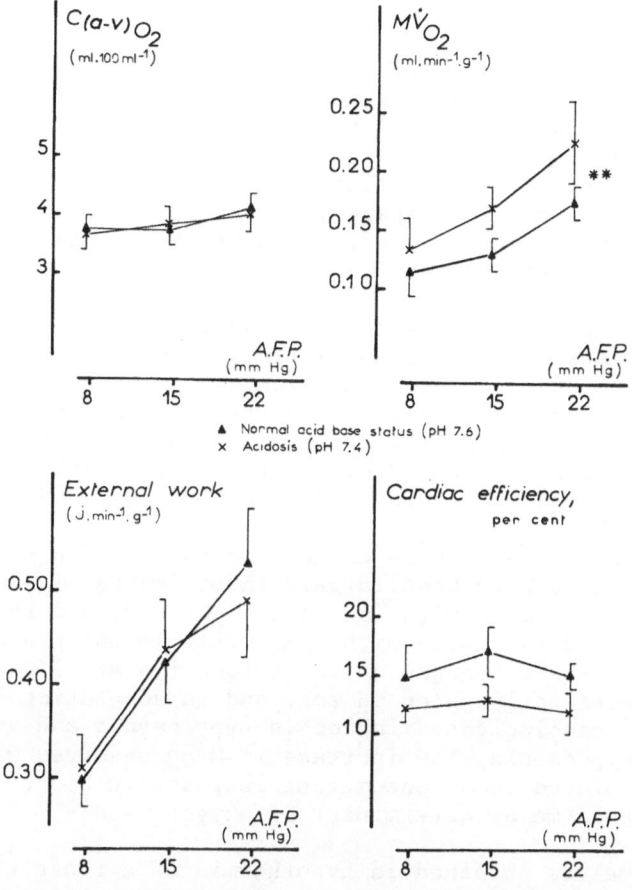

Fig. 2   Effect of pH on external work and oxygen utilization of
the blood perfusated isolated working rat heart.
A.F.P.: atrial filling pressure.

pH levels and was not influenced by perfusate pH. For the highest
atrial filling pressure, as coronary flow was significantly higher
at pH 7.4, $M\dot{V}_{O2}$ was also significantly increased. Both $M\dot{V}_{O2}$ and
external work increased with increasing workload without any change
in cardiac efficiency. Since coronary flow raised at pH 7.4, cardiac
efficiency tended to be lower at this pH level but no significant
change was exhibited.

From these results, it appears that, in moderate hypothermia,
the working heart was able to increase its oxygen consumption in
response to increased workload indicating that O_2 supply-to-demand
ratio was adequately adjusted.

DISCUSSION

The present study describes the effects of blood acid-base changes on the function and oxygen utilization of isolated heart in moderate hypothermia. Our data demonstrate that moderate variations in extracellular acid-base status during hypothermia did not impair either myocardial function or the O_2 supply-to-demand ratio. Hypothermic heart had the capacity to resist noticeable changes in blood pH with no deleterious effect on its functional characteristics even at high workloads.

The blood perfused working isolated rat heart was chosen for these experiments since this model provided a good means for perfusion control through a tissue in which small changes in blood oxygen delivery would be critical to its function. By reconstituted blood perfusate it was possible to satisfy myocardial oxygen demand[3,6] and to investigate the adaptation of heart in hypothermia to acid-base changes involving modifications in blood oxygen release.

The effects of acid-base changes on cardiac function and coronary vascular tone have been largely investigated. It was shown that contractility increased with increasing pH[7,8,9], and that coronary resistance varied inversely with P_{CO2}[10,11]. In the present work the effects of acid-base changes on heart function at 37°C resulted in heart rate acceleration when pH rose and in adaptation in coronary vascular tone causing vasodilation in hypercapnia and vasoconstriction in hypocapnia. The increase in $M\dot{V}_{O2}$ observed with increasing pH was related to a concomitant increase in heart rate, which is known to be a major determinant of oxygen need[12].

The pH values obtained in hypothermia were those that parallel the pH-temperature relationship of neutral water according to the theory of Rahn et al.[1]. Reducing temperature when normal acid-base status is preserved induced both a decrease in heart mechanical performance and $M\dot{V}_{O2}$. Cardiac output and heart rate were decreased. External work and $M\dot{V}_{O2}$ fell proportionately, to 68% of their values in normothermia, with no change in cardiac efficiency. The working isolated heart under hypothermic conditions preserves its capacity for vascular tone regulation since, as in normothermia, coronary flow decreased when pH increased. The increase of heart rate with pH was also observed but the amplitude of variation was less than in normothermia.

The heart works essentially in aerobic conditions, therefore an inadequate oxygen supply to cardiac muscle will induce a rapid fall in cardiac performance and the first criterion of adequate O_2 availability is the capacity of heart to do work. In our experimental model, the determinants of O_2 supply were modified with temperature and acid-base changes. $M\dot{V}_{O2}$ and external work were preserved even when both hypothermia and alkalosis occured, inducing a left shift of the ODC and a coronary flow decrease. These results suggest that cardiac activity was not impaired and oxygen demand was satisfied.

Results from studies undertaken to examine the consequences of pH adaptation to hypothermia using the concept of pH-temperature dependence[13,14,15] suggested that choice of blood acid-base equilibrium is crucial for cellular function and that the only optimum pH value is that which follows the pH-temperature relationship of neutral water. To further define the relationship between O_2 supply and consumption during acid-base changes in hypothermia, new investigations were performed on working hearts in circumstances where the oxygen demand was increased by increasing workload.

It was shown that hypothermic working hearts were able to respond to changes in filling pressure : cardiac output, external work and $M\dot{V}_{O2}$ increased with atrial filling pressure and the coronary vascular bed was capable of flow autoregulation (coronary flow rose in response to change in perfusion pressure). External work was not altered by pH change even at high workload. The only pH effect observed in this experimental group was an increase in coronary flow when pH decreased inducing an increase in $M\dot{V}_{O2}$ at the highest workload. The absence of pH effect on external work is in accordance with results obtained by Clancy and Gonzalez on cat papillary muscle[16]. They showed that the negative inotropic effect of acidosis observed at 38 and 30°C disappeared at 25°C. It remains that the absence of change in cardiac work should be the consequence of two antagonistic effects of pH changes. Whereas myocardial contractility is enhanced by alkalosis, this positive effect on cardiac work may be abolished by a limitation of oxygen delivery due to both decrease of coronary flow and left shifting of the ODC. No conclusion concerning intracellular oxygenation can be made from the present results. We would stress the interest of adding to these experiments the measurement of NADH/NAD ratio by laser fluorometry[17] for a better comprehension of cellular modifications induced by acid-base changes.

Valeri et al.[18] underlined that the poorer O_2 consumption of heart observed during hypothermia could be due to inadequate O_2 delivery in these conditions of left shifted ODC. It would seem reasonable to rule out this hypothesis since in the present work oxygen consumption of working hypothermic heart was able to increase with increasing workload.

In conclusion, these results provide informations for application in the management of organ preservation and the choice of cardioplegic solutions. Although the pH-temperature dependence of biological fluids is unquestionable, the hypothermic isolated organ has the capacity to resist somewhat noticeable changes in blood pH without functional damages. Even in conditions where the oxygen need was increased, no impairment in the O_2 supply-to-demand ratio was evidenced and cardiac work was not altered by pH changes.

REFERENCES

1. H. Rahn, R. B. Reeves and B. J. Howell, Hydrogen ion regulation, temperature and evolution, Am. Rev. Resp. Dis. 112:165 (1975).
2. R. B. Reeves, An imidazole alphastat hypothesis for vertebrate acid-base regulation : tissue carbon dioxide content and body temperature in bullfrogs, Respir. Physiol. 14:219 (1972).
3. M. A. Duvelleroy, M. Duruble, J. L. Martin, B. Teisseire, J. Droulez and M. Cain, Blood perfused working isolated rat heart, J. Appl. Physiol. 41:603 (1976).
4. M. Sinet, M. Muffat-Joly, D. Henzel, G. Renault and J. J. Pocidalo, Performance of hypothermic isolated rat heart at various levels of blood acid-base status, J. Appl. Physiol.: Resp. Environ. Exercise Physiol. 56: 1526 (1984).
5. R. C. Weast, S. M. Selby and C. D. Hodgman, "Handbook of Chemistry and Physics", Cleveland OH (1964).
6. J. L. Martin, M. Duvelleroy, B. Teisseire and M. Duruble, Effect of an increase in HbO_2 affinity on the calculated capillary recruitment of an isolated rat heart, Pfluegers Arch. 382:57 (1979).
7. N. C. Gonzalez, R. L. Clancy, Inotropic and intracellular acid-base changes during metabolic acidosis, Am. J. Physiol 228:1060 (1975).
8. J. R. Williamson, B. Safer, T. Rich, S. Schaffer and K. Kobayashi, Effects of acidosis on myocardial contractility and metabolism, Acta Med. Scand. Suppl. 587:95 (1976).
9. P. A. Poole-Wilson and C. A. Langer, Effects of acidosis on mechanical function and Ca^{2+} exchange in rabbit myocardium, Am. J. Physiol. 236:H525 (1979).
10. R. B. Case, A. Felix, M. Watcher, G. Kryakidis and F. Castellana, Relative effect of CO_2 on canine coronary vascular resistance, Circ. Res. 42:410 (1978).
11. T. Rooke and H. V. Sparks, Arterial CO_2, myocardial O_2 consumption and coronary blood flow in the dog, Circ. Res. 47/217 (1980).
12. K. T. Weber and J. S. Janicki, The metabolic demand and oxygen supply of the heart : physiologic and clinical considerations, Am. J. Cardiol. 44:722 (1979).
13. H. Becker, J. Vinten Johansen, G. D. Buckberg, J. M. Robertson, J. D. Leaf, H. L. Lazar and A. J. Manganaro, Myocardial damage caused by keeping pH 7.40 during systemic deep hypothermia, J. Thorac. Cardiovasc. Surg. 82: 810 (1981).
14. M. C. Blayo, Y. Lecompte and J. J. Pocidalo, Control of acid-base status during hypothermia in man, Respir. Physiol. 42/287 (1980).

15. J. N. Carter, F. N. White, G. M. Collins and N.A. Halasz, Studies of the ideal [H⁺] for perfusional preservation, Transplantation 30:409 (1980).
16. R. L. Clancy and N. C. Gonzalez, Influence of temperature upon inotropic effect of metablolic acidosis in cat papillary muscles, Proc. Soc. Exp. Biol. Med. 145:904 (1974).
17. G. Renault, E. Raynal, M. Sinet, M. Muffat-Joly, J. P. Berthier, J. Cornillault, B. Godard and J. J. Pocidalo, In situ double-beam NADH laser fluorometry : choice of a reference wave-lenght, Am. J. Physiol. 246:491 (1984).
18. C. R. Valeri, M. Yarnoz, J. J. Vecchione, R. C. Dennis, J. Anastasi, D.A. Valeri, L. E. Pivacek and H. B. Hechtman, Improved oxygen delivery to the myocardium during hypothermia by perfusion with 2,3 DPG-enriched red blood cells, Ann. Thorac. Surg. 30:527 (1980).

IN SITU NADH LASER FLUORIMETRY AND ITS

APPLICATION TO THE STUDY OF CARDIAC METABOLISM

Guy Renault, Elisabeth Raynal, Martine Sinet, Martine
Muffat-Joly, Jean Cornillault*, and Jean-Jacques Pocidalo

INSERM U13 Hopital Claude Bernard
75944 Paris, France
* Cilas-Alcatel, Marcoussis, France

INTRODUCTION

The in vivo fluorimetry of NADH has proven to be a very efficient
method for non-destructive investigation of organ metabolism. First
defined by Chance and his group(1) this method was subsequently
extended to numerous experimental models and provided important
information on challenging topics, such as the importance of the
border zone in myocardial infarction.

The continuous monitoring of the intratissular NADH level could
potentially be an important advance in the study of such diverse
fields of medicine and surgery as myocardial and cerebral ischemia
and the tissular viability of organs during transplantation or bypass surgery, among others.   However, few authors have considered
the clinical applicability of this method(2, 3)for several reasons.
Until now the microfluorimeters, being heavy, cumbersome and lacking
sensitivity and versatility, could only be used in experimental
research units. Moreover, blood circulation in living tissue
(hemodynamic artifact) disturbed the fluorescent measure. Therefore,
the studies were mainly performed on experimental models perfused
with blood-free solutions.

To overcome these obstacles, we developed an apparatus called
the laser fluorimeter, especially designed for studies of NADH level
in in situ and blood-perfused organs in an intact organism(4, 5, 6)
together with a new method of elimination of "hemodynamic artifact"(7).
The entire device has been successful experimentally on varied in vivo
and in situ experimented models and an industrial prototype is currently being developed for clinical applications.

PRINCIPLE OF THE DEVICE

We have thus developed a device(4)which includes (Fig.1) :
- a nitrogen laser
- an optical unit with a dye laser, an optical set-up and
  photoreceivers
- an optical probe
- an analog circuits unit
- a microcomputer

DESCRIPTION OF THE DEVICE

1 - We chose the nitrogen laser first because of its wavelength
(337 nm) which is very close to the absorption peak of NADH (reduced
nicotinamide adenine dinucleotide). It must be pointed out that, at
this wavelength, light absorption by this compound only occurs when
it is reduced (NADH) and not when it is oxidized (NAD$^+$). This absorption is followed by a fluorescent emission (peak 480 nm) from the
irradiated tissue which is proportional to the amount of excited
NADH and is thus a direct function of the intratissular NADH to NAD
ratio.

In addition to its wavelength, the nitrogen laser was advantageous
for three reasons : (i) its pulse repetition rate allows at least ten

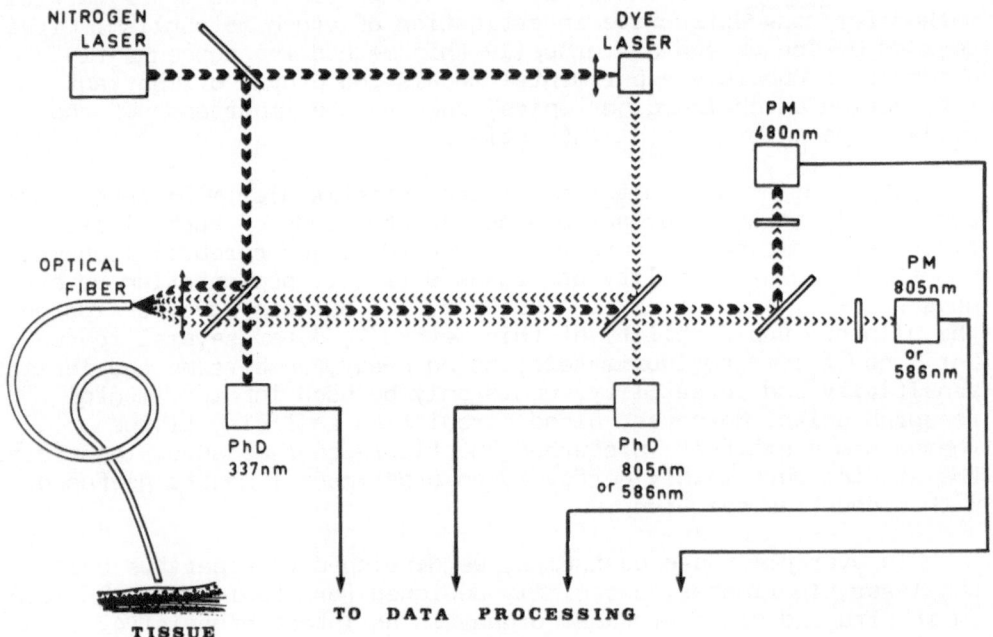

Fig.1: block diagram of optical system of laser fluorimeter

measurements during a single cardiac cycle, even on rat heart whose frequency is about 5-6 hz.(ii) pulsed light sources improve sensitivity of measurements in fluorimetry. (iii) its pulses last a very short time (about 3 ns) : this allows relatively high power to be emitted along with small average power deposition in the living tissue.

2 - The dye laser gives a reference light whose wavelength can easily be tuned by simply changing the dye. Our experiments led us to the choice of 586 nm as a reference wavelength, because its optical behaviour, especially relating to absorption by hemoglobin, is as close as possible to the optical behaviour of the fluorescence, without interfering with it (805 nm which we first used, did not prove to be accurate).

Furthermore, 586 nm is an isobestic point for hemoglobin,i.e the absorption by hemoglobin at this wavelength does not vary with its oxygenation state.

The back-scattering of the reference light by the tissue is thus only a function of the intra-tissular blood content and this signal can be used to compensate the signal of measured fluorescence for the variations induced by blood circulation into the tissue.

3 - An optical fiber F.O.I conducts the ultraviolet NADH excitation light and the reference light to the living tissue, and collects the back-scattered (I) and fluorescent (F) lights arising from this tissue.

This optical probe, which is 5 meters long and 400 microns in core diameter, has especially designed end faces, in order to cancel out parasitic lights at the two extremities of the fiber(5).

4 - Optical system and photoreceivers.

An optical system of lenses, mirrors, beam splitters and filters accurately focuses, reflects or conducts light beams from sources to the fiber and from the fiber to the photoreceivers (two photodiodes phD and two photomultipliers PM).

5 - Analogic circuit.

The aim of this electronic system is to give a signal proportional to the recorded energy with every impulse by the photomultiplier, while compensating the influence of possible variations of laser source intensities and while performing the gating of parasitic impulses.

6 - Microcomputer.

Analogic data (F and I) are continuously displayed on a chart recorder, after 5 Hz filtering, and are simultaneously converted into digital data for introduction into a HP 85 (Hewlett-Packard) microcomputer. The fluorescence signal is then processed in order to cancel the effects of variations in intratissular blood content on the fluorescence measure (hemodynamic artifact) by using the reference signal and an accurate relationship between I and F established in vivo (see below). The signal given by this processing is Fo, which is a linear function of the intratissular concentration of NADH (see below).

The digital processing of data (together with the use of a single optical fiber) gives the system great versatility.

BIOLOGICAL EXPERIMENTS

In Vitro Measurements

1) Measurements on test surfaces : absolute calibration. Up until now, in in vivo fluorimetry measurements of fluorescence and refection in absolute values were not possible and the results were expressed in relative values (%) of the baseline fluorescence, measured at the beginning of the experiment on a normoxic tissue. With our apparatus, as the geometry of the interface (tip of the fiber-observed tissue) was quite steady, such measurements could be carried out : at each experiment, calibration values of the fluorescence (F) and of the reflection (I) were measured on a neutral test card Kodak and were used to calibrate (in percentage) the values of F and I obtained from the biological model.

2) Measurements on non-perfused isolated tissues.

An experimental model 8 was developed to determine the optical properties of organ slices and diluted blood samples, in order to compute, from in vitro data, the coefficient K1/K2 of the relationship for compensation of hemodynamic artifacts in in situ NADH laser fluorimetry. The system used proved to be accurate, reliable and versatile for optical measurements on biological tissues. It allowed measurement of transmittance of rat liver and rat heart slices of 100, 200 and 500 um thickness and of diluted blood samples (2%, 4%, 6%) at the same thickness. Beer's law was demonstrated to apply to signal analysis in in situ NADH laser fluorimetry, at the wavelengths used in this technique : $\lambda 1 = 337$ nm, $\lambda 2 = 473$nm, $\lambda 3 = 586$ nm.

In Vivo Measurements

To assess the method, in vivo we used a system of isolated

perfused rat heart, with retrograde perfusion by the aorta, according to the Langendorff technique; we had the possibility of rapidly shifting the perfusate between the four permanently available perfusates (Fig.2) : KO2 oxygenated Krebs-Henseleit buffer, KN2 non-oxygenated Krebs-Henseleit buffer, BO2 oxygenated blood, BN2 non-oxygenated blood.

The "blood" was in fact a mixture of Krebs-Henseleit buffer and washed erythrocytes of pig, up to a hematocrit of 30%. The tip of the fiber was positioned against the middle part of the left ventricle with a micromanipulator and the mechanical artifact due to the wall motion was easily cancelled by exerting a slight pressure on the heart.

With this model, we established the relationship for compensating the fluorescence for the artifact induced by blood circulation into the tissue(7):

$$Fo = F (I/Io)^{- K1/K2}$$

This relation was established by eliminating the intratissular blood content N between the two exponential relations of the fluorescence and of the reflectance with N :

$$F = Fo\ e^{- K1N} \qquad I = Io\ e^{- K2N}$$

according to the application of Beer's law in the conditions of in situ fluorimetry.

Figure 3 shows a typical experiment performed on our isolated rat heart model with the variations of Fo (compensated fluorescence : upper panel), F (fluorescence : middle panel), I (reflectance : lower panel) during a sequence of four tests (anoxia, hematocrit shift and two combined tests).

Thus, anoxia is expressed by an increase in the measured fluorescence Fo (state 3 to state 5 transition); a change in hematocrit on an anoxic heart leads to marked decreases in F and I, but to a constant compensated fluorescence (state 5).

In Situ Measurements

1) Rats : surgical approach.

These experiments were performed on ventilated rats, anesthetized with pentobarbital. The chest was opened and the tip of the fiber was positioned against the wall of the middle part of the left ventricle with a device which allowed a good control of the incidence angle between optical fiber axis and heart surface, as well as a control of the pressure applied by the fiber tip on the

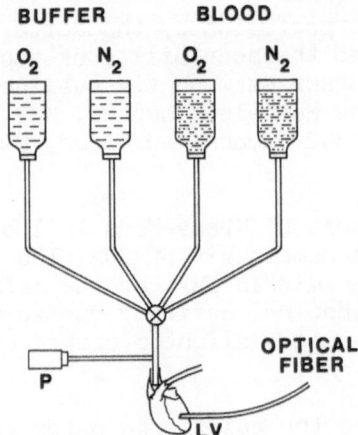

BUFFER   BLOOD

Fig.2 Experimental
model of isolated
perfused rat heart

T·

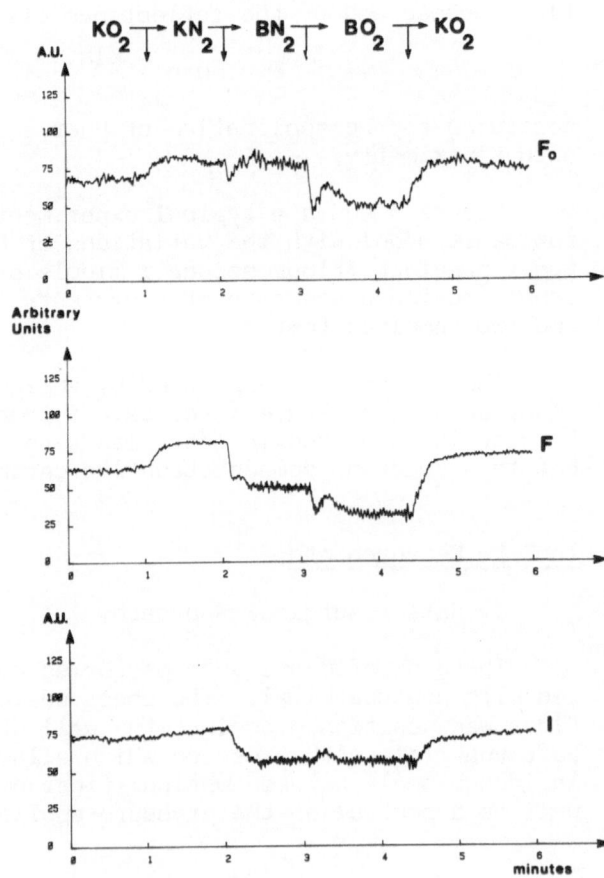

Fig.3 Typical experiment
in vivo on isolated
perfused rat heart

tissue. This device also allowed pressurization (for a short period) to be exerted by the fiber tip on the tissue surface, thus inducing a local ischemia in the examination zone.

With this device, we obtained the results presented in Figure 4 :

- in the "A" panel, on rat hearts anesthetized by slight doses of pentobarbital, 3 local ischemia tests gave a large increase in fluorescence and little increase in reflectance. The 3 tests were perfectly reproducible, and the energetic state of the heart was a state 3 of Chance's nomenclature.

- in the "B" panel, on animals which received large doses of pentobarbital, the same 3 ischemia tests did not give any increase in fluorescence or reflectance. The energetic state of the myocardium was a state 4 or 5 of Chance's nomenclature, explained by a direct inhibition of NADH dehydrogenase by pentobarbital(8).

- in the "C" panel, the same 3 tests performed after an anoxia period gave very large increases in fluorescence and reflectance. The compensated fluorescence was similar to that obtained in "A". The

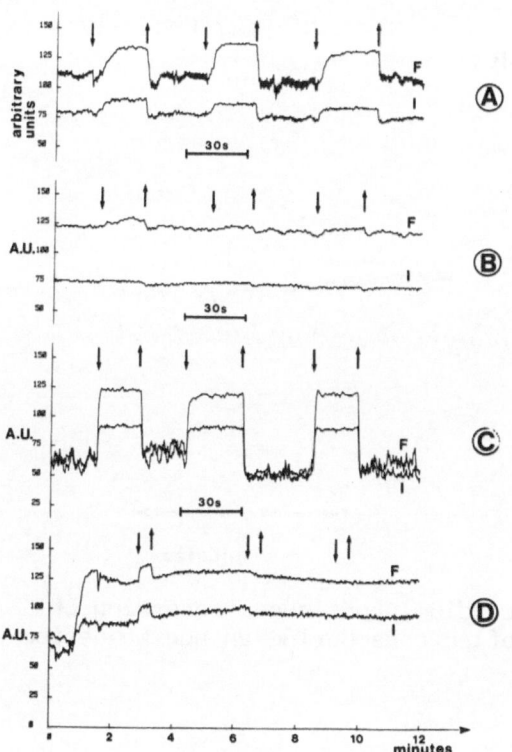

Fig.4 Pressurization test : continuous recording of F and I

A usual response.
   downward arrow :pressing
   upward arrow :loosening

B response on a tissue already at its maximal NADH reduction level

C response during an anoxia recovery period

D response after the death of the rat

energetic state was also a state 3 of Chance's nomenclature.

- last of all, in the "D" panel, the same 3 ischemia tests were
performed immediately after the animal's death by complete anoxia.
After the sudden rise in the NADH to NAD ratio due to anoxia, the
first ischemia test induced similar increases in fluorescence and
reflectance, due to the blood being expelled from the examination
zone. The tests which followed did not give any variation in fluorescence or reflectance, as the tissue was at its maximal reduction level
and was not perfused.

Thus, the local ischemia test by pressurization allows the
instantaneous determination of the maximal NADH reduction level
in the myocardium; this maximal level can then be used as a reference
for assessing the steady state level, obtained before and after the
test.

From this information (maximal level of NADH during pressurization compared to steady state level), it is possible to determine
whether ATP production in the zone of the tissue investigated is still
continuing, thereby preserving tissular viability, or has stopped.

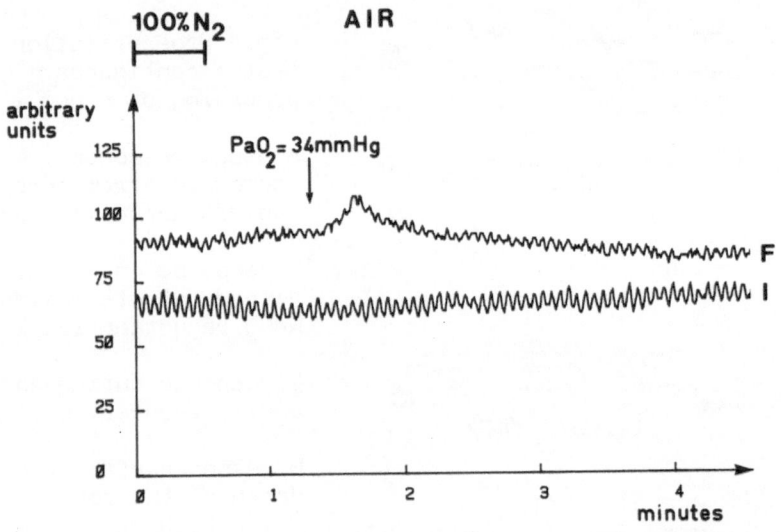

Fig.5 Dog right ventricle endocardium, continuous recording of
NADH fluorescence and 586 nm reflectance during an anoxia period

In this way, we think that this test can now be applied to the intraoperative on-line assessment of the adequacy of myocardial preservation during cardiac operation.

2) Dogs : heart catheterization.

To perform in situ studies of the (NADH) red/ox state of the left or right endomyocardium of the intact dogs, we used a modified Mobin-Uddin catheter. The modifications consisted in removing the distal capsule and in "rounding off" the new extremity. This catheter then allowed good control of the movements of the optical fiber inside the catheter and, with this experimental arrangement, we could measure fluorescence and reflectance from the right or left endocardial wall. Figure 5 shows the variations in the fluorescence and in the reflectance during a test of anoxia at the level of the apex of the right endomyocardium of an intact dog. This anoxia was achieved by having the dog breathe 100% nitrogen for a period of 30 seconds. The arterial PO2 just before the rising of the NADH to NAD ratio was 34 mmHg.

CONCLUSION

In conclusion, we have demonstrated the feasibility of measurement of NADH oxido-reduction state on line and in situ and we have developed the corresponding device. In this way, without any destructive sampling, we can obtain information on the in situ mitochondrial red/ox state. Such information can be of major clinical importance in that it should permit early diagnosis of potentially dangerous situations, in terms of myocardial viability, and thus enable proper clinical procedures to be undertaken. We also feel that this is a preferential method for studying the intracellular effects of cardiac-aimed drugs.

Finally, we should point out the ubiquitous nature of NADH, enabling this method to be equally applied to studies of cerebral, renal and hepatic metabolisms.

REFERENCES

1. B.Chance, J.R. Williamson, D. Jamieson, and B. Schroener, Properties and kinetics of reduced pyridine nucleotide fluorescence of the isolated and in vivo rat heart, Biochem.Z. 341 : 357-377 (1965).

2. S.Kobayashi, K.Nishiki, K.Kaede and E.Ogata, Optical consequences of blood substitution on tissue oxidation-reduction state microfluorometry, J.Appl.Physiol. 31 : 93-96 (1971).

3. S.A.Mills, F.F.Jöbsis and A.V.Seaber, A fluorimeter study of oxidative metabolism in the in vivo canine heart during acute ischemia and hypoxia, Ann.Surg. 186 : 193-200 (1977).

4. G.Renault, E.Raynal, M.Sinet, J.P.Berthier, B.Godard and J.Cornillault, A laser fluorimeter for direct cardiac metabolism investigation, Optics and laser technology 14 : 143-148 (1982).

5. G.Renault, E.Raynal, and J.Cornillault, Cancelling of Fresnel reflections in in situ double beam laser fluorimetry using a single optical fibre, J.Biomed.Eng 5 : 243-247 (1983).

6. G.Renault, M.Sinet, M.Muffat-Joly, E.Raynal, J.P.Berthier, R.L.Inglebert, J.Cornillault and B.Godard, In situ monitoring of living organs metabolism with a laser fluorimeter, SPIE proceedings 405 : 34-43 (1984).

7. G.Renault, E.Raynal, M.Sinet, M.Muffat-Joly, J.P.Berthier, J.Cornillault, B.Godard, and J.J.Pocidalo, In situ double-beam NADH laser fluorimetry : choice of a reference wavelength, Am.J. Physiol. 246 : H491-H499 (1984).

8. I.Kissin, D.F.Aultman and L.R.Smith, Effects of volatile anesthetics on myocardial oxidation-reduction status assessed by NADH fluorometry, Anesthesiology 59 : 447-452 (1983).

VARIABILITY OF INTERCAPILLARY DISTANCE ESTIMATED ON HISTOLOGICAL
SECTIONS OF RAT HEART

L. Hoofd, Z. Turek, K. Kubat[+], B.E.M. Ringnalda, and
S. Kazda[*]

Department of Physiology, University of Nijmegen
[+]Department of Pathol. Anatomy, University of Nijmegen
Nijmegen, The Netherlands
[*]Institute of Pharmacology, Bayer AG., Wuppertal, FRG

INTRODUCTION

The majority of models of O_2 supply to myocardial tissue are
based on the classical model of Krogh (1919). This model requires
the radius of the tissue cylinder as one of the crucial input data.
Usually, only its mean value has been considered, as derived on histological sections from the number of capillaries per mm^2. However,
for a realistic description, the full distribution of the radii of
the tissue cylinders has to be taken into account. Recently this
distribution was shown to be approximately log-normal (Renkin et al.,
1981; Turek and Rakusan, 1981), and thus to be fully defined by
median radius and logarithmic standard deviation (log SD), the latter
serving as an index of the variability.

Renkin et al. (1981) measured the distances between capillaries
by drawing a net of non-overlapping triangles. From this they derived
median and log SD of the radii of the tissue cylinders. However, the
majority of studies attempting to characterize the heterogeneity of
capillary spacing focused their attention on the distribution of
tissue at various distances from the nearest capillary (Loats et al.,
1978; Kayar et al., 1982). Such an approach does not provide directly
median and log SD. These, however, can be derived by an indirect procedure (Turek and Rakusan, 1981; Rakusan and Turek, 1984).

In the present paper we present a new computerized method for
the estimation of mean and log SD of the radius of tissue cylinder,

the method of capillary domains. Once the coordinates of the capillaries on a photomicrograph have been fed into the computer, using an
image analyzer, no further effort is required. Thus, the total time
needed does not differ much from that required for counting the capillaries only. This avoids the serious handicap of the previous
methods, the tediousness and great time demand.

METHODS

Five untreated rats with spontaneous hypertension (SHR), body
weight (b.w.; mean +S.D.) of 408 + 8 g, seven SHR rats treated with
Nifedipin 300 ppm daily for 20 weeks (NIF), b.w. of 390 + 11 g, and
five control rats of Kyoto-Wistar strain (KYW), b.w. of 400 + 8 g,
were used. SHR rats were chosen here, as from a previous study it
was to be expected that they develop a larger heterogeneity of myocardial capillary spacing than their controls (Rakusan et al., 1984).
Therefore they could provide a good material for checking the newly
developed method of capillary domains. The effect of Nifedipin on
capillarization was unknown. Small numbers of animals were judged
to be sufficient, as the primary purpose of this paper was to check
the new method rather than to study the pharmacological effects of
Nifedipin.

Immediately after sacrificing the animals the hearts were excised, weighed and transversely sliced through the ventricles. The
middle portions between apex and base were selected and frozen in
liquid nitrogen. The cryostat slices, 7 μm thick, were incubated for
30 minutes for the activity of alkaline phosphatase after Burstone
(Pearse, 1968), where Napthol AS-TR phosphate was used as a substrate
and Fast Blue B as a dye. Afther the incubation the slices were fixed
in 4% formaline overnight and the impregnation of reticulin fibres
was performed in a 5x diluted Ag-solution for 5 minutes. Due to the
latter procedure, the blue color marking the activity of alkaline
phosphatase turned rose to red.

Photomicrographs of the subendocardial region of the left ventricle were processed into a computer (PDP11-series) by using an
X-Y Tablet (Summagraphics), which feeds the location on the Tablet
into the computer as a pair of coordinates. A computer program
(TABLET) picks up and recalculates the data and stores them on a
disk. The following data were read in:

- First, the edge points of the photograph were stored to determine
  the dimensions and borders;
- Three points in the photograph were marked and stored as "marking
  points". If read in more than once, e.g. for both capillaries and
  open spaces, the correct placement of the photograph on both occasions could be checked from these marks;
- Hereafter, a series of coordinates was stored (see below);

- Data were saved under a unique 8-letter identification in a datafile on disk.

Four types of data could be stored for each photomicrograph under separate identifications:

1) The coordinates of each center of a capillary;
2) Open spaces: regions that appear to be void. These were stored as a series of coordinates located on the border of the region. A new series, for a different region, was marked by a point outside the photograph;
3) Connective tissue: a type of tissue that appears to be different from the rest of the tissue. Stored in the same way as for the open spaces;
4) Fibers: also stored as bounding coordinates.

An example of 1) and 2) is shown in Fig. 1a. Data of this kind were checked and processed in consecutive computer programs (see below); data of types 3) and 4) were not used here.

THEORY

The principle of the method of capillary domains, proposed here, is to allot to each capillary its surrounding area. Border lines between "central" and all neighboring capillaries were drawn at equal distance from both capillaries considered. These lines intersected and thus demarkated the region of the tissue enclosed around the "central" capillary. Coordinates are denoted x and y, coordinates of the "central" capillary of the domain to be determined are x_c and y_c, and coordinates of the neighboring capillary to be considered are x_n and y_n. Then we define the function:

$$L(x,y) = 2y(y_n-y_c) + 2x(x_n-x_c) + x_c{}^2 - x_n{}^2 + y_c{}^2 - y_n{}^2 \qquad (1)$$

Now the border line between both capillaries is given by the equation $L(x,y) = 0$; and that portion of the plane that is closer to the domain capillary is given by $L(x,y) < 0$. In this way, the total picture was subdivided into a number of adjacent polygonic domains around the capillaries (see Fig. 1b). The surface area of each domain was calculated and stored. Domains bordering on the side lines of the photomicrograph were marked; they can be excluded without biasing the population. If there were open spaces, also the domains that overlapped the open spaces were traced and marked.

One of the literature methods to characterize the capillary spacing in tissue is to impose a grid on the picture and determine, for each grid point, the distance to the nearest capillary ("closest-individual method"; Kayar et al., 1982). In our computer program, this type of treatment was applied too; we will refer to it as the "grid method". The grid is a square array, excluding a border zone with a width of the approximate mean intercapillary distance (see

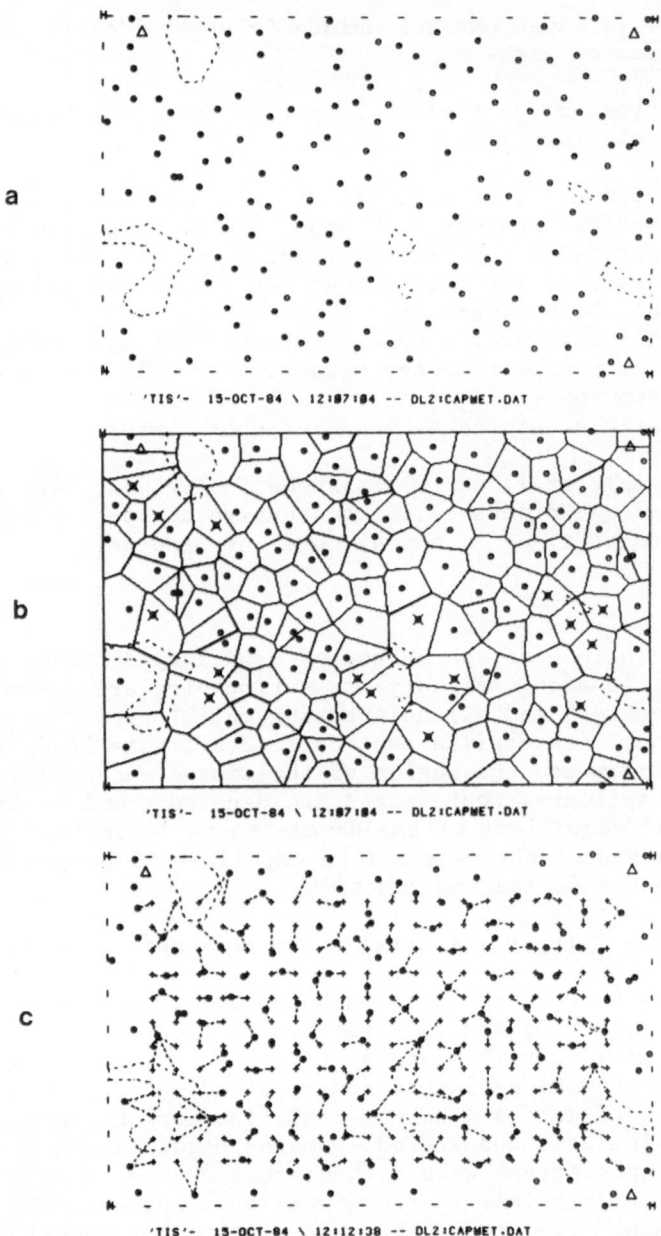

Fig. 1. Three steps of computer processing of one rat heart slice.
(a) Computer replot of stored data showing photomicrograph
side lines (H – – – H), marks (Δ), capillaries (Θ) and
open spaces (....); (b) The same with domains around each
capillary; capillaries crossed out indicate domains overlapping an open space ; (c) The same photograph with superimposed grid of 15 µm spacing; each grid point (+) is connected (---) to its nearest capillary.

Fig. 1c). If this border zone were not excluded, erroneous results might ensue. A grid point in the zone may or may not be closer to a capillary just outside the photomicrograph, and it is impossible to select which distance is correct and which is not. If only those grid points were omitted that were closer to the boundary than to a capillary, the population would become biased: grid points with a large distance from a capillary would be more likely to be excluded than grid points near a capillary. Only very occasionally a grid point was closer to the border line than to a capillary; these points were traced and marked by the computer program.

In the computer program for these calculations (TIS), also the input data could be corrected, as a forgotten or a doubly registered capillary leads to surface areas and/or grid point distances far from their correct values. For calculation of distribution of the data, such errors should be avoided.

A consecutive computer program (CTIS) allows the calculated data to be grouped into classes or fitted to a lognormal distribution (see below). Either one single or more photomicrographs together could be sampled. Here the data were handled in the following way:

- From the domain areas, the equivalent radii of a Krogh cylinder with the same surface area were calculated as a measure of intercapillary distance.
- From the grid point distances, the distribution of intercapillary distances was calculated according to Turek and Rakusan (1981) and Rakusan and Turek (1984);
- The results of both methods were fitted to a lognormal frequency distribution:

$$f(R) = \frac{\log(e)}{\sigma R \sqrt{2\pi}} \ \exp \left[-\frac{1}{2} \left\{ \frac{\log(R) - \log(R_m)}{\sigma} \right\}^2 \right]$$

where R = Krogh radius, R_m = Median radius and σ = log Standard Deviation, which will be referred to as "heterogeneity index". Krogh radius should be equivalent to half the intercapillary distance.

RESULTS

Rats with spontaneous hypertension developed high mean arterial blood pressure (237 $\pm$ 12 mm Hg; mean $\pm$ S.D.) as expected. The treatment with Nifedipin decreased it significantly (169 $\pm$ 7 mm Hg) without, however, reaching the control values (130 $\pm$ 11 mm Hg). For the sake of simplicity, only values measured before sacrificing the rats are presented here. A similar trend was observed concerning the weight of the ventricular part of the heart. SHR rats had a pronounced cardiac hypertrophy (1247 $\pm$ 26 mg) as compared to SHR treated with Nifedipin (1125 $\pm$ 43 mg) and Kyoto-Wistar rats (992 $\pm$ 21 mg).

Photomicrographs of the subendocardium, covering a region of approximately 225 x 340 μm, of all three groups of rats were subjected to both methods described in Theory.

A typical example of a partial result of the method of capillary domains on one photomicrograph is shown on Fig. 1b. The surfaces of the domains indicated on the Figure were calculated and those of photographs belonging to one rat were stored separately and further processed as a unit. These data were directly gathered into a lognormal distribution to calculate median R_m and heterogeneity index σ too. From each surface area A, the equivalent Krogh radius could be obtained as $R = \sqrt{A/\pi}$. However, mainly for practical reasons, the lognormal distribution was fitted for the surface areas A. This can be recalculated easily in lognormal parameters for the Krogh radii R because of the linear relationship between log (A) and log (R):

$$\log (A) = \log (\pi) + 2 \log (R) \qquad (3)$$

Additionally, on each photomicrograph, a grid with a spacing of 15 μm was superimposed (see Fig. 1c). Distances between grid points and the center of the nearest capillary were calculated. Results of each rat were pooled. Subsequently they were gathered into classes with a width of 2 μm. The frequency distribution obtained in this way was fitted to a model of lognormally distributed capillaries according to Turek and Rakusan (1981) to yield values of median R_m and heterogeneity index σ.

For either group of rats and either calculation method, mean and standard deviation of both R_m and σ were calculated. Results are shown in Fig. 2. There is a distinct difference in both calculation methods in that the "grid method" yields somewhat lower values of the median radius R_m and much larger values of the heterogeneity index σ when compared to the method of capillary domains. Both differences are significant (t-test: $P < 2\%$ and $P \ll 0.1\%$ respectively).

Using the "grid method", no significant difference could be detected between the different groups of rats, neither in R_m nor in σ. With the "domain method", also no difference was found in the median radius R_m, but there was a difference in heterogeneity index σ between controls and hypertensive rats: weakly significant for groups KYW and NIF (t-test: $P < 5\%$), and more significant for groups KYW and SHR (t-test: $P < 2\%$). No difference could be detected between nontreated and treated hypertensive rats (SHR and NIF).

DISCUSSION

The "domain method" proposed here is an easy and visually appealing method to determine capillarization of a tissue slice. Values of the surface areas A of each domain can be directly gathered into a lognormal distribution. Although these domains are polygons and

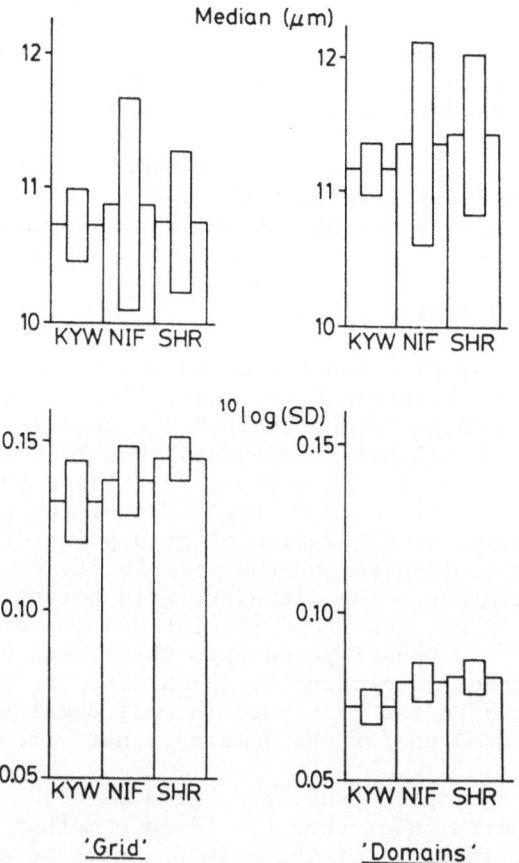

Fig. 2. Comparison of Median R_m (top half) and log Standard Deviation σ (bottom half) of Krogh cylinder radii for two methods of calculation and three groups of rats. Results shown on the left side of the figure were calculated using the "closest- individual method" (Kayar et al., 1982), results on the right by the "domain method" proposed here. Mean values (thick bars) are shown with their Standard Deviation (small bars) for groups KYW=Control group, NIF=hypertensive treated, and SHR=Hypertensive untreated.

not circles, the oxygen field may very well resemble the oxygen distribution in a Krogh cylinder. Even for domains where the capillary is not at a central place, less oxygen is needed for a region with a nearby boundary and consequently more oxygen will go into the region that is most remote, thus raising the oxygen pressure at the most distant boundary above that predicted from the Krogh-Erlang formula for such a distance. Therefore, we feel entitled in translating the area A into a Krogh cylinder radius R, to obtain median value R_m and log Standard Deviation σ for these radii.

Furthermore, the mean value of the domain areas is the inverse value of capillary density so that the method inclusively yields this quantity. We may recall here that, for a lognormal distribution as in eq. (2), the mean value $\bar{R}$ is related to R_m and σ according to:

$$\bar{R} = R_m \exp \{[\sigma \ln (10)]^2/2\} \qquad (4)$$

The most obvious difference between the results of both methods is the difference in heterogeneity index. Although there is also a difference in the median "Krogh radius" R_m, this is merely a consequence of eq. (4): capillarity index and thus $\bar{R}$ must be equal in both methods so that a different value of σ leads to different R_m and vice versa. The difference is explained by the non-circular shape of the domains. Recalculation of grid point distances into Krogh cylinder radii is based on the circularity of the cylinder. For a single domain not being circular, grid points will be distributed as if they originated from circular domains of different size. This heterogeneity is superimposed upon the tissue heterogeneity and will lead to a larger heterogeneity index. So, the difference between both methods is due to the fact that in most domains the capillary is not centrally located and/or the domain is not circular.

This reasoning implies that the "grid method" yields a different type of heterogeneity index than the "domain method". Therefore, it is not surprising that one of the methods leads to a significant difference between two groups of tissue while the other one does not. We may recall here that there is no contradiction: if a statistical method does not indicate a significant difference, this is no proof that there is no such difference. Although obvious, this fact tends to be overlooked easily.

The "domain method" indicated a significant difference in heterogeneity index between controls and hypertensive rats. One of the possible explanations may be found in an extension of the capillary network following hypertrophy of the hypertensive rat heart. As a first step, the intercapillary distances are increased due to hypertrophy of the muscle fibers. The next step then might be proliferation of capillaries in some places, so that the overall capillary distance is restored. These newly formed capillaries will decrease the intercapillary distance in their vicinity: altogether

246

the heterogeneity of capillary spacing will be accentuated.

REFERENCES

Kayar, S.R., Archer, P.G., Lechner, A.J. and Banchero, N., 1982, The closest-individual method in the analysis of the distribution of capillaries, Microvasc. Res., 24:326-341.

Krogh, A., 1919, The number and distribution of capillaries in muscles with calculations of the oxygen pressure head necessary for supplying the tissue, J. Physiol. (London), 52:409-415.

Loats, J.T., Sillau, A.H., and Banchero, N., 1978, How to quantify skeletal muscle capillarity, in: "Oxygen Transport to Tissue-III", I.A. Silver, M. Erecińska, and H.I. Bicher, eds., Adv. Exper. Med. Biol., Vol. 94, Plenum Press, New York and London, pp. 41-48.

Pearse, A.G.E., 1968, "Histochemistry", Vol. 1, J. & A. Churchill, London, p. 732.

Rakusan, K., and Turek, Z., 1984, A comparison of the methods for assessment of myocardial capillarity, in: "Oxygen Transport to Tissue-V", D.W. Lübbers, H. Acker, E. Leniger-Follert, and T.K. Goldstick, eds., Adv. Exper. Med. Biol., Vol. 169, Plenum Press, New York and London, pp. 411-418.

Rakusan, K., Hrdina, P.W., Turek, Z., Lakatta, E.G., Spurgeon, H.A., and Wolford, G.D., 1984, Cell size and capillary supply of the hypertensive rat heart: quantitative study, Bas. Res. Cardiol., 79:389-395.

Renkin, E.M., Gray, S.D., Dodd, L.R., and Lia, B.D., 1981, Heterogeneity of capillary distribution and capillary circulation in mammalian skeletal muscles, in: "Underwater Physiology", Vol. 7, A.J. Bachrach and M.M. Matzen, eds., Undersea Medical Soc., Bethesda, pp. 465-474.

Turek, Z., and Rakusan, K., 1981, Lognormal distribution of intercapillary distance in normal and hypertrophic rat heart as estimated by the method of concentric circles: its effect on tissue oxygenation, Pflügers Arch. 391:17-21.

MYOCARDIAL CAPILLARITY OF RATS EXPOSED TO SIMULATED HIGH ALTITUDE

Z. Turek, L.J.C. Hoofd, B.E.M. Ringnalda, K. Rakusan

Department of Physiology, Faculty of Medicine, University
of Nijmegen, The Netherlands, and Department of
Physiology, School of Medicine, University of Ottawa
Ottawa, Ontario, Canada

INTRODUCTION

The main purpose of the present study was to apply our new
method of computerized evaluation of "capillary domains" to practical problems dealing with capillarization of hearts from rats adapted to high altitude. The method itself is described in detail in another contribution to this volume (Hoofd et al., 1985). It is a convenient way to obtain not only the average radius of the Krogh
tissue cylinder but also the degree of heterogeneity in capillary
spacing. Both of these parameters are important determinants of
tissue oxygenation. The former is included in the Krogh-Erlang equation while the latter has been only recently reported as a factor
influencing tissue oxygen supply (Turek and Rakusan, 1981).

In spite of traditional "textbook" descriptions of increased
capillarization in mammalian hearts in animals adapted to high altitude, there is a growing number of reports which failed to find such
a response or which even reported a decreased capillarization following adaptation to this environment. Therefore, we decided to re-
examine this question using more advanced morphometric techniques
which yield not only the average capillarity of the myocardial
tissue but also the heterogeneity of the capillary spacing.

METHODS

Fourteen male rats of Wistar strain, 30 days old, were divided
into two equal groups. Experimental animals were placed in a low
pressure chamber which was maintained automatically at a barometric
pressure corresponding to an altitude of 3500 m. The exposure was
as continuous as possible with breaks necessary for cleaning, food

249

and water supply taking about half an hour every second day. The remaining rats served as controls and were kept in the same room outside the chamber in order to expose both groups to similar temperature and level of noise. This regime was kept for 85 days. Afterwards the rats were anesthetized with Nembutal (40 mg per kg body weight). Blood samples were taken from the abdominal aorta for the estimation of hematocrit and hemoglobin concentration using standard methods.

Hearts were fixed in a mixture of 1.5 per cent glutaraldehyde buffered to pH 7.4 with sodium cacodylate administered by a retrograde aortic perfusion at a pressure of 100 mm Hg. Hearts were removed after 20 minutes of perfusion, ventricles were separated from atria, the ventricular part of the heart was divided into right ventricle and left ventricle plus septum (Rakusan et al., 1984 a), and weighed. Cubical sections were taken from the mid-wall and subendocardial location of each ventricle. They were oriented in order to obtain tissue sections perpendicular to the long axis of the muscle fibers. Subsequently, the samples were post-fixed with 2 per cent OsO_4 and 150 mmol sodium cacodylate, washed overnight, dehydrated and embedded in Epon. Photomicrographs of 1 µm thick toluidine-stained sections were taken from each location (five to six photomicrographs per region, each having an area of 28 500 $µm^2$).

Our morphometric approach was described in detail by Hoofd et al. (1985). It consists of estimating the distribution of capillary domains and comparing the results with those obtained by the closest-individual method (Kayar et al., 1982). First, the position of each capillary was recorded using an image analyzer and stored in the memory. From the number of capillaries and the surface area, capillary density was derived (the number of capillaries per mm^2). Then the surface area surrounding each capillary, the capillary domain, was determined as follows: Each capillary was connected with a set of neighboring capillaries and lines perpendicular to these connections were drawn through the midpoints. These new lines intersected and thus defined a polygon, the domain of the "central" capillary. Surface areas of all domains were stored. Their distribution was approximately log-normal. Therefore, not only their arithmetic values but also the median and the logarithmic standard deviation (log SD) were calculated. Log SD serves as an index of the heterogeneity of the distribution of capillary domains. Afterwards, the median, mean and log SD of the radius of the tissue cylinder were calculated, R (domain), assuming a cylindrical shape and central location of capillaries.

On the same photomicrographs, the distribution of distances between square-array-grid points and the center of the nearest capillary was also determined. This corresponds to the distribution of tissue at various distances from the center of the nearest capillary. Kayar et al. (1982) called this approach the closest-individual

250

method. The computer program generated the grid and used the capillary coordinates already recorded and stored during the previous procedure. These data served as a source for an alternative way of characterization of the capillary spacing and its heterogeneity. Mean and median of the radius of the Krogh cylinder, R (closest), as well as log SD were calculated as described previously (Turek and Rakusan, 1981; Rakusan and Turek, 1984).

Differences between groups were evaluated using Student's t-test.

RESULTS AND DISCUSSION

Our basic data summarized in Table I are in agreement with previous reports. Rats exposed to simulated high altitude had significantly lower body weight and left ventricular weight, while the right ventricular weight was increased. At the same time, significantly increased hematocrit and hemoglobin concentration were found.

Table II contains data on myocardial capillarization. Indices of myocardial capillarization were similar in both groups. The only exception was the mid-wall section of the left ventricle in rats exposed to hypoxia, where an increased capillary density and a smaller median of the tissue cylinder radius were found. In similar studies on rats born at sea level and later exposed to simulated high altitude, Miller and Hale (1970) observed an increase of capillary density in both ventricles; Friedman et al. (1973) and Moravec et al. (1983) studied the capillarization only in the left ventricle and also found an increase. Contrary to this, Clark and Smith (1978) described a decrease in the right ventricle and in the midzone of the left ventricle without any change in the subendocardial zone of the left ventricle. Our present results are also at variance with previous reports from our own laboratory. In that study (Turek et al., 1972) we found an increase of capillary density in the right and no change in the left ventricle. It should be mentioned that the same low pressure chamber, the same altitude and the same strain of rats were used in both our studies. At the present time we have no plausible explanation for this discrepancy. We may only point out that in the present study the person using the image analyzer and computer was not aware of the origin of the photomicrograph. This was impossible in our previous work, where the capillaries were counted under a microscope and the hypertrophy of the right ventricle characterizing the high altitude group was clearly visible. However, we have no reason to assume that the person actually counting the capillaries was biased. The discrepancy is not unique for rats. In the left ventricle of guinea pigs native to high altitude, Rotta (1943) found a decrease of myocardial capillarization, Valdivia (1962) observed an increase of capillary-fiber ratio and Rakusan et al. (1981) did not find any change in any index of myocardial capillarization.

Table I. Body weight, cardiac ventricular weight, hemoglobin concentration and hematocrit of control and high-altitude exposed rats (mean + S.D.). RV= right ventricle, LB+SE= left ventricle plus septum, TVW= total ventricular weight, N.S.= not significant; number of animals in parenthesis.

	Body weight (g)	Cardiac weight (mg)			Hb. conc. (m.mol/l)	Hct (%)
		RV	LV+SE	TVW		
Control	411 +12 (7)	212 +30 (7)	1009 +73 (7)	1221 +88 (7)	8.95 +0.40 (5)	42.7 +2.0 (5)
Low pressure chamber	374 +22 (7)	351 +47 (7)	873 +104 (7)	1223 +113 (7)	10.23 +0.50 (5)	49.0 +2.9 (5)
P	< 0.01	<0.001	<0.05	N.S.	<0.01	<0.01

Table II. Data on myocardial capillarization of control and high-altitude exposed rats (mean $\pm$ S.D.). LV= left ventricle, RV= right ventricle, MC= mid-wall section, SC= subendocardial section, C.D.= number of capillaries per mm^2, R (domain)= radius of the Krogh cylinder estimated by the method of capillary domains, R (closest)= radius of the Krogh cylinder derived from data obtained by the closest-individual method. Asterisk indicates a statistically significant difference against control results at P<0.05; n= number of animals.

		C.D. (mm^{-2})	R (domain)			R (closest)		
			Mean (µm)	Median (µm)	log SD	Mean (µm)	Median (µm)	log SD
CONTROL (n = 7)								
LV	MC	2967 +206	10.3 +0.4	10.1 +0.4	0.059 +0.005	10.2 +0.4	9.9 +0.4	0.105 +0.005
LV	SC	3501 +421	9.6 +0.6	9.4 +0.6	0.058 +0.006	9.6 +0.6	9.3 +0.5	0.104 +0.011
RV	MC	3030 +480	10.2 +0.9	9.9 +0.9	0.064 +0.008	9.9 +0.9	9.6 +0.8	0.118 +0.111
RV	SC	3007 +495	10.2 +0.7	10.0 +0.7	0.061 +0.005	9.8 +0.7	9.5 +0.6	0.111 +0.006
LOW PRESSURE CHAMBER (n = 7)								
LV	MC	3567* +645	9.5 +0.9	9.3* +0.9	0.063 +0.007	9.5 +0.8	9.4 +0.7	0.107 +0.011
LV	SC	3477 +220	9.5 +0.2	9.3 +0.3	0.067 +0.018	9.3 +0.3	9.0 +0.3	0.118 +0.022
RV	MC	2963 +382	10.3 +0.6	10.1 +0.6	0.067 +0.005	10.1 +0.5	9.8 +0.5	0.117 +0.009
RV	SC	2898 +437	10.4 +0.7	10.2 +0.6	0.062 +0.005	10.3 +0.6	9.9 +0.6	0.112 +0.011

To our knowledge there is only one paper dealing with the heterogeneity of myocardial capillary spacing in high altitude animals. Rakusan et al. (1981) studied the hearts from Andean guinea pigs and found no difference in log SD of the radius of the Krogh cylinder derived from percentage of tissue at various distances to the wall of the nearest capillary. This is in agreement with our present results.

Median radius of tissue cylinder and the degree of its heterogeneity were similar in the right ventricles of both groups. Since the right ventricle of rats exposed to high altitude was hypertrophied, this suggests that in the enlarged ventricle capillary proliferation occurs without changing the spatial pattern of their distribution. In contrast, cardiac hypertrophy occurring in rats with arterial hypertension is characterized by an increased heterogeneity of the capillary spacing. This increase is usually but not always accompanied by an enlarged median radius of the tissue cylinder (Rakusan et al., 1984 a,b; Hoofd et al. 1985). As an increased heterogeneity of capillary spacing impairs tissue oxygenation (Turek and Rakusan, 1981; Rakusan et al., 1985), its absence may be a bonus for rats with high altitude-induced hypertrophy.

CONCLUSION

We found no important difference in myocardial capillarization between control rats and rats exposed to simulated altitude of 3500 m. The median and the heterogeneity of the radius of the tissue cylinder were similar in both groups. This suggests that capillary proliferation occurs in the hypertrophied right ventricle of rats adapted to altitude, without changing the spatial pattern of capillary distribution.

Supported by the Ontario Heart Foundation.

REFERENCES

Clark, D.R., and Smith, P., 1978, Capillary density and muscle fibre size in the hearts of rats subjected to simulated high altitude. Cardiovasc. Res., 12:578-584.

Friedman, I., Moravec, J., Reichart, E., and Hatt, P.Y., 1973, Subacute myocardial hypoxia in the rat. An E.M. study of the left ventricular myocardium. J. Mol. Cell. Cardiol., 5:125-132.

Hoofd, L., Turek, Z., Kubat, K., Ringnalda, B.E.M., and Kazda, S., 1985, Variability of intercapillary distance estimated on histological slides of rat heart, in: Oxygen Transport to Tissue-VII, F. Kreuzer, S.M. Cain, Z. Turek and T. K. Goldstick, eds., Plenum Press, New York and London, in press.

Kayar, S.R., Archer, P.G., Lechner, A.J., and Banchero, N., 1982, The closest-individual method in the analysis of the distribution of capillaries. Microvasc. Res. 24:326-341.

Miller, A.T., and Hale, D., 1970, Increased vascularity of brain, heart and skeletal muscle of polycythemic rats. Am. J. Physiol., 219:702-704.

Moravec, J., Cluzeaud, F., Rakusan, K., and Turek, Z., 1983, Capillary supply and utilization of intracellular oxygen in the left ventricular myocardium from rats adapted to high altitude, in: Oxygen Transport to Tissue-IV, H.I. Bicher and D.F. Bruley, eds., Adv. Exper. Med. Biol., Vol. 159, Plenum Press, New York and London, pp 243-252.

Rakusan, K., and Turek, Z., 1984, A comparison of the methods for assessment of myocardial capillarity, in: Oxygen Transport to Tissue-V, D.W. Lübbers, H. Acker, E. Leniger-Follert, and T.K. Goldstick, eds., Adv. Exper. Med. Biol., Vol. 169, Plenum Press, New York and London, pp 411-418.

Rakusan, K., Turek, Z., and Kreuzer, F., 1981, Myocardial capillaries in guinea pigs native to high altitude (Junin, Peru, 4,105 m). Pflügers Arch. 391:22-24.

Rakusan, K., Hoofd, L.J.C., and Turek, Z., 1985, The effect of cell size and capillary spacing on myocardial oxygen supply, in: Oxygen Transport to Tissue-VI, D.F. Bruley et al., eds., Plenum Press, New York and London, in press.

Rakusan, K., Hrdina, P.W., Turek, Z., Lakatta, E.G., Spurgeon, H.A., and Wolford, G.D., 1984, Cell size and capillary supply of the hypertensive rat heart: quantitative study. Bas. Res. Cardiol. 79:389-395.

Rakusan, K., Korecky, B., Sarkar, K., and Turek, Z., 1984 b, Merits and pitfalls in morphological assessment of cardiac growth. Fed. Proc., in press.

Rotta, A., 1943, Peso del corazon y numero de capillares cardiacos en cobayos de diferentes alturas. Revista Argent. Cardiol. 10:186-199.

Turek, Z., Rakusan, K., 1981, Lognormal distribution of intercapillary distance in normal and hypertrophic rat heart as estimated by the method of concentric circles: its effect on tissue oxygenation. Pflügers Arch., 391:17-21.

Turek, Z., Grandtner, M., and Kreuzer, F., 1972. Cardiac hypertrophy, capillary and muscle fiber density, muscle fiber diameter, capillary radius and diffusion distance in the myocardium of growing rats adapted to a simulated altitude of 3 500 m. Pflügers Arch., 335:19-28.

Valdivia, E., 1962, Total capillary bed of the myocardium in chronic hypoxia. Fed. Proc., 21:221.

THE EFFECT OF HETEROGENEITY OF CAPILLARY SPACING AND O_2 CONSUMPTION - BLOOD FLOW MISMATCHING ON MYOCARDIAL OXYGENATION

Karel Rakusan and Zdenek Turek

Department of Physiology, School of Medicine, University of Ottawa, Ottawa, Ontario, Canada, and Department of Physiology, Faculty of Medicine, University of Nijmegen Nijmegen, The Netherlands

Previously we demonstrated the importance of the heterogeneity of the capillary spacing for the oxygen supply to the myocardial tissue (Turek and Rakusan, 1981). The computed percentage of anoxic myocardial tissue turned out to be a better index of tissue oxygenation than the mean myocardial P_{O_2}. This was especially apparent in situations associated with myocardial hypoxia. The percentage of anoxic myocardial tissue depends not only on the average values of the traditional oxygen determinants included in the Krogh-Erlang equation but also on their variability. In our previous report we analyzed the dependence of myocardial oxygenation on the degree of heterogeneity of capillary spacing for a single value of the mean tissue radius (R) in two situations with respect to blood flow distribution. In the first situation (A) the volume blood flow was perfectly matched to the size of tissue cylinder supplied by a given capillary resulting in uniform end-capillary P_{O_2}. In the second situation (B) identical blood flow was assumed for all capillaries resulting in varying end-capillary P_{O_2}. If uniform oxygen consumption is assumed, then in this situation the O_2 consumption and blood flow must be seriously mismatched. In most cases the real situations obviously lie between these two extreme conditions. In the present communication we analyze the same relationship for various sizes of the tissue cylinders and for various degrees of mismatching between myocardial oxygen consumption and capillary blood flow.

First, we calculated the percentage of anoxic myocardial tissue as a function of heterogeneity in capillary spacing. In contrast to our previous computations, in which a single value of the radius of the tissue cylinder was used, this time we applied the values of the cylinder radii ranging from 8 to 18 μm. This range corresponds to realistic values expected from the histological measurements in the mammalian myocardium (Rakusan, 1971). Krogh's formula was used for calculation of the percentage of anoxic tissue as described previously (Turek and Rakusan, 1981; Rakusan et al., 1985). The average values of the myocardial oxygen determinants corresponding to the situation in the human heart used as the entry data for our computer program were as follows: arterial P_{O_2} = 100 mm Hg, arterial P_{CO_2} = 40 mm Hg, pH = 7.4, blood O_2 capacity = 20 ml/100 ml, P_{50} = 27 mm Hg, Q_{O_2} = 0.10 ml/min/g, blood flow = 1 ml/min/g, capillary radius = 3.2 μm. The distribution of intercapillary distances may be approximated by a log-normal distribution in which the spread is characterized by a single parameter, namely the log standard deviation. Hence, the log SD R served as an index of heterogeneity in capillary spacing. The effect of log SD R on myocardial oxygenation for various tissue cylinder radii (R) is displayed in Fig. 1.and summarized in Table 1. As may be expected, the percentage of anoxic tissue increases with both increasing heterogeneity of capillary spacing and increasing size of the tissue cylinder. However, less obvious are the quantitative aspects of this relationship. As follows from the table, the degree of

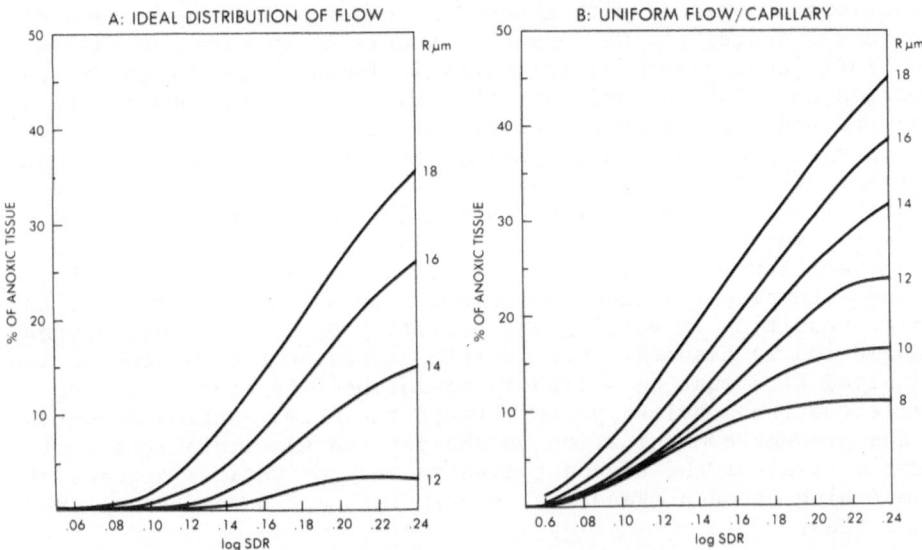

Fig. 1. The effect of heterogeneity of capillary spacing (log SDR) and diffusion distance (R) on myocardial oxygenation.

Table 1. Percentage of anoxic tissue as a function of Krogh's radius R and an index of heterogeneity in capillary spacing (log SD R).

log SD R	Rμm 8	10	12	14	16	18
.06	0.0- 0.2	0.0- 0.2	0.0- 0.2	0.0- 0.3	0.0- 0.5	0.1- 1.2
.08	0.0- 1.2	0.0- 1.1	0.0- 1.2	0.1- 1.6	0.1- 2.4	0.5- 4.1
.10	0.0- 2.9	0.0- 2.9	0.0- 3.2	0.1- 4.0	0.6- 5.6	2.0- 8.5
.12	0.0- 5.2	0.0- 5.4	0.1- 6.0	0.6- 7.4	2.1-10.0	5.0-13.8
.14	0.0- 7.4	0.0- 8.3	0.6- 9.5	2.0-11.7	4.8-15.0	9.3-19.5
.16	0.0- 9.0	0.0-11.2	1.4-13.4	4.3-16.3	8.7-20.4	14.5-25.3
.18	0.0-10.1	0.0-13.6	2.5-17.1	7.5-21.1	13.4-25.8	20.3-31.1
.20	0.0-10.6	0.0-15.2	3.4-20.3	10.7-25.6	18.3-30.9	26.1-36.5
.22	0.0-10.8	0.0-16.2	3.6-22.6	13.4-29.2	22.9-35.4	31.5-41.3
.24	0.0-10.8	0.0-16.5	3.1-23.9	15.1-31.9	26.4-39.0	36.8-45.3

Both situations A (= ideal distribution of flow) and B (uniform flow/capillary) included.

heterogeneity of capillary spacing becomes a very important myocardial oxygen determinant with increasing size of the tissue cylinder. Let us consider a theoretical situation in which an average radius of the tissue cylinder is rather large (R = 18 μm) and the remaining parameters are within normal range. In this case the percentage of anoxic tissue can vary from zero to forty-five per cent depending on the degree of heterogeneity of capillary spacing and blood flow distribution.

In the second part, we present a more detailed analysis of the mismatching of myocardial oxygen consumption and capillary blood flow. Instead of the two situations considered above (A,B), a more gradual range has been used. The following assumptions were adopted:
1) The ratio of oxygen consumption to blood flow (Q_{O_2}/F) is log-normally distributed and its variability can be described by its own log SD.
2) The Q_{O_2}/F distribution follows the distribution of R, so that the thickest cylinders have the highest Q_{O_2}/F and vice versa. The intention was to simulate a "lagging" of the adaptive changes in capillary flow to compensate for the size of tissue cylinders.
3) As above, the oxygen consumption per volume of myocardial tissue was assumed to be uniform.

It should be stressed that in all our considerations which
follow, the oxygen consumption as well as blood flow per gram of
tissue remained the same as shown in the entry data. Hence, the
overall ratio of these two parameters also remained the same. It
was the degree of mismatching between these two which varied and
more pronounced mismatching was expressed by a higher value of log
SD Q_{O_2}/F. Therefore, with log SD Q_{O_2}/F equal to zero, we obtained
the situation in which the flow is ideally matched to the size of
tissue cylinder (situation A), as considered above. It goes without
saying that even this rather complex approach involves many simplifications. For instance, we assumed that in cylinders of identical
radii capillary flow per tissue cylinder is also identical. This
assumption is probably not true and the real distribution of Q_{O_2}/F
with respect to the distribution of tissue cylinder radii is
unknown. However, this approach results in a substantial saving of
the computing time as Q_{O_2}/F and consequently the flow of each
cylinder can be calculated during the same integrating procedure as
the frequency of the radii of the tissue cylinders.

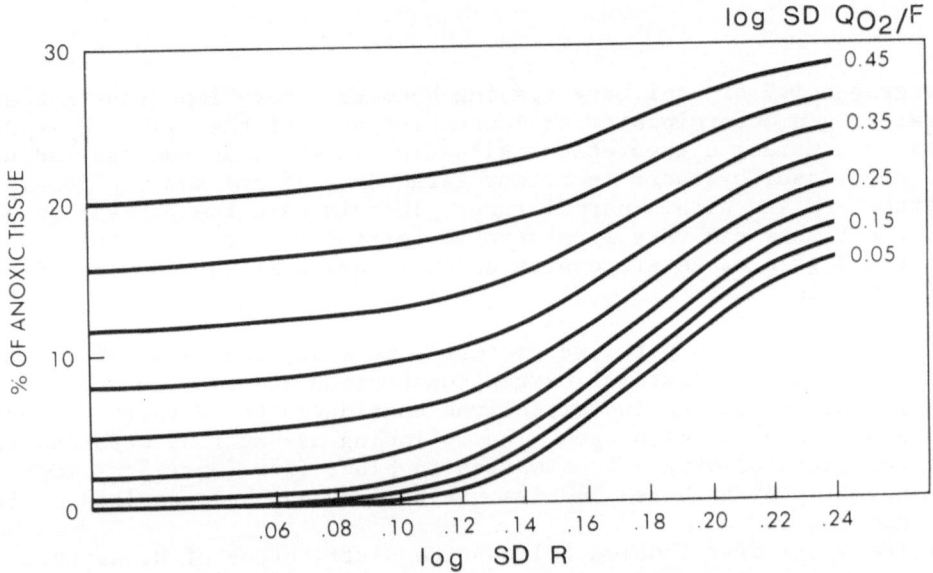

Fig. 2. The effect of heterogeneity of capillary spacing (log SD R)
and log SD Q_{O_2}/F on myocardial oxygenation. Mean R equals
12 μm.

The results of our calculations are summarized in Figure 2. In this graph, the percentage of anoxic myocardial tissue is expressed as a function of log SD R and log SD Q_{O_2}/F. It appears that the mismatching of myocardial oxygen consumption and blood flow has an effect on the myocardial oxygenation which is independent of heterogeneity of the myocardial spacing. It is, however, potentiated by the latter if log SD R increases to over 0.1.

The aim of our computations was twofold. First, we hoped to provide an experimentalist with readily available simplified charts of the dependence of myocardial oxygenation on some morphological and physiological parameters which are often measured or estimated in various experimental and clinical situations. Second, we wanted to demonstrate the limits of averages of oxygen determinants when they are not accompanied by estimates of their variability. For instance, in a hypothetical situation in which we consider the tissue with an average cylinder radius of 16 μm and log SD R of 0.06, the morphological conditions for the oxygen supply are probably better than in a tissue with half the average radius but double log SD R. This conclusion is contrary to the expected results based on the traditional approach of average oxygen determinants from the Krogh-Erlang equation. Our results clearly demonstrate that both heterogeneity in capillary spacing and in Q_{O_2}/F are important and independent tissue oxygen determinants irrespective of the mean values of these parameters. Therefore, they should be included in any future evaluations of the oxygen supply to tissue.

SUMMARY

The effect of heterogeneity of capillary spacing on myocardial oxygenation was estimated for various sizes of tissue cylinder radii ranging from 8 to 18 μm, which are the values expected from the histological measurements. Similarly, the effect of mismatching between myocardial oxygen consumption and capillary blood few was analyzed. The results are summarized in charts which demonstrate that both heterogeneities are important independent tissue oxygen determinants irrespective of the mean values of these parameters. Therefore they should be included in any future evaluation of the oxygen supply to tissue.

Supported by the Medical Research Council of Canada.

REFERENCES

Rakusan, K., 1971, Quantitative morphology of capillaries of the heart, in: Functional Morphology of the Heart, E. Bajusz and G. Jasmin, eds., Karger, Basel, pp 272-286.

Rakusan, K., Hoofd, L.J.C., and Turek, Z., 1985, The effect of cell
    size and capillary spacing on myocardial oxygen supply, in:
    Oxygen Transport to Tissue-VI, D.F. Bruley et al., eds.,
    Plenum Press, New York and London, in press.
Turek, Z., and Rakusan, K., 1981, Lognormal distribution of inter-
    capillary distance in normal and hypertrophic rat heart as
    estimated by the method of concentric circles: Its effect
    on tissue oxygenation. Pflügers Arch., 391:17-21.

MULTICOMPONENT ANALYSIS OF REFLECTION SPECTRA FROM THE GUINEA PIG
HEART FOR MEASURING TISSUE OXYGENATION BY QUANTITATIVE DETERMINA-
TION OF OXYGEN SATURATION OF MYOGLOBIN AND OF THE REDOX STATE OF
CYTOCHROME aa_3, c, AND b

L. Caspary, J. Hoffmann, H.R. Ahmad, and D.W. Lübbers

Max-Planck-Institut für Systemphysiologie
Rheinlanddamm 201, 4600 Dortmund 1, FRG

The oxygen saturation of myoglobin can be used as a quantitative indicator of the cellular oxygen supply[3,11] as well as of
the intracellular oxygen pressure[12]. On the hemoglobin free
perfused Langendorff-heart preparation such measurements can be
carried out non-invasively by reflection fotometry[4,6,9,10,12].
However, our investigations have shown, that under such conditions
the usually applied two wavelength method may yield erroneous
results 1) because of the superposition of the spectra of myoglobin
and cytochromes and 2) the complicated optical conditions during
reflection within the tissue[4,5]. Therefore a larger spectral
range is monitored and a new multicomponent evaluation method
applied which considers scattering using the two-flux theory of
Kubelka and Munk (two-flux evaluation method for multicomponent
systems: TEMMS[5]). The aim of the following experiments was
to test the new method under relatively simple and reproducible
conditions. These were achieved by arresting and cooling the
heart. The results demonstrate quite good applicability of
the new evaluation method.

MATERIALS AND METHODS

Preparation

Hearts were taken from guinea pigs weighing 250 - 300 g, fed
at libitum. The animals were killed by a blow on the head, then

bled. The thorax was opened and a canula directly inserted into the aortic arch. The heart was immediately perfused with 37° C warm Krebs-Henseleit modified Ringer solution containing 119.7 $mmol \cdot l^{-1}$ NaCl, 4.7 $mmol \cdot l^{-1}$ KCl, 1.25 $mmol \cdot l^{-1}$ $CaCl_2$, 1.2 $mmol \cdot l^{-1}$ KH_2PO_4, 24.9 $mmol \cdot l^{-1}$ $NaHCO_3$, 0.3 $mmol \cdot l^{-1}$ $MgSO_4$, 5.5 $mmol \cdot l^{-1}$ $C_6H_{12}O_6 \cdot H_2O$, 2.0 $mmol \cdot l^{-1}$ $C_3H_3O_3Na$.
The preparation procedure took approximately 90 to 120 sec. Afterwards the heart was removed and fixed on the perfusion apparatus, both of the venae cavae ligated and a canula put into the right ventricle through the pulmonary truncus. The left auricle was cut of and a latex balloon introduced into the left ventricle. The balloon was used to measure intraventricular pressure with a statham pressure transducer[2].

Equipment

Our perfusion system allowed both pressure and volume-constant perfusion of the left ventricle according to the Langendorff technique. The perfusate was equilibrated with gas mixtures produced by gasmixing pumps (Fa. Wösthof, Bochum). The medium was not recirculated. Coronary flow was measured by an electromagnetic flowmeter. Venous Po_2 was determined by a Clark Po_2 electrode in the perfusate drained by a catheter inserted in the pulmonary truncus. The Po_2 on the heart surface was determined by an 8 wire platinum electrode[7].

The electrode was fixed on a perpendicular lever and balanced so that the electrode touched the lateral surface of the ventricle. During steady state the weight of the electrode did not exert any pressure on the tissue; it was held in place only by capillary forces. The electrode followed the heart movements. Reflection spectra were recorded by the Rapid Spectrofotometer[8], stored on a HP-computer and evaluated by TEMMS[5]. The analysis simultaneously yielded the O_2 saturation of myoglobin and the redox state of cytochrome aa_3, c, and b. Additionally the parameter for the relative concentration of the components and a scattering index of the optical system was obtained.

For our experiments hearts were selected that achieved a ventricular pressure of at least 60 mm Hg, had a steady state coronary flow of less than 12 ml/min and a reactive hyperemia after a two-minute-ichemia that was more than twice that of the resting flow. The hearts were arrested by adjusting the perfusate to 25 $mmol \cdot l^{-1}$ KCl and cooled down to 22° C. During the experiments the Po_2 of the perfusate was reduced stepwise by adjusting the pump to an oxygen concentration value of 30, 10, 3, 1, 0.3 and zero percent in nitrogen. After setting the pump 8 - 12 minutes were needed until the surface and outflow

Po_2 values reached constant levels (jugded from the traces on the recorder, usually after 8 - 12 min: steady state).

RESULTS

The surface Po_2 values of the KCl arrested (25 mmol · 1^{-1}) and cooled (22° C) heart were smaller than the Po_2 of the gas mixture used for equilibration. The venous outflow corresponded well to the mean surface Po_2. After reaching steady state conditions the mean Po_2 value for the eight wire electrode was calculated for one second measuring time. The ends of the bar parallel to the Po_2 axis (Fig. 1) show the lowest and the highest surface Po_2 value measured by the 8 wire electrode. The Fig. 1 shows that under steady state conditions there is still a Po_2 gradient, mostly relatively small. Sometimes a larger gradient occurs without recognizable cause. At the same time the reflection spectra (recording time for a single spectra 10 ms) was measured for a period of 4 sec and the multicomponent analysis performed. The corresponding variation of myoglobin saturation is shown by the bar parallel to the myoglobin saturation axis.

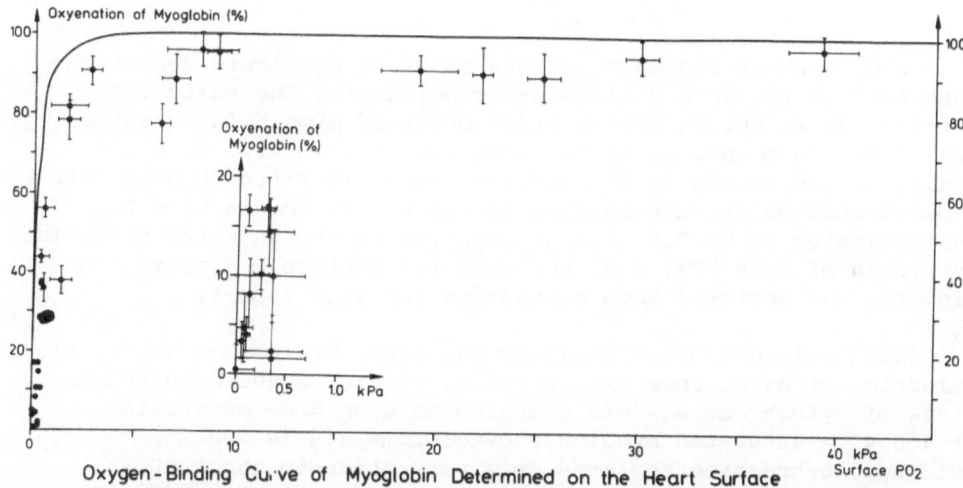

Oxygen-Binding Curve of Myoglobin Determined on the Heart Surface

Fig. 1.   Myoglobin O_2 saturation within the Langendorff heart during perfusion with medium equilibrated with different O_2 mixtures. The bar parallel to the Po_2 axis shows the span between the lowest and the highest Po_2 value measured simultaneously by the eight wire electrode. The bar parallel to the MbO_2 saturation axis denotes the variation of the MbO_2 saturation in the four second interval in which the Po_2 was measured. The insert shows the lower range in a larger scale. The solid line was calculated for a myoglobin solution of 20° C[1].

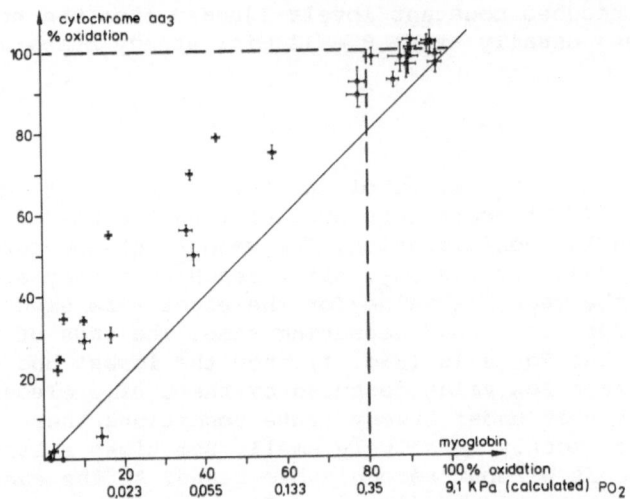

Fig. 2. Degree of cytochrome aa_3 oxidation vs O_2 saturation
of myoglobin.

Fig. 1 shows the mean O_2 saturation of myoglobin versus the
mean surface Po_2 from 5 different experiments. The solid line
corresponds to the O_2 dissociation curve of myoglobin in vitro
(20° C^1). The points measured experimentally in vivo have a
similar shape as the O_2 dissociation curve in vitro. However the
experimental points are shifted to the right. The in vivo P_{50}
was estimated to be 0.94 kPa as compared to the in vitro value for
myoglobin of 0.09 kPa, i.e. the measured surface Po_2 seems too
high for the measured MbO_2 saturation (or vice versa).

With multicomponent analysis one also obtains the degree of
oxidation of cytochrome aa_3, c and b. In Fig. 2 the mean redox
state of cytochrome aa_3 was compared to mean MbO_2 saturation.
At 100 % O_2 saturated myoglobin cytochrome aa_3 is 100 %
oxidized. Decreasing the mean MbO_2 saturation to about 80 %,
resulted in a mean surface Po_2 decreased from 30 kPa to 2 - 3
kPa (see Fig. 1). During this decrease the mean redox state of
cytochrome aa_3 remained unchanged. When the O_2 saturation of
myoglobin was further reduced the reduction of cytochrome aa_3
began. Although the values of the redox state of cytochrome aa_3
scattered considerably, the decrease of cytochrome aa_3 oxidation
was approximately parallel to the decrease of MbO_2 saturation
down to a MbO_2 saturation level of 10 - 20 %. The decrease did
not occur in a 1:1 manner. Fig. 3 shows that cytochrome c and
cytochrome aa_3 behaved similarly: the oxidation values scatter
around the identity line.

Cytochrome b behaved differently (Fig. 4). At 100 % oxidation of cytochrome aa_3 the maximum oxidation of cytochrome b was about 70 %. At a 70 to 80 % reduction of cytochrome aa_3 cytochrome b was already totally reduced.

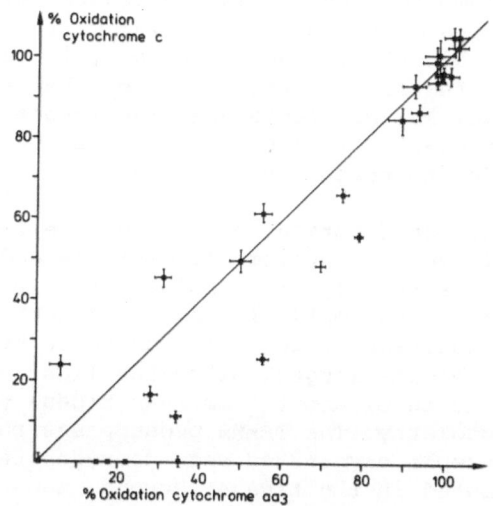

Fig. 3.   Degree of cytochrome c oxidation vs oxidation of cytochrome aa_3.

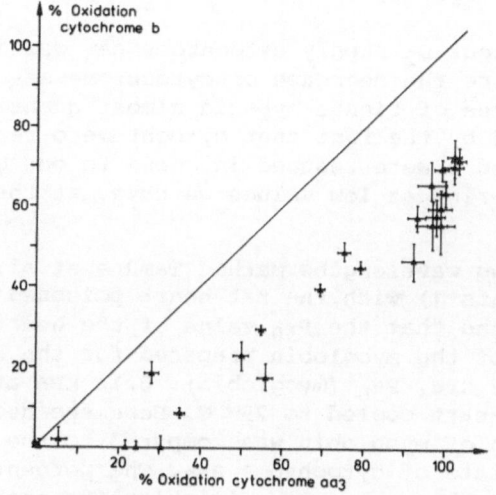

Fig. 4.   Degree of cytochrome b oxidation vs oxidation of cytochrome aa_3.

DISCUSSION

The multiwire Po_2 electrode fixed on a lever approximately parallel to the heart surface was easy to apply, did not cause tissue damage and gave stable and reproducible readings. Although O_2 consumption was distinctly reduced after application of KCl and decrease of temperature to 22° C, there were still Po_2 gradients within the tissue. Therefore, in saline perfused, respiring hearts the surface Po_2 is higher than that of the underlying tissue. Po_2 gradients are also favored by the anatomical structure of the heart. After switching to a new gas mixture 8 - 12 min were needed to reach a new steady state.

Under steady state optical conditions the two-flux evaluation method for multicomponent systems (TEMMS) yielded reproducible results. To improve the signal to noise ratio 16 spectra (ca. 0.8 s) were averaged. If the optical conditions changed (for example by changing the position of the light guide or by formation of an edema) the error became larger. Since the light beam penetrates the tissue to a depth of about 1 mm mean tissue values are obtained by reflection fotometry. The TEMMS presupposes that cellular pigments, for example oxygenated and deoxygenated myoglobin are randomly distributed in the tissue. Strong, non-random local variations of pigment concentrations may cause evaluation errors.

Since the Po_2 measured on the surface is always higher than the corresponding mean Po_2 of the underlying tissue, it is understandable that the P_{50} of the O_2 dissociation curve of myoglobin in vitro was smaller than the P_{50} measured in our experiments (see Fig. 1).

With sufficient O_2 supply cytochrome aa_3 was 100 % oxidized. Therefore the decrease of cytochrome aa_3 oxidation reflects the degree of tissue hypoxia almost quantitatively. This is supported by the fact that cytochrome c reacted similarly. Cytochrome aa_3 and c were reduced in a one to one manner. For the larger scattering at low values we have, at the moment, no explanation.

Using the two wavelengths method Tamura et al.[12] performed similar experiments 1) with the rat heart poisoned with 1 mmol $\cdot$ 1^{-1} KCN. They found that the P_{50} value of the heart was very similar to that of the myoglobin prepared for the rat heart (P_{50} (rat heart): 0.32 kPa, P_{50} (myoglobin): 0.16 kPa at 25° C) and 2) with the rat heart cooled to 25° C. Here the deoxygenation and reoxygenation of myoglobin was compared to the simultaneously measured redox state of cytochrome aa_3. The percental changes of myoglobin and cytochrome aa_3 were identical to each other and resulted in a straight line plot (see also[6]). This behaviour was explained by the existence of steep Po_2 gradients within the tissue. Our experiments did not show a straight line relationship between MbO_2 saturation and cytochrome aa_3 oxidation, probably because of the smaller Po_2 gradients in our preparation.

Cytochrome b shows a different behaviour. It was never more than about 70 % oxidized. The reason for this may be that cytochrome b is a mixture of the two components which are involved separately in the NADH and the succinate oxidation.

Considering the systematic error of the surface Po_2 measurement, the fotometricly measured MbO_2 saturation values demonstrate that results obtained by the application of TEMMS are quite reliable.

REFERENCES

1. E. Antonini, Interrelationship between structure and function in hemoglobin and myoglobin, Physiol. Rev. 45:123-170 (1965).

2. R. Bünger, F. J. Haddy, and A. Querengässer, An isolated guinea pig heart preparation with in vivo like features, Pflügers Arch. 353:317-326 (1975).

3. H. Fabel, and D. W. Lübbers, Measurements of reflection spectra of the beating rabbit heart in situ, Biochem. Z. 341:351-356 (1965).

4. H. R. Figulla, J. Hoffmann, and D. W. Lübbers, Evaluation of reflection spectra of the isolated heart by multicomponent spectra analysis in comparison to other evaluation methods, in: "Oxygen Transport to Tissue V," D. W. Lübbers, H. Acker, E. Leniger-Follert, and T.K. Goldstick, eds., Plenum Press, New York (1984), pp. 821-830.

5. J. Hoffmann, U. Heinrich, H. R. Ahmad, and D. W. Lübbers, Analysis of tissue reflection spectra obtained from brain or heart using the two flux theory from non-constant light scattering, in: "Oxygen Transport to Tissue VI," D. F. Bruley et al., eds., Plenum Press, New York (1984), in press.

6. H. Kanaide, R. Yoshimura, N. Makino, and M. Nakamura, Regional myocardial function and metabolism during acute coronary artery occlusion, Am. J. Physiol. 242:H980-989 (1982).

7. M. Kessler, and D. W. Lübbers, Aufbau und Anwendungsmöglichkeit verschiedener Po_2-Elektroden, Pflügers Arch. 291:R82 (1966).

8. D. W. Lübbers, and N. Niesel, Ein Kurzzeitspektralanalysator zur Registrierung schnell verlaufender Änderungen der Absorption, Naturwissenschaften 44:60 (1957).

9. D. W. Lübbers, H. H. Figulla, J. Hoffmann, and R. Wodick, The effect of hypoxic and histotoxic hypoxia on contractility and blood flow of the Langendorff guinea pig heart preparation, in: "Oxygen Transport to Tissie IV," H. I. Bicher, and D. F. Bruley, eds., Plenum Press, New York (1983), pp. 225-230.

10. N. Makino, H. Kanaide, R. Yoshimura, and M. Nakamura, Myoglobin oxygenation remains constant during the cardiac cycle, Am. J. Physiol. 245:H237-243 (1983).

11. G. A. Millikan, Experiments on muscle haemoglobin in vivo: the instanteous measurement of muscle metabolism. Proc. Roy. Soc. 123:218-241 (1937).

12. M. Tamura, N. Oshino, B. Chance, and I. A. Silver, Optical measurements of intracellular oxygen concentration of rat heart in vitro, Arch. Biochem. 191:8-22 (1978).

OXYGEN DIFFUSION IN A HEART MUSCLE FIBRE

D.L.S. McElwain

Department of Mathematics
Statistics and Computer Science
University of Newcastle, N.S.W. 2308, Australia

INTRODUCTION

The role of myoglobin in the function of muscle fibres has been the subject of many investigations. For many years it was thought that its main function in muscle is to act as a resevoir for oxygen with which it combines reversibly. In the 1960's, however, there were a number of papers which suggested that myoglobin is involved in intracellular oxygen transport.

In order to investigate this phenomenon, Wyman (1966) developed a theoretical model to study the transport of oxygen in the presence of either haemoglobin or myoglobin. Wyman considered two geometries in his paper. In the first, the transport is one-dimensional and models experiments which measure the flux of oxygen across a slab containing one of the proteins. The second geometry considered by Wyman is an infinitely long circular cylinder and is used to develop a theory of transport of oxygen into muscle fibres including myoglobin-facilitated oxygen diffusion. Wyman showed that the presence of myoglobin can act to increase the diffusional flux of oxygen and Wittenberg (1970) reviews experimental data which supports this theory.

In a series of papers Murray (1971, 1974, 1976; Mitchell and Murray, 1973; Taylor and Murray, 1977) analyzed the Wyman formulation in detail and developed general principles under which myoglobin can make a significant contribution to the diffusion flux. The two important conditions are (a) that the affinity of the carrier molecule for oxygen is such that the carrier is only partially saturated in some part of the system and (b) the reaction between the carrier and oxygen must be fast in comparison with

271

diffusional transit times.   A number of other theoretical investigations of the slab geometry have been published (see, for example, Kreuzer and Hoofd, 1970; Rubinow and Dembo, 1977).

In this paper, we consider a mathematical model for oxygen transport into a single cardiac muscle fibre including myoglobin-facilitated diffusion, and here we outline some of the characteristics of these fibres.

Like skeletal muscle, cardiac muscle consists of bundles of approximately parallel fibres each of about the same diameter.   In skeletal muscle each fibre has a radius of about 25 μm whereas in the human heart the corresponding radius is about 10 μm (Folkow and Neil, 1971).   In both cases the blood supply is in the form of fine capillaries which run alongside the fibres, but the density of these capillaries differs significantly in the two situations.   Folkow and Neil (1971) report that there are about 400 capillaries/mm² of skeletal tissue whereas the corresponding figure for cardiac muscle is about 2500 capillaries/mm². Wittenberg (1970) reports a value of 3300 for the capillary density of the human left ventricle. With this density, the fibre-capillary ratio is quite close to unity in the adult human heart, and each fibre is supplied by about four capillaries as depicted in Figure 1.   This geometry is confirmed by Wearn (1940) and Folkow and Neil (1970).   A similar structure is found in skeletal muscle. However, at any given time, not all of the capillaries are open, and the estimate given by Wittenberg (1970) is that about 0.57 of the capillaries are "normally operative".   In the hypertrophied heart, the fibres increase in diameter without any corresponding increase in the number of capillaries (Wearn, 1940).

The structure illustrated in Figure 1 leads to the idea of developing a mathematical model of facilitated diffusion in muscle fibres which accounts for the non-uniformity of the oxygen concentration at the surface of the fibre.

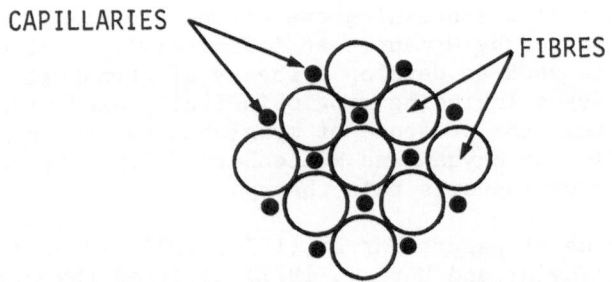

Fig.1.   A diagram illustrating the relationship between capillaries and fibres in the myocardium.   Each fibre has a radius of about 10 μm.

MATHEMATICAL MODEL

We model a single fibre as a long cylinder surrounded by m equally spaced capillaries. We adopt the notation used by Murray (1974) and let c_p denote the concentration of myoglobin in the fibre and let Y denote the fractional saturation, so that the concentration of bound oxygen is $c_p Y$. Let c denote the concentration of free oxygen and R denote the radius of the fibre.

The reversible reaction between myoglobin and oxygen is assumed to be represented by

$$O_2 + Mb \underset{k'}{\overset{k}{\rightleftarrows}} MbO_2 \qquad (1)$$

This reaction occurs at a rate ρ in favour of a decrease in free oxygen. k and k' are the on and off rate constants so that ρ is given by

$$\rho = k\, c_p (1-Y)c - k'\, c_p Y \quad .$$

Assuming a steady state and no longitudinal diffusion, the concentrations of free and bound oxygen are given by the diffusion equations

$$D_c \left\{ \frac{1}{r} \frac{\partial}{\partial r} \left[r\, \frac{\partial c}{\partial r} \right] + \frac{1}{r^2} \frac{\partial^2 c}{\partial \theta^2} \right\} = \rho + q \qquad (2)$$

and

$$c_p D_p \left\{ \frac{1}{r} \frac{\partial}{\partial r} \left[r\, \frac{\partial Y}{\partial r} \right] + \frac{1}{r^2} \frac{\partial^2 Y}{\partial \theta^2} \right\} = -\rho \quad . \qquad (3)$$

D_c and D_p are the diffusion coefficients of free oxygen and oxymyoglobin respectively and both are assumed to be constant. q is the local rate of consumption of oxygen while r and θ are the radial and angular coordinates respectively. Taylor and Murray (1977) discuss the use of a Michaelis-Menten form for the oxygen consumption rate and show that under typical conditions a good approximation can be obtained by assuming q is constant and we also do so here.

Equations (2) and (3) can be combined to give

$$\frac{1}{r} \frac{\partial}{\partial r} \left[r\, \frac{\partial Z}{\partial r} \right] + \frac{1}{r^2} \frac{\partial^2 Z}{\partial \theta^2} = q \qquad (4)$$

where $Z = D_c c + D_p c_p Y$.

At the surface of the cylinder, the concentration of free oxygen and the saturation of myoglobin are maximal at a position corresponding to the middle of a capillary, while they are minimal at the centre of the intercapillary section of the surface.

Between these two extreme values we assume that $c(R,\theta)$ and $Y(R,\theta)$ are given by

$$c(R,\theta) = c_0 + c_1 \cos m\theta \qquad (5)$$

and

$$Y(R,\theta) = Y_0 + Y_1 \cos m\theta \qquad (6)$$

for

$$s(\theta_1 + \theta_2) \leqslant \theta \leqslant (s+1)(\theta_1 + \theta_2)$$

where $s = 0,1,\ldots,m-1$ and θ_1 and θ_2 are the angles subtended at the centre of the cylinder by a capillary and the intercapillary space respectively.

The assumptions implicit in the expressions (5) and (6) model the effect of angular diffusion around the cylinder. We denote the maximum and minimum values of the surface concentration by c_c and c_t respectively where the subscripts denote the capillary and tissue while the corresponding maximum and minimum saturation values for myoglobin are Y_c and Y_t respectively. From equations (5) and (6) we can then establish the following relations

$$c_0 = (c_c + c_t)/2, \quad c_1 = (c_c - c_t)/2$$
$$Y_0 = (Y_c + Y_t)/2, \quad Y_1 = (Y_c - Y_t)/2 \ ,$$

and it then follows that

$$Z(R,\theta) = D_c[c_0 + c_1 \cos m\theta] + c_p D_p[Y_0 + Y_1 \cos m\theta] \quad (7)$$

If we now solve equation (4) subject to this boundary condition, using the method of separation of variables, we obtain

$$Z(r,\theta) = D_c c + D_p c_p Y$$
$$= D_c c_0 + c_p D_p Y_0 + q(r^2 - R^2)/4$$
$$+ (r\,R)^m (D_c c_1 + c_p D_p Y_1) \cos m\theta \ . \quad (8)$$

This expression can now be used to eliminate Y from ρ in equation (2) to give an equation involving only the free oxygen concentration c. If we introduce the dimensionless variables $c_* = c/c_c$ and $r_* = r/R$ this equation becomes

$$\frac{1}{r_*}\frac{\partial}{\partial r_*}\left[r_*\frac{\partial c_*}{\partial r_*}\right] + \frac{1}{r_*^2}\frac{\partial^2 c_*}{\partial \theta^2} = \alpha + \beta r_*^2 + \gamma r_*^m \cos m\theta$$
$$+ (\delta + \mu r_*^2 + \nu r_*^m \cos m\theta)c_*$$
$$+ \omega c_*^2 \qquad (9)$$

The dimensionless parameters are given by

$$\alpha = \frac{R^2 q}{D_c c_c} - \frac{k'R^2}{2D_p}\left(1 + \frac{c_t}{c_c}\right) - \frac{k'R^2 c_p (Y_a + Y_b)}{2 c_c D_c} + \frac{k' q R^4}{4 c_c D_c D_p}$$

$$\beta = - \frac{k' q R^4}{4 c_c D_c D_p} \quad ,$$

$$\gamma = \frac{-k'R^2}{2D_p}\left(1 - \frac{c_t}{c_c}\right) - \frac{k'R^2 c_p (Y_a - Y_b)}{2 c_c D_c} \quad ,$$

$$\delta = \frac{k_c c_p R^2}{D_c} + \frac{k'R^2}{D_p} - \frac{k_c R^2 (c_c + c_t)}{2 D_p}$$

$$- \frac{k_c R^2 c_p (Y_a + Y_b)}{2 D_c} + \frac{k_c R^4 q}{4 D_c D_p} \quad ,$$

$$\mu = - \frac{k_c R^4 q}{4 D_c D_p} \quad ,$$

$$\nu = - \frac{k_c R^2 (c_c - c_t)}{2 D_p} - \frac{k_c R^2 c_p (Y_a - Y_b)}{2 D_c} \quad ,$$

and

$$\omega = \frac{k_c R^2 c_c}{D_p} \quad .$$

Table 1 shows typical values for the parameters which are required for the model. With these values, $\alpha \approx -28$, $\beta \approx -0.2$, $\gamma \approx -9$, $\delta \approx -1.6 \times 10^3$, $\mu \approx -11$, $\nu \approx -5.5 \times 10^2$ and $\omega \approx 2.1 \times 10^3$. We introduce a small parameter $\varepsilon = 10^{-3}$ and write $\alpha = A/\varepsilon$, $\beta = B/\varepsilon$, $\gamma = G/\varepsilon$, $\delta = D/\varepsilon$, $\mu = M/\varepsilon$, $\nu = N/\varepsilon$ and $\omega = W/\varepsilon$ where A, B, D, G, M, N and W are order 1 or less. Equation (9) then becomes

$$\varepsilon \left\{ \frac{1}{r_*} \frac{\partial}{\partial r_*}\left(r_* \frac{\partial c_*}{\partial r_*}\right) + \frac{1}{r^2} \frac{\partial^2 c_*}{\partial \theta^2} \right\} = A + Br_*^2 + Gr_*^m \cos m\theta$$

$$+ (D + Mr_*^2 + Nr_*^m \cos m\theta)c_*$$

$$+ Wc_*^2 \qquad (10)$$

and this is subject to the boundary conditions

$$c_*(1,\theta) = \tfrac{1}{2} + \frac{c_t}{2c_c} + \tfrac{1}{2}\left(1 - \frac{c_t}{c_c}\right) \cos m\theta$$

$$\text{for} \quad s(\theta_1 + \theta_2) \leqslant \theta \leqslant (s+1)(\theta_1 + \theta_2)$$

$$s = 0,1,\ldots,m-1.$$

Table 1. Typical Values for Constants

c_p	1.1×10^{-7}	mol cm^{-3}	(Wittenberg, 1970)
c_0	1.7×10^{-7}	mol cm^{-3}	(at 37°C, 100 mm)
k	2.4×10^{10}	mol^{-1} cm^3 s^{-1}	(Murray, 1976)
k'	65 sec^{-1}		(Murray, 1976)
q	7×10^{-8}	mol cm^{-3} s^{-1}	(Folkow & Neil, 1971)
D_p	1.86×10^{-6}	cm^2 s^{-1}	(Murray, 1976)
D_c	2×10^{-5}	cm^2 s^{-1}	(Murray, 1976)
R	1×10^{-3}	cm	(Folkow & Neil, 1971)

The solution of equation (10) represents a singular perturbation problem, where the terms on the right hand side are order 1
or less while the derivatives on the left hand side are multiplied
by a small parameter ε. Singular perturbation problems in general
involve the existence of a boundary layer which would in this case
be at the boundary of the cylinder. However, on the basis of
physical reasoning and the theory developed by Mitchell and Murray
(1973) we assume that <u>no</u> such layer exists in which case the
solution given by putting the left hand side of Equation (10) to
zero gives a zeroth order approximation to the solution in the
whole cylinder. This being the case we impose the boundary conditions on the solution to the resulting equation, namely,

$$A + Br_*^2 + Gr_*^m \cos m\theta + (D + Mr_*^2 + Nr_*^m \cos m\theta)c_* + Wc_*^2 = 0 \quad (11)$$

The advantage of this approach is that now, for given values
of the coordinates (r,θ) we have to solve only a quadratic equation
to obtain an approximate solution. Using the conditions
$c_*(1,0) = 1$ and $c_*[1,(\theta_1 + \theta_2)/2] = c_t/c_c$ yields values for Y_a and
Y_b, namely

$$Y_a = \frac{q + k\, c_p c_c}{k' c_p + k\, c_p c_c} \quad , \quad Y_b = \frac{q + k\, c_p c_t}{k' c_p + k\, c_p c_t} .$$

The appropriate non-negative root of Equation (11) is

$$c_*(r_*,\theta) = (-P + \sqrt{P^2 - 4\omega Q} \qquad (12)$$

with
$$P = \delta + \mu r_*^2 + \nu r_*^m \cos m\theta,$$

and
$$Q = \alpha + \beta r_*^2 + \gamma r_*^m \cos m\theta.$$

RESULTS AND DISCUSSION

The results obtained using the model are shown in Table 2, which displays the scaled oxygen concentration at the centre of the fibre and the critical oxygen consumption under various conditions both with and without myoglobin-facilitated diffusion. The critical oxygen consumption is that value of q which gives a zero oxygen concentration at the centre of the fibre. In the case where we assume only two capillaries are open we have taken the minimal surface oxygen concentration, c_t, to be half the maximal value, c_c, whereas when four capillaries are open we have assumed that the minimum value is 9/10 of the maximum, except in the last case where $c_t = c_c/2$. The lower set of values for the surface oxygen concentration correspond to the situation at the distal end of a capillary where as much as 70% of the oxygen may have been removed (Folkow and Neil, 1971). We have also taken two values for the fibre radius, the larger one corresponding to a fibre in a hyper-trophied heart where the fibre radius may increase by about 40% (Wearn, 1940). The last case in the Table reflects a most extreme case where the oxygen consumption is 10 times "normal", where the fibre is enlarged, the surface oxygen concentration reduced and the myoglobin concentration in the muscle increased by 1.5 fold, corresponding to a suggestion by Wittenberg (1970) that myoglobin is excluded from the mitochondria.

In all the cases examined here the myoglobin-facilitated oxygen transport is negligible, and the critical oxygen consumption is well above physiological values. Several recent experiments have led to similar conclusions. Cole et al. (1978) report that "the conditions necessary for significant myoglobin facilitated transport are not present" in the isolated fluorocarbon-perfused dog heart. Jones and Kennedy (1982) conclude that there is no role for myoglobin in oxygen transport in cardiac myocytes in rats. Perhaps, as suggested by Stokes (1976), the main function of myoglobin in muscle is to allow efficient capillary autoregulation.

An apparent defect of the model is that it fails to take into account the mechanical interference to blood flow during heart muscular contractions. However, work on oxygen transport in the perfused rat heart by Tamura et al. (1978) appears to indicate that the oxygenation of myoglobin actually occurs during systole, so that contraction ischaemia may well be less important than originally thought.

ACKNOWLEDGEMENTS

This work was undertaken with Louise Morris, who obtained her Master of Mathematics degree at the University of Newcastle.

277

Table 2. Model Results Under Various Conditions

No. of capill.	Fibre radius μ	O_2 consumption mol cm^{-3} s^{-1}	Surface concentration mol cm^{-3}		Myoglobin content mol cm^{-3}	Centre concentration		Critical O_2 consumption mol cm^{-3} s^{-1}
			max.	min.		facil.	non-facilitat.	
2	10	7×10^{-8}	1.7×10^{-7}	8.5×10^{-8}	1.1×10^{-7}	0.7449	0.7447	9.9×10^{-6}
2	14	7×10^{-8}	1.7×10^{-7}	8.5×10^{-8}	1.1×10^{-7}	0.7399	0.7398	5.3×10^{-6}
4	10	7×10^{-8}	1.7×10^{-7}	1.5×10^{-7}	1.1×10^{-7}	0.9949	0.9949	1.2×10^{-5}
4	10	7×10^{-8}	5×10^{-8}	4.5×10^{-8}	1.1×10^{-7}	0.9327	0.9325	4.1×10^{-6}
4	14	7×10^{-8}	5×10^{-8}	4.5×10^{-8}	1.1×10^{-7}	0.9161	0.9157	2.2×10^{-6}
4	14	7×10^{-7}	5×10^{-8}	2.5×10^{-8}	1.65×10^{-7}	0.4185	0.4070	2.0×10^{-6}

REFERENCES

Cole, R.P., Wittenberg, B.A., and Caldwell, P.R.B., 1978, Myoglobin function in the isolated fluorocarbon-perfused dog heart, Am.J.Physiol., 234:H567.

Folkow, B., and Neil, E., 1971, "Circulation", Oxford University Press, New York.

Jones, D.P., and Kennedy, F.G., 1982, Intracellular O_2 gradients in cardiac myocytes. Lack of a role for myoglobin in facilitation of intracellular O_2 diffusion, Biochem.Biophys. Res.Comm., 105:419.

Kreuzer, F.,and Hoofd, L.J.C., 1970, Facilitated diffusion of oxygen in the presence of hemoglobin, Resp.Physiol.,10:542.

Mitchell, P.J., and Murray, J.D., 1973, Facilitated diffusion: The problem of boundary conditions, Biophysik, 9:177.

Murray, J.D., 1971, On the molecular mechanism of facilitated oxygen diffusion by haemoglobin and myoglobin, Proc.Roy.Soc. Lond.B., 178:95.

Murray, J.D., 1974, On the role of myoglobin in muscle respiration, J.Theor.Biol., 47:115.

Murray, J.D., 1976, On the functional role of myoglobin in skeletal muscle, Tiré à part, Myoglobin, Colloquium on Myoglobin, Brussels, Université Libre de Bruxelles.

Rubinow, S.I.,and Dembo, M., 1977, The facilitated transport of oxygen by hemoglobin and myoglobin, Biophys.J., 18:29.

Stokes, A.N., 1976, Capillary auto-regulation and the role of myoglobin, Microvasc.Res., 11:261.

Tamura, M., Oshino, N., Chance, B. and Silver, I.A., 1978, Optical measurements of intracellular oxygen concentration of rat heart in vitro, Arch.Biochem.Biophys., 191:8.

Taylor, B.A., and Murray, J.D., 1977, Effect of the rate of oxygen consumption on muscle respiration, J.Math.Biol., 4:1.

Wearn, J.T., 1940, Morphological and functional alterations of the coronary circulation, Harvey Lect.Series, 35:243.

Wittenberg, B.A., Wittenberg, J.B., and Caldwell, P.R.B., 1975, Role of myoglobin in the oxygen supply to red skeletal muscle, J.Biol.Chem., 250:9038.

Wittenberg, J.B., 1970, Myoglobin-facilitated oxygen diffusion: Role of myoglobin in oxygen entry in muscle, Physiol.Rev., 50:559.

Wyman, J., 1966, Facilitated diffusion and the possible role of myoglobin as a transport mechanism, J.Biol.Chem.,241:115.

MYOCARDIAL ISCHEMIC INJURY AND β-ADRENERGIC RECEPTORS

IN PERFUSED WORKING RABBIT HEARTS

H. M. Rhee and L. Tyler

Department of Pharmacology
Oral Roberts University School of Medicine
Tulsa, Oklahoma 74171

INTRODUCTION

Adrenergic nerve system modulates a host of diverse physio-logical functions in health and diseases.[1-4] Recent advances in the study of adrenergic receptors have contributed greatly to an understanding of both alpha- and beta-adrenergic receptors and their subtypes. Availability of radioactive agonists and antago-nists in high specific activity allowed to access directly the density and property of the receptors. However, their role in acute effect of myocardial ischemia on cardiac metabolism and function is poorly understood.

Early ischemic myocardial injury is biochemically reversible as are the physiological functional aspects upon reperfusion of the affected ischemic area.[5-7] Unrelieved ischemia for a certain point induces an irreversible biochemical and physiological alteration, which leads to permanent cell necrosis and myocardial infarction.[5-7] Little is known about the exact alteration of the beta-adrenergic activity and its receptor property during the irreversible ischemic injury. The studies presented here provide information on the density of beta-adrenergic receptors and receptor affinity in ischemic heart in relation to myocardial function.

Methods

Isolated working rabbit hearts were perfused and subjected to ischemia as described.[5,8] To apply a uniform work load, the hearts were paced 20% above their intrinsic rate by a stimulator which delivered square wave pulses of 5 msec duration. Cardiac

contractile force was measured directly by a strain-gauge arch
sutured on the left ventricle to quantitate the cardiac mechanical function.[5-8]

At the end of control or ischemic perfusion, the hearts were
used to prepare β-receptor according to Alexander et al.[9] with
modifications. Homogenation (10% instead of 20%) was carried out
by a Brinkmann polytron (PT 20 generator) three times for 5
seconds at half maximal speed. [-]-^{3}H-Dihydroalprenolol (DHA)
binding assay was carried out by incubating the receptor with
1 μc of DHA (sp. act. 100 ci/mmol) in a final volume of 1 ml
medium containing 75 mM Tris-HCl and 25 mM MgCl$_2$ at 37°C. At the
indicated time an aliquot was rapidly filtered through Whatman
glass filters (GF/C). Nonspecific binding was assayed in the
presence of 10^{-6} M propranolol.

Results

Figure 1 illustrates the effect of ischemia on cardiac left
ventricular pressure (LVP), perfusion pressure (PP), contractile
force (CF) and electrocardiogram (ECG). Onset of ischemia
(closed arrow of fig. 1) reduced perfusion pressure, which
reduced left ventricular pressure, and contractile force within 5
to 10 seconds. In 3 min the parameters were reduced to 10 to 20%
of the control values without any significant changes in electrical activity. The first gross electrocardiographic alteration
was noted in 9 min after the onset of ischemia, characterized by
numerous conduction blocks. Reperfusion of the ischemic heart
(e.g., 15 min after onset of ischemia, open arrow in fig. 1)
restored most of the parameters to control. Delayed reperfusion
usually produced cardiac arrhythmias and contractile force was
not restored to even 50% of the control value (data not shown),
suggesting the ischemic procedure is responsible for an irreversible alteration of cardiac function.

In order to understand the role of β-adrenergic receptors in
ischemic hearts, either control or 60 min ischemic hearts were
used to characterize the β-receptor, using [-]-^{3}H-dihydroapreno-
lol (DHA). Fig. 2 shows DHA concentration dependent drug binding
to the receptors in the control heart. The total DHA was increased as a function of drug concentration. Especially, the
nonspecific DHA binding, which was assayed in the presence of
10^{-6} propropanolol, was linearly increased up to 10 mM DHA
tested. The extent of the nonspecific DHA binding was usually
under one third of the total binding (fig. 2). The specific
binding (0-0), which is calculated from the difference between
the total and nonspecific binding shows a saturability of the DHA
binding. At saturation there were approximately 200 fmol of DHA
bound per mg of β-receptor (mean of five experiments).

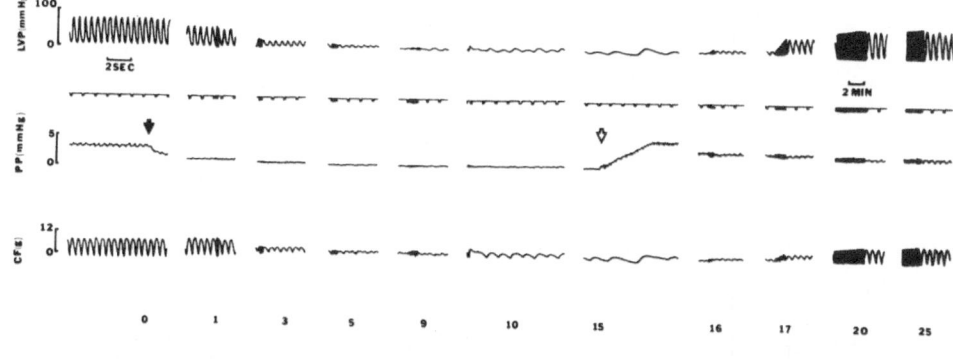

Fig. 1. A typical ischemic effect on cardiac function in isolated
working rabbit heart. An isolated rabbit heart was perfused with
Krebs-Henseleit solution as described under Methods and recorded
left intraventricular pressure (LVP), perfusion pressure (PP),
contractile force (CF) and electrocardiogram (ECG). Ischemia was
produced as described under Methods at the closed arrow and
reperfusion was initiated at the open arrow. The numbers between
CF and ECG indicate time after onset of ischemia.

   To characterize further the potential alteration of β-receptor as a result of ischemia, the data obtained from the DHA
binding study were analyzed by the Scatchard method[10]. As
illustrated in figs. 3 and 4, Scatchard plots obtained from the
DHA binding studies were monophasic straight lines, which suggest
DHA binding sites were rather homogeneous. In the control heart,
Scatchard plot (correlation coefficient, -0.932) indicates the
maximum number of DHA binding sites appeared to be $0.432 \pm$
0.033 pmol of DHA per mg protein, and dissociation contrast (Kd)
was 8.44 ± 1.03 nM in eight experiments (fig. 3). In ischemic
heart (fig. 4) Scatchard analysis indicates that Bmax was $0.342 \pm$
0.037 pmol/mg protein, which is significantly lower than Bmax of
the control heart. Kd for the ischemic hearts was also significantly less than the Kd obtained from the control heart as

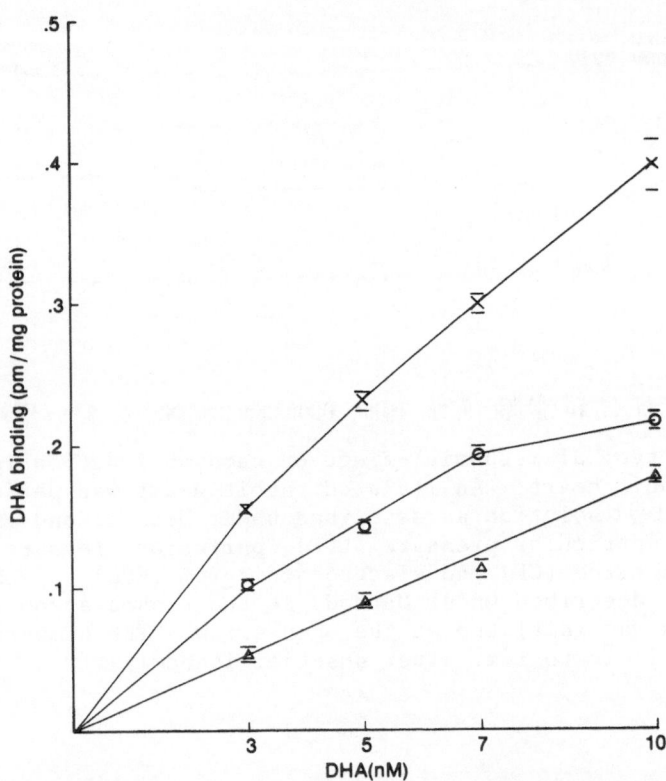

Fig. 2. Dihydroalprenolol (DHA) concentration dependent DHA binding in rabbit heart. From the homogenate of the control heart β-receptors were prepared and assayed for DHA binding to the receptor as described in Methods. Indicated concentrations of carrier-free ^{3}H-DHA were incubated with 102 μg of the receptors for 10 min and an aliquot of the incubation mixture was rapidly filtered and washed with 10 ml of the incubation medium. The DHA specific binding (0-0) was calculated from the difference between the total binding (X-X) and nonspecific binding (Δ-Δ), which was assayed in the presence of 10^{-6} M propranolol. Each point represents mean ± S.E. of at least 5 determinations from 5 animals.

summarized in Tab. 1. The table also shows that the yield of β-receptor as mg protein was significantly reduced in the ischemic heart (1.420 ± 0.129 vs. 0.745 ± 0.063 mg protein/g heart, wet weight).

Discussion

Biochemical and functional alterations during the experimental ischemia are reversible upon timely reperfusion of the ischemia region. Unrelieved ischemia beyond a certain point produces an irreversible myocardial injury leading to cell death and myocardial infarction. Although we do not know the exact dominant factor that determines the point of the irreversibility of myocardial injury, we have a wealth of information on biochemical metabolic characteristics of myocardial ischemia.[1-3]

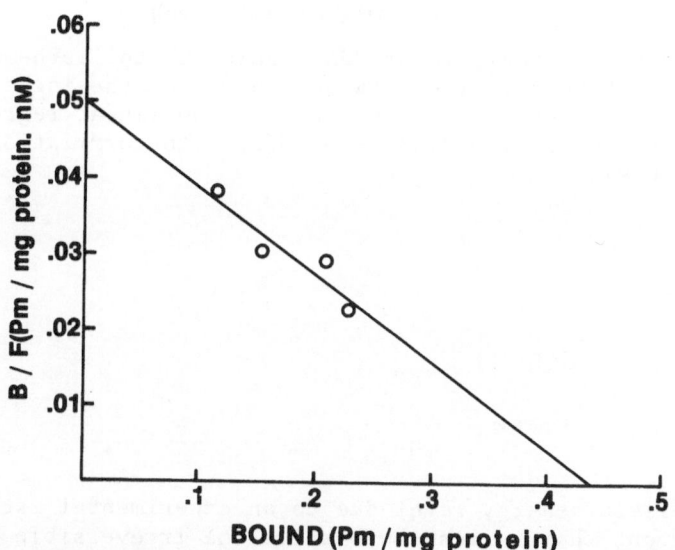

Fig. 3. Scatchard analysis of DHA binding to the control perfused rabbit heart. The data presented in fig. 2 were analyzed according to the principle of Scatchard[10]. Using least square method the linear regression line, y = 0.050 - 0.1139x, was obtained with correlation coefficient, R = 0.932.

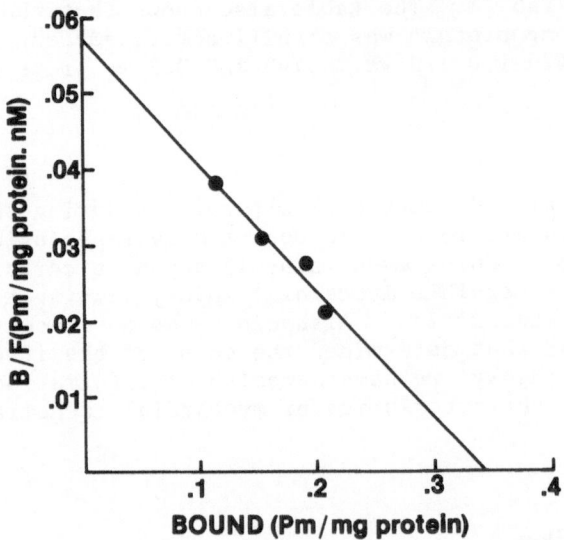

Fig. 4. Scatchard analysis of DHA binding to the ischemic perfused rabbit heart. The data obtained from the ischemic hearts were also analyzed as in fig. 3. The linear regression line has function of y = 0.057 - 0.167x, with correlation coefficient, R = 0.973.

Reduced cellular energy level due to an experimental ischemia may be a key event that is responsible for the irreversible nature of ischemia. However, there is a poor temporal correlation between a rapid reduction in contractile force (fig. 1) and rather slow reduction cellular ATP content.[11]

Recently, potential alteration of the plasma membrane structure as a result of ischemia was examined using ^{3}H-ouabain in the membrane bound Na^+,K^+-ATPase labelling technique. Reduced ouabain binding in ischemic heart is a generally accepted fact[5,12,13] which may be in agreement with Jennings et al.[14], who considered a possible sarcolemmal defect as a primary cause of irreversible myocardial injury. Thus, one of the major objectives of this paper was to examine potential alteration of membrane bound β-receptor during the ischemia.

In our study, ischemia caused a reduced yield of β-receptor protein (Tab. 1) and the characteristics of DHA binding to the β-receptors were similar to those of other systems.[9,15] The finding that Bmax was reduced significantly from the control value was expected because of reduced β-receptors protein yield after 60 min ischemic insult (figs. 2, 3, and tab. 1). However, a decrease in Kd (an increased affinity) was not expected in the ischemic heart (fig. 3) since myocardial ischemia is usually associated with an increase in serum and urine catecholamines. However, in the isolated heart perfused with blood-free physiological solution, catecholamines stored in the heart will be washed quickly upon stimulation. A continuous underperfusion which caused a decrease in β-receptor concentration (fig. 4 and tab. 1) may increase the DHA affinity of β-receptors. Many other speculating explanations may be possible, but our data support the contention that alteration of membrane structure and function induced by ischemia may be the crucial events leading to permanent myocardial damage and infarction.

Table 1. Parameters obtained from the normal and ischemic rabbit heart.[1]

Treatment	N	β-Receptor Yield (mg protein per g heart)	Bmax (pm DHA per mg protein)	Kd (nM)
Control	8	1.420 ± 0.129	0.432 ± 0.033	8.44 ± 1.03
Ischemic	8	0.745 ± 0.063^{2}	0.342 ± 0.037^{2}	5.89 ± 1.69^{2}

1. Each value is expressed as mean ± S.E., representing at least five determinations in each animal. N is the number of animals.
2. Indicates $p < 0.05$.

Acknowledgements

This work was supported in part by ORU Institutional Intramural Grant.

References

1. B. B. Hoffman and R. J. Lefkowitz, Ann. Rev. Physiol. 44:475-84 (1982).
2. J. B. Martins, R. E. Rekerber, M. L. Marcus, D. L. Laughlin, and D. M. Levy, Cardiovasc. Res. 14:116-124 (1980).
3. P.R.J. Burch, Cardiovas. Res. 14:307-338 (1980).
4. B. B. Hoffman and R. J. Lefkowitz, New Eng. J. Med. 302:1390-1396 (1980).
5. H. M. Rhee, and J. Cooper, Functional alteration of membrane integrity during global ischemic injury in perfused rabbit heart. in: "Oxygen Transport to Tissue, vol. v." D. W. Lubbers et al., ed., Plenum Publising Corp., New York, 1984.
6. R. B. Jennings, H. K. Hawkins, J. E. Lowe, M. L. Hill, M. S. Klotman, and K. A. Reimer, Am. J. Pathol. 92:187-214 (1978).
7. J. R. Neely, M. J. Rovetto, J. T. Whitmer, and H. E. Morgan, Amer. J. Physiol. 225:651-658 (1973).
8. W. Huang, H. M. Rhee, R. H. Chiu, and A. Askari, J. Pharmacol. Exp. Ther. 211:571-582 (1979).
9. R. W. Alexander, L. T. Williams, and R. J. Lefkowitz, Proc. Natl. Acad. Sci. USA 72:1564-1568 (1975).
10. G. Scatchard, Ann. N.Y. Acad. Sci. 51:660-672 (1949).
11. R. B. Jennings and C. E. Ganote, Cir. Res. 34 and 35 (Suppl. III):156-172 (1974).
12. G. A. Beller, J. Conroy, and T. W. Smith, 57:341-350 (1976).
13. B. E. Hopkins and R. R. Taylor, J. Mol. Cell. Cardiol. 36:902-907 (1973).
14. R. B. Jennings, C. E. Ganote, and K. A. Reimer, Amer. J. Pathol. 81:179-198 (1975).
15. R. J. Lefkowitz, C. Mukherjee, M. Coverstone, and M. G. Caron, Biochem. Biophys. Res. Comm. 60 (#2):703-709 (1974).

SKELETAL MUSCLE

AN UPPER BOUND ON THE MINIMUM PO_2 FOR O_2 CONSUMPTION IN RED MUSCLE

R.J. Connett, T.E.J. Gayeski, and C.R. Honig

The University of Rochester
School of Medicine and Dentistry
601 Elmwood Avenue
Rochester, New York 14642

INTRODUCTION

At a certain PO_2 the rate of O_2 consumption ($\dot{V}O_2$) becomes limited by O_2 availability rather than energy demand. This PO_2 may be defined as the critical PO_2 ($PcritO_2$) for the corresponding rate of cytochrome turnover. $PcritO_2$ sets the minimum PO_2 which convective and diffusive transport must defend. To date there have been no estimates of $PcritO_2$ for $\dot{V}O_2$ in vivo, though the influence of O_2 on redox ratios has been studied extensively in heart, liver and brain. Some contend that cytochrome a,a3 is highly reduced in tissue over the entire physiologic range of O_2 tensions.[1,2] Such reduction implies that tissue respiration should be strongly O_2 dependent and that there should be no $PcritO_2$ for $\dot{V}O_2$ in vivo. Chance and associates studied O_2 binding to cytochrome a, a3 in brain in the presence and absence of CO.[3] They interpret their data to mean that cytochrome a, a3 is almost fully oxidized in vivo and in vitro. Lubbers and associates found cytochrome a, a3 more than 95% oxidized in rat heart (personal communication). Highly oxidized a, a3 suggests that $\dot{V}O_2$ depends solely on redox and phosphorylation potentials above a PO_2 negligible for O_2 transport. The observations to be described resolve the above uncertainty with respect to myoglobin-containing muscle: If a $PcritO_2$ for $\dot{V}O_2$ exists it is <0.5 torr at the maximum rate of O_2 consumption ($\dot{V}O_{2\ max}$).

METHODS

Hound-type mongrels were anesthetized with pentobarbital, 30 mg/kg body wt. The gracilis muscle was isolated, wrapped in an O_2 barrier, and maintained at 37°C.[4] The distal tendon was attached to an isometric force transducer. Twitch contraction was induced with supramaximal square-wave monophasic pulses 0.1 ms in duration applied to the obturator nerve at 0.5-10 Hz. These frequencies cover the range from 5-100% of $\dot{V}O_{2\ max}$. Gracilis blood flow was measured by timed collection of venous outflow at rest. During exercise flow was read from a calibrated recording.

Venous and arterial samples were collected simultaneously and analysed with an Instrumentation Laboratories system programed for canine blood. The error of the hemoglobin (Hb) concentration and Hb saturation measurements was <0.1%. $\dot{V}O_2$ per g bulk muscle was determined by use of the Fick principle. In relating $\dot{V}O_2$ to local PO_2 we make the assumption that $\dot{V}O_2$ is uniform throughout the muscle. Absence of white fast glycolytic fibers and uniform distribution of mitochondria in electron photomicrographs are consistent with that assumption. The dog gracilis consists of about equal numbers of uniformly distributed slow oxidative and fast oxidative glycolytic fibers.

Tissue Samples and Biochemical Assays

Muscles were frozen in situ with a copper heat sink (5 x 5 x 5 cm) cooled to -196°C in liquid N_2 and applied to the muscle at 0.1 kg/cm^2. The cube was kept immersed in liquid N_2 until 2 s before use. Approximately 10 ms were required to reach 0°C 100 μm from the surface. The rate of freezing is sufficient to trap intra-and intercellular O_2 gradients.[5] Error in Mb saturation due to O_2 loading or unloading during freezing is <0.1%.[6] The muscle sample was excised while still in contact with the copper cube. The sample was trimmed and stored under liquid N_2. The muscle was fractured into blocks about 1 x 2 x 0.5 cm while under liquid N_2, and a freshly cleaved cross section prepared. A block was transferred to the microscope cold stage at -110 °C. At this temperature Mb spectra are stable for more than 5 h. The optical properties of frozen tissue depend mainly on the size of the ice crystals. Crystals in two samples averaged 0.75 μm. Such crystals limit the effective depth of penetration of light to about 2 μm.[7]

Mb saturation was determined on 10 cells selected at random from each block. Frequency distributions of saturation and PO_2 were constructed for each muscle based on 5 blocks, hence 50 cells. To account for microcirculatory heterogeneity each cell sampled was at least 500 μm from any other. All measurements were made at the cell center. Cell diameter was about 70 µm. The size of the measuring diaphragm averaged 5 x 5 µm. When spectroscopy was completed, the outermost 0.5 mm of muscle was broken into 1-to 5 mg chips. Chips from several blocks (i.e., macroscopic regions of the same gracilis) were pooled, weighed and extracted in perchloric acid.

Tissue metabolites were analyzed on neutralized aliquots of the perchloric acid extracts. All compounds with the exception of free creatine were assayed using enzymatic reactions coupled to the production or consumption of reduced pyridine nucleotides. Lactate and pyruvate were measured using the fluorometric assay of Lowry and Passonneau.[8] Metabolic measurements are expressed as micromoles per gram wet tissue or as concentration ratios.

Spectroscopy

Mb saturation was computed with a four-wavelength method for a nonisosbestic point at 578 nm.[7] A ratio of light intensities at the three isosbestic wavelengths (547, 568, and 588 nm) provided a check on system performance. The overall error for Mb saturation measurement was <5%. PO_2 was determined from Mb saturation and the oxymyoglobin dissociation curve. The P_{50} for canine Mb measured in this laboratory is 5.3 torr at 37°C.

RESULTS

Role of O_2 Delivery

If respiration were sensitive to O_2 at all O_2 tensions then the PO_2 in equilibrium with myoglobin ($PmbO_2$) should be a major determinant of $\dot{V}O_2$ in exercise. This is not the case; see Fig. 1. Each filled circle represents the median $PmbO_2$ for 50 cells in one muscle. The bars and open circles denote mean $\dot{V}O_2$ at each frequency, ±SEM. $\dot{V}O_2$ increases with twitch frequency through 8/s. In contrast, $PmbO_2$ is poorly correlated with work rate or $\dot{V}O_2$. Notice that the median $PmbO_2$ can be 4-6 torr at all frequencies (∿5-100% $\dot{V}O_2$ max). At a particular frequency $\dot{V}O_2$ varies 10-15%, whereas $PmbO_2$ varies 4-8 fold. The relation between $\dot{V}O_2$ and the minimum PO_2 encountered in each muscle is qualitatively the same as shown for median $PmbO_2$. Similarly, we find no correlation between O_2 delivery and either median or minimum $PmbO_2$. Poor correlation of $PmbO_2$ with $\dot{V}O_2$ and O_2 delivery is incompatible with the view[1,2] that the electron transport chain is highly reduced and hence O_2-sensitive in tissue. As further evidence to this point, the slopes of regressions of $PmbO_2$ on twitch frequency or on $\dot{V}O_2$ are significantly less than zero. The negative slopes are

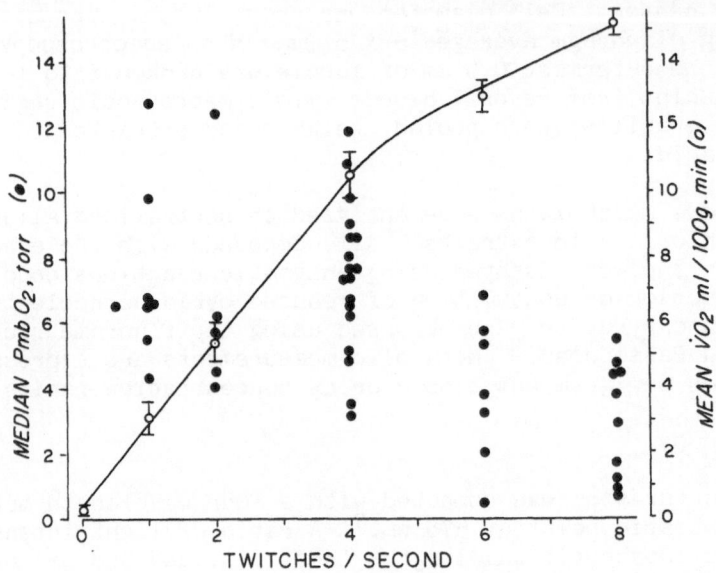

Fig. 1. Each filled circle indicates median PO_2 in one muscle based on 50 randomly sampled cells.

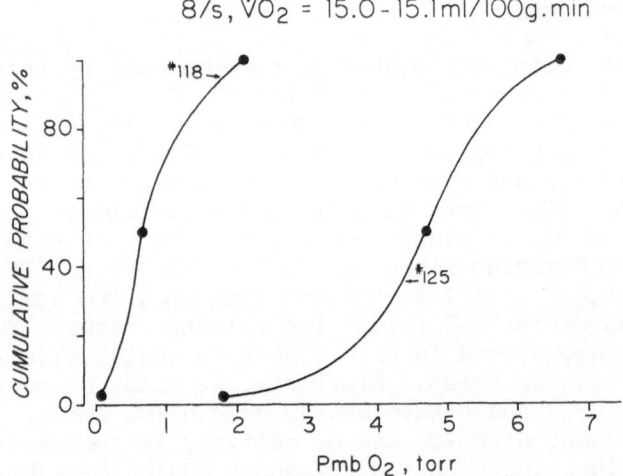

Fig. 2. Probability densities for $PmbO_2$ in two muscles working near $\dot{V}O_{2\ max}$. Filled circles indicate, minima, maxima, and medians. n = 50 cells/muscle.

the reverse of those expected if $PcritO_2$ were in the range of capillary PO_2. Absence of functional relation between $PmbO_2$ and $\dot{V}O_2$ is consistent with studies showing that $\dot{V}O_2$ is unchanged in heavily working dog gracilis if O_2 delivery is increased or decreased.[4,9]

Probability Densities for $PmbO_2$

Ogives for $PmbO_2$ in two muscles frozen after 3 min of twitch contraction at 8/s are shown in Fig. 2. $\dot{V}O_2$ in both muscles was at or near the maximum set by their enzyme capacities; see Table 1. The median $PmbO_2$ was 0.65 and 4.7 torr for muscles 118 and 125, respectively, a 7-fold difference despite equal O_2 flux. The lowest $PmbO_2$ found was 0.1 torr, and all tensions at or above the 5th percentile could be clearly distinguished from zero. (The transform from saturation, the measured quantity, to $PmbO_2$ is most precise below 3 torr because of the steep slope of the oxymyo-globin dissociation curve.) Thus no totally anoxic loci could be identified. Hypoxia may be defined as O_2-limited electron trans-port. Were hypoxic loci present? $\dot{V}O_2$ for muscles 118 and 125 was within 1% of the mean $\dot{V}O_2$ at 8/s and only 10% less than the highest $\dot{V}O_2$ we[4] or others[9] have encountered in dog gracilis during twitch contraction at any frequency. Therefore a large population of severely hypoxic loci could not have been present. In accord with this logic, the **maximum** PO_2 in muscle 118 was 2.1 torr, a value less than the lowest 5th percentile for muscle 125, despite equal and near maximal O_2 flux. Therefore, $PcritO_2$ must have been considerably less than 2.1 torr.

To obtain a more realistic upper bound let us assume that 30% the cells in muscle 118 were O_2-limited to some extent. Then $PcritO_2$ = $PmbO_2$ at cumulative probability 30%, = 0.45 torr. Further assume that the $\dot{V}O_2$ of muscle 118 in absence of an O_2 limit would have been 16.3 ml/100 g·min, the highest $\dot{V}O_2$ observed in gracilis muscles of random source dogs. If the average $\dot{V}O_2$ of cells below the 30th percentile had been 10% or 20% less than 16.3, the $\dot{V}O_2$ for the whole muscle would have been 15.5 or 14.7 ml/100 g·min. These values are not different from that measured. Had we set the average diminution in the $\dot{V}O_2$ of hypoxic cells at more than 20%, and/or set total $\dot{V}O_2$ equal to the population mean rather than the population maximum, it would be necessary to decrease the proportion of O_2 limited cells to <30% in order to remain consistent with the observed $\dot{V}O_2$. Thus a conservative upper bound on $PcritO_2$ in maximally respiring dog gracilis is 0.5 torr. This upper bound must be scaled downward as $\dot{V}O_2$ decreases from $\dot{V}O_{2\ max}$. Two additional muscle pairs comparable to the pair in Fig. 2 have been found at 8/s, as well as one pair at 6/s. $\dot{V}O_2$ at 6/s was 13.8 ml/100 g·min, the same as the mean $\dot{V}O_2$ at 6/s and only 10-15% less than $\dot{V}O_{2\ max}$ at 8/s. The median for the muscle with the lower $PmbO_2$ at 6/s was 0.4 torr. Since the maximum possible decrease in $\dot{V}O_2$ was 15%, respiration could not have been O_2-limited in half the cell population. Consequently, $PcritO_2$ was <0.4 torr.

Determinants of $\dot{V}O_2$

O_2 concentration, mitochondrial redox, and phosphorylation potential constitute the driving force for O_2 consumption. The relative importance of these determinants depends on O_2 flux and O_2 concentration.[10] If $PcritO_2$ is in fact <0.5 torr, $\dot{V}O_2$ should depend only on phosphorylation potential and redox above 0.5 torr. Table 1 confirms this for the muscles shown in Fig. 2. The ratios phosphorylcreatine (PCr) to free creatine (Cr_f) and ATP to ADP are identical, indicating that the two muscles were at the same phosphorylation potential. Since the steady-state $\dot{V}O_2$ was the same for both muscles the transmitochondrial redox gradient should have been about the same and intramitochondrial redox should have paralleled cytosolic redox. The cytosolic redox ($[NADH]\ [H^+]/[NAD]$) is reflected by the ratio of lactate (LA) to pyruvate (PYR) since lactate dehydrogenase is close to equilibrium in these steady-state muscles. The LA/PYR ratios for muscles 118 and 125 are not significantly different. In contrast median $PmbO_2$ and minimum $PmbO_2$ differ 7 fold and 18 fold respectively. Since phosphorylation potential, redox, and O_2 flux were the same, the enormous difference in PO_2 indicates PO_2 could not have been a significant determinant of cytochrome turnover. The muscles were somewhat energy depleted, as shown by the relatively low concentration of ATP. This depletion was no less for muscle 125, however, despite a much higher $PmbO_2$. Since twitch tension was well maintained by both muscles the observed [ATP] was adequate for the actomyosin cross-bridges.

Table 1. Metabolic data for muscles shown in Fig. 2. PO_2 is median of 50 cells. [ADP] calculated on the assumption that creatine phosphokinase is near equilibrium.

I.D.	$\dot{V}O_2$ ml / g·min	PO2 torr	PCr / Crf	ATP / ADP	ATP	LA μmol/g wet wt.	PYR	LA / PYR
118	0.151	0.65	0.09	21	1.5	19.7	0.10	189
125	0.154	4.7	0.09	20	1.7	21.2	0.09	236

Data comparable to those in Table 1 were obtained on 16 muscles at $\dot{V}O_2$ from 10-100% $\dot{V}O_2$ max. Multiple regression of $\dot{V}O_2$ on PCr/Cr_f, LA/PYR and median $PmbO_2$ resulted in a correlation coefficient (r^2) of 0.75. Though median $PmbO_2$ ranged from 0.4-12 torr, r^2 did not change if $PmbO_2$ was omitted from the regression, as expected if $PcritO_2$ were below 0.5 torr. The same result was obtained if the median $PmbO_2$ was replaced by minimum $PmbO_2$. A regression based on 7 muscles at 80-100% $\dot{V}O_2$ max also failed to identify a significant effect of median or minimum $PmbO_2$, indicating that data points at low O_2 flux did not obscure a relation between $\dot{V}O_2$ and PO_2. Tests of interaction and analysis of residuals suggest that the cytosolic redox and phosphorylation potentials contribute separable components to the control of $\dot{V}O_2$.

DISCUSSION

The principal findings we report are: 1) Almost all mitochondria function above 0.2 torr during exercise, even near $\dot{V}O_2$ max. 2) If O_2 delivery is normal $\dot{V}O_2$ can be fully accounted for by phosphorylation and redox potentials; O_2 per se is neither a limiting nor a controlling reactant. 3) A conservative upper bound on the PO_2 in vivo at which O_2 begins to limit respiration and energy turnover is 0.5 torr at $\dot{V}O_2$ max. This upper bound must be scaled downward at the lower work rates characteristic of normal exercise. 4) The $PcritO_2$ which the circulation must defend is extremely small relative to the O_2 tensions required for diffusive transport.

Comparison with Mitochondria In Vitro

Biochemists express $PcritO_2$ as the apparent K_m, i.e. the $[O_2]$ at half-maximal respiration. Published values for muscle mitochondria in state 3 measured at room temperature cluster about 0.03 torr.[11,12,13,14] Though the K_m is a convenient descriptor of in vitro data it is difficult to apply to organ function. Physiologists therefore define $PcritO_2$ as the $[O_2]$ at which a just detectable decrease in $\dot{V}O_2$ - say 10% - is observed. Data of Cole et al.[13] suggest $PcritO_2$ so defined is 2-3 times K_m for skeletal muscle mitochondria, or ∿0.1-0.2 torr at 25°C. Measurements of the effect on mitochondrial function of raising the temperature to 37°C suggest that although the rate increases ∿3 fold the oxygen dependence is very similar (D. Wilson personal communication). Thus 0.2 torr is a reasonable value with which to compare our upper bound for $PcritO_2$. In 6 muscles working at or near $\dot{V}O_2$ max only 10 of 300 cells were below 0.2 torr. We conclude that $PcritO_2$ is the same order of magnitude in vivo and in vitro. This conclusion is in accord with the fact that $\dot{V}O_2$ max for dog gracilis is almost exactly the same as $\dot{V}O_2$ max for isolated mitochondria when normalized to equal temperature and mitochondrial protein.[15] Measurements of NADH and flavoprotein fluorescence on the same muscles used for this report provide further evidence that the properties of mitochondria are the same in vivo and in vitro (unpublished observations with Olgin, Haselgrove, and Chance).

The reverse of the above conclusion was reached by Jöbsis and associates on the basis of reflectance spectrophotometry of cerebral cortex of cats and rabbits.[1,2] Cytochrome a,a3 was considered to be highly reduced, whereas it is 98-99% oxidized in mitochondria in vitro.[11,12,16] Cerebral redox and presumably $\dot{V}O_2$ were sensitive to O_2 even at partial pressures in the range of capillary PO_2! Highly reduced cytochrome a,a3 has also been reported in red muscle.[17] According to Jöbsis and associates one must distinguish between the binding of O_2 and the interaction of the O_2-cytochrome a,a3 complex with H^+ and electrons in the process of forming water. In their view the O_2 binding constant of cytochrome a,a3 could be much greater than the O_2 binding constants of Hb and Mb, even if cytochrome a,a3 were highly reduced. However, the subsequent electron transfer step would require a different reaction mechanism from that generally accepted.

Several technical factors could account for the spectroscopic observations of Jöbsis and associates. These include poor correlation of tissue PO_2 with PIO_2 and PaO_2, interference from Hb or Mb, an effect of hypoxemia on light scattering (Lubbers, personal communication), and most importantly inadequate spatial resolution. Light was collected from a tissue volume of ~ 4 mm^3. Such a volume is enormous on the scale of microcirculatory heterogeneities, and could contain poorly perfused loci. If half the mitochondria were anoxic and half normoxic the cytochrome spectrum would be the same as if cytochrome in a single mitochondrion were 50% reduced. Thus inferences about individual mitochondria cannot be drawn from potentially heterogeneous populations. In vitro, with no O_2 delivery system to contend with, measurements on populations should be acceptable.

Significance of PcritO_2 for O_2 Transport

Recent experiments identify the red-cell capillary system as a functional O_2 barrier.[5,18,19,20] The large transcapillary gradient results in low PO_2 in the interstitium and cytosol. Nature can achieve a large O_2 flux despite a small PO_2 gradient for extracapillary diffusion by creating short diffusion distances. The subsynaptic mitochondria in brain are an example. An alternative strategy is to use Mb as an O_2 carrier.[21] The Mb-facilitated O_2 flux increases as the percent Mb saturation and cell PO_2 decrease. We find $\dot{V}O_2$ unchanged at 10% saturation of Mb. Therefore, the critical PO_2 for cytochrome turnover must be less than 0.5 torr. Low Mb saturation and low critical PO_2 allow the cell to make full use of the Mb-facilitated O_2 flux.

ACKNOWLEDGEMENT

We thank Drs. A. Clark and P. Clark for stimulating discussions. This research was supported by grants HLB 03290, HLB 18208, and GM 07136 from the United States Public Health Service.

REFERENCES

1. F.F. Jobsis, J.H. Keizer, J.C. LaManna, and M. Rosenthal, Reflectance spectrophotometry of cytochrome a a3 in vivo, J. Appl. Physiol., 43:858 (1977).
2. M. Rosenthal, J.C. LaManna, F.F. Jobsis, J.E. Levasseur, H.A. Kontos, and J.L. Patterson, Effects of respiratory gases on cytochrome A in intact cerebral cortex: Is there a critical PO_2?, Brain Res., 108:143 (1976).
3. C.L. Bashford, C.H. Barlow, B. Chance, and J. Haselgrove, The oxidation-reduction state of cytochrome oxidase in freeze-trapped gerbil brains, FEBS Lett., 113:78 (1980).
4. C.R. Honig, C.L. Odoroff, and J.L. Frierson, Active and passive capillary control in a red muscle at rest and in exercise, Am. J. Physiol., 243:H196 (1982).
5. C.R. Honig, T.E.J. Gayeski, W. Federspiel, A. Clark Jr., and P. Clark, Muscle O_2 gradients from hemoglobin to cytochrome; new concepts, new complexities, Adv. Exp. Med. Biol., 169:23 (1984).
6. A. Clark, and P.A.A. Clark, Capture of spatially homogenous chemical reactions in tissue by freezing, Biophys. J., 42:25 (1983).
7. T.E.J. Gayeski, A cryogenic microspectrophotometric method for measuring myoglobin saturation in subcellular volumes; Application to resting dog gracilis muscle. Ph.D. Dissertation, University of Rochester, Rochester, NY (1982).
8. O. Lowry, and J.V. Passoneau, "A Flexible System of Enzymatic Analysis," Academic Press, New York (1972).
9. D.H. Horstman, M. Gleser, and J. Delehunt, Effects of altering O_2 delivery on $\dot{V}O_2$ of isolated, working muscle, Am. J. Physiol. 230:327 (1976).

10. D.F. Wilson, C.S. Owen, and A. Holian, Control of mitochon-drial respiration: A quantitative evaluation of the roles of cytochrome C and oxygen, Arch. Biochem. Biophys., 182:749 (1977).

11. B. Chance, and G.R. Williams, Respiratory enzymes in oxida-tive phosphorylation, J. Biol. Chem., 217, 383 (1955).

12. B. Chance, N. Oshino, T. Sugano, and A. Mayevsky, Basic prin-ciples of tissue oxygen determination from mitochondrial signals, Adv. Exp. Med. Biol., 37:277 (1973).

13. R.P. Cole, P.C. Sukanek, J.B. Wittenberg, and B.A. Witten-berg, Mitochondrial function in the presence of myoglobin, J. Appl. Physiol. 53:1116 (1982).

14. H. Starlinger, and D.W. Lubbers, Polarographic measurements of the oxygen pressure performed simultaneously with opti-cal measurements of the redox state of the respiratory chain in suspensions of mitochondria under steady state conditions at low oxygen tensions, Pfluger's Arch., 391:15 (1973).

15. R.J. Connett, T.E.J. Gayeski, and C.R. Honig, Lactate produc-tion in a pure red muscle in absence of anoxia, Adv. Exp. Med. Biol., 159:327 (1984).

16. B. Chance, Molecular basis of O_2 affinity for cytochrome oxi-dase, in: "Oxygen and Physiological Function," F.F. Jobsis, ed. Professional Information Library, Dallas, TX USA (1977).

17. I.E. Hassinen, and K. Hiltunen, Respiratory control in isolated perfused rat heart. Role of the equilibrium relations between the mitochondrial electron carriers and the adenylate system, Biochim. Biophys. Acta., 408, 319 (1975).

18. E.A. Rasio, and C.A. Goresky, Capillary limitation of oxygen diffusion in the isolated rete mirabili of the eel (Anguilla anguilla), Circ. Res. 44:498 (1979).

19. B.A. Wittenberg, and T.F.R. Robinson, Oxygen requirements, morphology, cell coat and membrane permeability of calcium-tolerant myocytes from hearts of adult rats, Cell Tissue Res. 216:231 (1981).

20. A. Clark, W. Federspiel, P.A.A. Clark, and G.R. Cokelet, Oxygen delivery from red cells, Biophys. J., in press.

21. B.A. Wittenberg, J.B. Wittenberg, and P.R.B. Caldwell, Role of myoglobin in the oxygen supply to red skeletal muscle. J. Biol. Chem. 250:9038 (1975).

WASHOUT OF A DILUENT BOLUS FROM CANINE HINDLIMB AS AN INDEX

OF RED CELL TRANSIT TIME[*]

S. Cain, Z. Turek, L. Hoofd, C. Chapler, and
F. Kreuzer

Depts. of Physiology, Univ. of Alabama in Birmingham
U.S.A., Univ. of Nijmegen, The Netherlands, and
Queen's Univ., Kingston, Ont., Canada

Our goal was to identify heterogeneity of blood flow
distribution in the canine hindlimb, particularly with onset of
hypoxia. The red blood cells served as a non-diffusible tracer
with the washout of a diluent bolus from the region. We used 2.5
ml of saline and recorded the wash-in and washout curves in
flowing blood as changes in hematocrit. To do this, the blood
flowed freely through an optical cuvette placed next to the
vessel. The light source was a fiberoptic cable carrying light
filtered for maximum transmission at 548 nm, an isobestic point
for hemoglobin. The detector was a phototransistor opposed to the
light source across a 2 mm light path. The output was linearized
by a log amplifier and calibrated against hematocrit. This
relatively simple system was adequately sensitive, stable, and was
not affected by hemoglobin saturation or by flow rate. The fact
that only a 2.5 ml bolus was used avoided potential problems of
recirculation and changing baseline values because of the
insignificant change in the whole body hematocrit.

The distribution of red cell transit times described by the
washout curve was fitted with a gamma density function for the
purpose of quantifying increased heterogeneity as increased
skewness of the curve. A generic form of this function is shown
in the box in Fig. 1. A measure of the variance in such curves
can be calculated as $1/\sqrt{\alpha}$ which has been called the "gamma"-index

---

[*] Supported by grants HL 14693 and HL 26927 from National Heart,
Lung, and Blood Institute, and by grants from MRC of Canada and
ZWO of The Netherlands.

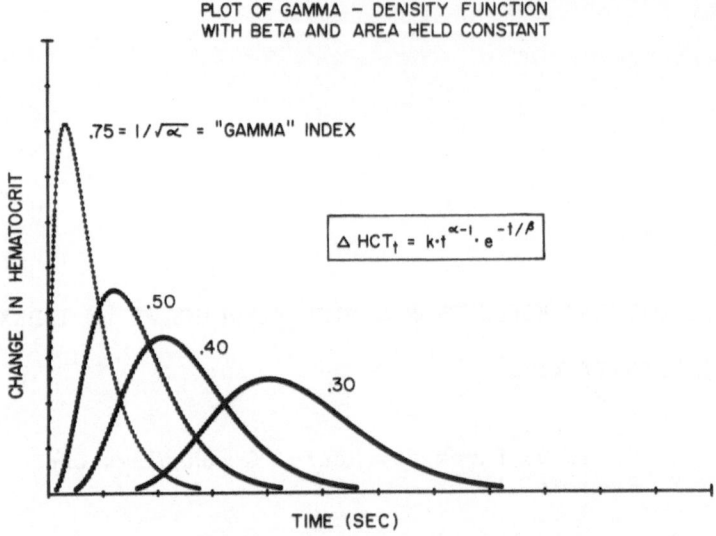

PLOT OF GAMMA – DENSITY FUNCTION
WITH BETA AND AREA HELD CONSTANT

$.75 = 1/\sqrt{\alpha} =$ "GAMMA" INDEX

$\Delta HCT_t = k \cdot t^{\alpha - 1} \cdot e^{-t/\beta}$

.50

.40

.30

CHANGE IN HEMATOCRIT

TIME (SEC)

Fig. 1.   Plot of the gamma density function with β and area under
the curve kept constant.

by Tomita and his associates (1983). This index, therefore,
quantifies the departure from normal distribution or skewness in
these curves and can be interpreted as a spatial dispersion of
transit times of the indicator particles, the red cells in this
case. As shown in this figure with beta and area under the curve
held constant, an increasing "gamma"-index denotes an increase in
skewness or, for our purposes, an increase in heterogeneity of
transit times through a regional circulation.

In the experimental preparation, the entire venous outflow of
the left hindlimb of anesthetized dogs was redirected through the
femoral vein by two tourniquets inserted through the limb at the
groin. The paw circulation was excluded by a third tourniquet. A
loop with two channels was inserted into the femoral artery and
one hematocrit sensor was placed in line distally. One channel
contained a measured volume of 2.5 ml of saline that was washed
into the limb at the prevailing perfusion pressure when two tubing
clamps were repositioned to the other channel where blood flowed
continually until that moment. A second hematocrit sensor was
placed in the venous outflow with a cannulating flow probe
proximal to it. For each trial, the arterial and venous
hematocrit and flow curves were sampled at a rate of 4/sec and
stored in digital form.

302

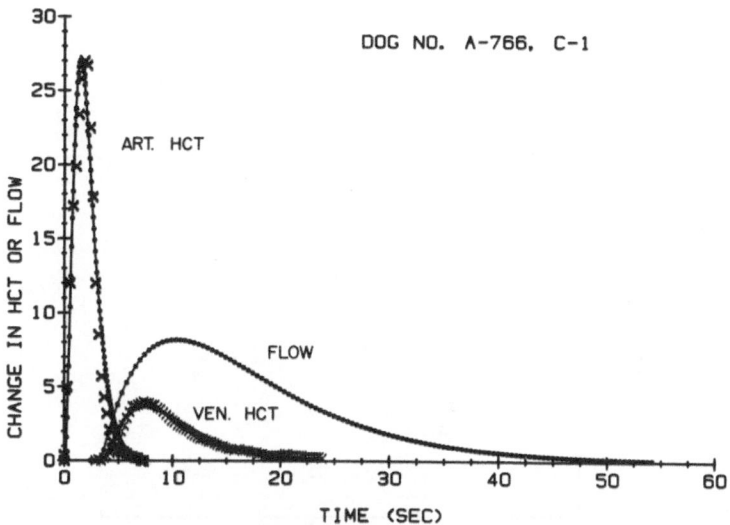

Fig. 2. Representative control curves for the change in hematocrit with venous washout, and for the change in limb blood flow

An example of the three curves that were recorded for each wash-in of diluent can be seen in Fig. 2. The individual data points are indicated by the "x"s and the fitted curves by connected dots. In most cases, a very good fit was obtained with correlation coefficients generally in excess of 0.95. One other phenomenon that was invariably associated with the wash-in of diluents was the transient increase in flow shown in the figure. We thought at first that this was due to the much lesser viscosity of saline relative to blood. High molecular weight Ficoll or dextran in saline made no difference, however. Mammalian Ringers solution or the animal's own plasma also had the same effect.

We do not believe that the flow transient importantly affects the interpretation of the "gamma"-index. As Fig. 3 shows, there was no relationship between the mean increase in flow and the dispersion of transit times as reflected by the "gamma"-index. For the two experiments illustrated, the flow increase tended to be much larger in one than the other but the range for the "gamma"-index was nearly the same in both. As Tomita et al (1983) pointed out, the "gamma"-index is entirely dependent on the complexity of the tissue model and was unaffected by flow rate variations even over a five-fold range.

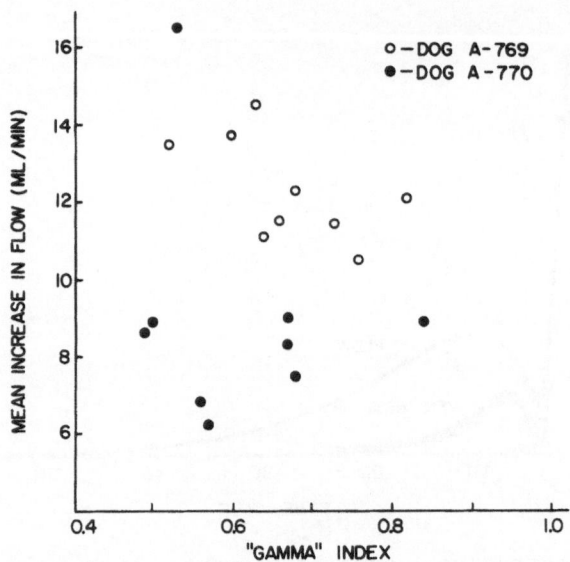

Fig. 3. The mean increase in flow shown in relation to the "gamma"-index for two experiments.

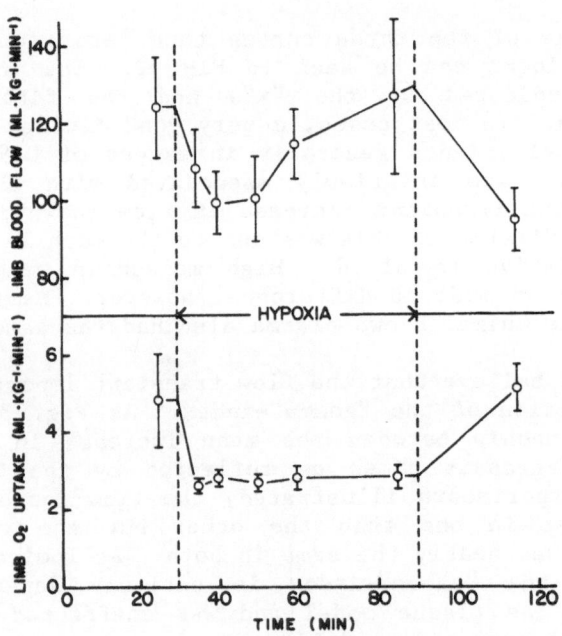

Fig. 4. Mean values (±SE) for limb blood flow and limb O_2 uptake.

We wished to see how the distribution of red cells transit times would be altered by a physiologic intervention such as severe hypoxia. Seven anesthetized dogs were paralyzed and pump-ventilated with room air for 30 min, then with 9% O_2 in N_2 for 60 min, followed by a 30 min recovery period in which they were ventilated once again with room air. Washout curves were recorded every 10 min during control, at 5, 10, 20, 30, and 55 min during hypoxia, and after 25 min of recovery. As shown in Fig. 4, this level of hypoxia was sufficient to decrease the limb O_2 uptake significantly throughout the entire 60 min period of hypoxia. During hypoxia, arterial PO_2 averaged about 25 mmHg and femoral venous PO_2 decreased from 21.2 mmHg at 5 min of hypoxia to 11.8 mmHg by the end of hypoxia. Limb blood flow, the upper part of Fig. 4, tended to be decreased during the first 20 min of hypoxia while limb peripheral resistance was significantly increased.

Fig. 5 illustrates the sequential changes in the venous washout curve. C3 is the last control and the 5 hypoxia curves at 5, 10, 20, 30, and 55 min are labelled H1 through H5. Once again, the "x"s are the sampled data points and the connected dots show the fitted curves. The "gamma"-index is indicated above the tail of each curve. This particular experiment followed the overall pattern very well. There was an increase in the heterogeneity of red cell transit times during the first 20 min of hypoxia with a

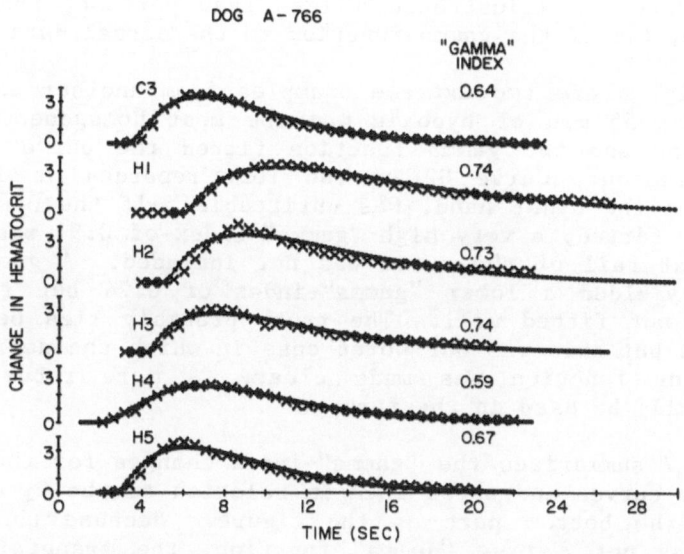

Fig. 5. Sequential changes in venous washout curves from control (C3), and 5, 10, 20, 30, and 55 min of hypoxia.

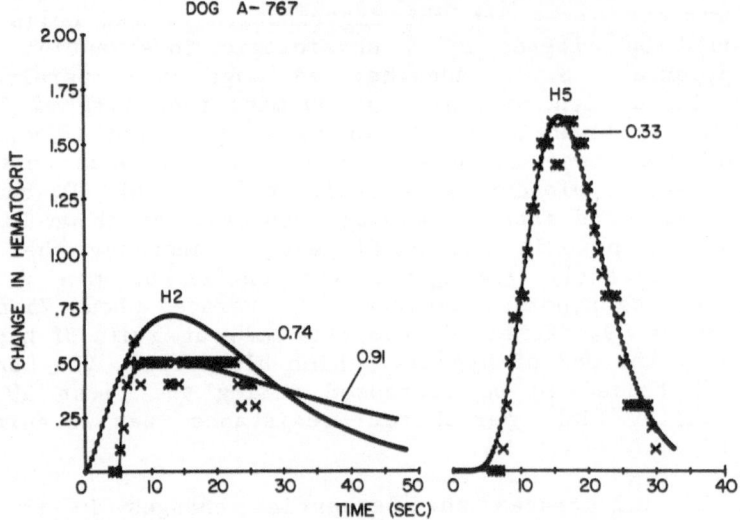

Fig. 6. Venous washout curves recorded at 10 and at 55 min of hypoxia in one experiment.

more homogeneous pattern returning further into the hypoxic period. Curve H2 illustrates a less than perfect, though still quite good, fit of the gamma function to the actual data.

In Fig. 6 are two extreme examples from another experiment. Curve H5 at 55 min of hypoxia was the most homogeneous pattern that we saw and the gamma function fitted the curve in nearly perfect fashion. Curve H2 on the left recorded at 10 min of hypoxia, on the other hand, was unfittable. If the onset of the change was fitted, a very high "gamma"-index of 0.91 was obtained but the fat tail of the curve was not included. A good fit for the tail yielded a lower "gamma"-index of 0.74 but the abrupt onset was not fitted well. The truth probably lies between the two values but this was our worst case in which the deficiency of the fitting function was made clear. A more robust fitting function will be used in the future.

Fig. 7 summarizes the "gamma"-index changes for the arterial and venous curves and shows them in relation to the O_2 extraction ratio in the bottom part of the figure. Because the arterial wash-in was not a true "delta" function, the transfer function should have been obtained by deconvoluting the two curves. Unfortunately, we have not yet had time to adapt a deconvolution program to the Apple microcomputer. Fortunately, the "gamma"-index

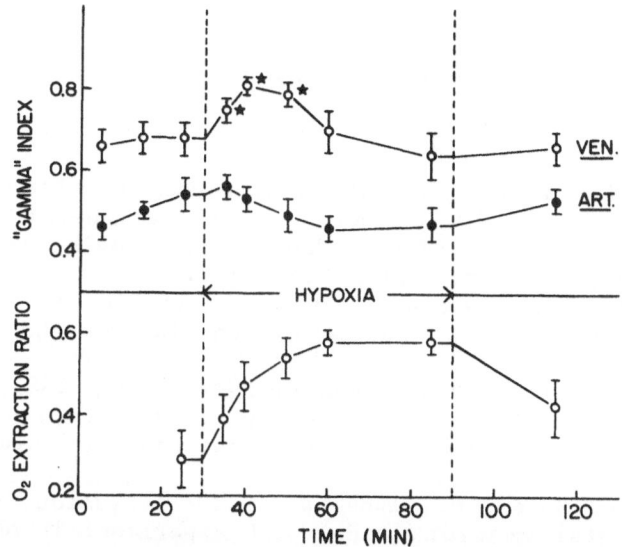

Fig. 7. Mean values (±SE) of the "gamma"-index for venous and arterial curves and for limb O_2 extraction ratio.

for the arterial wash-in did not change significantly with hypoxia. The significant increase in the "gamma"-index of the venous washout curves during the first 20 min of hypoxia, therefore, denotes an increased heterogeneity of perfusion. This occurred despite the fact that O_2 extraction was increasing and O_2 uptake was limited by availability at this time.

Past evidence has strongly suggested that an increase in O_2 extraction is associated with an increase in effective capillary surface area (Kvietys et al, 1983). Furthermore, the increase in capillary surface area is a function of precapillary vessels that are more sensitive than resistance vessels to tissue hypoxia (Granger et al, 1976). An increase in heterogeneity of perfusion with the onset of hypoxia would imply, therefore, that there was also a heterogeneous pattern of O_2 uptake reduction in the hindlimb musculature. In other words, all areas of this regional circulation may not have generated equal intensities of metabolic stimuli in response to the tissue hypoxia. As metabolic vasodilation became sufficiently strong to oppose the vasoconstrictor tone later in hypoxia, the "gamma"-index indicated a more homogeneous pattern of washout. We already knew from the work of Renkin et al (1981) and Piiper and Meyer (1984) that very large variability could exist in microvessel perfusion of resting skeletal muscle. Cerretelli et al (1979) have presented evidence that this can even be the case in contracting muscle. Our observations indicate that the early adjustment to tissue hypoxia actually involves an exaggeration of the existing heterogeneous pattern of perfusion.

REFERENCES

Cerretelli, P., Pendergast, D.R., Krasney, J., Plewes, J., and Rennie, D.W., 1979, Central and peripheral blood flow adjustments to exercise in dogs. Physiologist 22:18.

Granger, H.J., Goodman, A.H., and Granger, D.N., 1976, Role of resistance and exchange vessels in local microvascular control of skeletal muscle oxygenation in the dog. Circ. Res. 38:379–385.

Kvietys, P.R., Perry, M.A., and Granger, D.N., 1983, Intestinal capillary exchange capacity and oxygen delivery-to-demand ratio. Am. J. Physiol. 245 (Gastrointest. Liver Physiol. 8):G635–G640.

Piiper, J. and Meyer, M., 1984, Diffusion-perfusion relationships in skeletal muscle: model and experimental evidence from inert gas washout. In: Oxygen Transport to Tissue V. (Adv. Exp. Med. Biol. 169), edited by D.W. Lubbers, H. Acker, E. Lehniger-Follert, and T.K. Goldstick. New York, Plenum Press, pp. 457–466.

Renkin, E., Gray, S.D., and Dodd, L.R., 1981, Filling of micro-circulation in skeletal muscle during timed India ink perfusion. Am. J. Physiol. 241 (Heart Circ. Physiol. 10):H174–H186.

Tomita, M., Gotoh, F., Amaro, T., Tanahashi, N., Kobari, M., Shinohara, T., and Mihara, B., 1983, Transfer function through regional cerebral cortex evaluated by a photoelectric method. Am. J. Physiol. 245 (Heart Circ. Physiol. 14):H385–H398.

OXYGEN EXCHANGES BETWEEN BLOOD AND RESTING SKELETAL

MUSCLE: A SHUNT-SINK HYPOTHESIS

P. Grieb, P.C. Pape, R.E. Forster,
C.W. Goodwin, S. Nioka, and L. Labbatte

Department of Physiology
University of Pennsylvania
Philadelphia, PA   19104

Prevously we have reported the use of oxygen-18
isotope and double indicator dilution methodology to
measure the exchanges of eoxygen between blood and brain
tissues (Grieb et al., 1983).   In the present experiments
we used the same technique for the study of a canine
hind limb preparation.   To our knowledge, oxygen isotopes
have not been used to study the features of oxygen delivery to muscles, with the exception of preliminary
studies of Forster, el al. (1976) and Rose and Goreski
(1982).   More is known about the distribution of inert
diffusible tracers in muscle preparations; (eg. Aukland
and Leraand, 1960; Paradise et al., 1971; Piiper and
Meyer, in press; Sparks and Mohrman, 1977; Tonnesen and
Sjersen, 1967), and such data are sometimes extrapolated
to oxygen.

METHODS
Dogs were anesthetized with pentobarbital,
paralyzed with gallamine and mechanically ventilated
with air.   In most of the experiments arterial blood
was continuously withdrawn from the aorta and
propelled by a peristaltic pump through a plastic
tube, volume approximately 250 ml, into the exposed
femoral artery distal to a ligation.   The perfusion
rate was within the range of 50 - 120ml/min,
corresponding to 7 - 15 ml/100g tissue x min.
Pressure at entry into the femoral artery was higher

than the animal's own arterial pressure, eliminating other sources of blood flow into the limb. The leg was skinned and wrapped in a moist cloth, and temperature loss controlled by infrared heating.

Blood for injection was labelled with oxygen-18 and chromium-51 (reference label bound to erythrocytes) as described previously. In some experiments, inert diffusible tracers, acetylene and/or tritiated water (THO) were also added to injectate.

During the experimental run two to five ml of injectate were rapidly introduced into the femoral artery. Anaerobic sampling of the femoral venous outflow was performed in a non-obstructive manner using a 1.7 mm indwelling catheter and a peristaltic pump. Branches that might have added venous blood from tissue regions not supplied by the femoral artery were tied. Sampling rate did not exceed 30% of the perfusion rate. Up to 35 samples were taken within 60-90 s following the injection of the labelled blood. No recirculation occurs by this time.

Oxygen-18 and acetylene, chromium-51 and tritium were measured with a mass spectrometer, a gamma-counter and a liquid scintillation counter, respectively. Arterial and femoral venous oxygen content and PO_2 were measured before and after each sampling run.

RESULTS

Fig. 1 shows an example of a typical set of indicator-dilution curves. The fractions of the injected labelled species escaping from the tissue per unit of time, h(t), are plotted in a semi-logarithmic scale. Figs. 2 and 3 show the extraction plots. Extraction of a tracer is defined as

$$E(t) = 1 - h_{tracer}/h_{reference}$$

All recorded sets of curves seem to share the following common characteristics:
1. Labelled oxygen curves are either only slightly delayed behind the reference curves, or not delayed at all. The difference between oxygen-18 and chromium-51

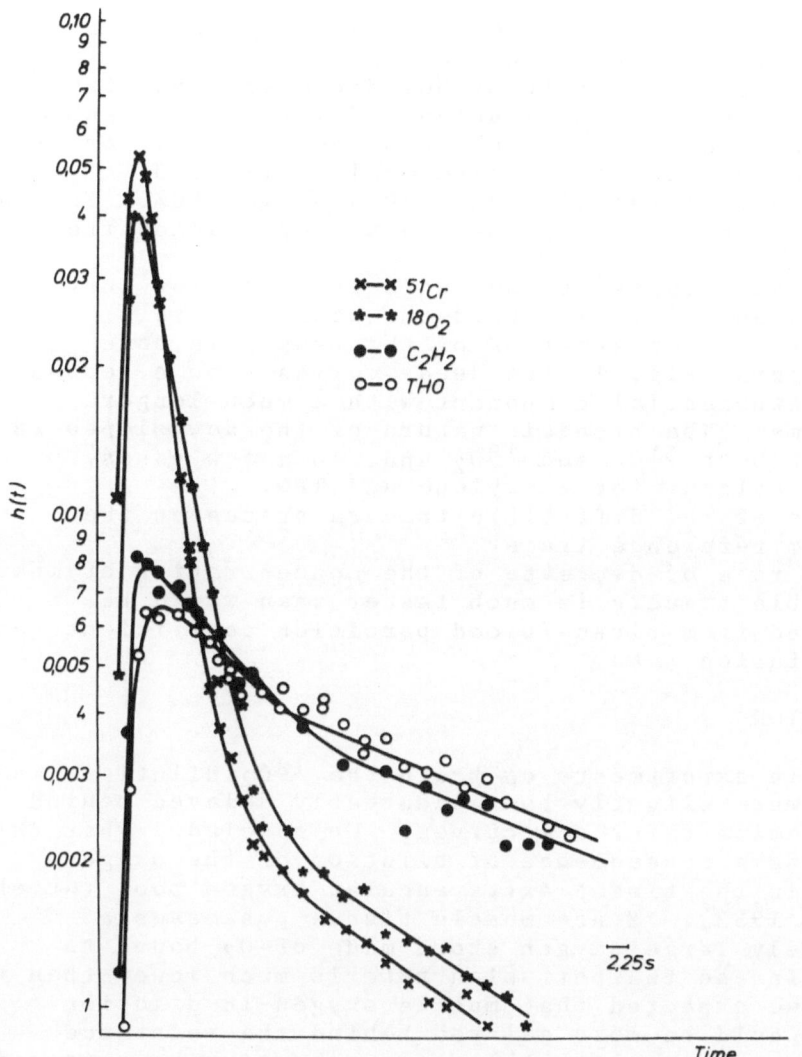

Fig. 1.   Indicator-dilution curves of four tracers
           plotted in a semilogarithmic scale.

mean transit times, calculated as

$$\frac{{}_0\int^\infty t\,C(t)\,dt}{{}_0\int^\infty C(t)\,dt}$$

ranged from 0.2 to 6.0 s.

2. The extraction of $^{18}O_2$ at the beginning of a pulse of indicators is higher than extraction of elemental O_2. Later it either decreases, showing the evidence of a small amount of labelled oxygen returning from tissue back to blood (Fig. 2), or it joins the extraction of elemental O_2 (Fig. 3). Initial extraction of oxygen-18 averages 60%. Initial extraction of inert diffusible tracers ranges from 85 to 95%.

3. The downslopes of the indicator dilution curves are exponential from behind the peak down to a concentration of about 5% of the peak. In some experiments (Fig. 1) the decay curves show a second slower exponential component with a much longer half-time. The biphasic nature of the downslopes is seen for both ^{51}Cr and $^{18}O_2$ and, in a few cases, is also evident for acetylene and THO.

4. None of the diffusible tracers precesses the chromium reference tracer.

5. The rate of decrease of the concentration of inert diffusible tracers is much faster than would be predicted from tissue/blood partition coefficients and the perfusion rate.

DISCUSSION

In experiments on brain the $^{18}O_2$ dilution curves were slightly but measureably delayed behind the chromium reference curves. We concluded that this delay was a consequence of dilution of the oxygen tracer in the tissue extravascular oxygen pool (Grieb et al., 1983). Since muscle tissue possesses a relatively large oxygen store made of O_2 bound to myoglobin and the perfusion rate is much lower than in brain, we expected that muscle oxygen-18 dilution curves would be more delayed behind the reference dilution curves, with the oxygen-chromium mean transit time difference in the range of half a minute. We never obtained a result even close to this expectation.

A lack of precession of inert gas curve compared to the tagged erythrocyte curve speaks against the presence of a significant diffusional

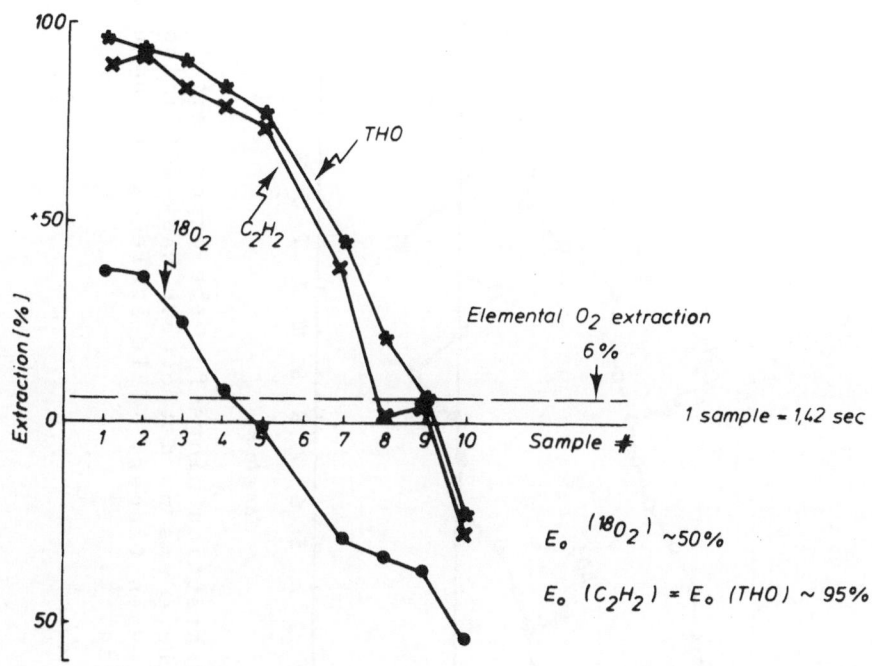

Fig. 2.   Extraction plots for the experiment shown
on Fig. 1.

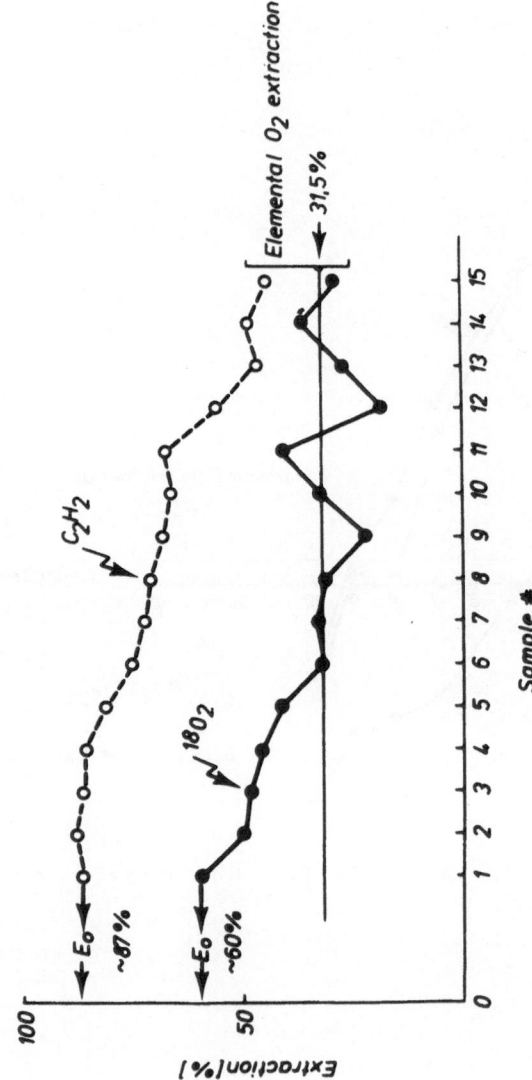

Fig. 3.   Extraction plots for the experiment in which
there was no detectable back-diffusion of the
oxygen tracer.   Tile scale is the same as in
Fig. 2.

shunting in our preparation. The concept of a barrier to oxygen penetration into the tissue also fails to explain our findings. If such were the case, the extraction of oxygen-18 should have a plateau at the beginning of the venous outflow curve. Extraction of the labelled oxygen at the very beginning of tracer profiles was the highest, and it had started to decline before the peak of the chromium curve. However, the present results can be explained by tissue perfusion heterogeneity.

Muscle tissue perfusion heterogeneity

Muscles are capable of increasing their resting oxygen consumption by a factor of up to 100 times. Therefore, the muscle vascular bed must be capable of delivering both quite small and very large quantities of oxygen, depending on demand. Presumably in heavy exercise all available capillaries are continuously perfused with blood. At rest, however, only a small number of capillaries may be open at a time. Some experimental estimates of the fraction of capillaries open to flow in a feline resting muscle are as low as 20% for sartorius (LaLone and Johnson, 1979), or 10% for gracilis and tenuissimus (Honig et al., 1970; McDonagh et al. 1982).

Consider that 10% of capillaries are open at a time. Such is a static, "snapshot" picture. We expect that tissue resistance vessels open and close in a cyclic manner. If the mean time for a capillary to be open to flow is 5 s, the average time a capillary stays closed may be above one minute.

Renkin et al. (1981) performed timed infusions of an intravascular tracer (India ink) into the arterial supply of a resting rabbit hind limb. They found that the fraction of capillary network which filled with the tracer increased progressively with the infusion time. After 3.5 s only 12 - 19% of capillaries were filled with ink, whereas after 60 - 90 s this fraction rose to 58 - 80%. This result may be interpreted as an evidence for capillary transit times ranging from less than 3 s to more than 30 s. The mechanism responsible for such a marked heterogeneity of muscle capillary transit times is not known. Analysis performed by Renkin et al. (1981) shows that the phenomenon cannot be fully explained by the distribution of capillary lengths, thus it must be related to varying flow velocities in different parts of the capillary network. Intermittency of flow in some capillaries may be a reasonable explanation here.

It has been hypothesized that two parallel vascular pathways exist in a skinned hind limb preparation, both located in muscle tissue (Renkin, 1955; 1971). These pathways were thought to be exchange capillaries with similar permeability characteristics, but varying in the ratio of blood flow to tissue volume. Our present observations may be explained by such a "double circulation" phenomenon, possibly involving capillary intermittent flow. Per analogiam to Renkin's "Nutritional-Shunt-Flow" hypothesis we describe such a hypothetical mechanism for oxygen distribution to resting muscle tissue as the "Nutritional-Shunt-Sink".

The Nutritional-Shunt-Sink model of oxygen supply to a resting muscle

Consider the possibility that arterial blood flowing into the resting muscles follows two very different routes. Of an element volume of blood, flow x dt, entering tissue, a fraction f flows through a part of the capillary network which at the moment is open to flow, its mean transit time in the range of seconds. The remaining fraction 1-f enters regions of capillary network in which flow is much slower. This fraction is "trapped" in tissue for a longer time, in the range of minutes. These two routes, the "fast" channel and the "slow" channel, are referred to as a "shunt" and a "sink".

Blood flowing through the "fast" channel ("shunt") may exchange substances with a small volume of tissue. Therefore, it is not a "perfect" shunt but a "shunt" with some, if small, exchanging capability. The remaining large volume of tissue equilibrates with blood trapped in the capillaries for a much longer time (the sink). If we then consider the oxygen exchange, we find that much more oxygen is withdrawn from blood flowing through the "slow channel", compared to the blood flowing through the "fast" channel. Here, analogously, the "slow" channel is not a "perfect" sink for oxygen, but a "sink" which

316

permits some, if a small, amount of oxygen to excape the "trap", even if it lasts a minute or longer.

Labelled erythrocytes and oxygen-18 are distributed between the "fast" and the "slow" flow channels in the same proportion. Blood leaving the "sink" region has almost all its oxygen removed, labelled or unlabelled as the case may be. It therefore acts to dilute the blood passing through the "shunt" region, which reduces both unlabelled and labelled oxygen in the mixed venous outflow in the same proportions. There is no lag in the transit of oxygen-18; the shape of the oxygen indicator dilution curve is almost the same as the reference chromium curve reduced by the proportion, venous elemental O_2 content/arterial elemental O_2 content. Chromium-labelled cells from the "sink" region are delayed, their transit time through the tissue is very long, so these cells may not be seen until the later parts of the venous curve. The inert diffusible tracers in the "sink" region diffuse into the surrounding tissue. Thus these species show delayed washout in the venous curve.

The shape of a particular set of dilution curves depends on the actual value of f, and on the degree of imperfectness of "shunt" and "sink". Some of our results seem quite close to the "perfect shunt-sink" situation, whereas others deviate substantially. But the overall pattern seems to be explainable, qualitatively at the moment, in terms of our hypothesis.

Dilution curves of intravascular tracers

It is commonly accepted, after Hamilton, et al. (1928), that the downslopes of intravascular indicator dilution curves are monoexponential. Such an outflow pattern is a common experience, related perhaps to the short recording time. Usually a deviation from mono-exponentiality would have been obscured by and/or attributed to the tracer recirculation. However, Effros and Weissman (1979) published a semilogarithmic plot of the dilution curves of several indicators in a perfused feline leg preparation, recorded up to 5 min after the injection. In that experiment the double-exponential nature of the tail of the intravascular tracer (radioiodinated albumin) dilution curve is evident. The other tracers used (Na^+ and bicarbonate) exhibit qualitatively similar behavior. The half-time of the slow component of the intravascular indicator outflow curve seems to be almost one minute, compared to approx. 4 s for the fast part. The difference is, therefore, fifteen-fold. The slow component shows up at a tracer concentration below 5% of the peak. Nevertheless, when extrapolated to time infinity, the area under the slow part of the curve may contribute about 30% of the total area.

Some of our records also show evidence of a slow component appearing at the tail of the chromium curve (Fig. 1). The oxygen-18 profile deviates from the monoexponential shape in a similar manner.

Dilution curves of inert diffusible tracers

Washout curves of inert diffusible tracers from muscle preparations are generally multi-exponential, displaying two or three components (eg. Aukland and Leraand, 1960; Piiper and Meyer, in press; Tonnesen and Sjersen, 1967). This multi-exponentiality has been interpreted as a consequence of flow heterogeneity (Sparks and Mohrman, 1977), or diffusional shunting (Aukland and Leraand, 1967). Recently Piiper and Meyer (in press) reported recordings of washout of two inert gases of differing diffusivity, CH_4 and SF_6, from the canine hind limb at rest and during exercise. These authors found the washout of the less diffusible gas (SF_6) faster than the washout of the more diffusible gas (CH_4). This was explained by assuming countercurrent veno-arterial exchange of gases in the hind limb circulation. However, we may also assume that the more diffusible gas penetrates more deeply into tissue structures, equilibrating with a larger volume of tissue, and thus its outflow is slower. In our experiments we did not see such a difference between acetylene and water indicators. However, the scatter in the data could have accounted for this.

We may also note another striking feature of the data of Effros and Weissman (1979). These authors used tritiated water as one of the indicators. The labelled water curve in that experiment does not show a multiexponential tail, but the half-time of its decay is as short as 3 min, which is only 3 times longer than $t_{1/2}$ for the slow component of intravascular indicator. Taking into account that the steady state tissue/blood partition coefficient of water is about 1, we must conclude that water equilibrated with only a very small volume of tissue. Presumably, the slow component of the water outflow curve did not show up within the recording time.

Tissue oxygen tension

A remaining unexplained observation is that tissue and intracellular PO_2 in resting muscle seem to be much lower than venous PO_2. This has been shown by direct measurements of PO_2 with microelectrodes (Whalen, 1971). Also, studies of myoglobin (Mb) oxygenation by a carbon monoxide/oxygen equilibrium method (Coburn and Mayers, 1971) showed that in resting muscle Mb is approximately 65% oxygenated. Since P_{50} for myoglobin is about 6 mmHg, these results translate to a mean tissue PO_2 of less than 10 mmHg. Cryophotometric measurements of MbO_2 in resting muscle (Gayeski and Honig, 1978) indicate a higher myoglobin oxygenation, 77 - 91%. However, the distribution of MbO_2 appears to be bimodal, with a broad peak corresponding to PO_2's of 14 - 35 mmHg, and a narrow peak at saturations indicating PO_2's of above 84 mmHg.

Both low PO_2's and their bimodal distribution can be explained by tissue perfusion heterogeneity of the degree mentioned above. Low PO_2 measurements would be found in tissue which is perfused very slowly (low perfusion to metabolism ratio). High PO_2 values would be found in tissue surrounding capillaries with fast (uninterrupted) flow.

We should mention a calculation of red cell velocity in canine hind limb muscle, reported by Honig and Gayeski (1982). These authors obtained an estimate of mean capillary transit time of 30 s, which would result in O_2 extraction of 100% in some capillaries. The result has been criticized, but it might be explained by the present hypothesis.

The evidence available at the moment to support the "Shunt-Sink" concept may be regarded as circumstantial. Nevertheless, the hypothesis of a "double circulation" in muscles, and the possibility of capillary intermittency and blood "trapping" in tissue should perhaps be considered along with other proposals, such as diffusional shunting, counter-current veno-arterial exchange and diffusional barriers (Grunewald and Sowa, 1977), in the interpretation of experimental data concerning the distribution of gases, including oxygen, between blood and muscle tissues.

Our ability to measure oxygen-18 dilution curves is limited by the resolution threshold of the mass spectrometric technique. A verification of our hypothesis could be provided, at least in part, by more systematic studies of the outflow patterns of intravascular indicators, particularly after their concentration in the venous outflow has fallen to below 5% of the peak.

REFERENCES

Aukland, K., and Leraand, S., 1960, Arteriovenous counter-current exchange of hydrogen gas in skeletal muscle. J. Clin. Lab. Invest., Suppl. 93:72-75.

Coburn, R.F., and Mayers, L.B., 1971, Myoglobin O_2 tension determined from measurements of carboxymyoglobin in skeletal muscle, Am. J. Physiol. 220: 66-74.

Effros, R.M., and Weissman, M.L., 1979, Carbonic anhydrase activity of the cat hind leg, J. Appl. Physiol.47: 1090-1098.

Forster, R.E., Goodwin, C.W., and Itada, N., 1976, A new approach to the experimental measurement of mean tissue PO_2, in: Oxygen Transport to Tissue-II, Adv. Exp. Med. Biol. 75: 41-46.

Gayeski, T.E.J., and Honig, C.R., 1978, Myoglobin saturation and calculated PO_2 in single cells of resting gracilis muscles, in: Oxygen Transport to Tissue-III, Adv. Exp. Med. Biol. 94: 77-84.

Grieb, P., Forster, R.E., and Pape, P.C., 1983, Oxygen indicator dilution curves of the canine cerebral circulation, in: Oxygen Transport to Tissue-IV, Adv. Exp. Med. Biol. 159: 103-117.

Grunewald, W.A. and Sowa, W., 1977, Capillary
structures and O_2 supply to tissue, Rev.
Physiol. Biochem. Pharmacol. 77:149-209.

Hamilton, W.F., Moore, J.W., Kinsman, J.J., and
Spurling,R.G., 1928, Simultaneous
determination of the greater and lesser
circulation time, of the mean velocity of
blood flow through the heart and lungs, of
the cardiac output and an approximation of
the amount of blood actively circulating in
the heart and lungs, Am. J. Physiol. 85:
337-345.

Honig, C.R., Frierson, J.L., and Patterson, J.L.,
1970, Comparison of neural controls of
resistance and capillary density in resting
muscle, Am. J. Physiol. 218: 937-942.

Honig, C.R., and Gayeski, T.E.J., 1982, Correlation
of O_2 transport in the micro and macro
scale, Int. J. Microcirc. Clin. Exp.
1:367-380.

LaLone, B.J., ad Johnson, P.C., 1979,
Arteriolar-capillary network analysis in
resting cat sartorius muscle, Microvasc. Res.
17:S19 (Abstract).

McDonagh, P.F., Gore, R.W., and Gray, S.D., 1982,
Perfused capillary surface area in postural
and locomotor skeletal muscle, Microvasc.
Res. 24: 142-157.

Paradise, N.F., Swayze, C.R., and Fox, I.J., 1971,
Perfusion heterogeneity in skeletal muscle
using tritiated water, Am. J. Physiol. 220:
1107-1115.

Piiper, J., and Meyer, M., 1984,
Diffusion-perfusion relationships in skeletal
muscle: models and experimental evidence
from inert gas washout, in: Oxygen Transport to
Tissue-V, Adv. Exp. Med. Biol! 169:457-465.

Renkin, E.M., 1955, Effects of blood flow on
perfusion kinetics in isolated, perfused
hindlegs of cats: A double circulation
hypothesis, Am. J. Physiol. 183: 125-131.

Renkin, E.M., 1971, The Nutritional-Shunt-Flow
hypothesis in skeletal muscle circulation,
Circ. Res. 28/29, Suppl.: 121-125.

Renkin, E.M., Gray, S.D., and Dodd, L.R., 1981,
Filling microcirculation in skeletal muscles
during timed India ink perfusion, Am. J.
Physiol. 241: H174-H186.

Rose, C.P., and Goreski, C.A., 1982, Barrier-limited
    transport of oxygen in the coronary
    circulation, Fed. Proc. 41: 1252 (Abstract).
Sparks, H.V., and Mohrman, D.E., 1977,
    Heterogeneity of flow as an explanation for
    the multiexponential washout of inert gas
    from skeletal muscle, Microvasc. Res.
    13: 181-184.
Tonnesen, K.H., and Sjersen, P., 1967, Inert gas
    diffusion method for measurement of blood
    flow, Circ. Res. 20: 552-564.
Whalen, W.J., 1971, Intracellular PO_2 in heart and
    skeletal muscle, Physiologist 14: 69-82.

ACKNOWLEDGEMENTS

    This research was supported in part by
Program Project Grant HLB 19737 from the NIH.
    P. Grieb was on leave of absence from the
Department of Neurophysiology, Polish Academy of
Sciences Medical Research Centre, Warsaw, Poland.
    Current address of C.W. Goodwin, Director, Burn
Center New York, Cornell Medical Center, New York, NY
10021.

EFFECTS OF INTERMITTENT CAPILLARY FLOW ON OXYGEN TRANSPORT

IN SKELETAL MUSCLE STUDIED BY DYNAMIC COMPUTER SIMULATION

Masakazu Fukuoka, Masahiro Shibata*, and Akira Kamiya*

Dept. of Physiology, Kyorin University and
Research Inst. of Applied Electricity, Hokkaido Univ.*
6-20-2, Shinkawa, Mitaka-shi, 182 Tokyo, Japan

INTRODUCTION

Intravital observations of the microcirculation in various skeletal muscles have revealed that the red cell velocity in the capillaries at the resting state is neither steady nor uniform. It often fluctuates rhythmically so that capillaries alternate in their extent of opening periodically (Cardon et al., 1970; Prewitt and Johnson, 1976; Lindbom et al., 1980). Fig.1 shows an example of red cell velocity changes measured at a capillary in the rabbit tenuissimus muscle suffused with oxygenated Tyrode solution (Shibata et al., 1983). Under physiological conditions of the ambient oxygen tension (PO_2, 30-50 mmHg) and pH (7.3-7.4), the frequency of cyclic velocity changes was in the range of 0.05 -0.2 Hz which was slower than the respiration rate of the animal.

Fig.1 Capillary red cell velocity measured in the rabbit tenuissimus muscle. Note the periodic changes in red cell velocities of 0.05-0.1 Hz which is much slower than the breathing rate as observed from the respiratory fluctuations of the arterial pressure simultaneously measured.

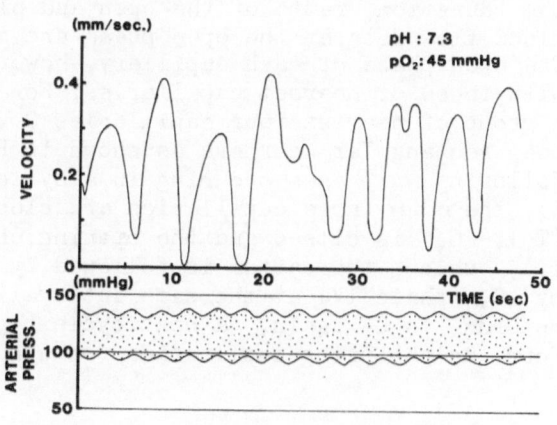

Although the mechanism inducing such periodic velocity changes is not completely clear, it is obvious that this phenomenon directly affects the gaseous transport and other nutrient supply to the tissue. For instance, tissue PO_2 in the skeletal muscle has been reported to fluctuate with a similar frequency (Whalen and Nair, 1967). Nevertheless, the physiological significance of this phenomenon in transcapillary substance exchange has not been well investigated yet. The purpose of this study is to elucidate the possible role of the periodic or intermittent capillary blood flow in O_2 transport to tissue by means of a dynamic computer simulation.

To perform such a simulation of dynamic oxygen transport, it is necessary to introduce a new model, instead of conventional steady state ones represented by the Krogh cylinder model. In this study, we use a dynamic model of intermittent capillary flow, in which each of the uniformly distributed capillaries repeats the open and closed states in the same frequency but with a different phase to any neighbouring capillaries.

MATHEMATICAL MODEL AND COMPUTATIONAL PROCEDURES

It is anatomically well known that most capillaries in the mammalian skeletal muscles run in parallel to the straight muscle fibers. Various physiological findings also indicate that only 1/4 to 1/3 of the total capillaries are open to pass blood flow in the resting skeletal muscle (Mellander and Johansson, 1968). To simulate such a situation, we use a symmetric model of capillary-tissue arrangement in this study as schematically illustrated in Fig.2 (a). In this model, 1/4 of the uniformly distributed capillaries are open at regular intervals while the remainders are closed at any moment. In each capillary, a regular cycle of intermittent flow is repeated in such a way that a state of constant flow continues during a certain period (open phase) and is then followed by a state of no flow (closed phase) which is 3-fold longer than the open phase. The frequency of the cycle, the duration ratio of the open and closed phases (1:3) and the blood flow rate at the open phase are common in all capillaries. The open phase of each capillary, however, has discrete time lags with those of nearest capillaries. For an instant, if one notices a group of nearest four capillaries C_1, C_2, C_3 and C_4 located at the rectangular corners as shown in Fig.2 (b), one finds the following 4 phases occuring in a cycle: When C_1 is open (phase I), the other three capillaries are closed. After a certain period (To), C_1 is closed and the opening channel moves to C_2 (phase II), which thereafter is followed by C_3 (phase III) and finally by C_4 (phase IV) at the same interval. When the open channel returns to C_1 again, a next cycle begins. Every group of such four neighbouring capillaries repeats the same cyclic change so as to maintain the symmetric pattern of open capillary distribution. This mode of a cyclic alteration in open capillaries provides a most uniform blood flow supply to the tissue in an intermittent flow pattern with duration ratio 1:3.

The symmetric geometry of the open capillary distribution in Fig.2 (b) indicates that if the group of capillaries C_1, C_2, C_3 and C_4 are located far enough from the tissue edge, there exist 4 planes of symmetry for the tissue space cornered with these capillaries at any moment; they are the planes parallel to the capillaries (perpendicular to the cross-section of the muscle fiber) and are passing on the lines C_1C_2 (from C_1 to C_2), C_2C_3, C_3C_4 and C_4C_1. If the mode of intermittent flow has been repeated sufficiently long, these planes may be regarded as the barrier for O_2 diffusion because there must be no O_2 tension gradient built up across these planes. Therefore, the minimum tissue region to be analysed is the rectangular space surrounded with these walls of diffusion barrier as shown in Fig.3 (a). This space of tissue is supplied O_2 from capillary C_1 across a quarter of the surface facing to it at phase I, from C_2 at phase II, from C_3 at phase III and from C_4 at phase IV as shown in Fig.3 (b).

Mathematical formulations for the dynamic simulation of O_2 exchange in this rectangular paralleropiped model necessitates a rectangular space co-ordinate x, y and z as shown in Fig.3 (a). The origin O of the coordinates is set at the arterial end of the capillary C_1, x axis along the line C_1C_2, y axis along the line C_1C_4 and z axis along C_1 itself. Relevant biophysical phenomena including O_2 diffusion across the capillary wall and in the tissue space as well as the O_2 convection by capillary blood flow are expressed by the following differential equations in terms of PO_2 changes in the open capillary (Pc) and in the tissue space (Pt) with time t respectively;

$$\partial Pc/\partial t = -Vc(\partial Pc/\partial z) + D(\alpha_t/\alpha_c)(2/Rc)(grad*P) + D\partial^2 Pc/\partial z^2$$

(1)

$$\partial Pt/\partial t = D(\partial^2 Pt/\partial x^2 + \partial^2 Pt/\partial y^2 + \partial^2 Pt/\partial z^2) - \dot{Q}t/\alpha_t$$

(2)

where Vc is the capillary red cell velocity, D the O_2 diffusion coefficient, α_c and α_t the O_2 solubility in blood and in tissue fluid (or in plasma) respectively, Rc the capillary radius and $\dot{Q}t$ the O_2 consumption rate in the tissue. The term grad*P indicates the PO_2 gradient across the capillary wall. The first term in the right side of Eq.(1) represents the O_2 convection by capillary blood flow, the second term the O_2 diffusion across the capillary wall and the last term the O_2 diffusion along z axis. Eq.(2) indicates the three dimensional O_2 diffusion in the tissue space with uniform O_2 consumption rate $\dot{Q}t$.

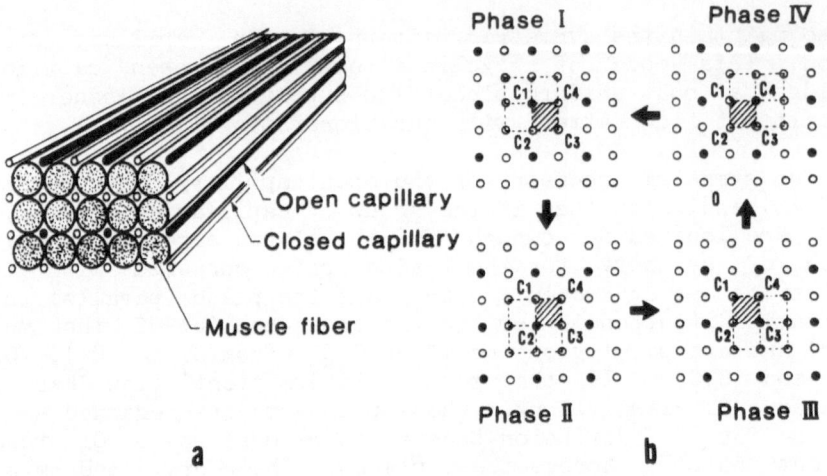

Fig.2 Schematic illustration of the capillary distribution in a resting skeletal muscle (a) and the uniform mode of open channel alternation associating 4 different phases (b).

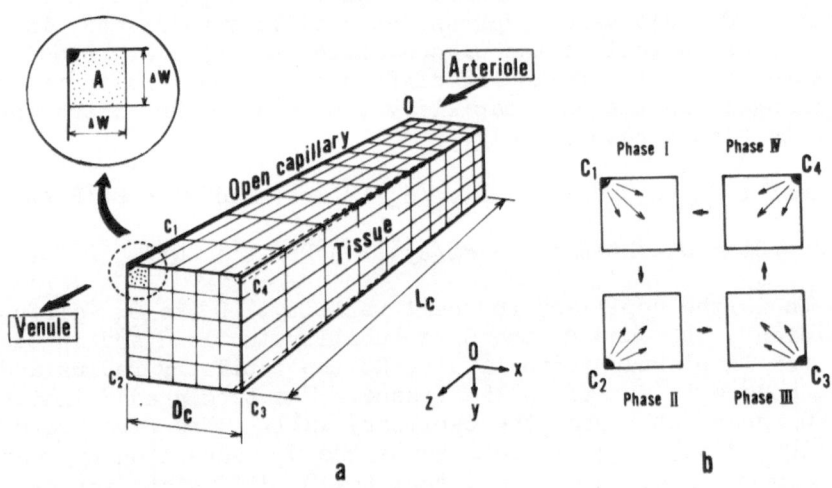

Fig.3 A rectangular parallelopiped model of the capillary-tissue system (a) and the cyclic mode of O_2 supply to the tissue from 4 capillaries by one open channel at each phase (b).

The boundary conditions for the above equations in this model are;

$$[\partial Pt/\partial x]_{x=0 \text{ and } x=Dc} = [\partial Pt/\partial y]_{y=0 \text{ and } y=Dc}$$

$$= [\partial Pt/\partial z]_{z=0 \text{ and } z=Lc} = 0 \qquad (3)$$

where Dc indicates the intercapillary distance and Lc the capillary length (see Fig.3).

The O_2 solubility coefficient in the capillary (α_c) is not actually constant but considerably PO_2 dependent because the O_2 dissociation curve of blood is markedly nonlinear. To simplify the simulation process in this study, the O_2 dissociation curve is approximated by two straight lines. It implies that we use two different solubility coefficients α_1 and α_2 separately for the PO_2 ranges higher or lower than 47 mmHg, as listed in Table 1. In addition, it is assumed that the O_2 dissociation of oxyhemoglobin occurs instantaneously because the reaction time of the dissociation process is reported to be much shorter than that of O_2 diffusion (Hyman et al, 1975).

To carry out the actual digital computation, the tissue spaces were divided into uniform rectangular compartments with the sides of Δx, Δy and Δz in length along the respective coordinates. The capillary channels are divided into the quartered columns with radius Rc and length Δz, as seen in Fig.3. Usually x and y axes of length Dc are divided into 5 sections and z axis of length Lc into 10 sections. Eqs.(1) and (2) were transformed into two difference equations respectively. For the sake of simplicity, the diffusion terms along z axis were neglected because the second derivatives, $\partial^2 Pc/\partial z^2$ and $\partial^2 Pt/\partial z^2$ were usually very small. According to these difference equations, PO_2 changes during a definite period of time Δt in the capillary columns and the tissue compartments were calculated. A special caution was taken to estimate grad*P between the open capillary column and the tissue compartment directly contactingt it.

The dynamic computor simulation was performed with the iterative method by calculating PO_2 changes in every column and every compartment during a discrete time interval Δt of 0.01 sec or less, consecutively. At the onset of the calculation, the open capillary column was assigned a linear PO_2 gradient from 95 mmHg at the arteriolar end to 40 mmHg at the venular end. The initial conditions of PO_2 distribution in the tissue compartments were given from the steady state solution of the Krogh-Erlang equation (Krogh, 1919).

The simulation of the intermittent capillary flow model was initiated from phase I and was continued in the order of phases

327

I–II–III–IV–I..., until numerical values of PO_2 distribution were converged into a certain cyclic mode. Even when the value of PO_2 in a tissue compartment became negative, the computation was continued with no special modifications. Values of physiological parameters used in the simulations are listed in Table 1. Most data are those measured in the skeletal muscles.

Besides the dynamic simulation, the steady state O_2 transport was simulated by fixing the open capillary channel to C_1 and by solving the difference equations obtained by letting $\partial Pt/\partial t = \partial Pc/\partial t = 0$ in Eq.(1) and (2). Both results of dynamic and steady state simulations under the same conditions of open capillary density, total blood flow supply and O_2 consumption were compared to elucidate the effects of the intermittent flow.

Table 1 Values of physiological parameters used in the computer simulations

Rc	capillary radius	2	(μm)
Lc	capillary length	1000	(μm)
Dc	intercapillary distance	30–80	(μm)
Vc	capillary red cell velocity	300–1500	(μm/s)
Pa	arterial O_2 tension	95	(mmHg)
α_{c1}	O_2 solubility in blood (pO_2 47mmHg)	38	(10^{-4}/mmHg)
α_{c2}	(pO_2 47mmHg)	58	(10^{-5}/mmHg)
	O_2 solubility in tissue	3	(10^{-5}/mmHg)
D^t	O_2 diffusion coefficient	1500	(μm²/s)
$\dot{Q}t$	tissue O_2 consumption	0.3–1.0	(ml/min/100g)
To	duration time of an open phase	5–20	(s)

RESULTS

Fig.4 (b) shows an example of the results obtained in the steady state capillary flow model. The figure indicates the PO_2 distribution upon the plane hatched in Fig.4 (a). The parameters used in this simulation are: intercapillary distance $Dc = 50$ μm, capillary red cell velocity $Vc = 1000$ μm/s, and O_2 consumption $Qt = 0.85$ ml/min per 100g tissue. The values of other parameters are as listed in Table 1. The region of the lowest PO_2 is located in the farthest corner from the venous end of the open capillary channel. In this region PO_2 often becomes lower than 0 mmHg (O_2 debt area) which is depicted in Fig.5 (b) as the darkly shaded area. This site of the poorest O_2 supply is often called "critical" or "lethal" corner because tissue most readily falls in necrosis. The area of O_2 debt in this corner increases as the tissue O_2 consumption ($\dot{Q}t$) increases or as the red cell velocity (Vc) decreases or as the intercapillary distance (Dc) increases.

Fig.5 shows an example of the results obtained in the

Fig.4 PO$_2$ distribution obtained in the steady capillary flow model (b) on the shaded plane in the rectangular tissue space in (a). See text for values of physiological parameters used in the simulation.

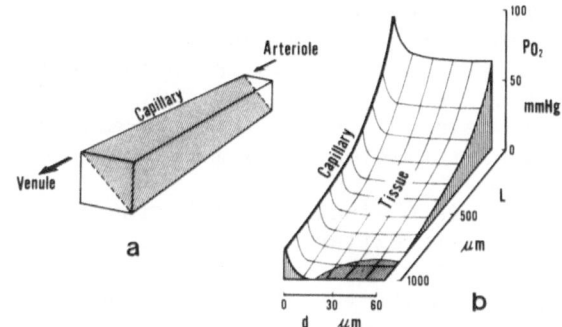

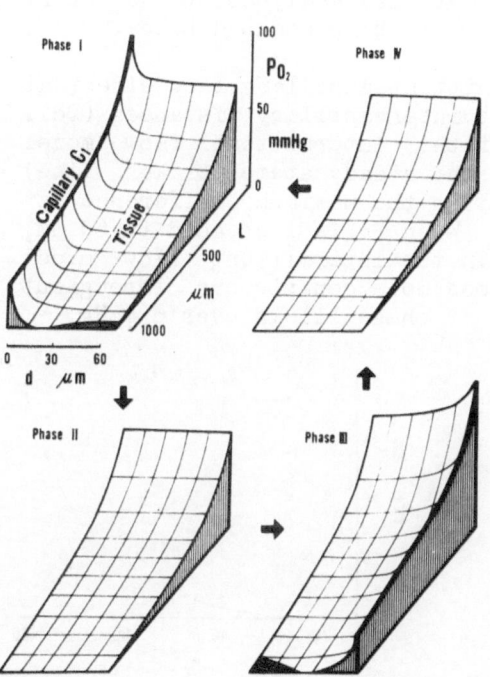

Fig.5 PO$_2$ distributions obtained at the end of the four phases in the intermittent capillary flow model on the same plane and with the same parameters as Fig.4.

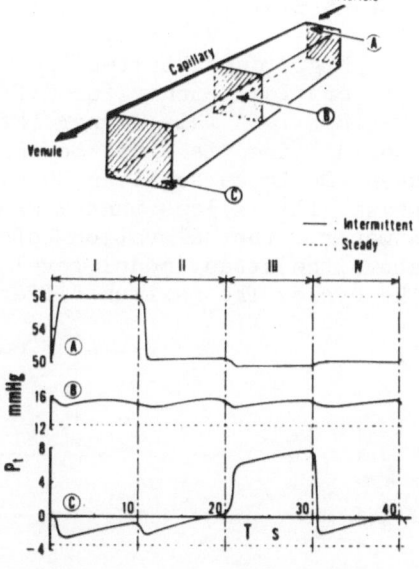

Fig.6 Cyclic changes in the tissue PO$_2$ (Pt) with time in the intermittent flow model (solid line) compared with the steady flow one (broken line) at the points A, B and C as indicated in the tissue space with arrows.

intermittent capillary flow model. Each figure indicates the PO_2 distribution upon the same plane as Fig.4 at the end of four phases. The values of the parameters Dc, Vc, $\dot{Q}t$ etc. are also the same as Fig.4. The duration of an open phase (To) is 10 sec. It is evident that as the open capillary moves according to the phase shift, the distribution varies the pattern conspicuously. It is also obvious that the area of O_2 debt becomes smaller in the intermittent flow model than that in the steady state model.

Fig.6 indicates the time courses of the tissue PO_2 (Pt) in the intermittent flow model obtained at the three points as designated by A, B and C in the tissue space (solid line) compared with the levels in the steady state model at the same points (broken line). The values of Dc, Vc and $\dot{Q}t$ are common in both simulation models. It is apparent that at point A (near the arteriolar end of capillary C_1), Pt level of the intermittent flow model is lower than in steady state, whereas at point C (near the venular end of C_3), the former is higher than the latter. These results suggest that the intermittent flow model has a specific effect to elevate Pt level at the critical corner in the steady state model. More detailed analyses of the intermittent flow effect at this corner will be presented below.

Fig.7 demonstrates the intermittent capillary flow effect at the critical corner for different intercapillary distances (Dc). The PO_2 at this corner (Ptl) of the intermittent flow model (solid line) is close to that of the steady state (broken line) when Dc is as small as 30 μm. Even the maximum difference at phase III is less than 2 mmHg. When Dc is increased to 60 μm, however, the elevation of Ptl in the intermittent flow model above the steady model level becomes more conspicuous throughout the cycle. The maximum difference at phase III is over 6 mmHg.

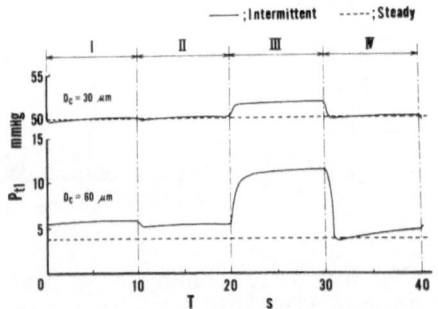 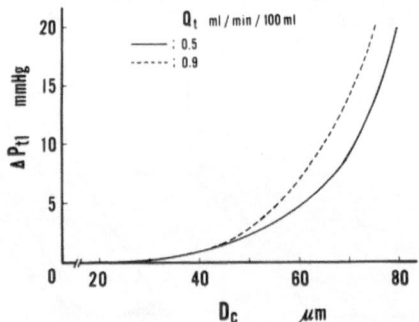

Fig.7 PO_2 at the critical corner (Ptl) for two different values of intercapillary distance (Dc).

Fig.8 Relationships of mean Ptl difference (ΔPtl) between intermittent and steady flow models vs. Dc.

The influence of the intercapillary distance (Dc) on the intermittent flow effect at the lethal corner (Ptl) is shown in Fig.8. Obviously, the effect increases as Dc is enlarged. It is also evident that as the tissue O_2 consumption Qt is elevated, the effect is augmented.

DISCUSSION AND CONCLUSION

In the resting skeletal muscles, blood flow rate is around 3-6 ml/min/100g tissue which is less than 1/10 of the flow rate during heavy exercise, corresponding to a marked reduction of O_2 consumption Qt to 1/10-1/5 of the maximum one during exercise (Mellander and Johansson, 1968). This low flow rate suggests that if all cappillaries were open at rest as they are during exercise, the capillary red cell velocity would become so slow that red cell aggregation or rouleau formation might frequently take place to plug capillary channels in various places. Actually, the red cell velocity is maintained at a higher level under physiological resting conditions by reducing the number of open capillaries to 1/3 or 1/4 of the total. The consequent increase in the intercapillary distance, however, results in enlargement of hypoxyic portions. Some of them may fall in a serious state, if open channels are fixed to certain capillaries as assumed in the steady flow model of this study. The present results of the dynamic simulation in the intermittent capillary flow model demonstrated that alternate perfusion of the tissue space from all the neighbouring capillaries is effective to relieve such hypoxyic portions without increasing blood flow supply. Since the primary role of circulation is to maintain the tissue under perfusion at the state of aerobic glycolysis, the predicted effect significantly elevating the lowest Pt is essential. To confirm the likelihood of the predicted results, however, the validity of the simulation model should be more closely examined.

The present model includes various assumptions to simplify the calculation process. It neglects the reaction time of hemoglobin for O_2 dissociation in the red cell and the O_2 diffusion along z-axis both in the tissue and capillary. It also assumes a uniform distribution of capillaries in the tissue space. and neglects the variations in it. The influence of these assumptions on the intermittent flow effect, however, seems to be rather limited because these factors are neglected both in the steady state and dynamic models.

The most important assumption to be examined here is the mode of open capillary alternation as seen in Fig.3. Our experiences in the intravital observations of the skeletal muscle microcirculation indicate that the periodic changes in red cell velocity often occur concomitantly in a group of capillaries coming out of the same arteriole (Shibata et al., 1983). It is rather rare to observe periodic capillary flow varying asynchronously with most adjacent capillaries. It should be noted, however, that such concomitant mode of intermittent capillary flow is observed only in the muscle under suffusion with Tyrode solution. It is necessary to confirm what kind of periodic flow pattern most frequently takes place under physiological resting conditions.

Furthermore, even if the concomitant stop-flow mode in such grouped capillaries is dominant, a similar effect as predicted in this study may be expected, because this principle is applicable to an extended model in which each group of adjacent capillaries is replaced by a single capillary in the present model. Therefore it may be concluded that the intermittent capillary flow can play an important role in the O_2 transport to tissue in the resting skeletal muscle.

REFERENCES

Cardon, S. Z., Oestermeyer, C. F. and Bloch, E. H., 1970, Effect of oxygen on cyclic red blood cell flow in unanesthetized mammalian striated muscle as determined by microscopy. Microvasc. Res., 2: 67-76.

Hyman, W. A., Grounds, D. J. and Newell, P. H., 1975, Oxygen tension in a capillary-tissue system subject to periodic occlusion. Microvasc. Res., 9: 49-63.

Krogh, A., 1919, Number and distribution of capillaries in muscles with calculations of oxygen pressure head necessary for supplying the tissue. J. Physiol. (London), 52: 409-415.

Lindbom, L., Tuma, R. F. and Arfors, K. E., 1980, Influence of oxygen on perfused capillary density and capillary red cell velocity in rabbit skeletal muscle. Microvas. Res., 19: 197-208.

Mellander, S. and Johansson, B., 1968, Control of resistance, exchange, and capacitance functions in the peripheral circulation. Pharmacol. Rev., 21, 117-196.

Prewitt, R. L. and Johnson, P. C., 1976, The effect of oxygen on arteriolar red cell velocity and capillary density in the rat cremaster muscle. Microvasc. Res., 12: 59-70.

Shibata, M. and Kamiya, A., 1983, Local and neural regulation of microcirculation in the rabbit tenuissimus muscle, in " Intravital Observation of Organ Microcirculation", M. Tsuchiya, H. Wayland, M. Oda and I. Okazaki, ed. Excerpta Medica, Amsterdam.

Whalen, W. J. and Nair, P., 1967, Intracellular PO_2 and its regulation in resting skeletal muscle of the guinea pig. Circ. Res., 21: 251-261.

EXERCISE REDUCES DIFFUSION DISTANCES IN SKELETAL MUSCLES OF

RABBITS FED AN ATHEROGENIC DIET

E.W. Kanabus and A.J. Merola

Departments of Physiology and Physiological Chemistry
Ohio State University
Columbus, Ohio 43210

INTRODUCTION

When work demands on skeletal muscles are increased, through
exercise or chronic electrical stimulation, metabolic advantage
lies in adaptations that shorten or at least maintain diffusion
distances for oxygen and other nutrients or metabolites. The
growth of new capillaries is one means to achieve this, and the
evidence for capillary proliferation in skeletal muscle in
response to higher functional demands has been reviewed elsewhere
(Hudlicka, 1982).

Cholesterol feeding has been shown to produce injury to
arterial endothelium in rabbits (Ehrhart and Holderbaum, 1977) and
chickens (Chvapil, et al., 1976), and hyperlipoproteinemia
disrupts endothelial repair, apparently distorting regenerating
endothelial cells in particular (Bowyer, 1978). If this
disruption of regenerative function occurs generally in vascular
endothelium, hyperlipoproteinemic animals may be less able to
respond to angiogenic factors invoked by long-term exercise.

We sought to test whether the capillary proliferative
response to long-term exercise occurs in animals on a high
cholesterol diet, and to evaluate its net effect on anatomic
diffusion distances within muscle tissue. Muscle vascularity has
most often been reported in terms of capillary density (capil-
laries/mm^2) or capillary/fiber ratio [(total capillaries) / (total
number of fibers)]. Since both quantities are affected by fiber
size, which also may change with increased work demands, the
vascular anatomic limitations to oxygen transport within exercised

333

muscles are best evaluated by measuring diffusion distances with a direct technique such as the closest individual method (Kayar et al., 1982).

METHODS

Four age-matched pairs of male New Zealand rabbits were obtained at weaning and maintained in standard vivarium housing throughout the study.

One of each pair was trained to run on an enclosed 4-foot long human treadmill, while the other served as a control. Initially, the runner was placed on the treadmill and allowed to familiarize himself with it. The treadmill was run at 1 m.p.h. with an incline of 10%. No electroshock was used. Once familiar with the treadmill, the animals ran of their own volition. Each runner ran two sessions a day, five days a week for 28 to 32 weeks. At the beginning of training they ran for five minutes each session. As their endurance increased, the time per session was extended gradually until, after 12 weeks, they could maintain this level of exercise for 17.5 minutes per session. This represented a final work rate of 7.9-10.0 kg-m/min (total work = 137-175 kg-m per session). The runners continued to exercise at this level for the remainder of the 30-week period. Sedentary control animals received the same degree of handling as the runners. During the final 14 to 16 weeks prior to sacrifice, all runners and controls received in their diet 0.3% cholesterol and 5% cottonseed oil.

At the end of the 30-week exercise program capillary densities, distributions around fibers, and diffusion distances for oxygen were evaluated by morphometric analysis of histological preparations from fast, slow, and intermediate hindlimb muscles. Rabbits were anesthetized with sodium pentobarbital (35 mg/kg, I.V.) and the tibialis anterior (TA), extensor digitorum longus (EDL), and soleus (SOL) muscles were dissected free and weighed. Steak sections of 1-mm thickness were obtained from the thickest part of each muscle and rapidly frozen in isopentane (2-methyl-butane) precooled to $-160^{\circ}C$ in liquid nitrogen. The frozen steaks were mounted on chucks using OCT compound, sectioned at 14 μm and stained for alkaline phosphatase to demonstrate capillary endothelium (Romanul and Bannister, 1962). Photomicrographs were analyzed with a Zeiss Videoplan system to evaluate the following anatomic parameters:
1. Capillary density (CD) was calculated from counts of the number of capillaries in 0.294 mm X 0.227 mm fields.
2. Diffusion distances for oxygen were measured by the closest individual method (Kayar, et al., 1982), wherein

a grid drawn on a transparent overlay was randomly placed over the photomicrograph, and measurements made of the distance between each grid point and the center of the nearest capillary (DtC). A grid with spacing of 14 μm, reflecting 45% of the mean intercapillary distance, yielded samplings with mean values reproducible to within 2%.

3. Capillaries per fiber (CpF) were evaluated as the number of capillaries touching each individual fiber.

Morphometric measurements from five fields in each muscle were pooled and differences evaluated by student's t test.

RESULTS

On the average, runners weighed 8% less than sedentary controls at time of sacrifice (3.21 $\pm$ 0.11 kg compared to 3.49 $\pm$ 0.15 kg), but this difference was not statistically significant (Figure 1). The lipid-enriched chow diet had no effect on the growth pattern of either group of animals, as no differences in body weight are evident between these cholesterol-fed animals and either runners or controls of comparable age in a later series of

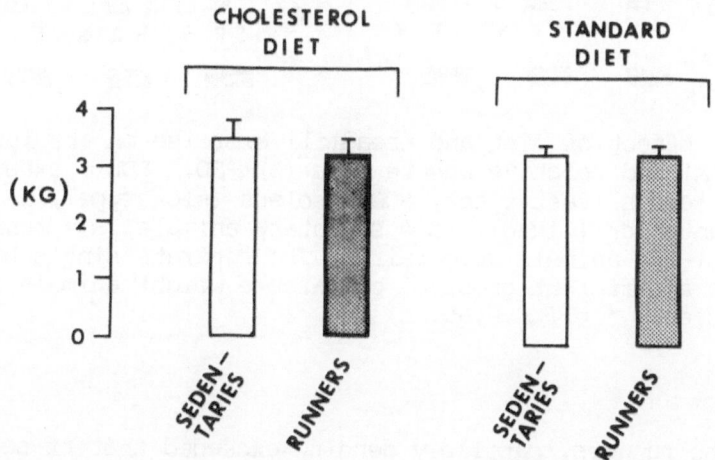

Figure 1. Effect of diet and treadmill exercise on body weights ($\pm$SD) of 34-38 week-old rabbits. Within each diet group animals were studied as age-matched pairs. No significant differences were found.

paired animals which received standard chow without lipid
supplementation (Figure 1). For all three muscles runners' and
sedentaries' muscle weights were similar (Figure 2A), but
normalization to body weight indicated a significant relative
increase in the mass of the runners' TAs (12%, P < 0.05) but not
of their EDLs or SOLs (Figure 2B). Comparison with muscles from
sedentary animals on normal chow diets indicates that the lipid-
rich diet _per se_ does not affect muscle development.

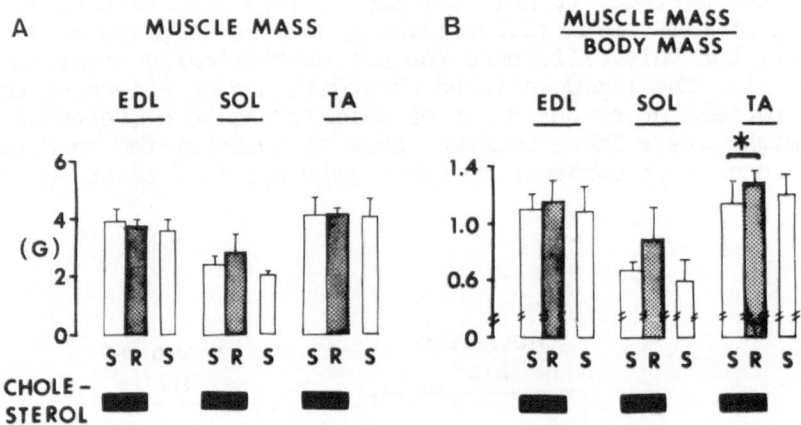

Figure 2. Effect of diet and treadmill exercise on absolute mass
in grams (A) and relative muscle mass (B) ±SD. EDL = extensor
digitorum longus (fast type), SOL = soleus (slow type), TA =
tibialis anterior (mixed). S = sedentary animals, R = runners.
Cholesterol-fed animals were paired. The separate single bar
represents a different group of comparable weight animals on
standard diet. * = P < 0.05.

In the runners, capillary density exceeded that of sedentary
controls by 49% and 32% in the EDLs and SOLs, respectively.
However, capillary density was identical in the TAs of both groups
(Figure 3A). Nevertheless, the number of capillaries adjacent to
individual muscle fibers (CpF) increased in all three muscles of
the runners (Figure 3B), indicating that growth of new capillaries
had occurred in TAs as well as in EDLs and SOLs. Diffusion

distances - as reflected by DtC, the distances from points within
the muscle cells to the nearest histologically demonstrable
capillary - were no different in the TAs of runners as compared to
the TAs of sedentary animals. EDLs and SOLs of runners, however,
showed 21% and 10% shorter diffusion path lengths as compared to
the same muscles from the sedentary animals (Figure 4).

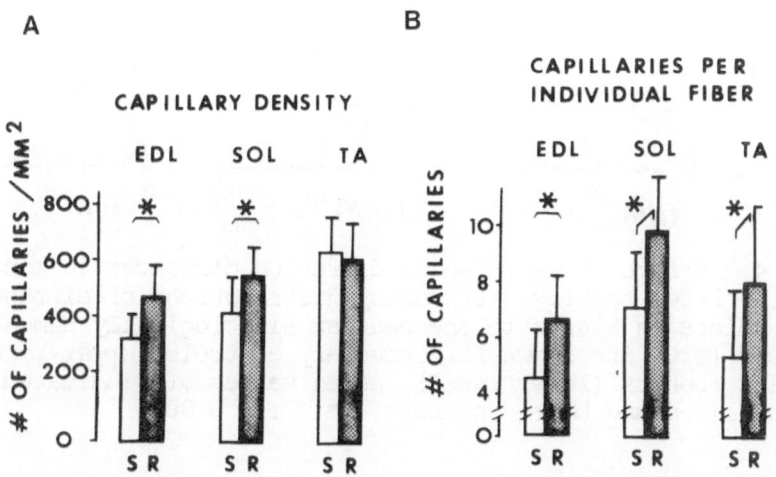

Figure 3. Effect of exercise on capillarity of skeletal muscles of
cholesterol-fed rabbits. Errors are standard deviations; * = P <
0.005. Abbreviations as in Figure 2.

DISCUSSION

The dietary lipid supplement was less than that which
produced endothelial disruption after 28 days of feeding in
rabbits of similiar age to our animals (Bowyer, 1978). However,
our rabbits received the high lipid diet 3 to 4 times longer.
This was sufficient to cause a 5-fold increase in sedentary
controls' plasma cholesterol over their pretreatment levels.

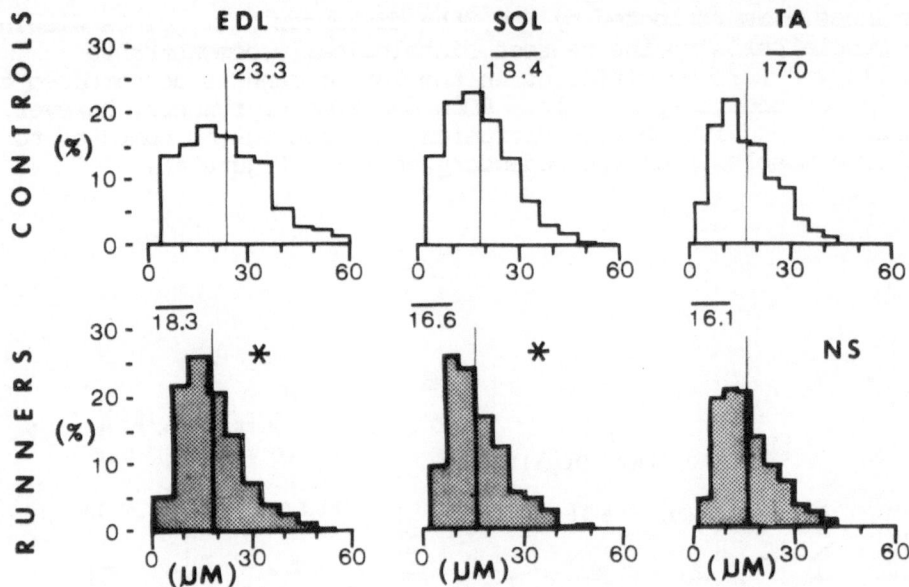

Figure 4. Effect of exercise on diffusion distances in muscles of cholesterol-fed rabbits. Frequency distributions of distance from random points in tissue to the nearest histologically demonstrable capillary (DtC) are shown for sedentary controls (upper panel) and treadmill runners (lower panel). Mean values are indicated by vertical lines and barred numbers. * = P < 0.005.

Because the runners' EDLs and SOLs did not increase in mass relative to body weight, we interpret the 12% increase in relative weight of their TAs as reflecting a true hypertrophy. Since the animals were in a rapid growth phase this represents a disproportionate acceleration in the accumulation of muscle mass. The lack of observed change in the runners' TAs may be due to fiber enlargement, which would be consistent with the hypertrophy. Fiber size was not measured, however.

The evidence that hyperlipoproteinemia impairs endothelial function suggests that high dietary lipid intake might hamper the endothelial cell proliferation that is necessary for new capillaries to form. We have shown here that under conditions of cholesterol feeding, diffusion distances need not be compromised when muscles are subjected to increased work loads over long periods of time. If anything, the anatomic constraints on oxygen transport are reduced as a result of capillary proliferation. Clearly, our measures only assess those limits to diffusion which are imposed by the configuration of vascular structures. They do not necessarily reflect functional diffusion distances, which are governed in vivo by physiological perfusion-regulating mechanisms.

It appears that the angiogenic stimulus of long term exercise can override potentially detrimental effects of a high cholesterol diet, permitting the formation of new capillary endothelium. However, the degree to which skeletal muscle angiogenesis may be affected by blood lipid levels is still to be established, by comparing these results with forthcoming data from exercising and sedentary animals on a normal diet.

ACKNOWLEDGEMENTS

We are grateful to Alice Cullen for exercising the animals. This study has been supported by grants from the Central Ohio Heart Chapter, Inc.

REFERENCES

Bowyer, D.E. Atherogenesis 13:12-36, 1978.

Chvapil, M., P.L. Stith, L.M. Tillema, E.C. Carlson, J.B. Campbell and C.D. Eskelson. Atherosclerosis 24:393-405, 1976.

Ehrhart, L.A. and D. Holderbaum. Atherosclerosis 27:477-485, 1977.

Hudlicka, O. Circ Res. 50:451-461, 1982.

Kayar, S.R., P.G. Archer, A.J. Lechner and N. Banchero. Microvasc. Res. 24:326-341, 1982.

Romanul, F.C.A. and R.G. Bannister. J. Cell Biol. 15:73-89, 1962.

SKELETAL MUSCLE CAPILLARITY IN HYPERTHYROID AND HYPOTHYROID RATS

A. H. Sillau

Department of Physiology and Biophysics
School of Medicine, University of Puerto Rico
San Juan, Puerto Rico 00936

INTRODUCTION

The capacity of the oxygen transport system to deliver O_2 to the muscle fibers depends, among other things, on the density and the geometric arrangement of the capillary network. Romanul (1965) and Myraghe (1978) have shown that the number of capillaries around the skeletal muscle fibers is directly correlated with the oxidative capacity of the fibers. On the other hand, Maxwell et al. (1980) and Zumstein et al. (1983) have presented evidence that runs counter to the above. Maxwell et al. (1980) studied different muscles from different animal species and muscle to muscle and species to species variability could have obscured the relationship between capillarity and oxidative capacity. In addition, both Maxwell et al. (1980) and Zumstein et al. (1983) reported their values of capillarity as capillary density and capillary to fiber ratio without taking into consideration the effect that fiber cross sectional area has on these parameters. It has been shown that this may lead to erroneous interpretations of the experimental results (Ripoll et al., 1979).

In this study we have analyzed the changes in capillarity in relation to the changes in oxidative capacity induced by hyperthyroidism and by hypothyroidism. We have studied muscles or areas of muscles made up of mostly fast glycolytic or slow oxidative fibers because it is known that the oxidative capacity of the slow oxidative fibers is significantly increased in hyperthyroidism while that of the fast glycolytic fibers is not affected (Winder and Holloszy, 1977). Also, we have measured maximal and mean diffusion distances and studied their relationship to the oxidative capacity of the muscle.

MATERIAL AND METHODS

Female Wistar rats (200-350g BW) were used in this investigation. Some of them were injected with triiodothyronine (300-400 ug/Kg BW) every other day for 7, 14, 21, 28 or 42 days. Others were injected with propylthiouracil (50 mg/Kg) every day for 21 or 42 days. Control animals received saline. At the end of the treatment periods the animals were killed and their muscles used for histochemical and biochemical studies. The soleus and gastrocnemius-plantaris muscles were excised, blotted dry and weighed. The soleus and the gastrocnemius medial head were cut transversely at the widest point of the belly and frozen in isopentane cooled to -140 C with liquid nitrogen. Portions of the soleus and the white area of the gastrocnemius medial head (from now on referred to as gastrocnemius) were separated and their fat and connective tissue removed. The muscle samples were minced with scissors and known amounts were homogenized in ice cooled buffers to determine the capacity of the homogenates to oxidize pyruvate plus malate (PM) and the activity of cytochrome c oxidase (CO) following the procedures of Winder et al. (1975) and Ferguson-Miller et al. (1976).

Thin cross sections (12-14um) of the frozen muscle samples were obtained in a cryostat and mounted on coverslips. The sections were treated histochemically to demonstrate ATPase activity after preincubation at pH 4.1 for 5 minutes (ATP 4.1). This procedure permits the easy visualization of capillaries by staining their endothelium (Sillau and Banchero, 1977).

Photomicrographs of the ATP 4.1 preparations were taken from the white area of the gastrocnemius. In the soleus, a more homogenous muscle, no specific area was selected to obtain the photomicrographs. The photomicrographs were projected onto tracing paper at a known magnification and capillary density (CD), fiber density and average fiber cross sectional area (FCSA) were obtained by direct count and by the point counting method (Weibel et al., 1966). The average number of fibers counted per animal was 423 in the gastrocnemius and 489 in the soleus. With this information capillary to fiber ratio (C/F) was calculated.

Photomicrographs of the ATP 4.1 preparations of the soleus and gastrocnemius muscle were also used to measure diffusion distances by the "closest individual" method (Kayar, et al., 1982). A grid of 9 points arranged in uniform rows and columns was laid at random over the projected microphotographs and the distance from each point to the nearest capillary was recorded. This procedure was repeated until a total of 200 distances was obtained for each

342

animal. Mean diffusion distance was taken as the arithmetic mean of the 200 distances measured. The distances were then ordered in ascending value and the 190th distance was taken as the maximal diffusion distance (Kayar et al., 1982)

RESULTS

Treatment with triiodothyronine (T3) induced an increase in the oxygen consumption of the animals, an increase in the capacity of liver homogenates to oxidize pyruvate plus malate, ventricular hypertrophy and higher levels of T3 in plasma. All this is compatible with the condition of hyperthyroidism. On the other hand administration of propilthyouracil (PTU) induced hypothyroidism as evidenced by lower oxygen consumptions, T3 plasma concentrations and smaller ventricular masses.

Animals treated with T3 lost weight during the first days but later on they grew normally. At the end of 14, 21, 28 or 42 days of treatment the hyperthyroid animals' BWs were not significantly different from those of the controls. The animals that received PTU lost weight while controls showed a slight increase in BW. However, the weight losses of the hypothyroid animals were small and after 21 or 42 days BWs of the experimental animals were not significantly different from the controls.

In the controls the capacity of the soleus muscle homogenates to oxidize PM was 112 ± 28ul $O_2/$(min. g wet weight) ($X \pm SD$). The capacity to oxidize PM was higher after 7 days of T3 administration and continued to increase, reaching a new plateau after 21 days of treatment (Fig. 1). In the hypothyroid animals the capacity to oxidize PM by the soleus homogenates was decreased to 50% of the controls after 21 days of PTU administration. Longer treatment with PTU did not result in additional decreases (Fig. 1). In the gastrocnemius of control animals, the capacity to oxidaze PM was 70 ± 14 ul $O_2/$(min. g wet weight) (Fig. 1). Treatment with T3 for up to 42 days did not increase while treatment with PTU resulted in a significant decrease in the capacity of the gastrocnemius homogenates to oxidaze PM.

Cytochrome c oxidase activity of the soleus homogenates of the controls was 1143 ± 244 ul $O_2/$(min. g wet weight) (Fig. 2). After 7 days of T3 treatment it was still the same but it became significantly higher than the controls after 14 days of T3 administration. After 21 days of treatment it reached a new plateau (Fig. 2). Treatment with PTU resulted in a lower activity of CO in the soleus of the experimental animals than in that of the controls (Fig. 2). The activity of CO of the gastrocnemius homogenates of the controls was 520 ± 118 (ul $O_2/$min. g wet weight). It did not change with T3 administration but was decreased by treatment with PTU (Fig. 2).

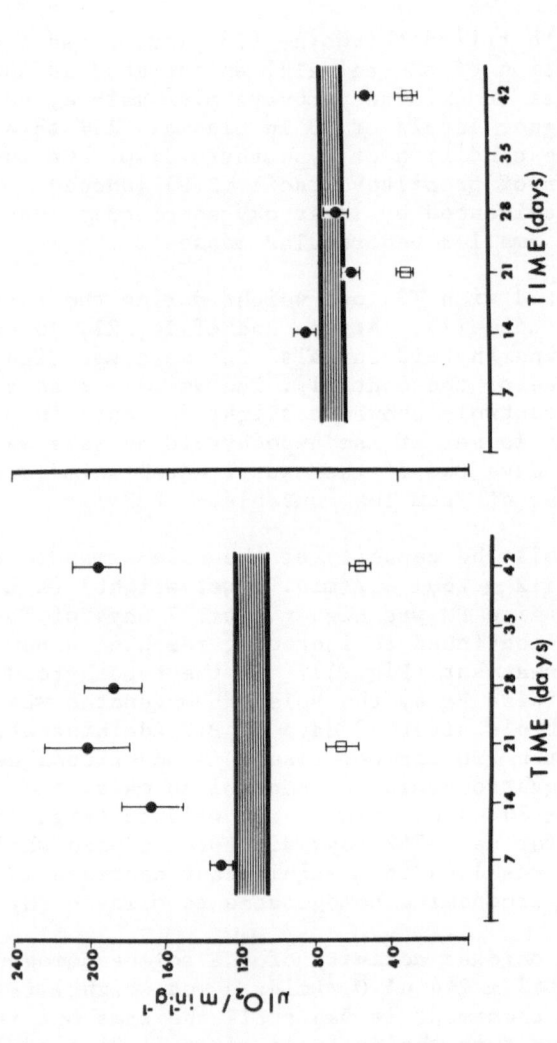

Fig. 1. Capacity to oxidaze pyruvate plus malate by soleus (left pannel) and gastrocnemius (right pannel) muscle homogenates of hyperthyroid (●) and hypothyroid (☐) rats. Symbols are means $\pm$ SE. Shaded areas limited by horizontal lines are 95% confidence intervals for mean control values.

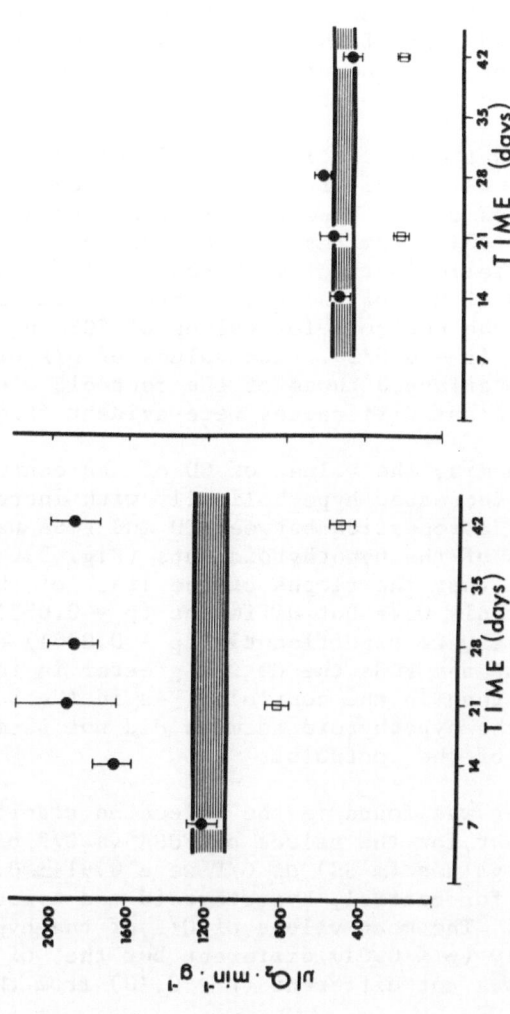

Fig. 2. Activity of cytochrome c oxidase in soleus (left pannel) and gastrocnemius (right pannel) muscle homogenates of hyperthyroid (●) and hypothyroid (□) rats. Symbols are means ± SE. Shaded areas limited by horizontal lines are 95% confidence intervals for mean control values.

In the soleus muscle of control and hyperthyroid animals CD decreased hyperbolically with increasing FCSA (Fig. 3). No significant correlation was found for the values of FCSA vs CD in the hypothyroid animals. Covariance analysis demonstrated that the slope of the line relating FCSA vs CD in the hyperthyroid animals was not different ($p = 0.705$) from that of the controls but that the adjusted altitudes of the two lines were different ($p = 0.0001$). Thus, at any FCSA the value of CD of the hyperthyroid animals was higher than that of the controls. On the other hand no clear differences existed between the values of CD of the hypothyroid animals and those of the controls.

Values of C/F in the soleus increased linearly with increasing FCSA (Fig. 4). Analysis of covariance demonstrated that the slopes of the lines of the hyperthyroid and hypothyroid values were different ($p = 0.003$) from that of the controls. Additionally, using Fieller's theorem (Zerbe et al., 1982), we found that the values of C/F of the hyperthyroid animals were higher than those of the controls for values of FCSA equal or greater than 2000 um. ($p = 0.033$). The values of C/F of the hypothyroid animals overlapped those of the controls over a wide range of FCSA and no clear differences were evident (Fig. 4).

In the gastrocnemius the values of CD of the control and hyperthyroid animals decreased hyperbolically with increasing FCSA (Fig. 5). No similar association between CD and FCSA was evident for the gastrocnemius of the hypothyroid rats (Fig. 5). Covariance analysis demonstrated that the slopes of the lines of the hyperthyroid and controls were not different ($p = 0.053$) and that the adjusted altitudes were significantly ($p = 0.0001$) different. This indicates that at any FCSA the CD was greater in the hyperthyroid animals than in the controls. As in the soleus muscle the values of CD of the hypothyroid animals did not seem to be different from those of the controls.

Contrary to what was found in the soleus no significant correlation was present for the values of FCSA vs C/F of the gastrocnemius. Mean values ($\pm$ SE) of C/F were 0.91 ± 0.04; 1.33 ± 0.04 and 0.78 ± 0.06 for control, hyperthyroid and hypothyroid animals respectively. The mean values of C/F of the hyperthyroid rats was significantly ($p < 0.01$) different but that of the hypothyroid animals was not different ($p > 0.10$) from that of the control rats.

Average values for mean ($\bar{R}$) and maximal (R95) diffusion distances are presented in table 1. In the soleus $\bar{R}$ and R 95 were not significantly affected by hypothyroidism. In the soleus and gastrocnemius of the hyperthyroid animals R was smaller ($p < 0.05$) but R95 was not different from that of the controls (Table 1).

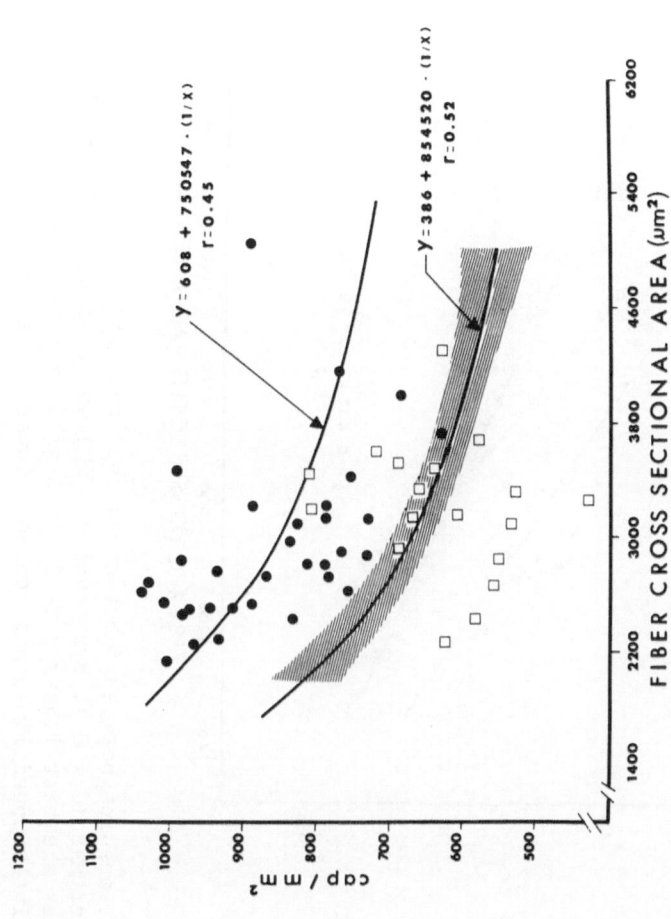

Fig. 3. Relationships between fiber cross sectional area vs capillary density in the soleus of hyperthyroid (●), hypothyroid (□) and control (individual values not shown) animals. Upper regression line is best hyperbolic fit for values from hyperthyroid rats. Lower regression line is best hyperbolic fit for values from control animals. Shaded area is 99% confidence interval.

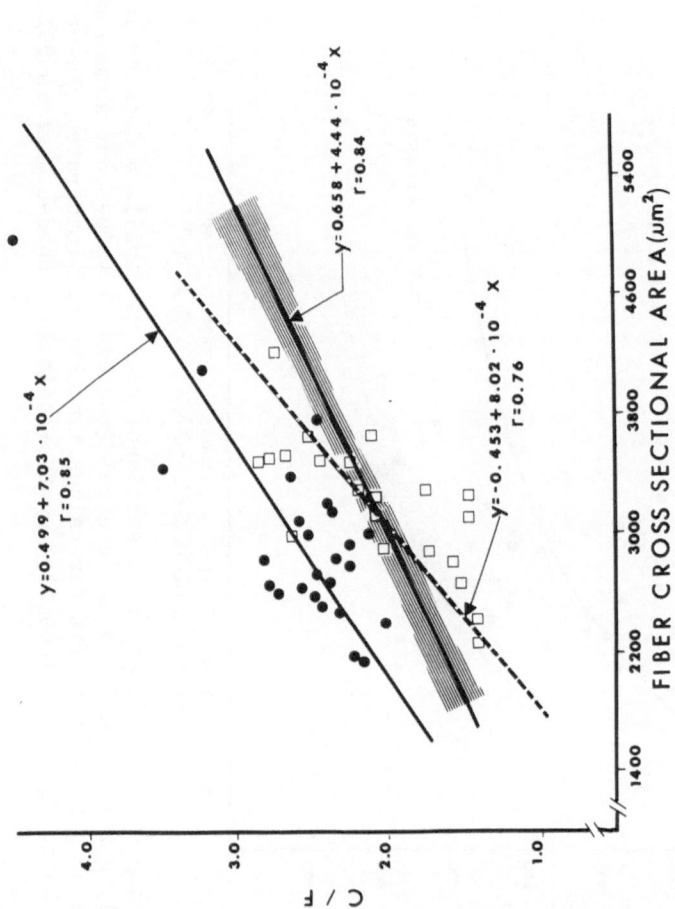

Fig. 4. Relationships between fiber cross sectional area vs capillary to fiber ratio in the soleus of hyperthyroid (●), hypothyroid (□) and control (individual values not shown) animals. Lines are best linear fits for values from hyperthyroid (upper continuous line), hypothyroid (interrupted line) and control (lower continuous line) animals. Shaded area is 99% confidence interval.

Values of $\bar{R}$ and R 95 in the control and hypothyroid animals were closer to the values predicted assuming a hexagonal distribution of capillaries. In the hyperthyroid animals these same values were closer to those predicted assuming a random array of capillaries. The shift of the capillary arrangement from a hexagonal towards a random array offsets part of the decrease in diffusion distances that theoretically would have occurred with a 38% and a 65% increase in CD in the soleus and gastrocnemius respectively (Table 1).

DISCUSSION

To determine whether a given treatment results in increased capillarity as a consequence of growth of new microvessels the evaluation of capillarity as CD or C/F has to take into consideration the important effect that FCSA has on these parameters (Ripoll et al., 1979; Aquin et al., 1980; Hudlicka, 1982). In the hyperthyroid animals values of CD or C/F at a given FCSA were higher than those of the controls. This permits us to conclude that treatment with thyroid hormones resulted in the growth of new microvessels. This conclusion, however, could be wrong if the treatment had resulted in a decrease of FCSA without a change in the number of capillaries. In this investigation this possibility seems unlikely. Our hyperthyroid animals grew normally with the exception of a few days at the beginning of the experiment. Furthermore, the magnitude of the changes in CD or C/F can not be explained by a simple reduction in FCSA.

Evidence of a positive correlation between oxidative capacity and capillarity in skeletal muscle has been presented by many workers (Romanul, 1965; Hudlicka, 1982). Also increases in the oxidative activity of muscle brought about by different experimental conditions are associated with increases in muscle capillarity (Sillau et al., 1980; Brown et al., 1976; Andersen and Henrickson, 1977). Others, however, have failed to find a clear correlation between capillarity and oxidative capacity (Maxwell et al., 1980). A significant positive correlation (r = 0.89) existed between CD and the activity of cytochrome c oxidase values of the control plus the hyperthyroid animals. However, this correlation coefficient dropped to r = 0.84 if the hypothyroid animals, in which the treatment induced a significant reduction in the activity of cytochrome c oxidase, were included in the analysis. Similar results were obtained when the values of CD were corrected to a common FCSA of 3000 um by using the equations of Fig. 3. This and the lack of correlation between CD and oxidative capacity in the gastrocnemius indicates that oxidative capacity is not necessarily associated with capillarity in skeletal muscle.

In the past diffusion distances or equivalent parameters have been approximated by simple extrapolation from the values of

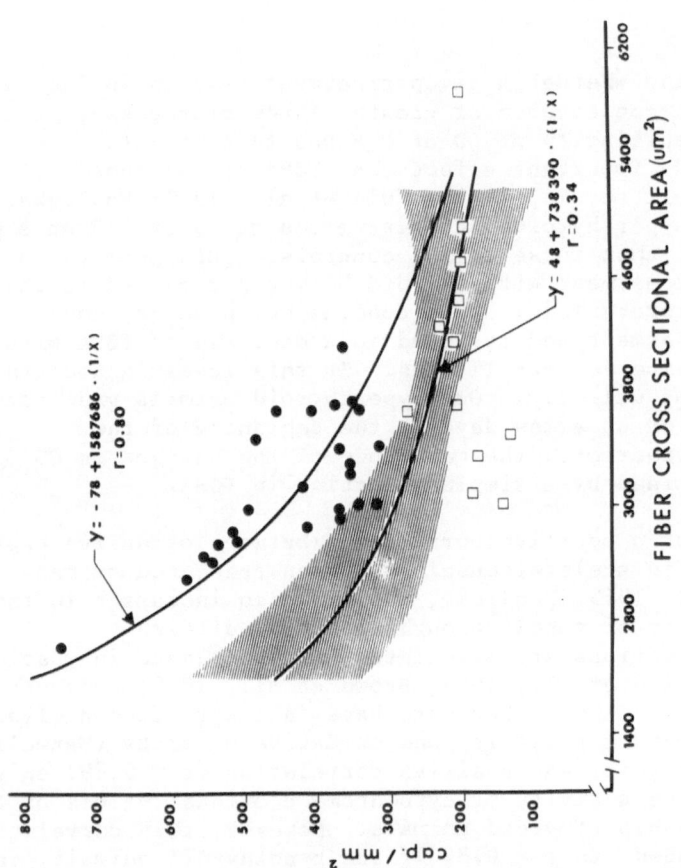

Fig. 5. Relationships between fiber cross sectional area vs capillary density in the gastroc-nemius of hyperthyroid (●), hypothyroid (□) and control (individual values not shown) animals. Upper line is best hyperbolic fit for the values of hyperthyroid animals. Best hyperbolic fit with 99% confidence interval for values from control animals is shown as lower line and shaded area.

TABLE 1

Mean ($\bar{R}$) and maximal (R95) diffusion distance in soleus and gastrocnemius of control (C) hyperthyroid (T3) and hypothyroid (PTU) rats.

		$\bar{R}$ (um)			R95 (um)		
		Measured	Predicted		Measured	Predicted	
			Hexagonal/Random			Hexagonal/Random	
SOLEUS	C (17)	16.64 ± 0.33°	15.36	19.03	31.11 ± 0.57	27.07	37.17
	T3 (11)	15.54 ± 0.41*	13.07	16.20	30.00 ± 0.76	23.03	31.63
	PTU (12)	16.74 ± 0.45	15.33	19.00	30.71 ± 0.65	27.03	37.12
GASTRO	C (12)	26.75 ± 0.80	24.78	30.71	48.88 ± 1.71	43.68	59.99
	T3 (8)	23.72 ± 0.76*	19.32	23.95	45.14 ± 1.13	34.05	46.77

° Values are means ± SE.

* Different from controls (p < 0.05).

Figures in parenthesis are number of observations.

351

capillary density (Tenney, 1974; Bassingthwaighte et al., 1974; Tomanek et al., 1982; Rakusan, 1971). In these approximations homogenous models of capillary distribution were assumed and the possibility that they could change if there were an increase in CD was not considered. This could be important because as shown by Kayar et al. (1982) identical values of CD could give different values of $\bar{R}$ and R95 if the arrangement of capillaries in the cross section is not the same. Our results indicate that a considerable part of the reduction in diffusion distances that would have occurred in the hyperthyroid rats is negated because of the change in the arrangement of the microvessels.

This is more clearly illustrated in the case of the values of R95 which were not significantly reduced in the hyperthyroid rats despite a 38% and 65% increase in CD. R95 values are particularly important because they represent tissue points which are more likely to become hypoxic. The lack of change in R95 is probably related to the fact that capillaries grow only in the peripheri of the fibers and maximal diffusion distances can only be reduced if the FCSA decreases or if the distribution of the capillaries changes to a more favorable arrangement (Kayar et al. 1982).

Diffusion distances, $\bar{R}$ or R95 were not correlated with the capacity to oxidize PM or with the activity of CO. This, plus the observation that the reduction of $\bar{R}$ and R95 in the soleus of the hyperthyroid rats were small or non-existant, probably indicates that in the conditions studied the increased CD serves the purpose of providing greater capillary surface area and/or capillary blood volume. It is not clear what is the role, if any, in terms of O_2 transport, of the increased capillarity of the gastrocnemius of the hyperthyroid rats.

ACKNOWLEDGEMENTS

This work was supported by National Institutes of Health: Grant RR 08102. The skillfull secretarial help of Ms. Iris Dalia Rivera is gratefully acknowledged.

REFERENCES

Andersen, P. and Henricksson, J. (1977). J. Physiol. 270:677.
Aquin, L.; Sillau, A. H.; Lechner, A. J.; and Banchero, N. (1980). Microvasc. Res. 20:41.
Bassingthwaighte, J. B.; Yipintsoi, T. and Harvey R. B. (1974). Microvasc. Res. 7:229.
Brown, M. D.; Cotter, M. A.; Hudlicka, O. and Vrbova, G. (1976). Pflugers Arch. 361:241.
Ferguson-Miller, S.; Brautigan, D. and Margoliash, E. (1976). J. Biol. Chem. 251:1104.

Hudlicka, O. (1982). Circulation Res. 50:451.

Kayar, S. R.; Lechner, A. J. and Banchero, N. (1982). Pflugers
    Arch. 394:124.

Maxwell, L. C.; White, T. P. and Faulkner, J. A. (1980). J. Appl.
    Physiol. 49:627.

Myrhage, R. (1978). Acta Physiol. Scand. 103:19.

Rakusan, K. (1977). Methods Achiev. Exp. Pathol. 5: 272.

Ripoll, E.; Sillau, A. H. and Banchero, N. (1979). Pflugers Arch.
    380:153.

Romanul, F. C. A. (1965). Arch. Neurol. 12:497.

Sillau, A. H. and Banchero, N. (1977). Pflugers Arch. 369:269.

Sillau, A. H.; Aquin, L.; Lechner, A.; Bui, M. V. and Banchero, N.
    (1980). Respir. Physiol. 42:233.

Tenney, S. M. (1974). Respir. Physiol. 20:283.

Tomanek, R. J.; Searls, J. C. and Lachenbruch. P. A. (1982).
    Circulation Res. 51:295.

Weibel, E. R.; Kistler, G. S. and Scherle, W. F. (1966). J. Cell
    Biol. 30:23.

Winder, W. W.; Baldwin, K. M.; Terjung, R. L. and Holloszy, J. O.
    (1975). Am. J. Physiol. 228:1341.

Winder, W. W. and Holloszy, J. O. (1977). Am. J. Physiol. 232:
    C180.

Zerbe, G. O., Archer, P. G.; Banchero, N. and Lechner, A. J.
    (1982). Am. J. Physiol. 242:R178.

Zumstein, A.; Matnier, O.; Howald, H. and Hoppeler, H. (1983).
    Pflugers Arch. 397:277.

ADAPTATION OF MUSCLE CAPILLARITY

Natalio Banchero

Department of Physiology
University of Colorado School of Medicine
Denver, Colorado 80262

INTRODUCTION

The single most important physiological factor affecting the capillarity of skeletal and cardiac muscle is normal growth. In both skeletal and cardiac muscle, increases in body size and weight are associated with increases in the cross sectional area of existing fibers and decreases in capillary density which result in longer diffusion distances (Aquin et al., 1980; Kayar et al., 1982). These normal decreases in capillary density occur despite increases in the total number of capillaries which are measured as increases in the capillary density to fiber density ratio (C/F). However, it is not clear what factors are involved in the development of new capillaries in muscle growth.

A number of physiological stresses, namely prolonged endurance training, chronic electrical stimulation of skeletal muscle and environmental insults such as hypoxia and cold may affect this normal progression and produce an increase in the capillarity of muscles. There is considerable disagreement, however, concerning the factors involved in the elicitation of capillary proliferation. Some investigators have postulated that increased muscle blood flow alone or in combination with greater metabolic needs are important in initiating the development of new capillaries (Hudlicka, 1982). The combination of these two factors is especially noticeable in muscles subjected to electrical stimulation. Others believe that a low PO_2 may be the sole factor regulating capillary growth. The relative contribution these mechanisms play towards explaining the experimental findings in skeletal and cardiac muscle is a topic of current interest.

NORMAL GROWTH — During normal growth the specific oxygen needs of the tissues and the blood flow per gram of tissue decrease. A direct linear relationship between muscle oxygen uptake and blood flow is known to exist (Stainsby and Otis, 1964). In guinea pigs the total oxygen uptake decreases with growth (Blake and Banchero, 1984). Hence, it is difficult to explain the growth-related increases in the total number of capillaries in muscle by using simultaneous increases in blood flow and oxygen uptake as an explanation. It is tempting to speculate that tissue PO_2 may be of paramount importance in eliciting the development of new capillaries in normal growing muscle. Increases in fiber cross sectional area push the capillaries apart, decreasing capillary density and increasing diffusion distances for O_2. This would cause some critical degree of tissue hypoxia which in turn would trigger the development of new capillaries. In the guinea pig, postnatal growth is accompanied by increases in body weight from 100 to 1200 grams. Linear increases in fiber cross sectional area of skeletal muscle from 500 to 3800 um^2, are concomitant with the normal gains in body weight (Aquin, et al., 1980). Simultaneous linear increases in C/F, indicative of development of new capillaries, accompany the increases in the size of the fibers; however, these newly formed capillaries are not sufficient to maintain a constant value of capillary density (Fig. 1). Despite these changes in the degree of capillarity, the oxygen supply to the muscle fibers is adequate to maintain normal muscle function because the O_2 needs of these tissues decrease with body weight.

It would seem logical that a similar mechanism, i.e., a low PO_2 of the tissues, could be important in the elicitation of changes in the capillarity of muscle in other physiological and experimental conditions. Let us examine the data on skeletal and cardiac muscle under different environmental conditions to ascertain the mechanisms involved in the adaptation of tissue capillarity.

HYPOXIA — Acclimation to hypoxia causes a significant increase in ventilation but does not cause changes in oxygen consumption or in cardiac output. Hemoglobin concentration and hematocrit increase significantly (Fig. 2). We have been unable to demonstrate an increase in skeletal muscle capillarity in rats and guinea pigs exposed to hypoxia equivalent to approximately 5000 meters above sea level. This level of stress represents a greater degree of hypoxia than that experienced normally by guinea pigs in the Andes. This is a key point in that it was in the Peruvian guinea pig of the Andes that Valdivia (1958) originally described an increased capillarity in skeletal muscle compared to sea level guinea pigs. In contrast, we did not observe any differences in skeletal muscle capillarity in guinea

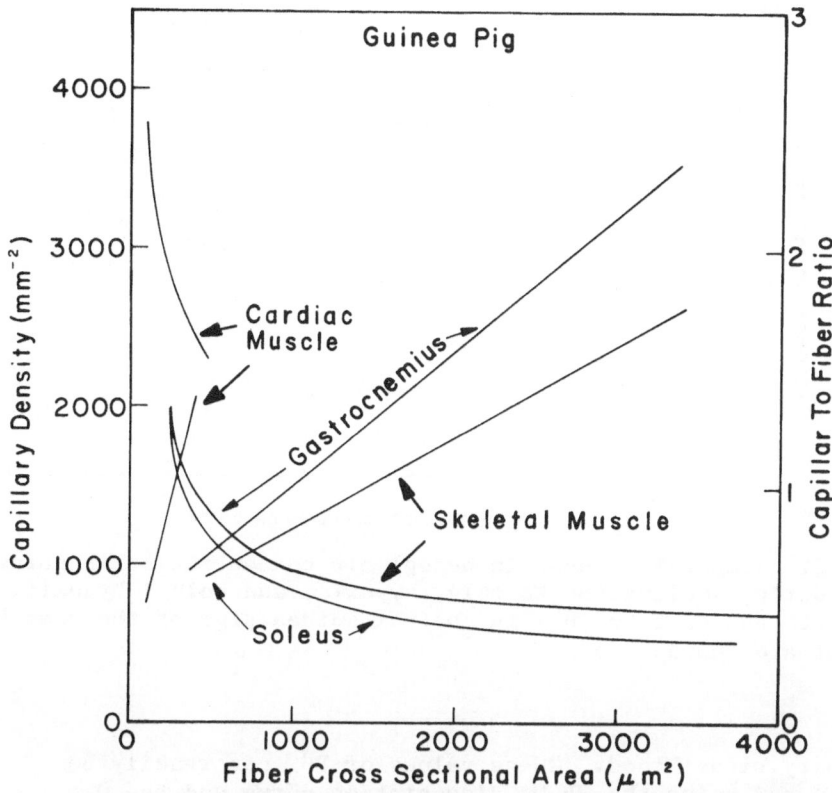

Fig. 1. Changes in muscle capillarity, i.e., capillary density and C/F, with fiber cross sectional area in the gastrocnemius and soleus of guinea pigs reared in normoxia. Capillary density decreases hyperbolically whereas C/F increases linearly with fiber size. Capillarity is always greater in cardiac than in skeletal muscle and it is greater in the gastrocnemius than in the soleus.

pigs native to the Peruvian Andes acclimatized to 3900 meters (Sillau and Banchero, 1979). Chronic exposure of young guinea pigs to hypobaric hypoxia produces increases in myocardial capillarity with decreases in oxygen diffusion distances (Kayar and Banchero 1984). However, this was not a sustained effect and the myocardial capillarity of the larger guinea pigs returned to normal (Fig. 3). These results have led us to conclude that the degree of hypoxia necessary to elicit changes muscle in capillarity is probably severe.

The PO_2 of the venous blood leaving a tissue is considered an index of the tissue PO_2 (Tenney et al., 1974). Thus, skeletal muscle PO_2 can be approximated by the mixed venous PO_2, whereas the cardiac muscle PO_2 can be approximated by the PO_2 of

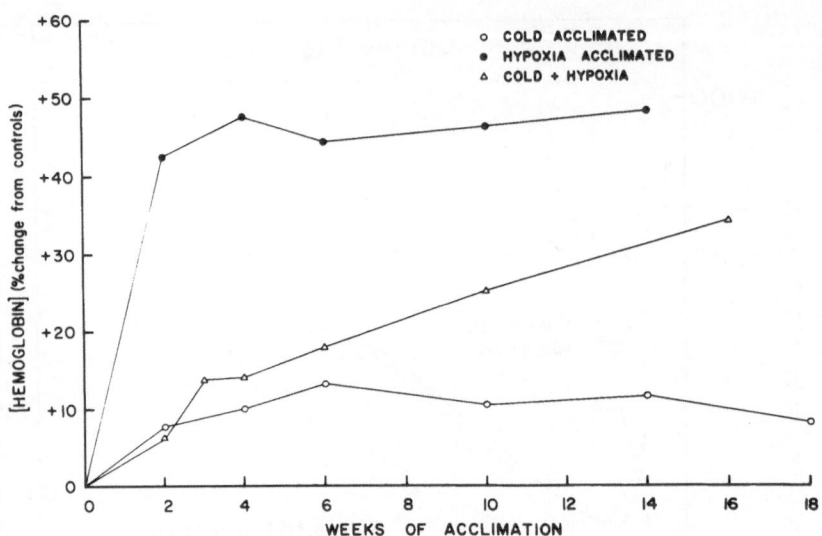

Fig. 2. Temporal changes in hemoglobin concentration in guinea
pigs during acclimation to cold, hypoxia, and cold + hypoxia.
Percent changes from [Hb] in control guinea pigs of the same body
weight are shown.

coronary sinus blood. These values of PO_2 can readily be
calculated using the $Hb-O_2$ dissociation curve and the O_2
content values. In hypobaric hypoxia equivalent to 4800 m the
S_aO_2 is 82% and the P_aO_2 is 50 torr. Hematocrit and
hemoglobin concentration measured in these guinea pigs under the
same environmental conditions need to be considered as these affect
the O_2 carrying capacity of blood. The O_2 transport system of
Hartley guinea pigs has not been adequately studied and data are
scarce. However, it is possible to approximate the blood gas
values (Fig. 4). The PO_2 of mixed venous blood (PvO_2)
calculated for guinea pigs at 4800 m is about 35 torr, which is
insufficient to increase skeletal muscle capillarity beyond normal
values; however, the PO_2 of coronary sinus blood is much lower,
about 25 torr after erythrocytosis has occurred. Coronary sinus
PO_2 is probably less than 20 torr in the early hours of exposure
while Q is high and hemoglobin concentration increases have not yet
occurred. This is apparently enough to increase the capillarity
of cardiac muscle in guinea pigs exposed to severe hypoxia.
Increased capillarity of cardiac muscle appears to occur as an
expression of the much lower PO_2 in the myocardium. The changes
in myocardial capillarity are more marked in the right ventricle
than in the left ventricle because of the increased pressure load
of the right ventricle in the presence of pulmonary artery arterial
hypertension.

358

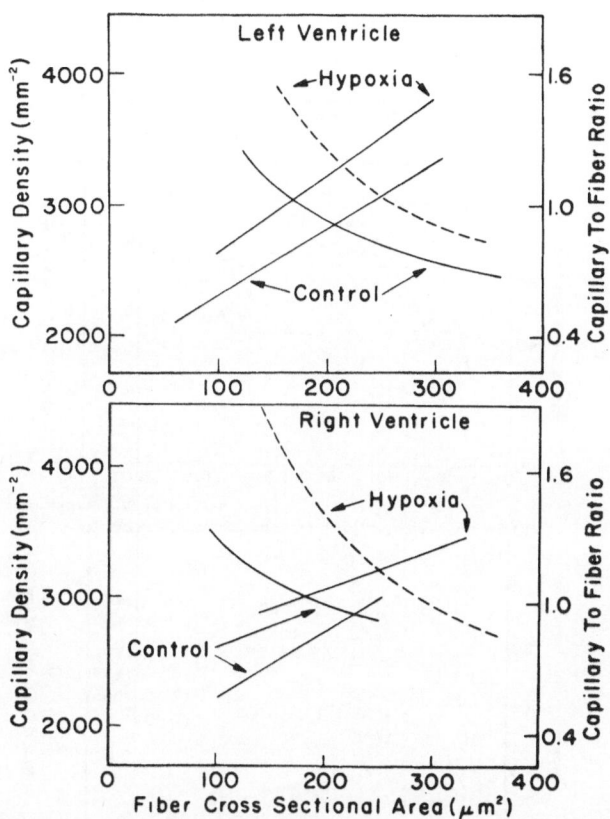

Fig. 3. Changes in myocardial capillarity, i.e., capillary
density and C/F, with fiber cross sectional area for the left and
right ventricles of normoxic guinea pigs and guinea pigs raised in
hypobaric hypoxia.

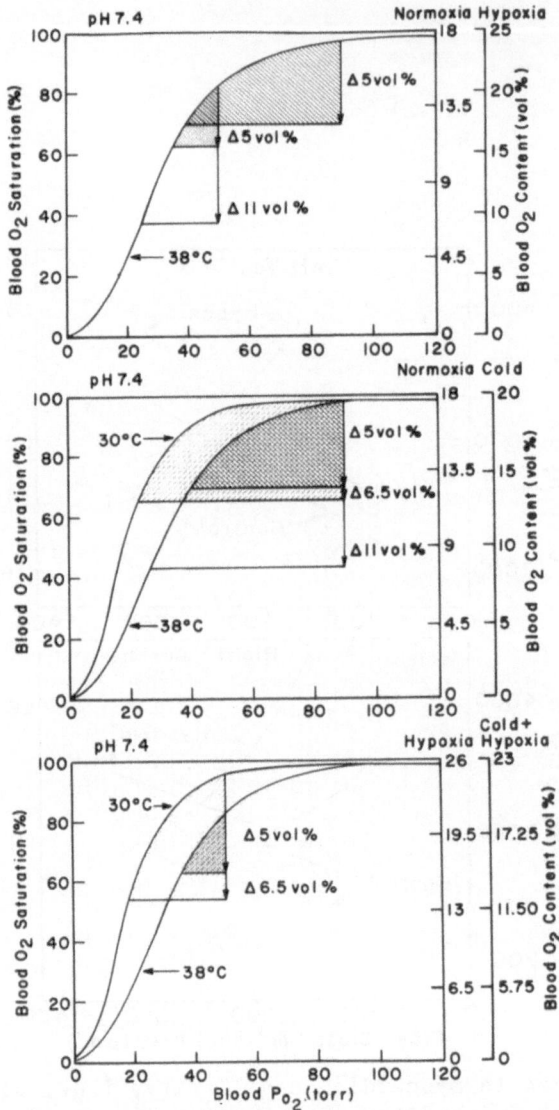

Fig. 4. Hemoglobin-oxygen dissociation curves for guinea pigs
acclimated to hypoxia, cold, and cold + hypoxia. Arterio-venous
oxygen differences of 5 vol% are shown for resting animals in
normoxia and hypoxia. In the cold- and cold + hypoxia-acclimated
guinea pigs an (a-v) O_2 of 6.5 vol% reflects greater O_2
extraction whereas for the myocardium an (a-v) O_2 of 11 vol% is
shown. Hb-O_2 affinity increases as blood is cooled to 30°C.
These are approximate values because no data on skeletal muscle
temperature or coronary blood flow are available.

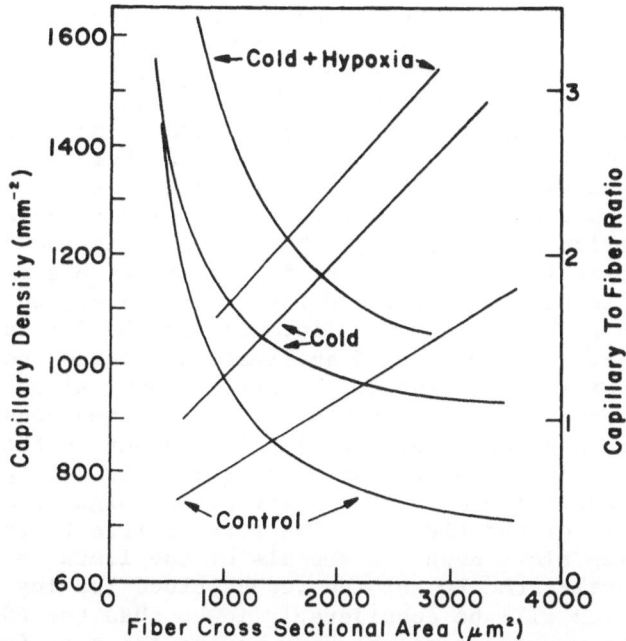

Fig. 5. Changes in the capillarity of the gastrocnemius with
fiber cross sectional area in guinea pigs acclimated to cold and
to cold + hypoxia, and in guinea pigs raised in normoxia.

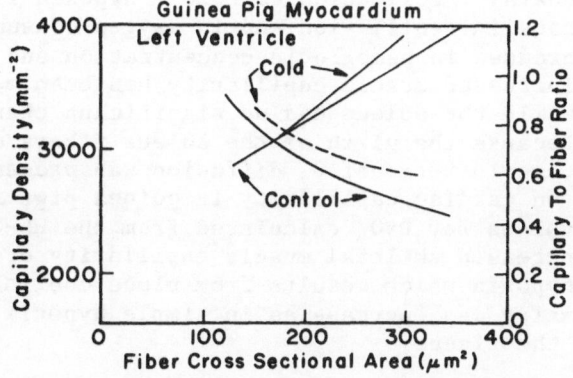

Fig. 6. Changes in left ventricular capillarity with fiber cross
sectional area in guinea pigs acclimated to cold and in animals
raised under normal laboratory conditions. No differences in
capillarity were measured between these two groups of guinea
pigs.

COLD ACCLIMATION. Rodents acclimated to severe cold, about 5°C, show a doubling of their oxygen consumption and their cardiac output while their core body temperature remains unchanged. Modest increases in hemoglobin concentration and hemocrit are measured in cold acclimated guinea pigs (Fig. 2). There is no disagreement concerning the effect of cold acclimation on skeletal muscle capillarity. Greater capillarity in skeletal muscle of rats and guinea pigs exposed to 5°C was reported by Heroux and St. Pierre (1957) and Sillau et al. (1980). The increase in the capillarity of these muscles is absolute (Fig. 5). A priori one may think that because in cold acclimation blood flow rate and oxygen consumption are increased the capillary proliferation may be due to their combined effect. However, cold acclimation produces no changes in myocardial capillarity, despite greater coronary blood flow rate and cardiac work which increases myocardial oxygen consumption [Fig. 6 (Kayar and Banchero, 1984)]. The answer to this apparent paradox may reside in the PO_2 at which these tissues operate. The $Hb-O_2$ dissociation curve for these guinea pigs is affected by the temperature of the tissues. The curve shifts to the left as the blood which flows down the vessels of the limbs is cooled (Fig. 4). Consequently, the PO_2 of the venous blood leaving the skeletal muscles will be considerably lower than the PO_2 of the blood from other muscles of the body having the same (a-v) O_2. A PvO_2 of 22 torr is much lower than the PO_2 at which these muscles normally operate and it is apparently enough to trigger the development of new capillaries in those muscles directly affected by the low temperature. Cardiac muscle, at normal body temperature, maintains normal capillarity because the coronary sinus PO_2 is not lower than in those tissues at normal temperature.

COLD + HYPOXIA. Acclimation to cold + hypoxia is accompanied by large increases in ventilation and in oxygen consumption but only modest increases in hemoglobin concentration and hematocrit (Fig. 2). An increased muscle capillarity has been measured in the gastrocnemius while the soleus had no significant changes (Fig. 6). However, because the girth of the soleus fibers was smaller, a relative advantage in terms of O_2 diffusion was present. There are no studies on cardiac capillarity in guinea pigs in cold + hypoxia. The values for PvO_2 calculated from the $Hb-O_2$ curve suggest that increased skeletal muscle capillarity occurs because of the severe hypoxia which results from blood cooling, whereas cardiac capillarity may increase as in simple hypoxia because of the low PO_2 of the tissue.

These data on skeletal and cardiac muscle suggest that changes in capillarity occur in response to a low PO_2 in the tissue. Therefore, the development of new capillaries in muscle in response to environmental insults may be similar to the development of new capillaries in wounds in that a certain

362

critical level of hypoxia is required for angiogenesis to occur. This mechanism for angiogenesis provides an explanation for the angiogenesis that accompanies normal growth and responses to environmental stresses in skeletal and cardiac muscle.

Supported by NIH grants HL-18145 and HL-28849. The author wishes to express his appreciation to Drs. A.H. Sillau, A.J. Lechner, S.R. Kayar, C.I. Blake and C.R. Jackson for their contributions to this project.

REFERENCES

Aquin, L., Sillau, A.H., Lechner, A.J., and Banchero, N., 1980, Growth and skeletal muscle microvascularity in the guinea pig, Microvasc. Res., 20:41-50.

Blake, C.I., and Banchero, N., 1984, Ventilation and oxygen consumption in the guinea pig, Respir. Physiol., (submitted).

Heroux, O., and St. Pierre, J., 1957, Effect of cold acclimation on vascularization of ears, heart, liver, and muscles of white rats, Am.J. Physiol., 188:163-168.

Hudlicka, O., 1982, Growth of capillaries in skeletal and cardiac muscle, Circ. Res., 50:451-461.

Kayar, S.R., Archer, P.G., Lechner, A.J., and Banchero, N., 1982, The closest individual method in the analysis of the distribution of capillaries, Microvasc. Res., 24:326-341.

Kayar, S.R., and Banchero, N., 1984, Myocardial capillarity in acclimation to hypoxia, Pflugers Arch., accepted for publication.

Sillau, A.H., and Banchero, N., 1979, Effects of hypoxia on guinea pig skeletal muscle, Proc. Soc. Exp. Biol. Med., 160:368-373.

Sillau, A.H., Aquin, L., Lechner, A.J., Bui, M.V., and Banchero, N., 1980, Increased capillary supply in skeletal muscle of guinea pigs acclimated to cold, Respir. Physiol., 42:233-245.

Stainsby, W.N., and Otis, A.B., 1964, Blood flow, blood oxygen tension, oxygen uptake, and oxygen transport in skeletal muscle, Am. J. Physiol., 206:858-866.

Tenney, S.M., 1974, A theoretical analysis of the relationship between venous blood and mean tissue oxygen pressures, Respir. Physiol., 20:283-296.

Valdivia, E., 1958, Total capillary bed in striated muscle of guinea pigs native to the Peruvian mountains, Am. J. Physiol., 194:585-589.

DISTRIBUTION OF LOCAL OXYGEN CONSUMPTION IN RESTING SKELETAL MUSCLE

Hans-Jürgen Meuer, Michael Ahrens, and Christine Ranke

Medizinische Hochschule Hannover
Zentrum Physiologie
D-3000 Hannover 61, FRG

INTRODUCTION

Skeletal muscle tissue is composed of muscle fibers of different metabolic types. Therefore, the oxygen consumption rate, $\dot{V}O_2$, is expected to vary within the tissue. An appropriate principle to determine these local differences is perfusion stop, because the tissue PO_2 drop, reflecting $\dot{V}O_2$, can be measured at sufficient high spatial resolution by oxygen microelectrodes.

In blood perfused tissue, however, oxygen demand during perfusion stop is not only met by oxygen physically dissolved, but also chemically bound to hemoglobin and myoglobin. Thus tissue PO_2 does not decrease at a constant rate, even if $\dot{V}O_2$ does not change with time. An example is given in Fig. 1 showing a typical PO_2 time course and the corresponding PO_2 decrease measured in the rat gracilis muscle during perfusion stop. It can be demonstrated that with different metabolic rates similar curves are obtained. The absolute readings, of course, depend on $\dot{V}O_2$, but also on hemoglobin and myoglobin content.

Our aim was to determine the local $\dot{V}O_2$ from the time course of the PO_2 decrease measured in tissue perfused by blood at physiological PO_2. By mathematical modelling we derived an equation allowing to calculate $\dot{V}O_2$ from the maximum PO_2 decrease occuring shortly after the beginning of perfusion stop (dotted line in Fig. 1). The validity of this method is demonstrated by experimental data.

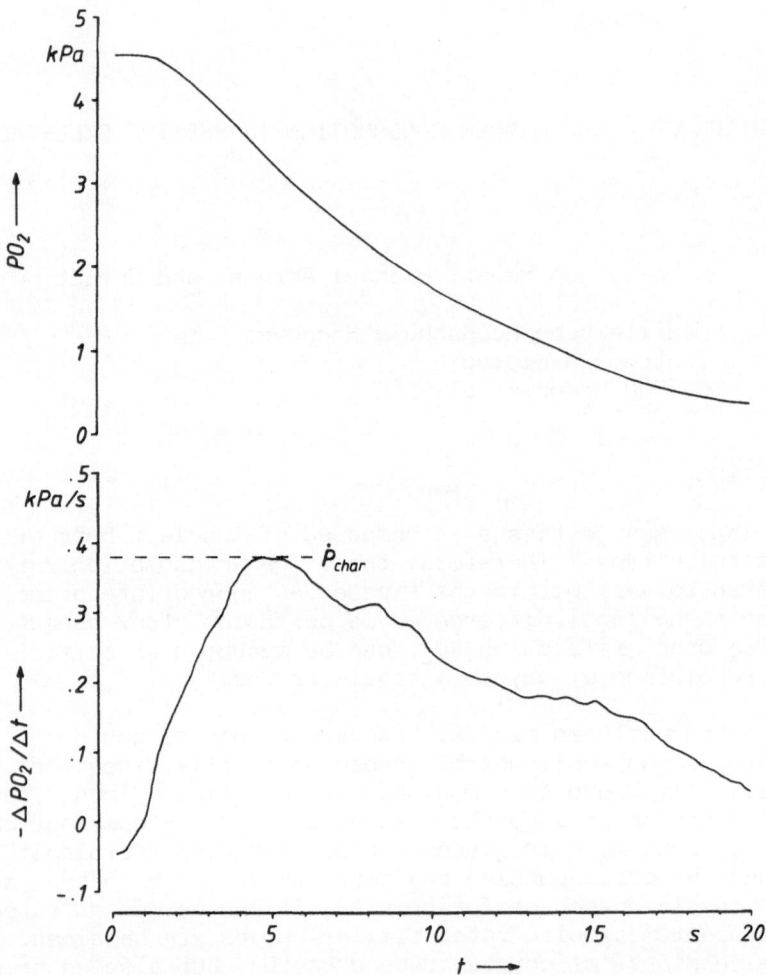

Fig. 1. Typical PO_2 time course and corresponding PO_2 decrease
measured in the rat gracilis muscle at rest. Perfusion was
interrupted at t = 1 s.

THEORETICAL METHOD

Perfusion stop was simulated using Krogh´s tissue model (Fig. 2). By numerical solution of the diffusion equation PO_2 time courses under different supply conditions were calculated. A typical result is shown in Fig. 3. In the upper part PO_2 vs. time curves are plotted refering to different distances, r, from the cylinder axis. The corresponding PO_2 decrease is given in the lower part. For the biological parameters values of the resting skeletal muscle were substituted.

In the initial phase after the beginning of perfusion stop the PO_2 decrease varies with the distance from the cylinder axis. These differences, however, decay rapidly until the PO_2 decrease is nearly the same from capillary wall to cylinder surface. Therefore, the maximum PO_2 decrease appearing at the cylinder surface represents the PO_2 decrease at any place in the tissue cylinder at the same time. This important feature does not only hold for the case presented in Fig. 3, but is also valid when in the model the values of the biological parameters influencing the PO_2 time course are varied within their physiological ranges. The maximum PO_2 decrease is therefore called the characteristic PO_2 decrease and abbreviated by $\dot{P}_{char}$.

The shape of the measured time course of PO_2 decrease (Fig. 1) accords best to the curve calculated for the cylinder surface (r = 32 μm). This has to be expected, because a microelectrode tip randomly injected into tissue is located with higher probability distant from capillaries than aside a capillary wall.

As predicted by the model the maximum PO_2 drop in a measured PO_2 time course occurs shortly after the beginning of perfusion stop Therefore, this value is assumed to be the characteristic PO_2 decrease and taken as a measure for the oxygen consumption rate.

In the model the characteristic PO_2 decrease depends not only on $\dot{V}O_2$, but also on the size of the tissue cylinder and on hemoglobin and myoglobin concentration and oxygen affinity. By varying

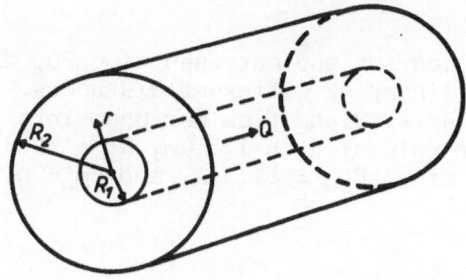

Fig. 2.   Krogh´s tissue cylinder used for mathematical modelling.

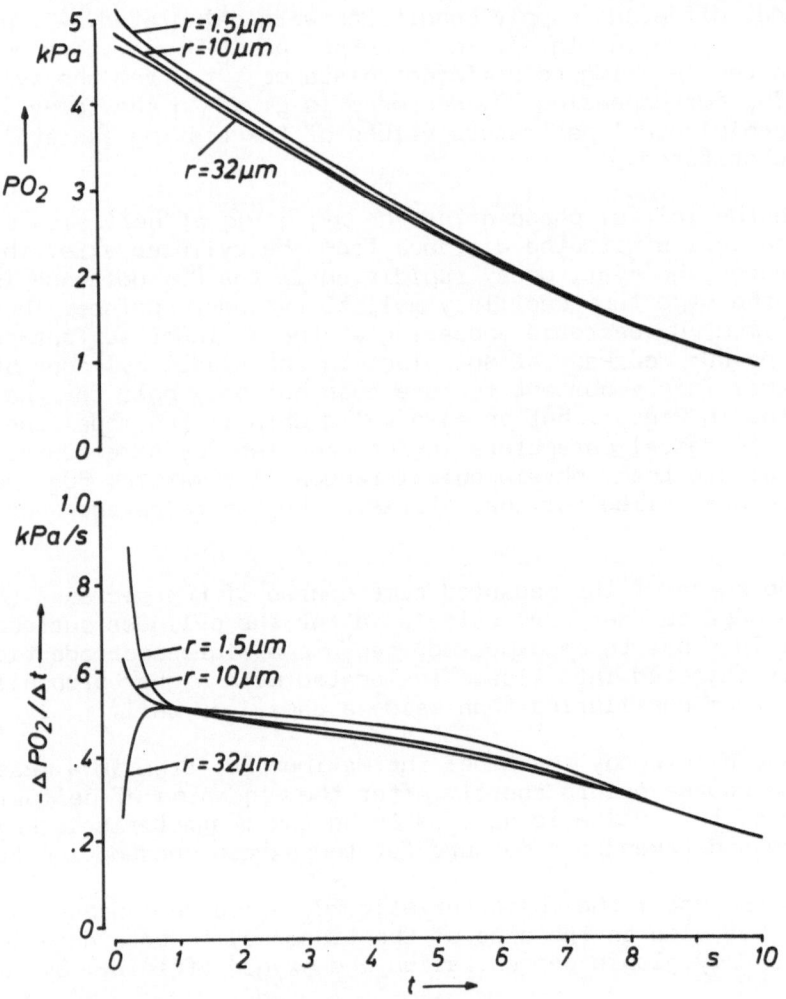

Fig. 3. PO_2 time courses and corresponding PO_2 decrease in a tissue cylinder at different distances, r, from the cylinder axis. Blood flow has been interrupted at t = 0. Parameter values: R_1 = 1.5 μm, R_2 = 32 μm, $\dot{V}O_2$ = 1 ml O_2/(100g min), C_{Hb} = 11.2 %, and C_{Mb} = 0.2 %.

the values of these biological parameters different supply conditions could be simulated. From the results of these calculations equ. (1) was derived describing mathematically the relationship between $\dot{P}_{char}$ und $\dot{V}O_2$.

$$\dot{V}O_2 = (S_t + m_{Mb} \; H \; C_{Mb} + m_{Hb \; max} \; H \; C_{Hb}/F^*) \; \dot{P}_{char} \qquad (1)$$

were S_t is the O_2 solubility coefficient in tissue, m_{Mb} is the slope of the normalized O_2-Mb-dissociation curve at tissue PO_2 equal to P_a (see Fig. 4), $m_{Hb \; max}$ is the maximum slope of the O_2-Hb-dissociation curve, H is Hüfner's number, C_{Mb} and C_{Hb} are myoglobin and hemoglobin concentration, and F^* is the ratio of tissue to capillary cross-section area. m_{Mb} can be expressed by

$$m_{Mb} = P_{50 \; Mb}/(P_a + P_{50 \; Mb})^2 \qquad (2)$$

and F^* by

$$F^* = (R_2/R_1)^2 - 1 \qquad (3)$$

Equ. (1) shows that $\dot{V}O_2$ is proportional to $\dot{P}_{char}$. The factor in parenthesis consists of three terms each representing one of the three oxygen pools covering the oxygen demand during perfusion stop. (Oxygen physically dissolved in blood is neglected in the

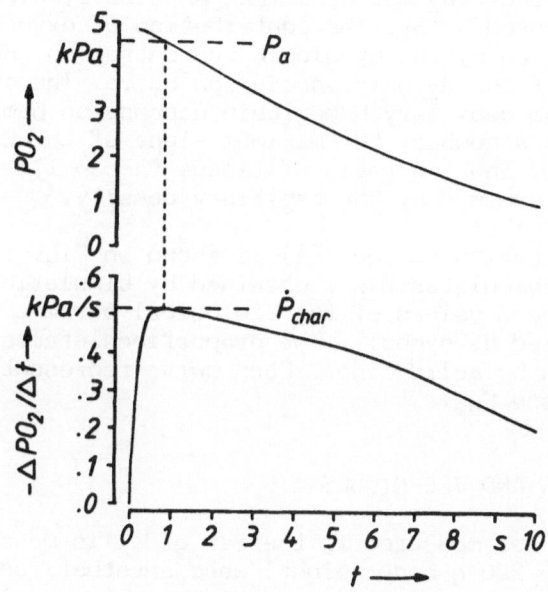

Fig. 4.   Determination of $\dot{P}_{char}$ and P_a from a measured PO_2 time course. $\dot{P}_{char}$ is the absolute value of maximum slope and P_a the tissue pressure corresponding to $\dot{P}_{char}$.

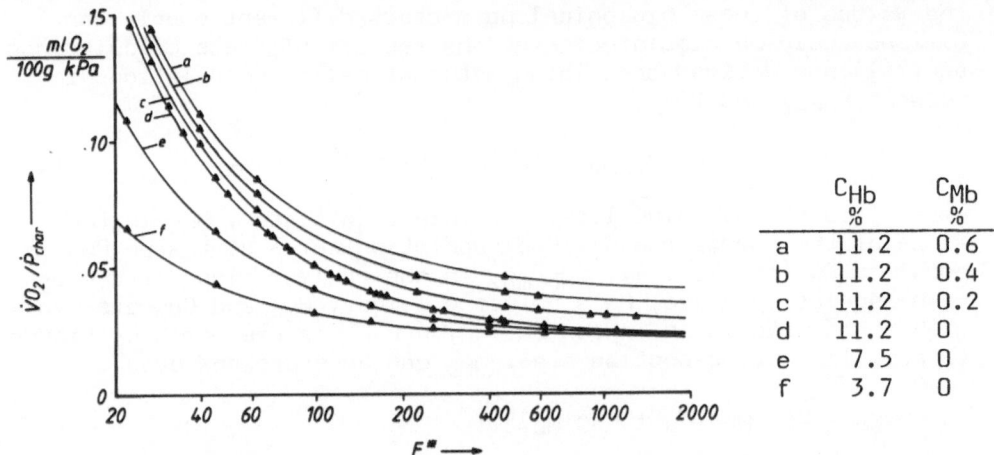

	c_{Hb} %	c_{Mb} %
a	11.2	0.6
b	11.2	0.4
c	11.2	0.2
d	11.2	0
e	7.5	0
f	3.7	0

Fig. 5.   Verification of equ. (1). Symbols denote the results of simulating perfusion stop for different values of the biological parameters. Solid lines are calculated by equ. (1). Each curve represents different myoglobin and hemoglobin concentrations.

model.) The part of $\dot{V}O_2$ met by oxygen physically dissolved in tissue is expressed by S_t. The contribution of oxygen released from myoglobin is given by the myoglobin concentration, Hüfner´s number, and the slope of the O_2-Mb-dissociation curve. The amount of oxygen originating from capillary hemoglobin depends on hemoglobin concentration, Hüfner´s number, the maximum slope of the O_2-Hb-dissociation curve, and the ratio of tissue to capillary cross-section area mainly determined by the capillary density.

The verification of equ. (1) is shown in Fig. 5. Ratios of given $\dot{V}O_2$ and calculated $\dot{P}_{char}$ obtained by simulating perfusion stop for different values of the biological parameters mentioned above are plotted by symbols. The proportional factor of equ. (1) vs. F^* is drawn by solid lines. Each curve represents different values of c_{Mb} and c_{Hb}.

INSTRUMENTATION AND TECHNIQUES

Local $\dot{V}O_2$ was measured in the rat gracilis muscle at rest. The animals (160 to 220 g body weight) were anesthetized with thiobutabarbital (0.1 g/kg b.w.). They respired spontaneously or were ventilated artificially, when paralysed by neuromuscular blocking agent. Central blood pressure, expiratory carbon dioxide fraction, and body temperature were monitored.

Tissue PO_2 was measured by recessed-tip oxygen microelectrodes of the Whalen type (Whalen et al., 1967; 1973) with an outer tip diameter of 3 to 5 μm and a sensivity of 1 to 3 pA/kPa. Perfusion stop was performed by clamping the femoral artery. After recording of the PO_2 drop the electrode tip position was marked by staining the tissue surface, and the muscle was shock-frozen. Serial cryostat sections of the tissue were stained for capillary endothelia by the ATPase reaction after preincubation at pH 4.3 (Sillau and Banchero, 1977) and for succinic dehydrogenase (SDH) by the method of Dubowitz and Brooke, 1973, with slight modifications. From these sections the density of perfused capillaries, CD, and the relative cross-section area consisting of muscle fibers with high activity of SDH (percentage of oxidative fibers) were determined. The ratio of tissue to capillary cross-section area F^* was calculated by equ. (4):

$$F^* = 1/(CD \ R_1^2 \ \pi) - 1 \tag{4}$$

The capillary radius R_1 was determined in previous experiments under perfusion stop conditions. Values of the other parameters $(S_t, C_{Mb}, P_{50 \ Mb}, m_{Hb \ max})$ required for calculating $\dot{V}O_2$ by equ. (1) were taken from literature with exception of C_{Hb}. This figure was estimated, because no data for the rat gracilis muscle were available. The error caused by a wrong number of C_{Hb} is small. For example, if C_{Hb} is overestimated by 50 % this affects the value of $\dot{V}O_2$ by about 10 %. The data used for the calculation of $\dot{V}O_2$ are listed in Table 1.

RESULTS

For $\dot{V}O_2$ measurements tissue areas had been selected with capillaries running parallel to muscle fibers and no major vessels being visible. With respect to capillary flow direction two types of tissue areas can be distinguished by microscopic observation: concurrent and countercurrent perfused areas. In concurrent per-

Table 1. Data used for the calculation of $\dot{V}O_2$ by equ. (1). Gas volumes are given in STPD.

Quantity, unit	Numerical value	Reference
S_t, 10^{-4} kPa^{-1}	2.2	Thews, 1960
$P_{50 \ Mb}$, kPa	0.43	Theorell, 1934
H, ml O_2/g	1.34	
C_{Mb}, %, concurrent	0.2	based on
countercurrent	0.25	Harms and Hickson, 1983
$m_{Hb \ max}$, kPa^{-1}	0.187	Bork et al., 1975
C_{Hb}, %	11.2	estimated
R_1, μm, perfusion stop	1.5	measured

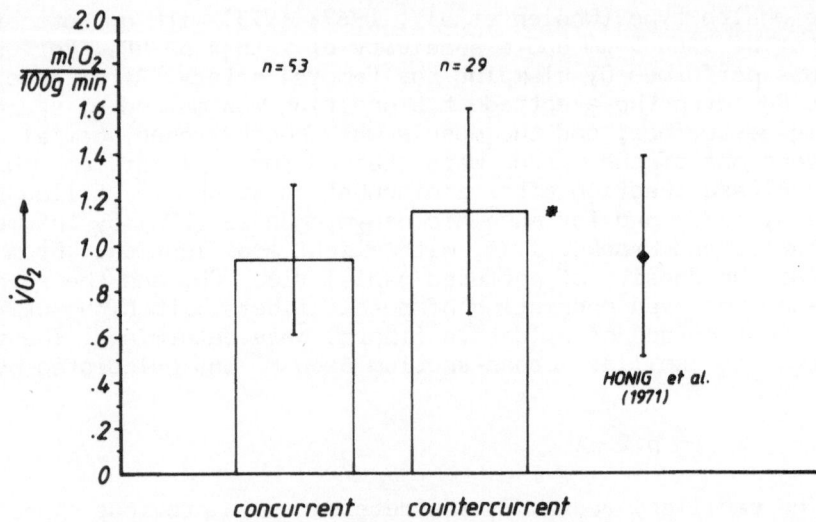

Fig. 6. Oxygen consumption rate of concurrent and countercurrent perfused areas of rat gracilis muscle, means +/-SD. For comparison the value of Honig et al., 1971, is given, who measured $\dot{V}O_2$ of the whole gracilis muscle using Fick's principle.

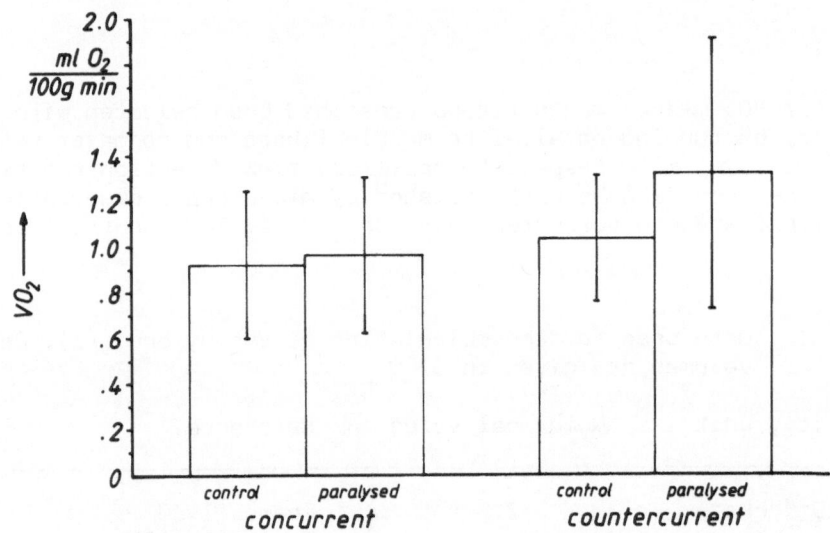

Fig. 7. Oxygen consumption rate of rat gracilis muscle paralysed by neuromuscular blocking agent. No significant difference exists in comparison to controls of the same group.

fusion flow direction of erythrocytes in adjacent capillaries is
the same, whereas in the countercurrent case erythrocytes in adjacent capillaries move in opposite directions. As these differences seem to indicate functional differences of the muscle cells,
measurements were performed in both types of tissue areas for
comparison.

As shown in Fig. 6, $\dot{V}O_2$ of countercurrent perfused areas was
significant higher than in concurrent perfused areas (1.15 +/-0.45
and 0.94 +/-0.33 ml O_2 STPD/(100g min), means +/-SD). Neuromuscular
blockade did not change these values significantly (Fig. 7). The
only data we found to compare with our results had been reported by
Honig et al., 1971 ($\dot{V}O_2$ = 0.95 +/-0.44 ml O_2/(100g min)), who
measured the oxygen consumption rate of the whole rat gracilis
muscle at rest using Fick´s principle.

Furthermore, differences between both types of perfusion were
also found in the number of perfused capillaries per cross-section
area, CD, and in the percentage of oxidative fibers identified by
strong SDH staining. In countercurrent perfused areas significantly
higher values of both figures were determined (CD = 554 +/-87 and
732 +/-151 mm^{-2}, percentage of oxidative fibers = 15.3 +/-5.9 and
23.6 +/-6.8 %, means +/-SD, concurrent and countercurrent,
respectively).

CONCLUDING REMARKS

The perfusion stop method has so far been applied only to $\dot{V}O_2$
measurements of muscle tissue perfused by hemoglobin-free solution
(Leniger-Follert and Lübbers, 1973) or by blood at an unphysiological high PO_2 (Becker et al., 1970). These experimental conditions
were required, because the amount of oxygen released from capillary
hemoglobin during perfusion stop was unknown. In this paper an
equation was presented improving the perfusion stop method essentially, as it now can be applied to normally perfused tissue too.
The experimental data obtained by the new method are comparable to
those determined in the conventional way using Fick´s principle.
This indicates that the differences between the tissue model and
the skeletal muscle mainly with respect to geometrical shape do not
seem to affect the characteristic PO_2 decrease substantially.
Furthermore, it has been shown by experiments that the perfusion
stop method is suitable for $\dot{V}O_2$ measurements at high spatial resolution (in the range of cell size), reflecting local $\dot{V}O_2$. Another
advantage is the applicability to even the smallest animals, where
Fick´s principle fails due to technical problems.

Our results demonstrate variations in $\dot{V}O_2$ within the same
muscle. A higher metabolic rate correlates with a more pronounced
vascularization and a greater portion of cells with high activity

of oxidative enzymes. This finding indicates that in the resting skeletal muscle the major part of energy (heat and possibly mechanical energy too) is produced by cells with aerobic metabolism, while glycolytic fibers are less active.

ACKNOWLEDGEMENT

This study was supported by the Deutsche Forschungsgemeinschaft.

REFERENCES

Becker, B., Rathscheck, W., Rathscheck, H., Müller, H., and Schroeder, W., 1970, Sauerstoffdruck, Sauerstoffverbrauch und Durchblutung in der Extremitätenmuskulatur des wachen Frosches, Pflügers Arch., 321:15

Bork, R., Vaupel P., and Thews G., 1975, Atemgas-pH-Nomogramme für das Rattenblut bei 37 $^{\circ}$C, Anaesthesist, 24:84

Dubowitz, V., and Brooke, M.H., 1973, "Muscle biopsy: a modern approach," Saunders, London

Harms, S.J., and Hickson R.C., 1983, Skeletal muscle mitochondria and myoglobin, endurance, and intensity of training, J. Appl. Physiol., 54(3):798

Honig, C.R., Frierson, J.L., and Nelson, C.N., 1971, O_2 transport and $\dot{V}O_2$ in resting muscle: significance for tissue-capillary exchange, Am. J. Physiol., 220(2):357

Leniger-Follert, E., and Lübbers, D.W., 1973, Determination of local myoglobin concentration in the guinea pig heart, Pflügers Arch., 341:271

Sillau, A.H., and Banchero, N., 1977, Vizualization of capillaries in skeletal muscle by the ATPase reaction, Pflügers Arch., 369:269

Theorell, H., 1934, Kristallinisches Myoglobin. V. Mitteilung: Die Sauerstoffbindungskurve des Myoglobins, Biochem. Z., 268:73

Thews, G., 1960, Ein Verfahren zur Bestimmung des O_2-Diffusionskoeffizienten, der O_2-Leitfähigkeit und des O_2-Löslichkeitskoeffizienten im Gehirngewebe, Pflügers Arch., 271:227

Whalen, W.J., Riley, J., and Nair, P., 1967, A microelectrode for measuring intracellular PO_2, J. Appl. Physiol., 23(5):798

Whalen, W.J., Nair, P., and Granfield, R.A., 1973, Measurements of oxygen tension in tissues with a micro oxygen electrode, Microvasc. Res., 5:254

PYRIDINE NUCLEOTIDE FLUORESCENCE MEASUREMENTS WITH SIMULTANEOUS

VISUALIZATION OF THE MICROCIRCULATION IN SKELETAL MUSCLE

Akos Koller and Paul C. Johnson

Dept. of Physiology, Univ. of Arizona
College of Med. Tucson, AZ 85724

Spectrophotometric and fluoro-reflectometric observations on different kinds of tissues have received great attention of physiologists over the past thirty years. Their studies were aimed at providing in vivo information about the metabolic events taking place in the tissue. One of these techniques is the in vivo observation of intracellular redox changes by means of pyridine nucleotide fluorescence, which is based on the fact that the light of the 350 nm region elicits fluorescence from only the reduced pyridine nucleotide at around 460 nm. This technique was introduced and developed by Chance, Jobsis, Legallais, Thorell and further improved by Harbig, Dora, Kovach and others [1,2,3,4,5]. These investigators made the fluoro-reflectometric measurements in a 1-2 mm diameter area. This approach gives an average tissue fluorescence change but does not spatially resolve such a change at the microcirculatory level and requires a strong correction for the changes of tissue blood content [4,5,6,12].

The purpose of our studies was to develop a microscope spectrofluorometer capable of monitoring the fluorescence and the absorbance of pyridine nucleotides in vivo at the microcirculatory level, and simultaneously to follow the diameter changes of the microvessels.

Methods

Fig. 1 shows the experimental arrangement. An Argon ion laser gives 357 nm wavelength excitation which is reflected by standing or scanning mirrors into a quartz objective to illuminate the tissue. The objective used gives a light spot of five microns diameter in vitro. Besides the laser spot excitation, the tissue is illuminated

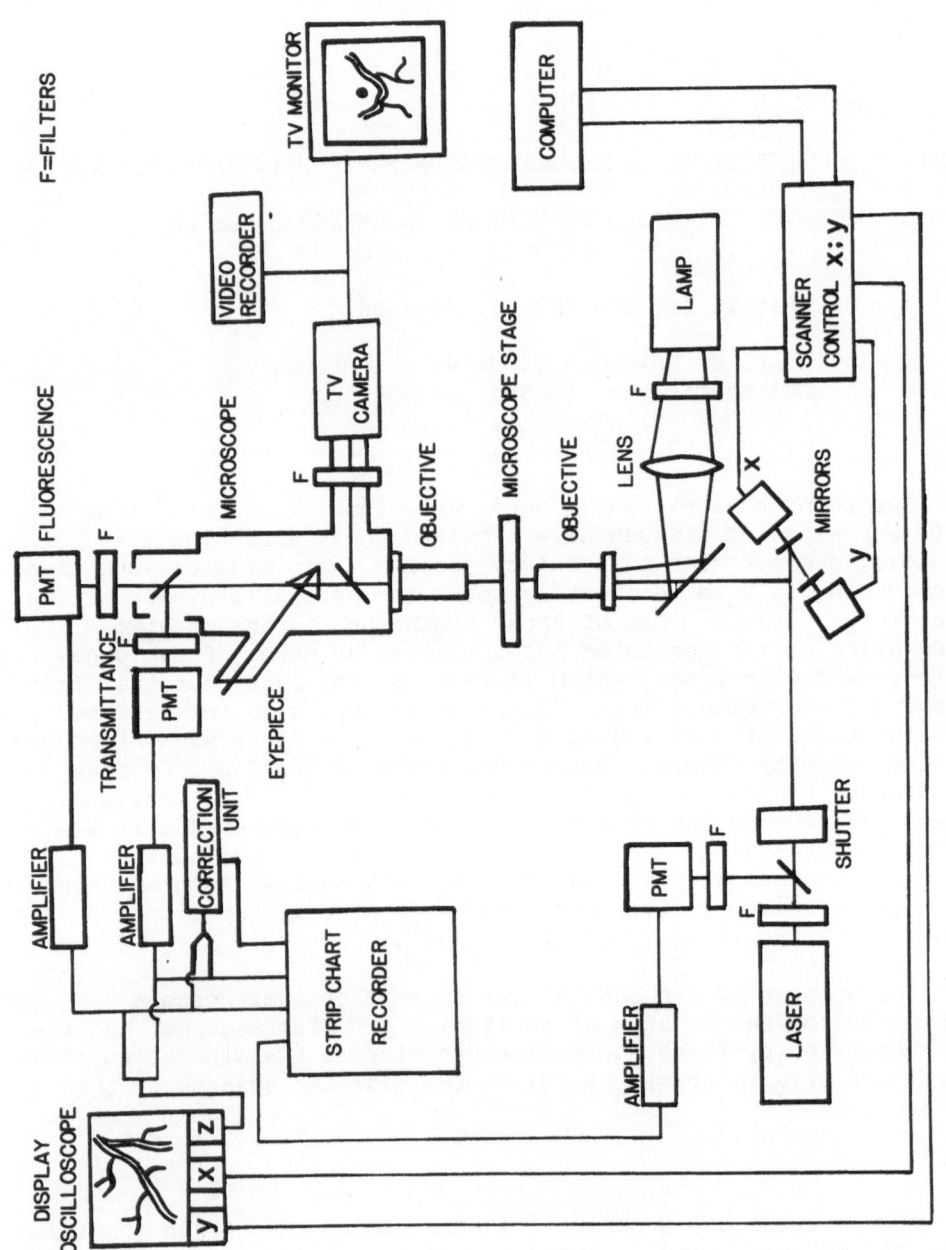

Figure 1. Experimental arrangement.

by 400 nm diffuse light and the image of the microcirculation formed by a Leitz H 32 X objective. The image is projected to an ISIT TV camera and recorded on a videorecorder. The transmitted (or reflected) excitation and the emitted fluorescence light are detected by photomultiplier tubes, (PMT) and spectral selectivity is achieved with appropriate filters. The output of the photomultiplier tubes are amplified and recorded on a chart recorder or displayed on a long persistence phosphorescent oscilloscope.

Spectral selectivity and sensitivity of the optical system.

The emission spectrum of in vivo muscle and of β-NADH solution, (placed under the microscope) were similar in shape and their maxima were around 470 nm wavelength. In the illuminated volume (which is about 2.3×10^{-11} liter) the number of reduced pyridine nucleotide molecules would be expected to change by around 10^9 or 10^{10} in different tissues under different conditions according to reports in the literature[7,8,9,10,11]. In comparison in vitro we could detect around 10^7 NADH molecules. Thus, spectral selectivity and sensitivity of this instrument seem appropriate to detect the expected changes in the number of reduced pyridine nucleotide molecules in muscle.

In vivo testing, reduced pyridine nucleotide fluorescence image.

To determine that we can detect fluorescence changes due to the increased number of reduced pyridine nucleotide molecules we have performed experiments with isolated saline perfused liver where the interference of the light signal by the blood was excluded[12]. We followed the changes in one spot during ischemia with epiillumination by recording in this case the reflected excitation and the emitted fluorescence. These results showed that only fluorescence emission was significantly changed, namely increased. We obtained the same result during topical application of KCN, which indicates that this optical system can detect fluorescence changes due to the reduced pyridine nucleotide changes in such a small volume. After this we began to use hamster cremaster and retractor muscles which have an intact blood supply.

Visualizing the tissue with 400 nm wavelength light illumination or scanning the tissue with the laser spot we were able to see the microvessels and select avascular areas to make measurements in one spot. These experiments gave quite comparable results to those found in liver when we applied KCN topically. Fluorescence greatly increased as shown in Fig. 2.

When we scanned the tissue with the laser spot we could see the image of the fluorescence of reduced pyridine nucleotide by viewing the PMT output on a long persistence phosphorescent oscilloscope (Fig. 3). Some differences in

fluorescent intensity in several avascular areas as well as the
absorption of fluorescence by blood in the microvessel can be seen
(Note: the bright spots are photomultiplier noise. The diameter of
the large vessel is 70-80 microns).

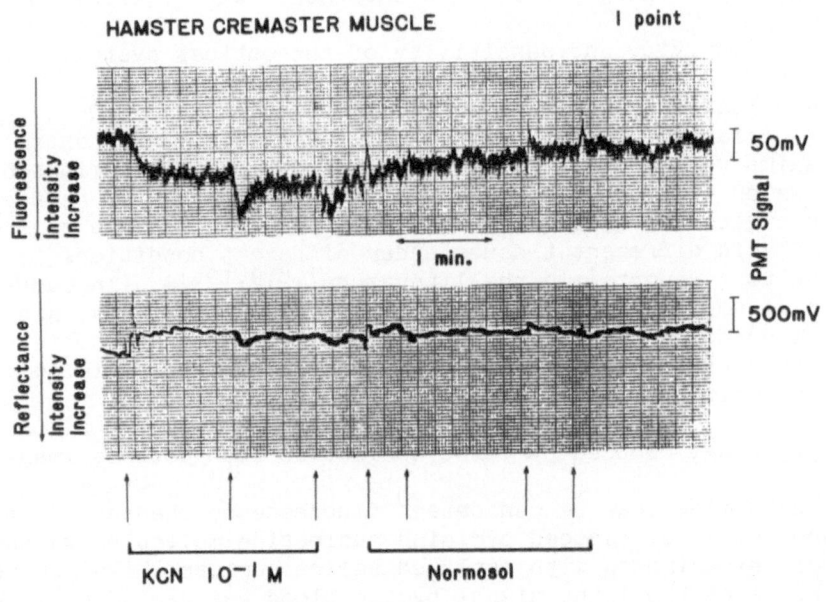

Figure 2. Effect of topical application of KCN on the in vivo
fluorescence of pyridine nucleotide in hamster cremaster muscle.

Correction for non-specific absorption

Our next step was to examine the possibility of correcting the
signals for non-specific absorption changes and thus obtain a
quantitative estimate of pyridine nucleotide changes in the tissue.
(The non-specific absorption changes include optical density
changes of the tissue, laser intensity changes etc., which could
effect the excitation energy intensity and absorption of the
wavelengths of interest.

For this procedure the illumination spot was set in a fixed
position. To simulate the effect of changing excitation light
intensity we changed the excitation energy in a step-wise fashion

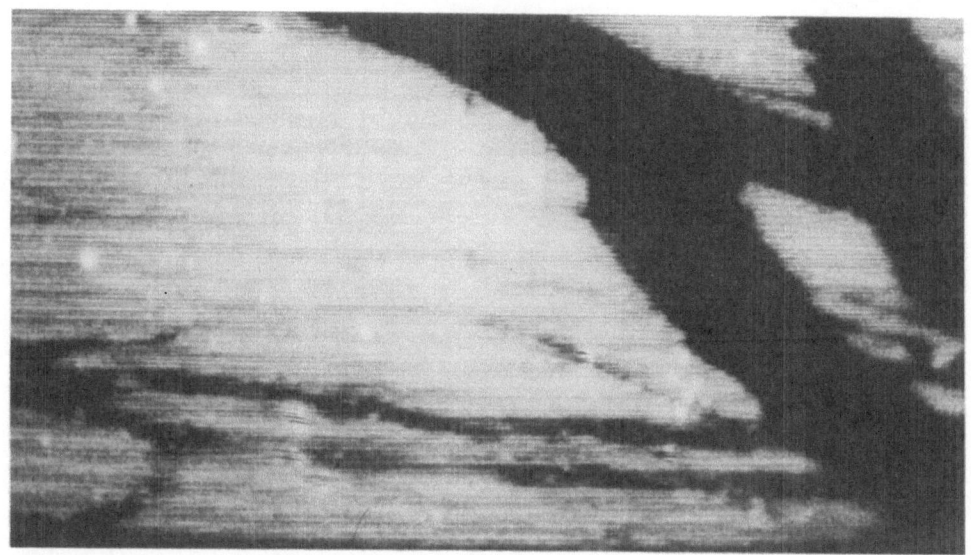

Figure 3. Pyridine nucleotide fluorescence image of hamster
cremaster muscle

and measured the transmitted excitation as well as the emitted
fluorescence light intensity of different concentrations of β-NADH
solution. The results showed that the relation between transmitted
excitation light and fluorescence is linear for any given
concentration (Fig. 4). So at a given concentration of β-NADH the
fluorescence signal is determined in a predictable manner by the
excitation intensity. We obtained the same result if we placed
neutral density filters before or after the sample, to achieve about
the same density level as our muscle preparation. These
measurements indicated that the changes in the light signals due to
changes in excitation intensity before or in the sample could be
corrected by measuring at the same time the transmitted excitation
light intensity and fluorescence of a given sample.

Fig. 5 shows how an analog circuit, calculating the ratio of F
over T (F/T), provides a corrected signal. We can change the ·
excitation energy intensity falling on the β-NADH solution without
causing changes in the corrected signal. But we see changes when
the concentration of the β-NADH solution was altered. In other
words we did not see changes when non-specific absorption occurred,
but did see changes when specific absorbance and fluorescence
changes took place due to the change in number of fluorescent
molecules. This indicated the possibility of comparing the in
vitro and in vivo corrected signals. The same results were obtained
in vivo. The light intensity changes in the light path before or
after the hamster retractor muscle did not affect the corrected
signal.

379

But we have seen changes when tissue ischemia was achieved with KCN 10^{-2} M (Fig. 6). The great increase in the corrected signal indicates a large increase in the number of reduced pyridine nucleotide molecules in the tissue. It is worth noting that during topical application of papaverine HCl (1 mg/ml, 0.4 ~ 4.0 ml) there was no change in this signal.

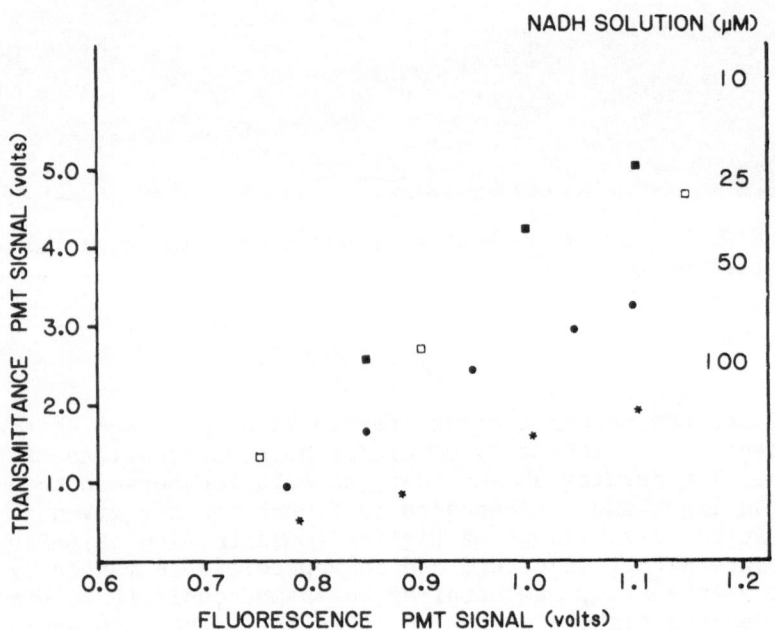

Figure 4. Effect of excitation light intensity changes on the fluorescence and the transmittance of known concentration of β-NADH solution.

Theoretical considerations, possibility of quantification

A simplified theoretical basis for characterizing the concentration changes of NADH quantitatively in different optical density environments by measuring the fluorescence and absorption changes of a given sample is shown below. Figure 7 shows how the excitation and the fluorescent light intensities could change through a given sample.

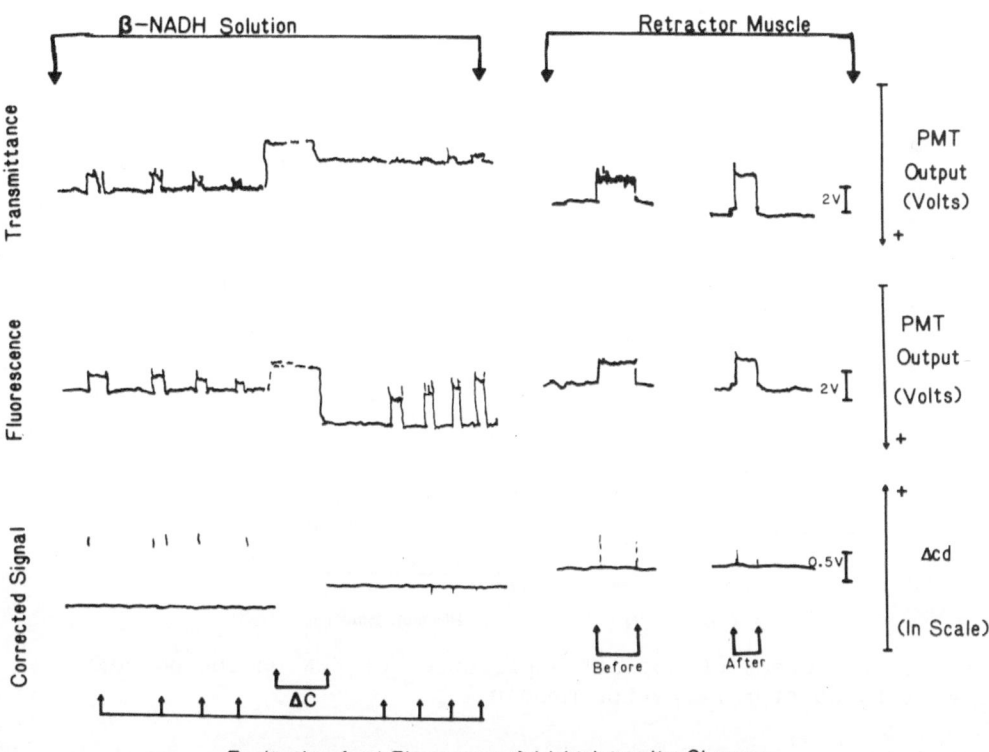

Figure 5. Effect of changes in excitation (and fluorescence) intensity on the transmittance, fluorescence and corrected signal of different concentrations of β-NADH solution and of hamster retractor muscle.

The equations are based on Beer's law. I represents the transmitted laser light and F the emitted fluorescence of the sample (in the transmitted position). We assume that a, the non-specific molar absorption coefficient, includes the non-specific absorption and reabsorption of the two wavelengths by the tissue and it is the same for both wavelengths. When we take the ratio of the two equations, F over I (F/I), we get the spectrofluorometric value.

According to this, the non-specific absorption part drops out from this equation. This means that if any light intensity changes occur in the sample, due to non-specific absorption, this does not affect the calculation of the concentration of a given sample, with known thickness. And if we fix the location of the measurements in the case of the tissue with an unknown thickness, the spectrofluorometric value could be expressed in terms of concentration distance product, or in terms of the number of

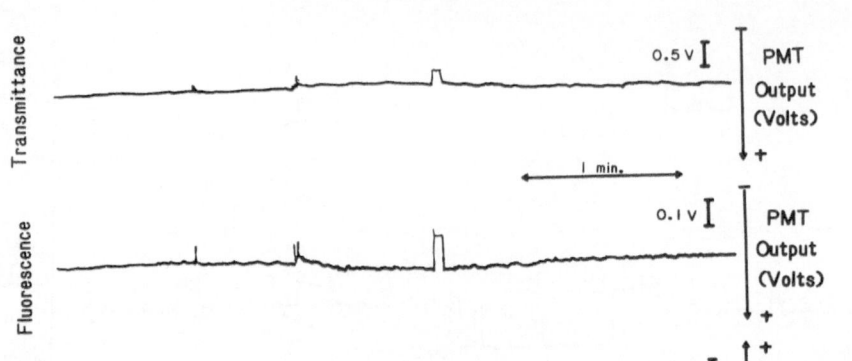

Figure 6. Effect of topical application of KCN on the corrected signal in hamster retractor muscle.

molecules. By measuring the thickness of the muscle optically or mechanically perhaps we can estimate the in vivo concentration changes of reduced pyridine nucleotide in that location.

Calibration of the system

The in vitro obtained calibration curve shows a linear relationship between the concentration and the logarithm of the corrected signal (CS) (Fig. 8).

To illustrate the possibility of quantifying the in vivo changes, we can use the calibration curve to estimate the reduced pyridine nucleotide concentration changes in vivo during topical application of KCN [10^{-2} M]. If we assume that the tissue thickness is about 150 microns[13] and that the fluorescence of the bound NADH is enhanced about 4-6 times[14], we can estimate actual concentration changes. By using the in vitro β-NADH-calibration curve, and the above mentioned data we estimated an increase of approximately 620 micromolar from normal (control) muscle to the muscle treated with KCN. In an other case, when the blood flow was stopped in the muscle, and we applied KCN topically, the

382

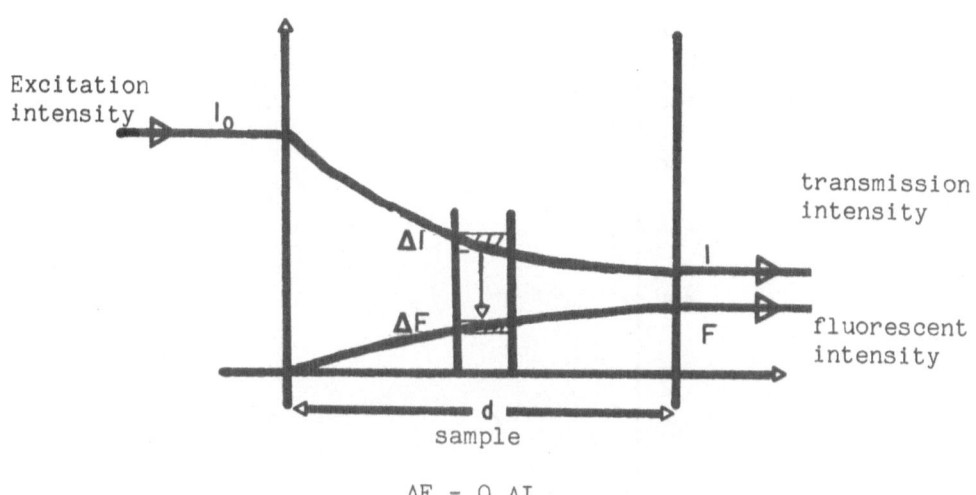

Excitation intensity

transmission intensity

fluorescent intensity

sample

$$\Delta F = Q \ \Delta I$$

$I = Io \ e^{-(ck+a)d}$

$F = Io \ Q \ [1-e^{-ckd}] \ e^{-ad}$

(note: neglect the fluorescence due to non-specific absorption)

Q = quantum yield of the fluorescent molecule
k = molar absorbance coefficient of the fluorescent molecule
c = concentration of the given molecule in the sample
a = non-specific molar absorption coefficient of the sample

SF = F/I = spectrofluorometric value

$SF = Q[1 - e^{-ckd}] \ /e^{-ckd}$ Note: e^{-ad} drops out
                                                (non-specific absorption)
and so

$c = 1/kd \ \ln[1 + F/QI]$

                            at fixed location with d = constant,
$cd = 1/k \ \ln \ [1 + F/QI]$

Figure 7.   Theoretical consideration.

estimate was around 150 micromolar increase in the concentration of reduced pyridine nucleotide. It is worth mentioning that the differences between the end values for the two KCN-treated muscle was around 27 micromolar. These estimated data are in agreement with the in vitro measured data found in the literature[8,11].

383

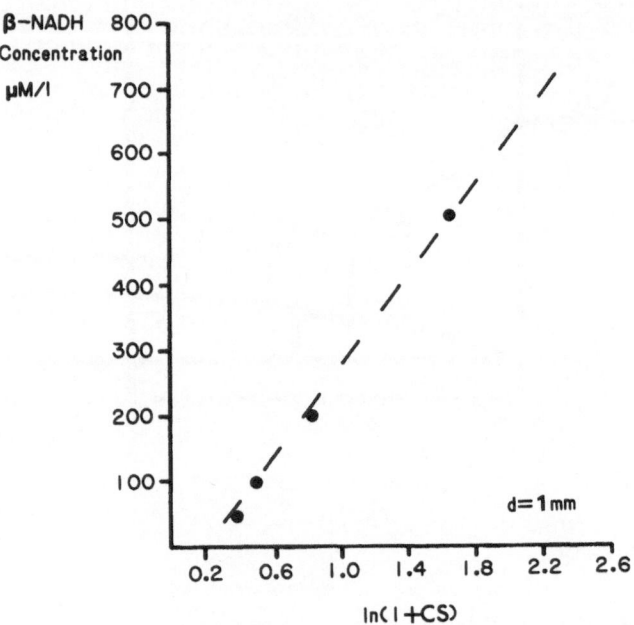

Figure 8. Relationship between the corrected signal (CS) and the concentration of β-NADH solution.

Conclusion

The fluorescence and transmittance of the tissue probably involves other sources than reduced pyridine nucleotide. However, the specific fluorescence and absorbance changes during ischemia, hypoxia, or during changes in metabolism is most likely due to changes in reduced pyridine nucleotide molecules in the tissue. Our results indicate that in this experimental condition the spectrofluorometric value or corrected signal is not affected by changes due to non-specific absorption in the tissue or excitation intensity changes. Further developments of this method may make it possible to quantify in vivo, changes of reduced pyridine nucleotide and relate it to local microcirculatory events in skeletal muscle. (Supported by NIH HL 17421 and HL 07249).

References

1. B. Chance and F. Jobsis, Changes in fluorescence in a frog sartorius muscle following in twitch. Nature No. 468, July 18, 1959.
2. B. Chance, and B. Thorell, Fluorescence measurements of mito-chondrial pyridine nucleotide in aerobiosis and anaerobiosis. Nature No. 4691, Sept. 26, 1959.
3. B. Chance and V. Lagallais. Differential microfluorometer for the localization of reduced pyridine nucleotide in living cells. Rev. Sci. Instr. 30: 732-735, 1959.
4. K. Harbig, B. Chance, A.G.B. Kovach and M. Reivich. In vivo measurement of pyridine nucleotide fluorescence from cat brain cortex. J. Appl. Physiol. 41(4):480-488, Oct. 1976.
5. E. Dora and A.G.B. Kovach. The problems of the correction and evaluation of in vivo NADH fluorescence measurements. In: Cardiovascular Physiology. Heart, Peripheral Circulation and Methodology, edited by A.G.B. Kovach, et al. Budapest: Pergamon, 1980. vol. 8, pp. 373-391, 1979.
6. S. Kobayashi, K. Nishiki, K. Kaede and E. Ogata. Optical consequences of blood substitution or tissue oxidation-reduction state microfluorometry. J. Appl. Physiol. 31(1):93-96, 1971.
7. F.F. Jobsis. Spectrophotometric studies on intact muscle. I. Components of the respiratory chain. J. General Physiol. 46:905-928, 1963.
8. J.R. Williamson, Gylcolytic control mechanisms. I. Inhibition of glycolysis by acetate and pyruvate in the isolated, perfused rat heart. J. Biological Chem. 240(6): June 1965.
9. E. Kohen, C. Kohen, B. Thorell and G. Wagener, Quantitative aspects of rapid microfluorometry for the study of enzyme reactions and transport mechanisms in single living cells. In: Fluorescence Techniques in Cell Biology, Edited by A.A. Thaer and M. Sernetz 1973, pp. 207-218, Springer Verlag, Heidelberg.
10. T.M. Sundt, Jr., R.E. Anderson and F.W. Sharbrough. Effect of hypocapnia, hypercapnia, and blood pressure on NADH fluorescence, electrical activity, and blood flow in normal and partially ischemic monkey cortex. J. Neurochem. 27: 1125-1133, 1976.
11. M.E. Tischler, D. Friedrichs, K. Coll, and J.R. Williamson, Pyridine nucleotide distributions and enzyme mass action ratios in hepatocytes from fed and starved rats. Arch. Biochem. and Biophys. 184, 222-236, 1977.

12. H. Schnitger, R. Scholz, Th. Bucher and D.W. Lubbers. Comparative fluorometric studies on rat liver in vivo and on isolated, perfused, hemoglobin-free liver. Biochemische Zeitschrift 344:334-339, 1965.
13. S.M. Sullivan and R.N. Pittman, Hamster retractor muscle: a new preparation for intravital microscopy. Microvasc. Res. 23:329-335, 1982.
14. R.W. Estabrook, Fluorometric measurement of reduced pyridine nucleotide in cellular and subcellular particles. Analytical Biochem. 4:231-245, 1962.

REDISTRIBUTION OF MICROCIRCULATION IN SKELETAL MUSCLE DURING HYPOXAEMIA

D.K. Harrison, S.K. Knauf, H. Vogel* H. Günther and
M. Kessler

Institut für Physiologie und Kardiologie der Universität
Erlangen-Nürnberg, Waldstrasse 6, D.8520 Erlangen / FRG
*Institut für Anaesthesiologie der Universität München

INTRODUCTION

Previous studies of tissue pO_2 in the sartorius muscle in dogs revealed that hypoxaemia induced a redistribution of local pO_2 in such a way that a lower mean value, but a very much narrower range of values was observed, without the appearance of partial pressures in the 0-5 mmHg range (Harrison et al.,1984). Preliminary measurements of capillary blood flow using the hydrogen clearance technique indicated that under these conditions a redistribution of microflow may occur.

The heterogeneity of the blood supply to muscles of different types has recently been reported by Armstrong and Laughlin (1983) after studies using microspheres in the hind limbs of rats. Even in the same muscle, resting blood flows differing by up to 700%, depending on the predominance of fibre-type, are reported. At the microcirculation level such heterogeneities in capillary flow (Lindblom, 1983) and tissue pO_2 (Rettig et al., 1984) are also found to be dependent on the prevailing physiological conditions.

In order,therefore, to investigate the relationship between the distribution of tissue pO_2 and microflow, and to gain some insight into the above-mentioned heterogeneities, histograms of both tissue pO_2 and microflow distributions in the same small area of the sartorius muscle in six anaesthetised mongrel dogs were compared under control and hypoxaemic conditions.

METHODS

The Hydrogen Clearance Technique

The use of a hydrogen electrode to record the washout of this
freely diffusible gas from tissue was first introduced by Aukland
et al., (1964) as a method for measuring blood flow. The technique
has since been developed in many forms (Baumgärtl and Lübbers, 1973;
Stosseck et al., 1974; Krumme et al., 1975). In these experiments
the basic technique of Krumme et al. has been applied in that a pre-
palladinised multiwire surface electrode (Kessler and Lübbers, 1966)
was used for the polarographic measurement of hydrogen. The modified palladinisation technique involved the following steps: 1)
Polishing of the electrode surface until absolutely flat and free
of grease. 2) Hydration for 1 hour in double distilled water. 3)
Electrolytic deposition of palladium from a solution of $PdCl_2$
(60.07% purity) in 0.1 M HCl onto the platinum cathodes with a
current density of 0.09 mA/mm^2 for 7 min at $45^\circ C$ using an annular
platinum anode. 4) Microscopic examination of the quality of the
palladium film. 5) Dry storage for at least 12 hours before use.
This palladinisation technique produced electrodes with a drift
of less than 5% per hour, a pH_2 sensitivity of 1 nA per 100 mmHg
and a 90% response time of less than 5 sec.

Three methods for introducing hydrogen into the area of measurement were investigated. The first, a bolus of physiological saline
saturated with hydrogen injected into the iliac aorta, needed to be so
large (20 ml) in order to record a reasonable pH_2 that arterial
flow changes were induced. The second, equilibration of the dog
to a constant tissue pH_2 (saturation) by addition of a given concentration of hydrogen to the inspired gas mixture and then abruptly turning the hydrogen off resulted in reproducible washout curves, but since each reaction lasted at least 30 min the method was
thus impractical for the purposes of microflow histogram measurements under constant conditions. The third method, and that used
throughout these experiments, involved the addition of pure hydrogen to a concentration of 30% in the inspired gas mixture for precisely 30 sec whilst keeping the inspired oxygen concentration
(FiO_2) constant (inspired bolus).

The clearance data were recorded using a Digital Equipment
PDP 11/34 computer and stored for further analysis (Brunner et al.,
1984). The curves could be plotted in their original (drift-correc-
ted) form (Fig.1a) or semilogarithmically (Fig.1b). Each curve was
measured at the muscle surface by the individual wires of the electrode. Since each wire has a hemispherical catchment zone with a
radius of only 35 μm, the respective curve represented the flow
only within this region.

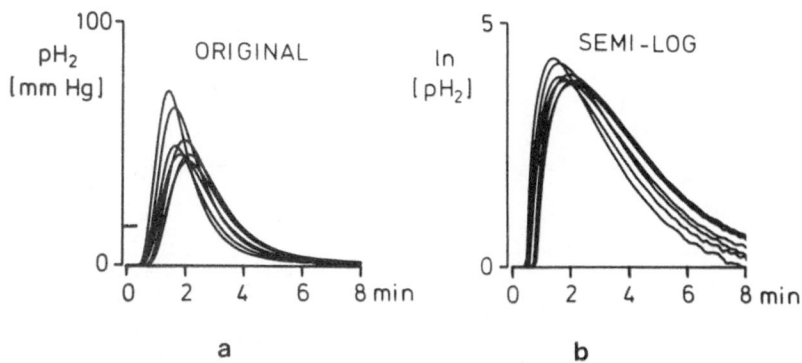

Fig.1a) Original and (b) semilogarithmic clearance curves measured
on skeletal muscle after administration of a 30 second inspired bolus

Microflow values (MF) were calculated from the maximum slope
of the semilogarithmic washout curve according to the formula:

$$MF = \frac{\Delta \ln(pH_2)}{\Delta t} \cdot 100$$

(see Aukland et al., 1964), again with the aid of the computer.
The maximum semilogarithmic slope was also recognisable as the most
linear part of the curve ($r > 0.95$), was always to be found at the
latest 1 minute after the peak pH_2 value had been reached, and
lasted about 2 1/2 minutes, thus indicating that any remaining component of the wash- in function could be neglected.

Experimental Procedure

Six mongrel dogs (25-30 kg) were anaesthetised initially with
a short-acting barbiturate and then maintained with piritrimide,
flunitrazepam and N_2O. Pancuronium was administered as a relaxant
and the dogs were ventilated at an FiO_2 of approximately 0.25 regulated so that consistent control arterial pO_2 (P_aO_2) values of
117 ± 6 mmHg were obtained. Throughout the experiments haemoglobin
concentration, haematocrit and blood gas/acid-base status (IL 1302)
were measured at regular intervals. Arterial pressure was measured
by means of a tip manometer (Miller) located in the iliac aorta,
and venous pressure measured with a Statham pressure transducer,
via a catheter located in the abdominal vena cava. Femoral artery
flow was measured using a Statham electromagnetic flowmeter. ECG,
pressures and femoral flow were recorded semi-continuously using
the PDP 11/34 computer.

389

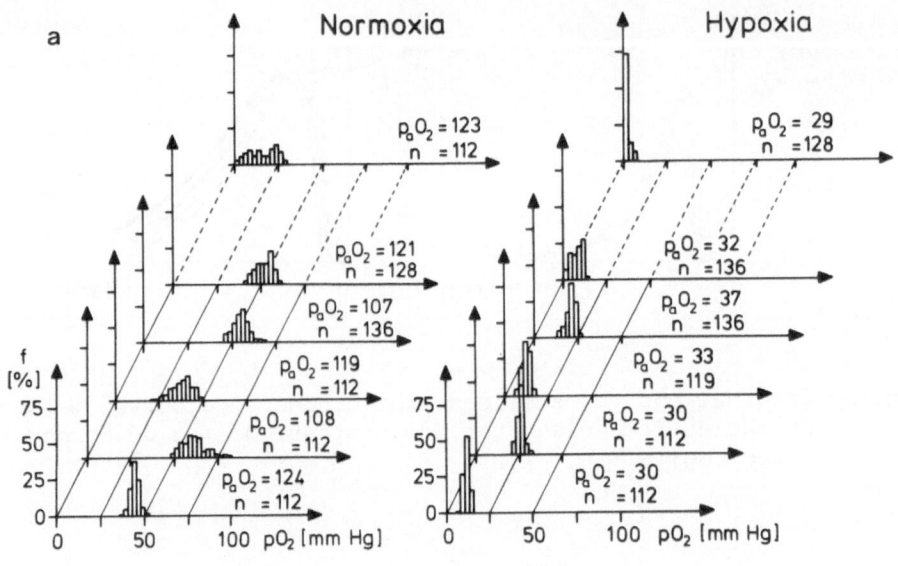

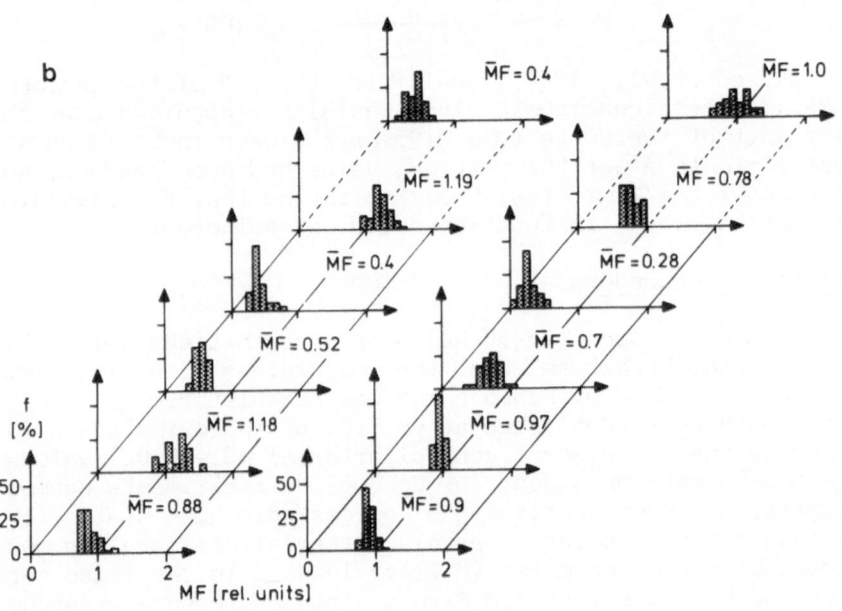

Fig.2a) pO_2 and (b) microflow histograms before and during hypoxaemia.

A small area of the sartorius muscle was carefully prepared and freed of fascia. A silicone rubber disc incorporating an "O"ring electrode holder, which allowed rotation of the pO_2 or pH_2 electrode about its own axis, was used to keep the respective electrodes in position on the muscle. In this way pO_2 and microflow histograms could be constructed over the same area of muscle. In the latter case, seven hydrogen clearances were performed, rotating the electrode between each clearance, in order to produce a microflow histogram of 49 values; pO_2 histograms were constructed from at least 100 values.

Hypoxaemia was induced by reducing the FiO_2 to approximately 0.1 and regulating it so that the p_AO_2 was held constant at 32 ± 3 mmHg. Measurements of global parameters, pO_2 and microflow histograms were carried out under control and hypoxaemic conditions. Continuous measurements of pulsatile parameters and tissue pO_2 were carried out during the switch to hypoxaemia.

RESULTS

The pO_2 and microflow histograms from all experiments are shown respectively in Figs.2 (a) and (b) during normal and hypoxic conditions. In considering these results, it should be borne in mind that both the pO_2 and microflow histograms are representations of the real distribution values within the tissue.

The pO_2 histograms displayed no values below 20 mmHg under normal conditions, with the exception of the uppermost experiment. During hypoxaemia no values were found in the region 0-5 mmHg in four experiments, in one 8% such values were found, and in the uppermost histogram 75% of the values lay within this range. The pO_2 histograms were, however, shifted to the left and were more homogeneous.

The microflow histograms (again with the exception of the uppermost experiment) displayed an overall slight decrease in mean value despite large increases in femoral artery flow (see Fig.4). This is shown more clearly in Fig.3 which is a plot of the changes in femoral artery flow and microflow over the course of one experiment. Although the femoral flow increased by 70% almost no change in microflow was observed.

The summary of haemodynamic results given in Fig.4 shows that the total range of microflow values was reduced by 50% during hypoxaemia. The same figure shows a mean decrease in peripheral resistance of 28%, an increase in arterial pressure of 15% and a mean increase of 61% in femoral blood flow.

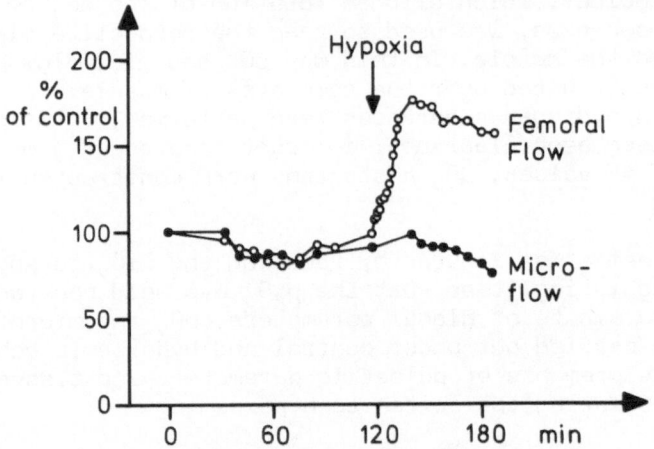

Fig.3. Femoral flow and microflow values before and during hypoxaemia.

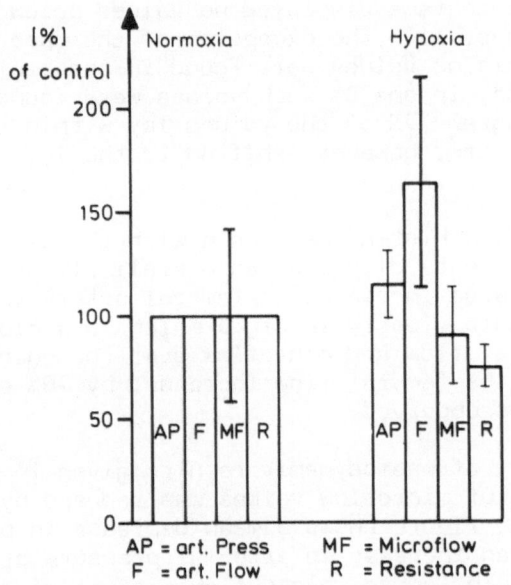

Fig.4. Summary of changes in haemodynamic parameters (± SD) and
microflow (± range) due to hypoxaemia.

The experiment illustrated in the uppermost histograms of Fig.2(a) and (b), as well as displaying atypical pO_2 distributions, demonstrated a mean increase in microflow (140%) proportional to that of femoral artery flow. The reactions of pressures and flow during hypoxaemia were the same as in the other experiments, but the disintegrated form of the control pO_2 histogram indicated the existence of a microcirculatory disturbance of the local tissue oxygen supply. This conclusion is confirmed by the appearance of 75% of tissue pO_2 values in the range 0-5 mmHg during hypoxaemia.

DISCUSSION AND CONCLUSIONS

The increase in femoral artery flow observed during hypoxaemia occured mainly as a result of remote-control by the peripheral chemoreceptors. A mean decrease in microflow (10%), however, was observed at the site of our measurements on the sartorius muscle. On the other hand a change in tonus of the arterial vessels was indicated by the decrease in peripheral resistance which, together with the 50% decrease in the range of microflow, demonstrated that redistribution of flow had occured. One possible argument concerning the discrepancy between femoral flow and microflow might be that the measurements of microflow at the surface of the sartorius muscle were not representative of capillary flow in other muscles or even to other parts of the same muscle. In the light of the enormous heterogeneities in muscle blood flows found by Armstrong and Laughlin (1983) quoted earlier, the question as to which muscle, or part thereof, is "typical" is probably somewhat academic. However, the fact that large increases (up to 150%) in microflow, in the absence of any increase in femoral artery blood flow, were observed in the same site (Fig.5) when the sartorius muscle was stimulated at different frequencies via the femoral nerve (see Harrison et al., 1984)

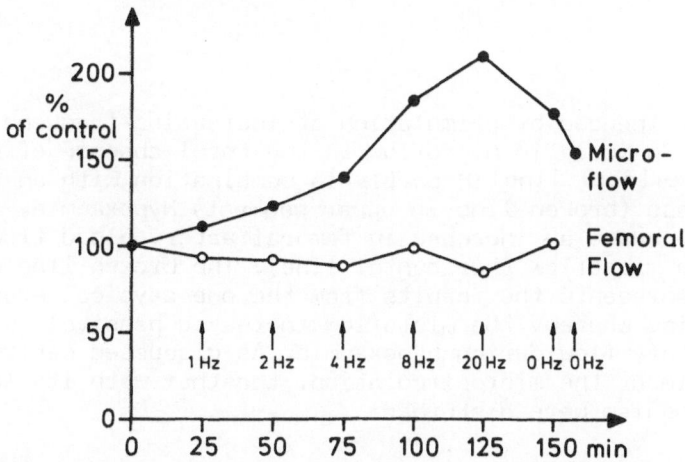

Fig.5. Femoral flow and microflow values during stimulation of the sartorius muscle via the femoral nerve (1.3V, 0.5 ms) at increasing frequencies.

certainly proves the existence of an active local regulation of microflow within the supply compartment studied in our experiments. It is interesting that the reaction illustrated in Fig.5 was almost an exact converse of that shown in Fig.3.

The two types of reaction are summarised in Fig.6 where changes in microflow (ordinate) are plotted _schematically_ against changes in femoral artery flow (abscissa). As shown in earlier experiments (Harrison et al., 1984) stepwise increase in local oxygen

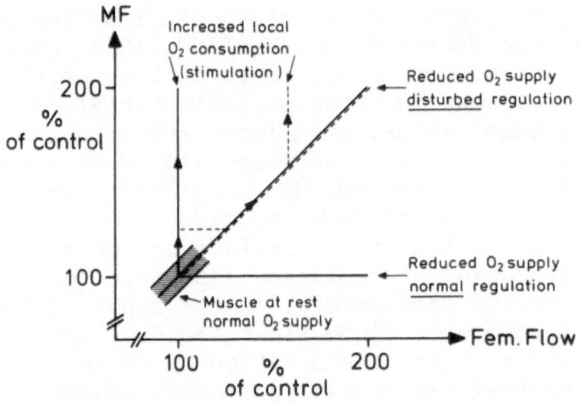

Fig.6. Schematic representation of the types of microflow vs flow reactions observed during hypoxia and stimulation (cf.Figs. 3 and 5).

consumption induced by stimulation at increasing frequencies can produce an increase in microflow in the total absence of femoral flow increase (vertical line) or partly in combination with an arterial flow increase (broken line in upper segment).Hypoxaemia, on the other hand caused an increase in femoral artery blood flow with no increase in microflow (horizontal line). The broken line below the 45° line represents the results from the one atypical experiment of our series whereby the microflow increased passively with the femoral artery flow during hypoxaemia. As discussed earlier, in this experiment the microcirculation, together with its local regulatory mechanism were disturbed.

The questions arising from Fig.6 are a) Where does the blood (upper segment) come from? b) Where does it (lower segment) go to? and c) What is the regulating mechanism?

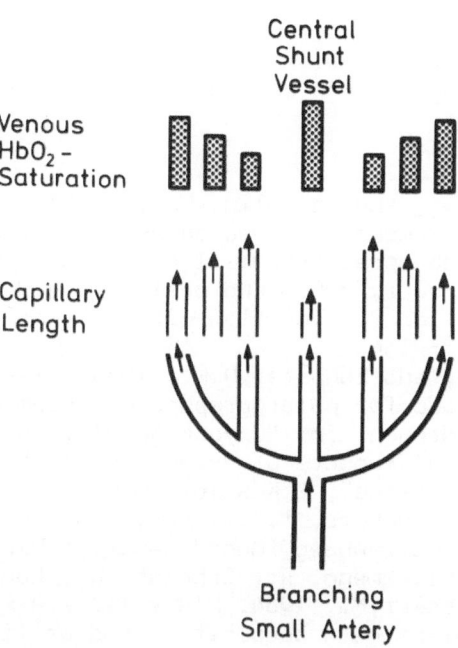

Fig.7. Schematic representation of high- medium- and low-flow
       capillaries.

Although our findings do not provide direct answers to these
questions, some clues are provided by the results of Piiper and
Meyer (1984) who, by use of inert gas clearance, found three flow
compartments in the resting gastrocnemius muscle in dogs: 7% tissue
volume is supplied by 35% of flow (fast compartment), 15% volume by
35% flow (medium) and 81% tissue volume by 31% flow (slow).

A schematic representation of this three compartment model
based on our own findings is given in Fig.7 (Kessler et al., 1984a).
A branching small artery feeds capillaries of different lengths.
The short central capillaries form the high-flow channels, whose
flow can be locally regulated to assure sufficient delivery of oxygen to the more peripheral medium length (medium flow) and long
(slow) capillaries. The relative haemoglobin oxygenations at the
venous ends of the respective capillaries are also illustrated.
This model is consistent with previous findings that regulation of
capillary flow is effected by local tissue chemoreceptors (cellular
signal oxidases) (Kessler et al., 1984b).

Under hypoxaemia flow is probably increased through the central
shunt vessels (as a result of the increased arterial flow, and as
suggested by the decrease in peripheral resistance) as a precautio-
nary mechanism which ensures that oxygenated blood is immediately
available through the local regulatory system should it be required
in order to prevent the occurence of tissue anoxia. In contrast,
during stimulation, oxygenated blood is probably diverted from the

high-flow channels to the peripheral capillaries in order to meet
the increased oxygen demand. However, further functional and anatomical investigations of such channels are required.

REFERENCES

Armstrong, R.B., and Laughlin, M.H., 1983, Blood flows within
and among rat muscles as a function of time during
high speed treadmill exercise, J.Physiol., 344 : 189

Aukland, K., Bower, B.F., and Berliner, R.W., 1964, Measurement
of local blood flow with hydrogen gas, Circ.Res.,
14 : 164

Baumgärtl, H., and Lübbers, D.W., 1973, Platinum needle electrode for polarographic measurement of oxygen and
hydrogen, in: "Oxygen Supply. Theoretical and Practical Aspects of Oxygen Supply and Microcirculation
of Tissue", M.Kessler, D.F.Bruley, L.C.Clark Jr.,
D.W.Lübbers, I.A.Silver, J.Strauss, eds.. Urban +
Schwarzenberg, München-Berlin-Wien.

Brunner, M., Ellermann, R., Scheidt, W., Günther, H., and
Kessler,M., 1984, DIG V 1.3 - a software package for
online data acquisition and offline processing: An
application for hemodynamic data, Proc. 7th Annual
Meeting of the German Microcirculation Society, in
press.

Harrison, D.K., Höper, J., Günther, H., Vogel, H., Frank, K.H.,
Brunner, M., Ellermann, R., and Kessler, M., 1984,
Microcirculation and pO_2 in skeletal muscle during
respiratory hypoxia and stimulation, in: "Oxygen
Transport to Tissue V", Adv.Exp.Med.Biol., Vol.169,
D.W.Lübbers, H.Acker, E.Leniger-Follert, and T.K.
Goldstick, eds., Plenum, New York and London.

Kessler, M., Harrison, D.K., Ellermann, R., Brunner, M., Frank,
K.H., and Höper, J., 1984a, Erfassung und Interpre-
tation von Mikrozirkulationsstörungen, Proc. 2nd
Erlangen Anaesthesiology Symposium, in press.

Kessler, M., Höper, J., Harrison, D.K., Skolasinska, K., Klöve-
korn, W.P., Sebening, F., Volkholz, H., Beier, I.,
Kernbach, C., Rettig, B., and Richter, H., 1984b,
Tissue O_2 supply under normal and pathological con-
ditions, in: Oxygen Transport to Tissue V", Adv.Exp.
Biol.,Vol.169, D.W.Lübbers, H.Acker, E.Leniger-Fol-
lert, and T.K.Goldstick, eds., Plenum, New York and
London.

Kessler, M., and Lübbers, D.W., 1966, Aufbau und Anwendungsmöglichkeiten verschiedener pO_2-Elektroden, Pflügers
Arch.Ges.Physiol., 291 : R 82.

Krumme, B.A., Strehlau, R., and Kessler, M., 1975, Hydrogen clearance measurements on the liver surface in situ with the multiwire electrode, Arzneim.-Forsch. (Drug. Res.). 25 : 1666.

Lindblom, L., 1983, Microvascular blood flow distribution in skeletal muscle, Acta Physiol.Scand. Suppl. 525.

Piiper, J., and Meyer, M., 1984, Diffusion-perfusion relation-ships in skeletal muscle: models and experimental evidence from inert gas washout, in: "Oxygen Transport to Tissue V", Adv.Exp.Med.Biol., Vol.169, D.W.Lübbers, H. Acker, E.Leniger-Follert, and T.K.Goldstick, eds., Plenum, New York and London.

Rettig, V. Baier,I., Ellermann, R., and Kessler, M., 1984, Topo-graphical aspects of local oxygen distribution (pO_2 and intracapillary HbO_2) in the skeletal muscle of the rat, Proc. 7th Annual Meeting of the German Microcir-culation Society, in press.

Stosseck, K., Lübbers, D.W., and Cotting, N., 1974, Determina-tion of local blood flow (microflow) by electrochemi-cally generated hydrogen, Pflügers Arch.Ges.Physiol., 348 : 225.

RELATIONSHIP BETWEEN OXYGEN DEFICIT AND OXYGEN DEBT IN EXERCISES OF DIFFERENT INTENSITY AND DURATION

R. Kubica, B. Wilk and J. Januszewski

Department of Human Physiology and Biochemistry, Academy of Physical Education, Al. Planu 6-letniego 62a, 31-571 Krakow, Poland

Krogh and Lindhard were the first who measured and described oxygen debt (R) and oxygen deficit (D) in 1913-1914. The theory of oxygen debt developed by Furusawa, Hill, Long and Lupton (1924-1925) based upon an observation that the oxygen uptake during recovery is higher than that in rest before exercise. The possible relationship between the increased O_2 consumption in recovery and the anaerobic processes during exercise was at that time suggested.

The question arises: is the measured oxygen debt during recovery (repayed O_2 debt) equal to the oxygen deficit during exercise (contracted O_2 debt)?

Asmussen (1946) found that the oxygen debt could be as high as 160% or 190% of the oxygen deficit depending on the experimental conditions. Christensen and Högberg (1950) noted oxygen debt twice as great as oxygen deficit. Also Alpert (1952) and Henry and De Moor (1956) confirmed significantly higher O_2 debt than O_2 deficit.

There were some attempts to calculate the theoretical value of R/D ratio. If we assume that the efficiency of anaerobic processes is 50% of aerobic reactions the R/D ratio should be 2 : 1.

Agnewik et al. (1969) found that during maximum exercise the above ratio was equal to 2.5 : 1 and there was a correlation between blood lactate concentration and both oxygen debt and oxygen deficit. Some other authors were not able to find the same correlation.

Furthermore, Lukin and Ralston (1962) on the basis of a great number of individual results ascertained a wide variability of R/D ratio (from 0.6 to 3.6).

Authors engaged in the above problem differed regarding to technics of measurements and kind of applied exercises. Some of them analysed the O_2 debt/O_2 deficit relationship during exercises of different duration but the same intensity. Others considered exertion of different intensity paying rather little attention to their duration.

In this context it seems to be purposeful to try to put in order the data about oxygen debt/oxygen deficit ratio taking into account the different intensity and duration of exercise.

METHODS AND TECHNICS

Forty-eight examinations were carried out on two physical education students. Before every exercise session during 30 minutes the resting values of pulmonary ventilation ($\dot{V}_E$), oxygen uptake (V_{O}), carbon dioxide output ($\dot{V}_{CO_2}$) and lactate blood concentration (La)[2] were evaluated.

Physical exercise was performed on bicycle ergometer, Zimmer-mann type. The following intensities and durations of exercise were applied: 50 W-duration of exercise from 1 to 7 min, 125 W-duration from 1 to 8 min, and 180 W-duration from 1 to 9 minutes.

Thus every subject performed 24 exercise sessions.

The values of $\dot{V}_E$, $\dot{V}_{O_2}$ were measured during the entire exercise (every 2 minutes) and recovery (in first 2 minutes, between 2-nd and 5-th minute, and then every 4 minutes till the resting level of the above parameters were reached). In recovery the blood lactate was analysed.

The following values were calculated: oxygen requirement (OR), oxygen deficit (D), oxygen debt (R) and oxygen cost ($\dot{V}_{O_2}$ E+R) as the net values; i.e. the rest levels of $\dot{V}_{O_2}$ were subtracted.

Thus we assume that the oxygen requirement (OR) is the average minute oxygen uptake ($\dot{V}_{O_2}$) in steady state multiplied by the minutes of exercise.

Oxygen deficit (D) expresses the difference between the total oxygen uptake during the exercise ($\dot{V}_{O_2}$ E) and the oxygen requirement (OR).

Oxygen debt (R) is the excess of oxygen uptake during the recovery i.e. above the rest values of $\dot{V}_{O_2}$.

Finally, the oxygen cost ($\dot{V}_{O_2}$ E+R) is treated as a sum of the total oxygen uptake during the exercise ($\dot{V}_{O_2}$ E) and the oxygen debt (R).

Pulmonary ventilation was measured by means of the Max Planck gasmeter. Oxygen and carbon dioxide concentrations in expired air were analysed by gaschromatography and by Godart capnograph, respectively.

Lactate blood concentration was analysed by the method described by Barker and Summerson (1941), modified by Ström (1949). Arterialized blood was drawn from the fingertip preheated in the water bath with the temperature of $45^{\circ}C$. During the recovery blood was drawn several times to evaluate the peak concentration of lactate.

Aerobic capacity ($\dot{V}_{O_2}$ max), evaluated with the direct method, was the same in both subjects. It amounts to 45.6 ml $\cdot$ kg^{-1} $\cdot$ min^{-1}.

RESULTS AND DISCUSSION

The oxygen cost of exercise was the greater the higher the intensity and the longer the duration of exercise session (Fig. 1, 2). However, in spite of the well-known simple relationship of the total energy uptake to the duration of exercise, their values oscillated from minute to minute during steady state.

The analysis of exercise oxygen consumption ($\dot{V}_{O_2}$) allows us to ascertain the steady state as early as after 2 min of the exercise at 50 W and 125 W and after 3 mins at 180 W. The lack of stability of the steady state was also visible in the O_2 level.

Oxygen debt and oxygen deficit increased with the elevation of work intensity whereas the duration of exercise after the steady state had been reached had no clear effect on their averages. The distinct fluctuations of R and D near this average level could be observed. It is reasonable to add that in one subject (A.M.) both oxygen debt and oxygen deficit values showed a close correlation with blood lactate but in the other subject the correlation was only slightly marked.

The differences between O_2 debt and O_2 deficit are variable in two subjects (Tab. I). In subject A.M. the differences are well-marked and statistically significant. They also gradually increase from the average value of 193 ml O_2 at the lowest intensity to 480 ml O_2 at the highest one. In the other subject (W.B.) the above differences are negligible and statistically not significant.

Consequently in the subject A.M. the ratio R/D is visibly higher than 1.0 and even reaches 2 at the 50 W exercise and it becomes lower and lower when the intensity of exercise is increasing. In the second subject the ratio is on an average close to 1.

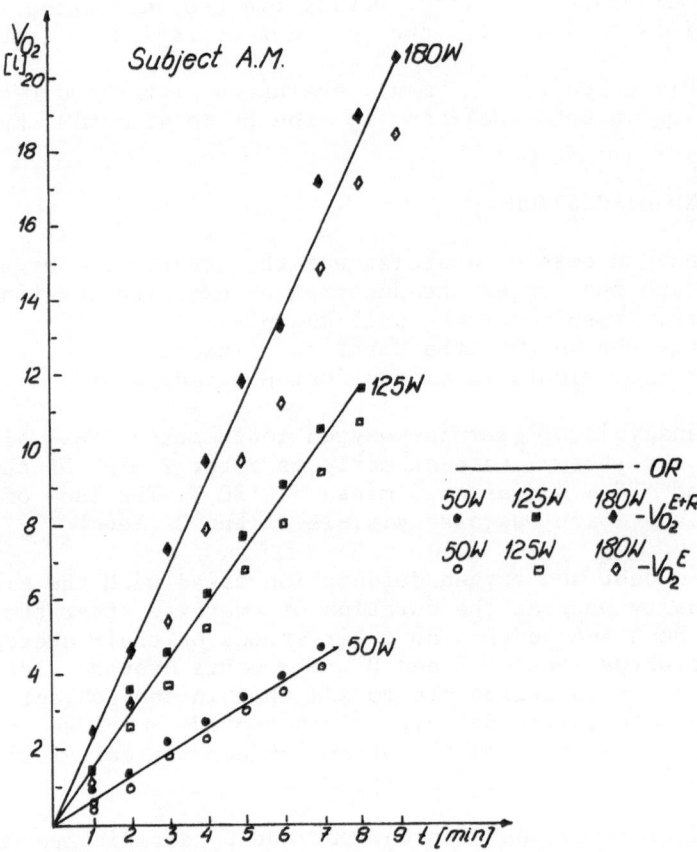

Fig. 1 Changes of oxygen requirement (OR), total oxygen uptake during exercise ($\dot{V}_{O_2}$ E) and oxygen cost ($\dot{V}_{O_2}$ E+R) in different exercise sessions (Subject A.M.).

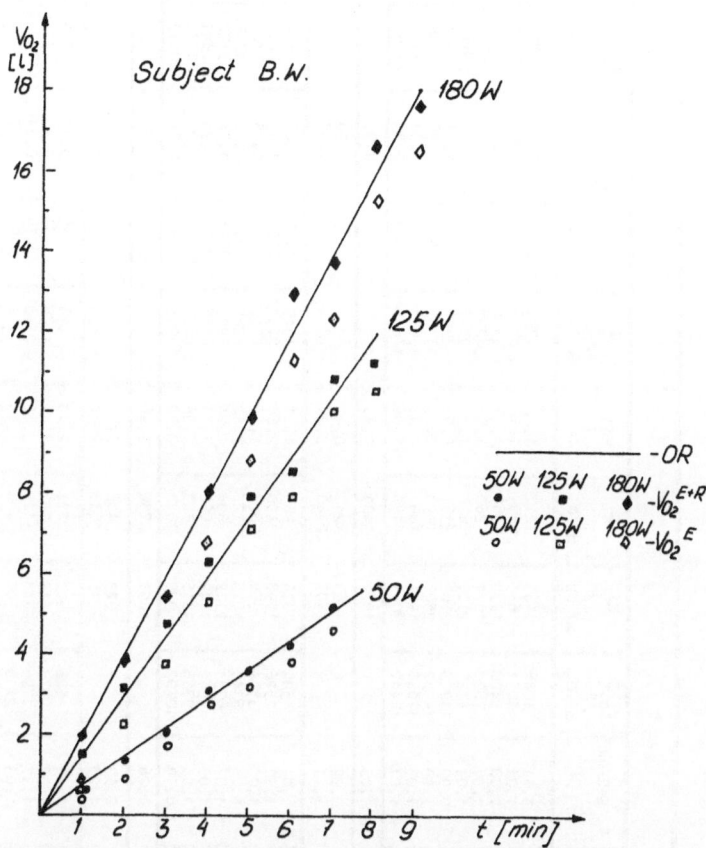

Fig. 2 Changes of oxygen requirement (OR), total oxygen uptake during exercise ($\dot{V}_{O_2}E$) and oxygen cost ($\dot{V}_{O_2}$ E+R) in different exercise sessions (Subject B.W.).

Table 1. Values of oxygen requirement (OR), total oxygen uptake during exercise ($\dot{V}_{O_2}$ E), oxygen cost ($\dot{V}_{O_2}$ ER), oxygen deficit (D), oxygen debt (R) and relationship[2] between oxygen deficit[2] and oxygen debt (R/D) in different exercise sessions. (Subjects A.M. and R.W).

Subjects			A. M							B. W						
Intensity of work	t (min)	V_{O_2} E+R (ml O2)	OR (ml O2)	V_{O_2} E+R/OR	V_{O_2} E (ml O2)	R (ml O2)	D (ml O2)	R/D	V_{O_2} E+R (ml O2)	OR (ml O2)	V_{O_2} E+R/OR	V_{O_2} E (ml O2)	R (ml O2)	D (ml O2)	R/D
180 W	1	2511	2265	1,11	1048	1463	1217	1,20	1998	2007	0,99	873	1125	1134	0,99
	2	4696	4530	1,04	3031	1665	1499	1,11	3856	4014	0,96	2720	1136	1294	0,88
	3	7339	6795	1,08	5408	1930	1387	1,39	5398	6021	0,90	4112	1285	1909	0,67
	4	9721	9060	1,07	7800	1921	1260	1,52	8008	8028	0,99	6786	1222	1242	0,98
	5	11832	11325	1,04	9725	2107	1600	1,32	9967	10035	0,99	8883	1084	1152	0,94
	6	13412	13590	0,99	11223	2189	2367	0,92	12983	12042	1,07	11303	1680	739	2,27
	7	17269	15855	1,09	14762	2507	1093	2,29	13762	14049	0,98	12376	1386	1673	0,83
	8	18969	18120	1,05	17067	1901	1053	1,81	16653	16056	1,03	15340	1313	716	1,83
	9	20503	20385	1,01	18442	2061	1493	1,06	17685	18063	0,98	16485	1200	1578	0,76
	x̄			1,05		1971	1491	1,40			0,99		1270	1271	1,12
	Bx̄			0,99; 1,11		1463; 2507	1217; 2363	0,92; 2,29			0,90; 1,07		1084; 1680	716; 1909	0,67; 2,27
125 W	1	1478	1467	1,01	502	976	965	1,01	1549	1499	1,03	611	938	888	1,06
	2	3618	2934	1,23	2526	1098	408	2,68	3161	2998	1,05	2223	938	775	1,21
	3	4552	4401	1,03	3584	968	817	1,18	4710	4497	1,05	3809	901	688	1,31
	4	6156	5868	1,05	5141	1015	727	1,40	6268	5996	1,05	5304	964	692	1,39
	5	7843	7335	1,07	6731	1112	604	1,84	7943	7495	1,06	7122	821	373	2,20
	6	9089	8802	1,03	7940	1149	862	1,33	8566	8994	0,95	7941	625	1053	0,59
	7	10581	10269	1,03	9366	1215	903	1,35	10837	10493	1,03	10021	816	472	1,73
	8	11632	11736	0,99	10703	929	1033	0,90	11215	11992	0,94	10549	666	1443	0,46
	x̄			1,06		1057	790	1,46			1,02		846	798	1,24
	Bx̄			0,99; 1,23		929; 1215	408; 1033	0,90; 2,68			0,94; 1,06		666; 964	373; 1443	0,46; 2,20
50 W	1	933	637	1,46	426	507	211	2,40	596	725	0,82	325	271	400	0,68
	2	1392	1274	1,09	979	413	295	1,40	1388	1450	0,96	901	487	549	0,89
	3	2240	1911	1,17	1796	444	115	3,86	2148	2175	0,99	1733	415	442	0,94
	4	2613	2548	1,03	2110	503	438	1,15	3114	2900	1,07	2787	327	113	2,89
	5	3406	3185	1,07	3012	394	173	2,28	3602	3625	0,99	3209	393	416	0,94
	6	3920	3822	1,03	3504	416	318	1,31	4286	4350	0,86	3831	455	519	0,88
	7	4683	4459	1,05	4112	571	347	1,65	5226	5075	1,03	4628	598	447	1,34
	x̄			1,13		464	271	2,01			0,96		421	412	1,22
	Bx̄			1,03; 1,46		394; 571	115; 438	1,15; 3,86			0,82; 1,07		271; 455	113; 549	0,68; 2,89

When we take into analysis all individual values it appears that the R/D ratio varied widely ranging from 0.46 to 3.86. Therefore, it seems to be almost impossible to predict the proper value for this ratio in any given exercise. A very similar range of R/D ratio was noticed by Lukin and Ralston (1962), i.e. from 0.6 to 3.6.

The question arises: what is the reason of such great discrepancies of the R/D ratio?

The "nonstability" of the steady state, as an effect of physiological fluctuations, could be emphasized as one of the important reasons. From the experiments carried out by Hubbard (1973) with lactate C^{14} we can conclude that the fluctuations could be an effect of the continuous production and utilization of lactate. This phenomenon can be noted even in the steady state.

The reason that is also mentioned can be the utilization of some amount of oxygen to produce heat only during recovery as an effect of elevation of the level of epinephrine circulation as well as to maintain the higher level of cardiocirculatory and pulmonary functions. This amount of oxygen can enlarge the measured oxygen debt.

The possibility of repayment of oxygen indebtedness already during the exercise is also considered. This might be the reason of lowering of the O_2 debt value.

Thus the oxygen debt measured in recovery (repayed) is a complicated value. In analysis of its magnitude one should take into account the necessity to repay some amount of oxygen which was derived from the body oxygen stores at the beginning of the exercise, i.e. desaturation of oxyhemoglobin and oxymyoglobin, reduction of oxidized coenzymes and decrease of the amount of oxygen dissolved in body fluids, etc. (maximum about 550 ml). This amount of O_2 increases the value of oxygen debt, because the restoration of these stores agrees with the period of repayment of alactic debt (Margaria et al., 1933).

Furthermore, now we know that the efficiency of chemical energy reactions during recovery (resynthesis) is only about 50% of those during the exercise (splitting reactions). Thus the oxygen debt (repayment) should be twice as high as oxygen deficit.

Some authors who took into account the reactions of high-energy phosphate compounds and lactate calculated a R/D ratio as high as 3 : 1.

As it was mentioned above there were significant differences between R/D ratio in two examined subjects. We tried also to find any relationship to the level of maximum oxygen consumption which gives us information about the capacity of mechanisms of oxygen supply. However, the level of $\dot{V}_{O_2}$ max was the same in the two subjects. Then we compared the relative intensity of exercise (expressed as % $\dot{V}_{O_2}$ max) and it was easy to notice that in one of them (A.M.) the values of % $\dot{V}_{O_2}$ max were lower indicating the higher degree of exercise ability. The meaning of this fact is rather difficult to explain at present.

At last it is important to emphasize that the inaccuracy of physiological methods we used for the determination of oxygen debt and deficit can be responsible for some errors.

CONCLUSIONS

1. The values of oxygen debt (repayment) and oxygen deficit (contracted debt) depend on the intensity of exercise whereas the duration of exercise does not affect them in the visible manner. The fluctuations similar to those of energy cost and total exercise O_2 consumption are marked.
2. The levels of R/D ratio vary in very wide range from 0.46 to 3.86.
3. The differences between oxygen debt and oxygen deficit seem to be an individual feature.

REFERENCES

Alpert N.R., 1952, Effect of acute tamponade upon respiratory metabolism of the dog, Amer.J.Physiol., 168:565.
Agnevik G., Karlsson J., Diamant B. and Saltin B., 1969, Oxygen debt, lactate in blood and muscle tissue during maximal exercise in man, in: "Biochemistry of Exercise Medicine and Sport", vol. 3, Karper, Basel/New York.
Asmussen E., 1946, Aerobic recovery after anaerobiosis in rest and work, Acta Physiol.Scand., 11:197.
Barker S.B. and Summerson W.H., 1941, The calorimetric determination of lactic acid in biological material, J.Biol.Chem., 138:535.
Christensen E.H. and Högberg P., 1950, Steady-state, O_2-deficit and O_2-debt at severe work, Arbeitsphysiologie, 14:251.
Furusawa K., Hill A.V., Long C.N.H. and Lupton H., 1924-1925. Muscular exercise, lactic acid and the supply and utilization of oxygen: Part VIII. Muscular exercise and oxygen requirement, Proc. Roy.Soc.B., 97:167.
Henry F.M. and De Moor J.C., 1956, Lactic and alactic oxygen consumption in moderate exercise of graded intensity, J.Appl.Physiol., 8:608.
Hubbard J.L., 1973, The effect of exercise on lactate metabolism, J.Physiol., 231:1.

Krogh A. and Lindhard J., 1913-1914, The regulation of respiration and circulation during the initial stages of muscular work, J.Physiol. /Lond./, 47:112.

Lukin L. and Ralston H.J., 1962, Oxygen deficit and repayment in exercise, Int.Z.Angew.Physiol.Einschl.Arbeitsphysiol., 19:183.

Margaria R., Edwards H.T. and Dill D.B., 1933, The possible mechanisms of contracting and paying the oxygen debt and the role of lactic acid in muscular contraction, Amer.J.Physiol., 106:689.

Ström G., 1949, The influence of anoxia as lactate utilization in man after prolonged muscular work, Acta Physiol.Scand., 17:440.

METABOLIC AND VENTILATORY RESPONSES TO EXERCISE IN PATIENTS WITH A DEFICIENT O2 UTILIZATION BY A MITOCHONDRIAL MYOPATHY

J.M. Bogaard, H.F.M. Busch*, W.F.M.Arts*,
M. Heijsteeg, H. Stam and A. Versprille

Department of Pulmonary Diseases and Neurology (*)
Erasmus University Rotterdam, The Netherlands

INTRODUCTION

Patients with an abnormal mitochondrial metabolism may become easily fatigued. In some of them severe exercise intolerance [1,2,6] is present. A lactic acidosis, occurring on low exercise levels then causes a specific response of ventilatory and metabolic variables when considered as a function of the oxygen consumption ($\dot{V}_{O_2}$) as a measure for the metabolic demand [1,4]. In this report exercise responses of three young patients with a mitochondrial myopathy are described. The exercise tests were repeated at regular time intervals. The responses during these tests were analyzed in relation to basic mechanisms in order to determine the effects of therapy.

EXERCISE RESPONSES AND CELLULAR METABOLISM

Wasserman [10] defined the anaerobic threshold (AT) during exercise as the level of $\dot{V}_{O_2}$ above which aerobic energy production is supplemented by anaerobic mechanisms. He explained the basis for this discrete change in cell metabolism via a schematic presentation of the metabolic pathways, leading to the production of adenosine triphosphate (ATP, fig. 1). A shuttle mechanism (the mitochondrial H+ shuttle) provides the reoxidation of reduced cytosol nicotinic adenine dinucleotide (NAD) in the mitochondrial compartment. At a certain exercise level the glycolytic component of the energy production may proceed at such a rate that cytosol NADH has to be reoxidised not only via the shuttle mechanism but partly within the cytosol. Pyruvate starts to act as a H+ receptor, oxidizes NADH and is converted to lactate, allowing glycolysis to proceed. The beginning of this process is defined as the anaerobic threshold

(AT). Specific changes of ventilatory and metabolic variables are accompanied by the sequence of intra- and extracellular processes starting at this point. Schematically this is shown in fig. 2. Lactic acid is buffered by HCO_3^- ions giving CO_2 as immediate byproduct. Cell lactate increases, HCO_3^- decreases and an anion exchange occurs, causing also blood lactate to increase and HCO_3^- to decrease. The normal responses of CO_2 production ($\dot{V}_{CO_2}$), respiratory minute volume ($\dot{V}_E$), respiratory quotient (RQ), lactate concentration in blood, ventilatory equivalent (VE) and heart rate(HR) are presented against $\dot{V}_{O_2}$ during exercise in fig. 3. Below the AT, $\dot{V}_{CO_2}$ and $\dot{V}_E$ approximate a linear increase with $\dot{V}_{O_2}$. RQ and lactate increase slightly. The VE decreases which is caused by a more efficient ventilation as associated with a better ventilation/perfusion equality because of a more equal perfusion of different parts of the lung [8].

Above the AT the increased CO_2 production causes an increase in venous CO_2 load which is usually accompanied by a progressive increase in $\dot{V}_E$, thereby keeping arterial P_{CO_2} (P_aCO_2) constant. Because $\dot{V}_{O_2}$ remains linearly related to work load, P_aO_2 and VE are increased by the extra ventilation. Excess $\dot{V}_{CO_2}$ with respect to $\dot{V}_{O_2}$ also causes the respiratory quotient (RQ) to increase. When at high work load levels the pH falls further the carotid bodies respond with a stimulus, causing $\dot{V}_E$ to increase more than $\dot{V}_{CO_2}$ and consequently also the RQ rise becomes steeper. The normal responses presented in fig. 3 are those of adult men [5], except the response of lactate which is from a group of boys, 12 to 15 years old [3]. The change in Base Excess (BE) appeared to be approximately equal and opposite to the change in lactate [9].

In fig. 3 also the responses of a 16-year-old boy with a mitochondrial myopathy (case 1, described in one of the next sections), are presented. Although also in his case the AT occurs at about half of maximal $\dot{V}_{O_2}$ lactate acidosis occurs much earlier causing at the same time a sharp increase of RQ, lactate, $\dot{V}_E$ and $\dot{V}_{CO_2}$ beyond that level.

METHODS

The exercise protocol was equal to that described by N.L.Jones et al. ([5], stage 2, 3 and 4 test, page 51). Data are collected in steady state. Usually power outputs were chosen corresponding to 1/4, 1/2, 3/4 of maximum. Each work load was sustained for 4 minutes and measurements made during the last minute. Expiratory flow was obtained with a pneumotachometer (Jaeger, Würzburg, Germany) and volumes were obtained by integration. Mixed expired gases were obtained via a mixing box with a volume of about 3 L. O_2 concentration was measured with a paramagnetic O_2 oxygen analysor (Taylor, Servomex) and CO_2 concentration with an infrared CO_2 analysor (Jaeger, Würzburg, Germany). In some cases arterial blood gases and blood pressure were obtained via an arterial line (brachial artery), in most cases only noninvasive measurements were performed.

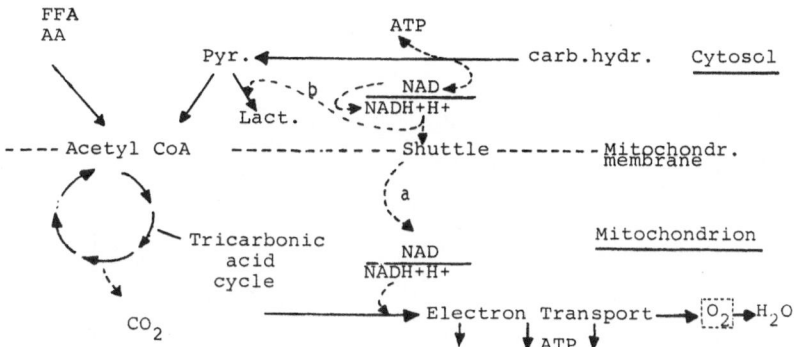

Fig. 1.   Schematic presentation of the biochemical pathways for gas
          exchange and production of ATP. The shuttle mechanisms
          (pathway a) reoxidize cytoplasmic NADH aerobically, allowing
          glycolysis to proceed without lactate production. Supplemen-
          tal anaerobic oxidation of cytoplasmic NADH by pyruvate
          (pathway b) results in generation of lactate.
          FFA, Free fatty acids; AA, Amino acids (from 10).

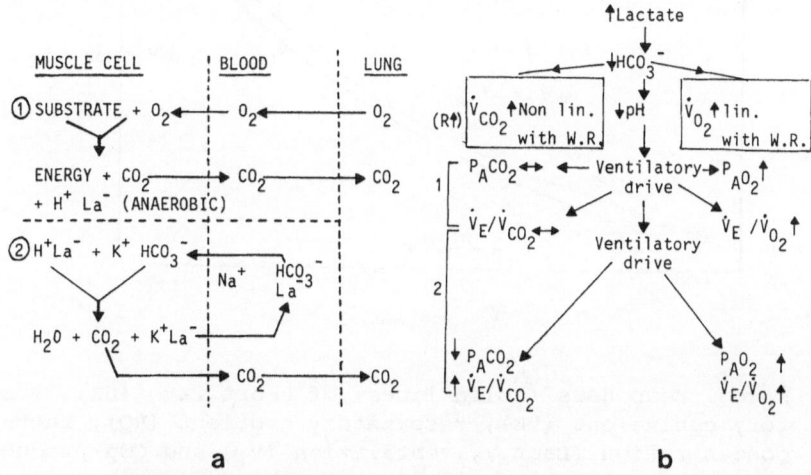

a   **b**

Fig. 2 a.   Chemical reactions, associated with the buffering of
            lactic acid by HCO_3.
      b.   Consequences of the anaerobic metabolism for some meta-
            bolic and ventilatory variables. Large arrows: mutual
            interactions. Small vertical arrows next to variables:
            increase or decrease. Further explanation in the text
            (from 10).

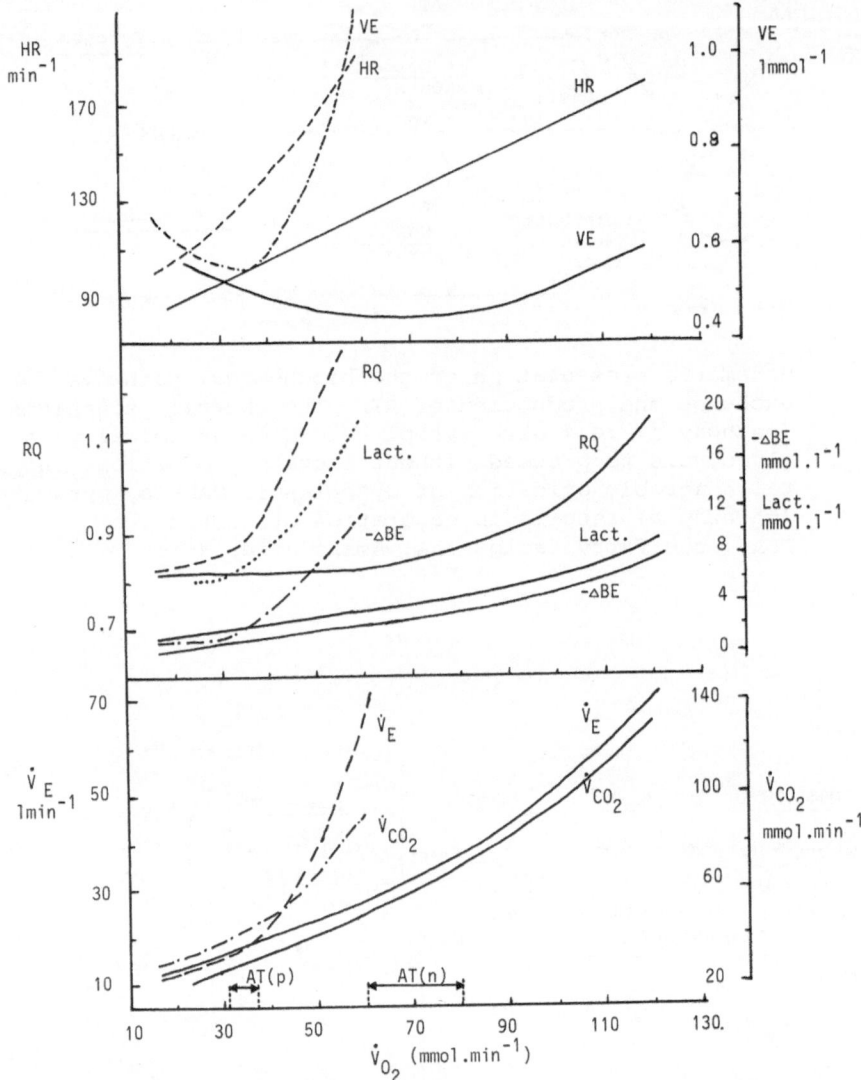

Fig. 3. Normal responses (solid lines) of heart rate (HR), ventilatory equivalent (VE), respiratory quotient (RQ), lactate
concentration (Lact.), ventilation ($\dot{V}_E$) and CO_2 production
($\dot{V}_{CO_2}$) as a function of oxygen uptake during exercise; ([5];
Lactate response, [3]). The interrupted lines present the
responses of a 16-year-old boy with a mitochondrial myopathy (case 1). For comparison with lactate response also
the change in Base Excess (BE) is presented. Note that BE
is opposite in sign to Lactate. The AT range for both the
normal (n) and patient (p) response is indicated.

In most cases the noninvasive measurements are completed by lactate determination in venous blood, obtained via a peripheral venous line. Our bicycle ergometer was of the hyperbolic type (Lode, Groningen, The Netherlands) giving a constant work load at a pedalling frequency of 40-80 per min.

RESULTS

Case 1

The first patient was a boy, 16 years old at the beginning of the tests (length 184 cm, weight 69 kg). From his 10th year he was easily fatigued, showing exercise intolerance and muscle weakness. Biochemical analysis of isolated muscle mitochondria (Dept. of Biochemistry, H.R.Scholte, Erasmus Univ., Rotterdam) showed a respiratory chain defect, recognized as a deficiency of the NADH-ubiquinone reductase complex. The mitochondrial myopathy is hereditary, his mother showing the same pathology which is described elsewhere [2].

A representative response is presented in fig. 3. His blood lactate concentration was already elevated at rest (4.4 mmol/l, normal 1-2 mmol/l). Three successive exercise tests at 4-and 9-month intervals (fig. 4) showed no improvement of his exercise performance, despite therapy. The mean $\dot{V}_{O2max}$ was 60.8 mmol.min^{-1} (SEM 2.2, 40% of reference) at a similar heart rate of 189 beats min^{-1}. This patient differed with respect to the other cases, not only because of a lack of improvement, but also because of his high blood pressures with respect to the normal response. Cardiological investigations did not reveal a relation to his primary disease.

Case 2

This patient was a girl, 13 years old at the beginning of the tests (length 160 cm, weight 51 kg) having progressive exercise intolerance with increased lactate production causing a severe metabolic acidosis already at low work loads.
At rest, her muscle strength was normal. The family history was negative. Biochemical analysis revealed a lesion at the level of NADH-CoQ reductase. Her pathology is reported elsewhere [1].
In her case a significant and sustained improvement has resulted from treatment with large doses of riboflavin. Numerical data are shown in table I. At a comparable heart rate, which was maximal for the patient's age, the improvement is characterized by lower values for BE, $\dot{V}_E$ and RQ at even increased values for $\dot{V}_{O2}$ and maximal work.
After a period of sustained improvement the exercise performance started to fluctuate. This fluctuation ranged between 60 and 80% of normal (A6, table I) during the same treatment, never reaching however the low tolerance before riboflavin therapy. For these fluctuations we have no explanation but possibly psychosomatic and conditional effects could be involved.

413

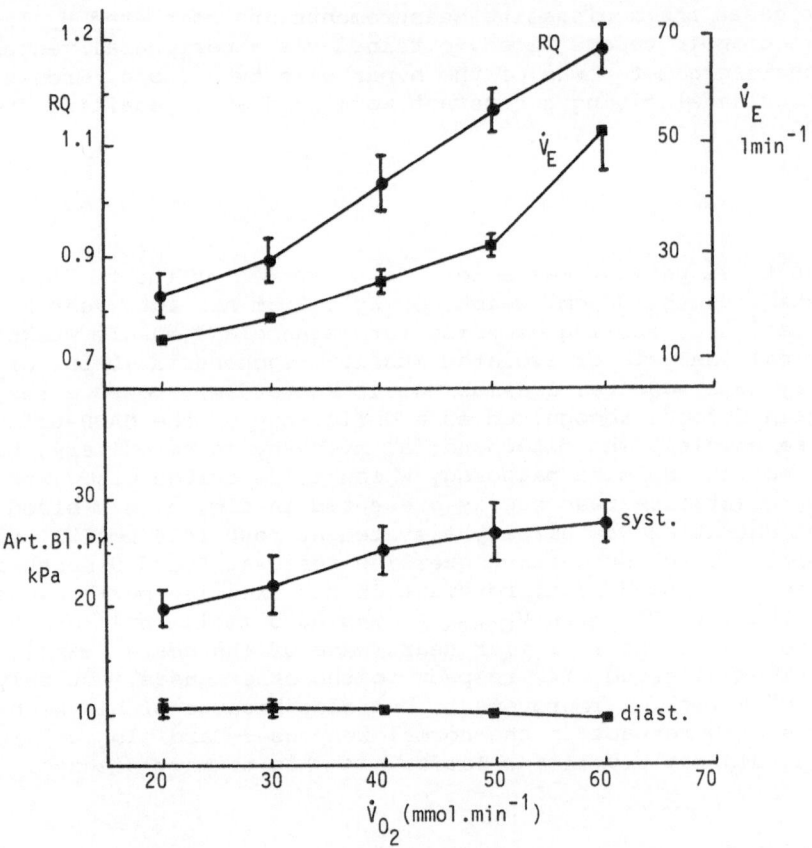

Fig. 4. Mean RQ, $\dot{V}_E$ systolic blood pressure and diastolic blood pressure responses from three exercise tests in patient 1. Also the SEM at 10 mmol.min^{-1} $\dot{V}_{O_2}$ intervals is presented.

Case 3

The third patient was a boy, 12 years old at the beginning of the tests (length 152 cm, weight 34 kg). In his case the diagnosis was the Kearns-Sayre syndrome.
Morphological and histochemical investigations suggested a mitochondrial myopathy but biochemically no lesion in the respiratory chain could be detected. The diagnosis is not yet firmly stated and the defect in mitochondrial function is possibly not primary. The boy was treated with carnitine (the carnitine level in his muscles was low) and Folic acid till two months before the last test. Three successive exercise tests with respectively a 9-and 7-month interval (fig. 5) showed nearly a doubling of the maximal $\dot{V}_{O_2}$ between the first and the third test at comparable heart rate.

Table I. Variables, obtained at rest and during maximal work capacity before (B) and 3 and 6 months (A3, A6) after riboflavin therapy in a 13-year- old girl with a mitochondrial myopathy (patient 2). For further explanation see text (from [1]).

	At rest			At maximal work capacity		
	B	A3	A6	B	A3	A6
Heart rate (min^{-1})	96	93	90	207	195	201
Max. work cap. (W.)	--	--	--	90	120	120
Resp.min.vol. (1 min^{-1})	6.5	5.3	6.5	54.6	46.3	47.4
O_2 uptake (mmol.min^{-1})	10.7	9.7	9.7	53.5	71.1	75.7
RQ	.74	0.85	.86	1.20	1.07	1.05
Base excess (mmol. 1^{-1})	0.0	0.0	0.0	-10.0	-7.5	-8.5

Although the increase of length and weight (147 - 152 - 155 cm and 32 - 34 - 35 kg) certainly has influenced the responses, the large improvement suggested a significant effect of therapy, that was also confirmed by the clinical picture. Changes in $\dot{V}_E$ and VE showed the AT to shift to higher work load levels. Although maximal RQ was even decreased between the second and the third test starting levels of RQ differed between 0.72 (third test) and 0.87 (first test), the responses of RQ being also different. We assume these differences to be real, based on careful calibration of our measuring system. Perhaps the different starting levels were associated with a different nutrition, while the variation of the RQ patterns may be associated with a varying ventilatory pattern (tidal volume versus frequency).

DISCUSSION AND CONCLUSIONS

In a recent review [10] Wasserman stated that there could be an increase in lactate during exercise, based on a deficiency of mitochondrial enzyme availability. We cite from his paper "although it is easy to envisage that a shortage of these enzymes might prevent adequate utilisation of pyruvate and thereby cause lactate to increase, there is no direct evidence for this unless the mitochondria are poisoned". We think our report gives this direct evidence because the exercise responses could be explained from biochemically detected lesions in two of the three cases. In our opinion the hypothesis of Wasserman as put forward in the second section about the oxygen availability/requirement concept is not in

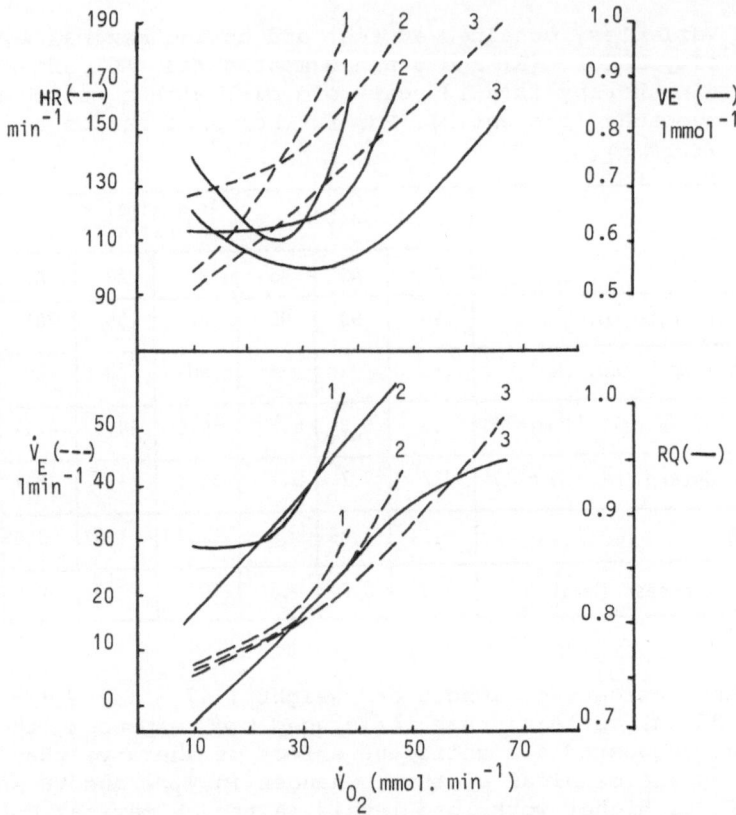

Fig. 5. heart rate, ventilation, RQ and ventilatory equivalent
responses at a 9 and 7 month interval (1, 2, 3 respectively) in patient 3. For further explanation see text.

contradiction to the enzyme availability concept. Changing the
first hypothesis by making the requirement partly dependent on mitochondrial reaction kinetics would be more realistic.
In our report we show how the disturbed cellular metabolism in mitochondrial myopathies may be associated with a change of exercise
responses with respect to normal. Although in a number of cases also
lactate and lactate/pyruvate ratios (as a measure for the redox
situation within the cytosol) were determined we have restricted
ourselves to the description of responses of mainly noninvasively
determined variables. In patients, certainly in children, we prefer
noninvasive measurements in cases of suspected myopathies leading
only to the addition of invasive measurements in cases of abnormal
responses. Mills and Edwards [7] for instance described investigative
strategies for muscle pain and found exercise testing to be one of
the important diagnostic tests. In our patient two the exercise
responses were leading to a biochemical analysis of isolated

mitochondria, defining ultimately the defect in the respiratory chain.

In conclusion we stress the diagnostic importance of exercise testing, both in suspected and well defined myopathies, giving quantitative information certainly if a therapy has to be evaluated.

REFERENCES

1. W.F.M.Arts, H.R.Scholte, J.M.Bogaard, K.F.Kerrebijn, I.E.M.Luijt-Houwen, NADH-CoQ Reductase deficient myopathy: successful treatment with Riboflavin. The Lancet, Sept. 3, 581-582 (1983).
2. H.F.M.Busch, H.R.Scholte, W.F.M.Arts, I.E.M.Luijt-Houwen, A mitochondrial myopathy with a respiratory chain defect and carnitine deficiency, in: H.F.M.Busch et al. eds, Beesterzwaag, The Netherlands, 207-211 (1981).
3. S.Gadhoke, N.L.Jones, The responses to exercise in boys aged 9 - 15 years, Clin. Sci., 37, 789-801 (1969).
4. R.D.Faihrster, J.Walters, K.Salness, M.Fox, V.Dinh Minh, A.F. Wilson, A comparison of incremental exercise tests during cycle and treadmill ergometry, Med. Sci. Sports Exerc., 15(6), 549-554 (1983).
5. N.L.Jones, E.J.Moran Campbell, R.M.T.Edwards, D.G.Robertson, Clinical exercise testing, W.B.Saunders Cie, (1975).
6. J.M.Land, J.M.Hockaday, J.Trevor Hughes, B.D.Ross, Childhood mitochondrial myopathy with ophthalmoplegia, J. Neurol. Sci., 51, 371-382 (1981).
7. K.R.Mills, R.H.T.Edwards, Investigative strategies for muscle pain, J. Neurol. Sci., 58, 73-88 (1983).
8. K.Wasserman, B.J.Whipp, Exercise physiology in health and disease, Am. Rev. Resp. Dis., 112, 33-63 (1975).
9. K.Wasserman, Coupling of external to internal respiration. Am. Rev. Resp. Dis., 129, Suppl S21-S24 (1984).
10. K.Wasserman, The anaerobic threshold measurement to evaluate exercise performance, Am. Rev. Resp. Dis., 129, suppl S35-S40 (1984).

REGULATION OF MUSCLE PO$_2$ IN RATS WITH PORTOCAVAL ANASTOMOSIS

R. Heinrich, C. Bayer, M. Günderoth-Palmowski, S. Dette,
N. Grein, W. Grauer, W. Fleckenstein and H. Schomerus

Medizinische Universitätsklinik Tübingen
Otfried-Müller-Strasse 10, 74 Tübingen (FRG)

Spontaneous portosystemic shunting as a consequence of liver
cirrhosis leads to a hypercirculatory syndrome as well as to changes
in blood distribution of different organs. These circulatory alterations, characterized by increased cardiac output, intrapulmonary
venous admixture, decreased peripheral vascular resistance and increased systolic ejection rate are also found in rats with portocaval
anastomosis (PCA), a well established experimental model (Herz et
al. 1972, Liehr et al. 1976). In previous studies we could demonstrate that also distribution of PO$_2$ in skeletal muscle of these
animals is influenced by a PCA. Under normoxic conditions mean
muscular PO$_2$ decreases after an initial rise, and reaches about 200
days after operation the level of control animals with persisting
signs of maldistribution (Heinrich et al. 1984, 1984). The following
experiments were done to evaluate whether late after PCA regulation
of muscle PO$_2$ is altered under hypoxic, hyperoxic and hypercapnic
conditions.

MATERIAL AND METHODS

Six female Sprague-Dawley rats, body weight 130-170 g, at
operation were subjected to end-to-side portocaval anastomosis by
the technique of Lee and Fisher (1961) under ether anesthesia. 12
Sprague-Dawley rats underwent sham operation (clamping the portal
vein for 10-15 min). Both groups were compared to 13 intact age-
matched controls. Rats with PCA and sham-operated and intact controls
were kept under constant environmental conditions: normal daylight
rhythm, feeding ad libitum, room temperature 26º C, constant air
humidity. The animals were kept in cages in groups of 2.

245 days after operation PO$_2$ measurements were done using a

multiwire platinum electrode according to Kessler and Lübbers (1966).

During the steady state of ether anesthesia PO_2 histograms were taken from the surface of the muscles of the abdominal wall. During the experiments the animals were allowed to breathe spontaneously ambient air over a period of 5'- 10 minutes, followed by 10 min exposition to a) hypoxic mixture (FiO_2 0.1), b) hyperoxic mixture (FiO_2 0.4), and c) hypercapnic mixture ($FiCO_2$ 0.05). At least a period of 20 min of ambient air was allowed between gas mixtures. Histograms were taken 5 min after onset of gas exposure and were pooled together. Arterial PO_2 was documented at the time of the PO_2 recording by taking blood from the cannulated abdominal aorta.

Fig. 1 shows the duration of the various exposures to the different gas mixtures as described above.

RESULTS

1. Intact controls

a) Blood gases
Under normoxic conditions mean arterial pH was in a narrow range of 7.40 - 7.42. Arterial PCO_2 was between 35 and 39 mm Hg. During hypoxia mean arterial pH was slightly increased to about 7.43, PCO_2 decreased to 26 - 33 mm Hg. Hyperoxia changed neither mean arterial pH nor mean arterial PCO_2. Hypercapnia decreased mean arterial pH to 7.27 - 7.31 and increased arterial PCO_2 to 43 - 49 mm Hg.

b) Tissue PO_2
Fig. 2 shows the cumulative histograms while breathing the various gas mixtures. Mean arterial PO_2 during exposures to the normoxic, hypoxic, hyperoxic and hypercapnic gas mixtures is shown on the left of each figure.

Mean muscle PO_2 during normoxia was 32 mm Hg, with a bell-shaped distribution. During hypoxia mean muscle PO_2 was 11 mm Hg, with left-shifted distribution and a great number of anoxic values. During hyperoxia and hypercapnia mean tissue PO_2 was 20 mm Hg. Histograms were nearly homogeneously distributed, having a small number of anoxic values.

2. Sham-operated animals

a) Blood gases
Under normoxia, hypoxia, hyperoxia and hypercapnia mean arterial pH and PCO_2 were nearly the same as in the intact controls.

b) Tissue PO_2
Fig. 3 shows the cumulative histograms while breathing the various gas mixtures.

Under normoxia mean muscle PO_2 was 25 mm Hg with a bell-shaped histogram. Hypoxia diminished mean muscle PO_2 to 11 mm Hg, there was a left-shifted histogram with a great number of anoxic values. During hyperoxia mean muscle PO_2 was 22 mm Hg, during hypercapnia 20 mm Hg. Both histograms had slightly increased numbers of anoxic values.

3. Rats with PCA

a) Blood gases
Under normoxia there was no difference in mean arterial pH and PCO_2 compared to intact and sham-operated animals. Hypoxia increased areterial pH to 7.45 and decreased arterial PCO_2 to 25 - 30 mm Hg. Hyperoxia increased mean arterial pH to 7.43 and decreased mean arterial PCO_2 to 36 mm Hg. Hypercapnia decreased mean arterial pH to 7.30 and increased arterial PCO_2 to 50 mm Hg.

b) Tissue PO_2
Under normoxic conditions PO_2 histograms were, as expected, inhomogeneously distributed, mean PO_2 was 32 mm Hg, there were no anoxic values. During hypoxia mean muscular PO_2 decreased to 15 mm Hg with a nearly bell-shaped configuration of the histogram including a small number of anoxic values. Under hyperoxic conditions mean musle PO_2 increased slightly to 35 mm Hg. The histogram was again inhomogeneously distributed. Hypercapnia decreased mean muscle PO_2 to 22 mm Hg, the histogram returned to a nearly bell-shaped configuration.

DISCUSSION

Portosystemic shunting in patients with liver cirrhosis leads to a number of hemodynamic alterations which are more life threatening than the alterations of liver function (Siegel et al. 1974). It is known that in patients with liver cirrhosis and spontaneous portosystemic shunting there is no adequate reaction of mean muscular PO_2 during hyperoxia. This inadequate reaction is not due to impaired pulmonary function, but may be a consequence of impaired muscular microcirculation (Fleckenstein et al. 1984).

Rats with PCA were investigated to study the effect of portosystemic shunting on PO_2 distribution in skeletal muscle. As we have already demonstrated, PCA including the associated liver changes which are not of a cirrhotic nature leads to a time-limited hyperperfusion of skeletal muscle. Late after PCA mean muscular PO_2 decreases and PO_2 distribution becomes inhomogeneous (Heinrich et al. 1984), corresponding to the PO_2 distribution in the muscle of patients with liver cirrhosis and spontaneous portosystemic shunting (Schomerus et al. 1984).

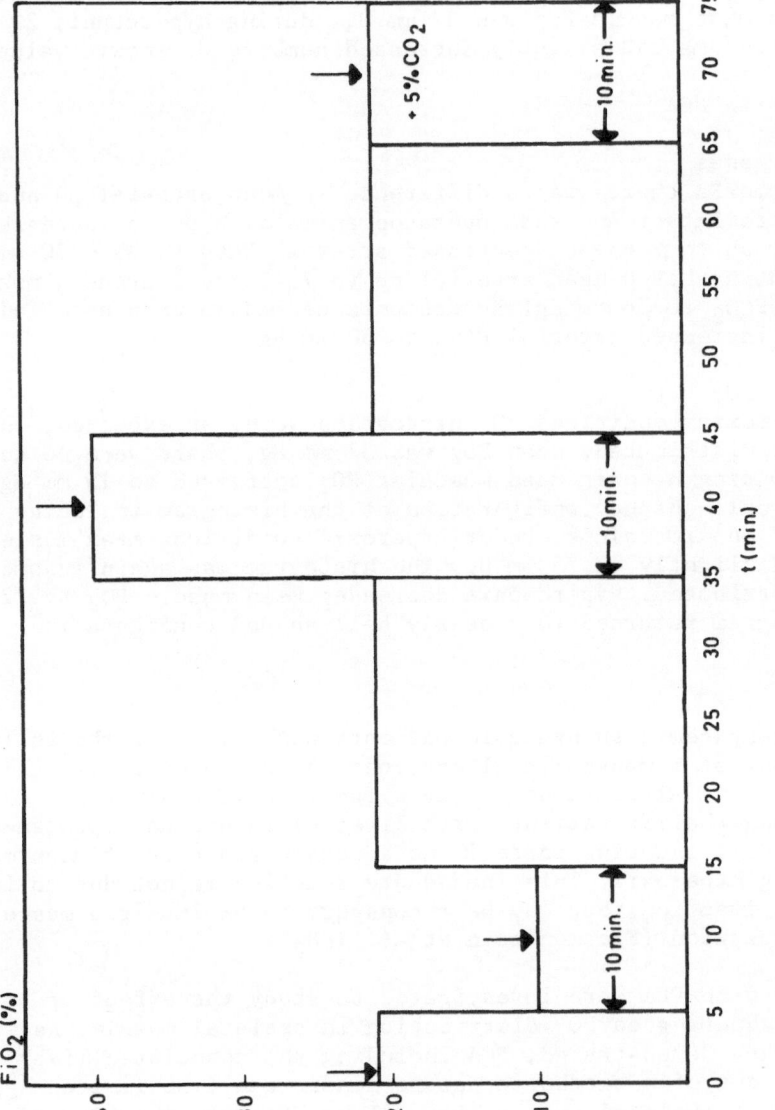

Fig. 1. Sequence and duration of exposures to the different gas mixtures
↓ = histogram taking

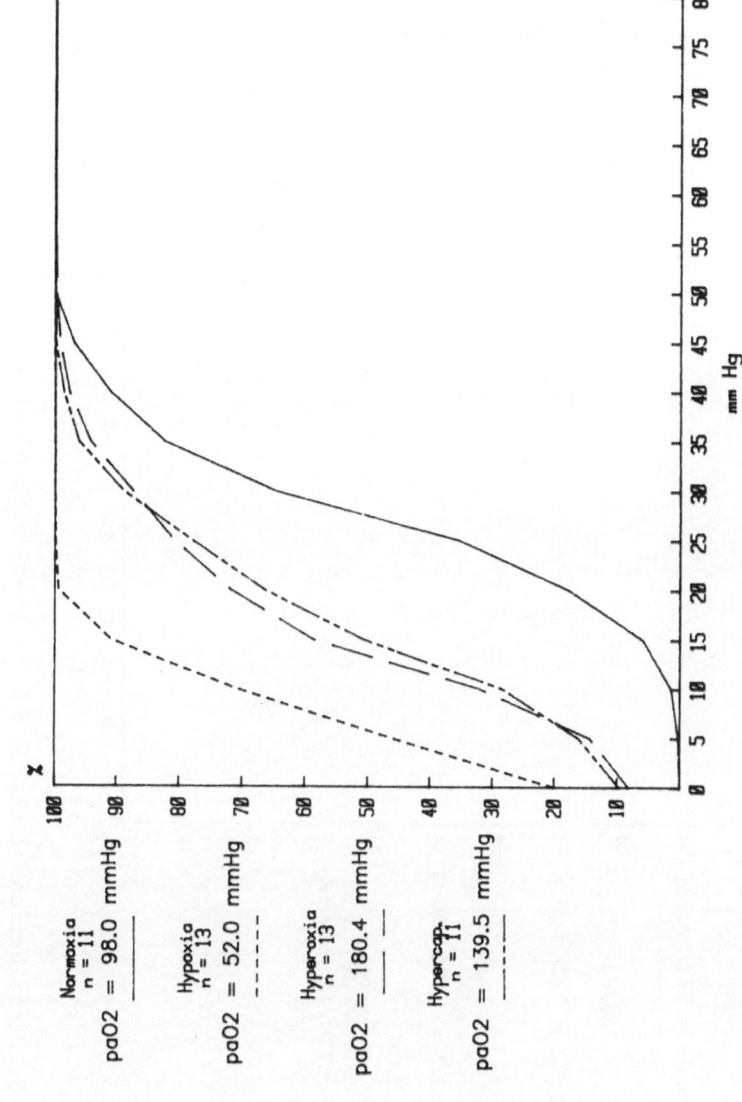

Fig. 2. Distribution of muscle PO_2 in intact rats under normoxic, hypoxic, and hyperoxic conditions as well as under hypercapnia

n = number of animals

paO_2 = arterial oxygen tension

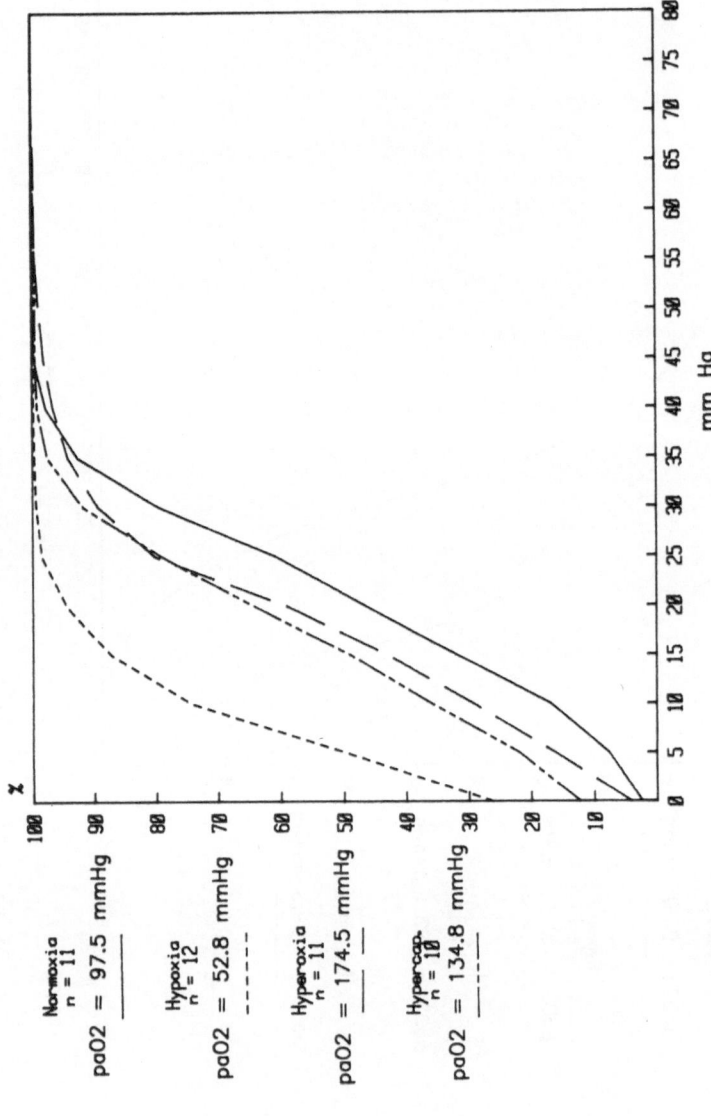

Fig. 3. Distribution of muscle PO$_2$ in sham operated rats under normoxic, hypoxic, and hyperoxic conditions as well as under hypercapnia

n = number of animals

paO2 = arterial oxygen tension

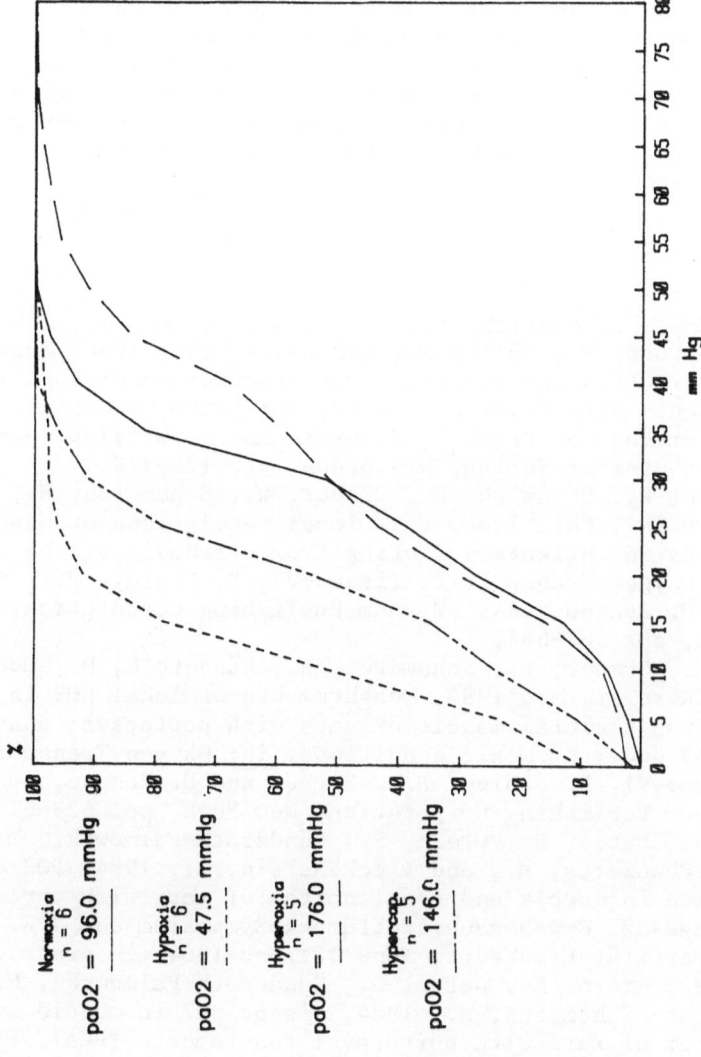

Fig. 4. Distribution of muscle PO_2 in rats with PCA under normoxic, hypoxic, and hyperoxic conditions as well as under hypercapnia

n = number of animals

paO2 = arterial oxygen tension

In controls, sham-operated rats and rats with PCA there was no difference in mean and distribution of muscular PO_2 under hypoxia and hypercapnia. During hyperoxia arterial PO_2 was in the same range in all investigated groups, but rats with PCA had a markedly higher mean muscular PO_2 compared to the other groups, and furthermore the distribution of PO_2 values was inhomogeneous.

The results show that a PCA in rats affects the regulation of muscular PO_2 under hyperoxia. Both the inhomogeneous distribution of muscle PO_2 during normoxia and its increase under hyperoxia might indicate that the hemodynamic effects of a PCA result in a disturbed microcirculation, similar to the findings in patients with liver cirrhosis. Further experiments are necessary to find out why PCA in rats alters regulation of muscle PO_2 under hyperoxia, but not under hypoxia or hypercapnia.

REFERENCES

Fleckenstein, W., Heinrich, R., Huber, A., Grauer, W., Schomerus, H., Günderoth, M., Dölle, W., and Weiss, Ch., 1984, Muscle pO2 distribution and pulmonary gas transfer conditions in patients with liver cirrhosis, in: "Atemgaswechsel und O2-Versorgung der Organe", J. Grote and E. Witzleb, eds., Franz Steiner Verlag, Wiesbaden, pp. 125-129.

Fleckenstein, W., Heinrich, R., Grauer, W., Schomerus, H., Dölle, W., and Weiss, Ch., 1984, Fast local regulations of muscle pO2 fields in patients suffering from cirrhosis of the liver, in: Oxygen Transport to Tissue-VI, D. Bruley, H.I. Bicher and D. Reneau, eds., Plenum Publishing Corporation, New York, pp. 687-694.

Heinrich, R., Grauer, W., Schomerus, H., Günderoth, M., Hoeper, J., and Kessler, M., 1984, Measurements of local pO2 in the resting skeletal muscle of rats with portocaval anastomosis (PCA) under normoxic conditions, in: Oxygen Transport to Tissue-VI, D. Bruley, H.I. Bicher and D. Reneau, eds., Plenum Publishing Corporation, New York, pp. 623-628.

Heinrich, R., Dette, S., Grein, N., Günderoth-Palmowski, M., Grauer, W., Schomerus, H., and Fleckenstein, W., 1984, PO2 distribution in muscle and renal cortex of rats with chronic liver changes, 2. Gewebesauerstoffdruck-Symposium der J.W. Goethe Universität Frankfurt, June 1st/2nd 1984 (in press).

Heinrich, R., Grein, N., Dette, S., Günderoth-Palmowski, M., Grauer, W., and Schomerus, H., 1984, Tissue pO2 in muscle and renal cortex of rats with portocaval anastomosis (PCA), Pflüg. Arch., Europ. J. Physiol., 400 (Suppl.) R 64.

Herz, R., Sautter, V., Robert, R., and Bircher, J., 1972, The Eck fistula rat: Definition of an experimental model, Europ. J. Clin. Invest., 2:390.

Kessler, M., and Lübbers, D.W., 1966, Aufbau und Anwendungsmöglich-
    keiten verschiedener pO2-Elektroden, Pflüg. Arch., 291:82.
Lee, S.H., and Fischer, B., 1961, Portocaval shunt in the rat,
    Surgery, 50:668.
Liehr, H., Grün, M., and Thiel, H., 1976, Hepatic blood flow and
    cardiac output after portocaval anastomosis in the rat,
    Acta Hepato-Gastroenterol., 23:31.
Schomerus, H., Heinrich, R., Grauer, W., Huber, A., Fleckenstein,
    W., and Weiss, Ch., 1984, Sauerstoffdruckverteilung im
    ruhenden Muskel und pulmonaler Gasaustausch bei Patienten
    mit Leberzirrhose. Verh. Dtsch. Ges. Inn. Med. 90:666.
Siegel, J.H., Goldwin, R.M., Farrell, H.J., Gallin, P., and
    Friedman, H.P., 1974, Hyperdynamic states and physiologic
    determinants of survival. Arch. Surg. 108:282.

This study was supported by grant HE 1293/1 from the Deutsche
Forschungsgemeinschaft.

SKELETAL MUSCLE PO$_2$ IN BURN SHOCK

A CLINICAL STUDY

G.I.J.M. Beerthuizen*, R.J.A. Goris*, A.J,v.d. Kley*,
H.P. Kimmich**, and F. Kreuzer**

*Department of General Surgery
**Department of Physiology
University of Nijmegen, The Netherlands

During the first 48 hours after a severe burn, the main clinical problem is development of burn shock. Patients are treated according to different protocols (Evans et al.,1952; Moore, 1970; Monafo et al., 1973). Large amounts of isotonic or hypertonic saline and/or colloids are administered. Diuresis is used as a parameter to control the infusion rate.
A parameter for assessment of the microcirculation is not available yet. It has been shown in a hypovolemic shock model that muscle PO$_2$ decreased before shock developed (v.d.Kley et al., 1983). Therefore we investigated the muscle PO$_2$ as a parameter of the microcirculation in patients with severe burns.

MATERIAL AND METHODS

13 Patients, 25-71 years old (mean 44.9 years), were studied. All patients suffered a severe burn (25-90% of body surface, mean 49%). During the first 48 hours after the burn, heart rate, arterial blood pressure, arterial blood gases, muscle PO$_2$, arterial pH, amount of infusion and diuresis/hour were recorded. Muscle PO$_2$ was measured in the m.quadriceps femoris using a polarographic needle electrode.

RESULTS

Eight patients were treated according to this protocol. During the period of investigation, heart rate and arterial blood pressure increased significantly. Arterial PO$_2$ did not change.

429

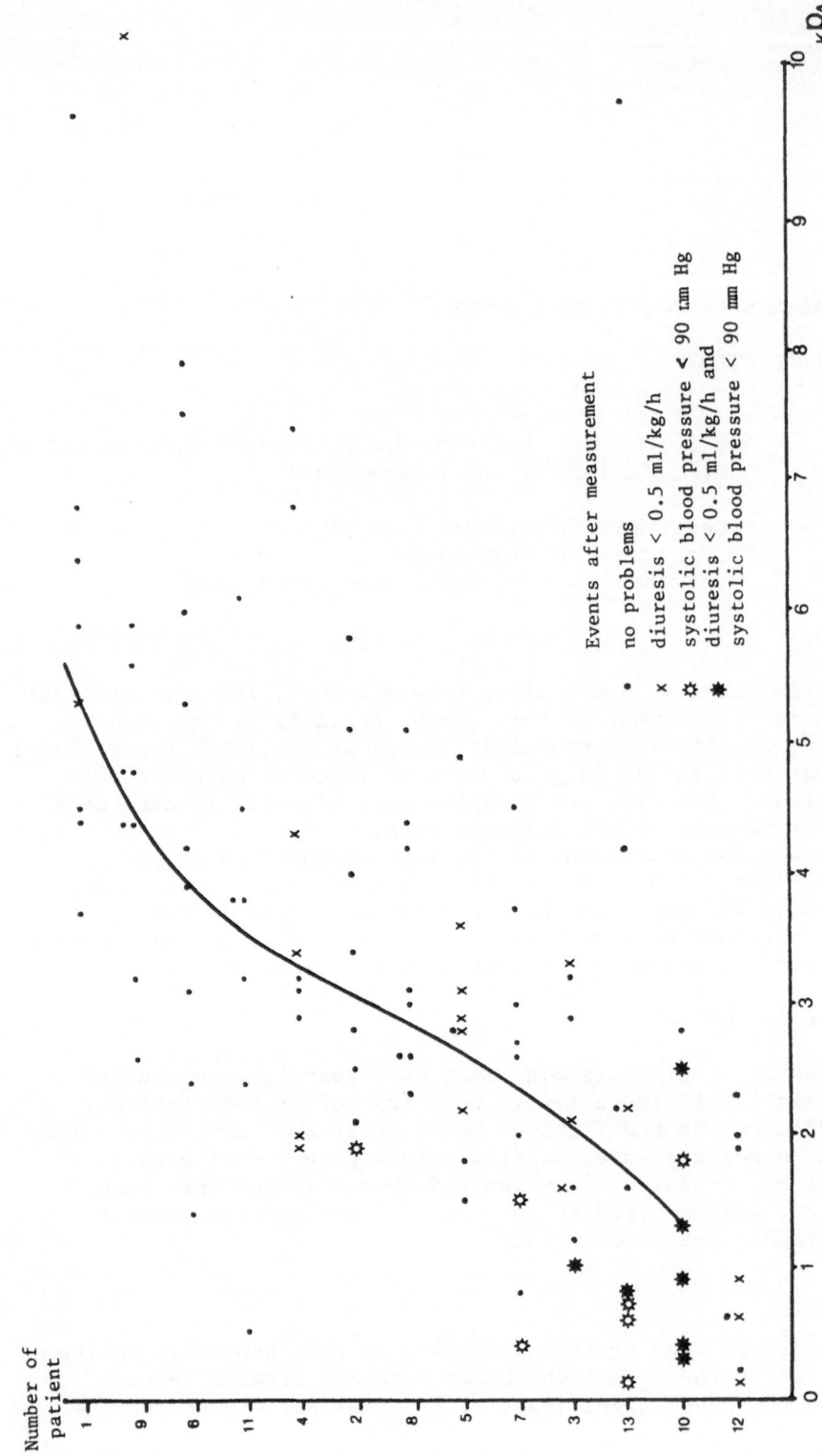

Fig.1. Patients arranged according to increasing muscle PO_2 values with associated resuscitation problems.

Muscle PO$_2$ was lower during the first 24 hours. Diuresis decreased between 18 and 24 hours postburn. In all 13 patients, muscle PO$_2$ prior to a period of shock (systolic blood pressure < 90 mm Hg)^2 was significantly lower than prior to a period without shock (Fig.1). If muscle PO$_2$ was above 3.0 kPa shock did not occur in the subsequent period. There was no relationship between muscle PO$_2$ and diuresis (Fig.1).

CONCLUSIONS

In severely burned patients muscle PO$_2$ is decreased prior to an episode of shock during the first 48 hours after a severe burn. During the first 24 hours after a severe burn intravascular plasma volume decreases. Hypoxia develops in the muscle tissue probably because of decreasing flow as a mechanism to maintain an adequate systemic arterial blood pressure. If resuscitation is not adequate shock develops. Muscle PO$_2$ assessment enables early detection of impending shock and is a valuable parameter to measure the effect of therapy during the first 48 hours after a severe burn.

REFERENCES

Evans, E.L., Purnell, O.J., Robinett, P.W., Batchelor, A., and Martin, M., 1952, Fluid and electrolyte requirements in severe burns. Ann. Surg., 135:804.
Kleij,van der, A.J., de Koning, J., Beerthuizen, G., Goris, R.J.A., Kreuzer, F., and Kimmich, H.P., 1983, Early detection of hemorrhagic hypovolemia by muscle oxygen pressure assessment: Preliminary report. Surgery, 93:518-524.
Monafo, W.W., Chuntrasakal, Ch., and Ayvazian, V.H., 1973, Hypertonic sodium solutions in the treatment of burn shock. Am. J. of Surgery, 126:778-783.
Moore, F.D., 1970, The body-weight burn budget: basic fluid therapy for the early burn. Surg. Clin. North. Am., 50:1249.

ELECTRIC POTENTIALS DUE TO CO_2 DIFFUSION IN MYOGLOBIN SOLUTIONS

L. Hoofd and W. van der Ven

Department of Physiology, University of Nijmegen
6525 EZ Nijmegan, The Netherlands

SUMMARY

The passage of CO_2 through water layers is attended by concurrent transport of (bi)carbonate. Since both bicarbonate and carbonate are charged molecules, their diffusion may evoke electric potentials and thus there will be interaction with all other ions present in the solution. Such effects have been described in the literature for weak acids and protein solutions of hemoglobin and albumin (Stroeve et al., 1985). Here, we present measurements of electric potential difference across layers containing 1.5 mmol/l myoglobin at 25° C and various amounts of Na^+ ions, where chemical equilibrium for the hydration reaction of CO_2 was achieved by adding carbonic anhydrase. Voltages measured ranged from up to 5 mV at zero cation concentration to 0.7 mV around 100-150 mmol/l $[Na^+]$. Contrary to hemoglobin and albumin, these voltages are lower, and even much lower, than theoretical predictions.

METHODS

The apparatus used for measuring potential differences in and across the layer is shown in Fig. 1. It is identical to the type originally described by Meldon et al. (1978). The layer of myoglobin solution is supported by a microporous membrane (CELGARD 2500, Celanese Plastics Comp.) which offers virtually no resistance to CO_2 diffusion. The layer holder is placed in a diffusion chamber where both top and bottom parts can be flushed separately with different gas mixtures at atmospheric pressure. Microelectrodes are attached to micrometers placed vertically upon the chamber so that electrodes can be moved upward and downward by turning the micrometer screw. This allows for the electrodes to be placed at a pre-

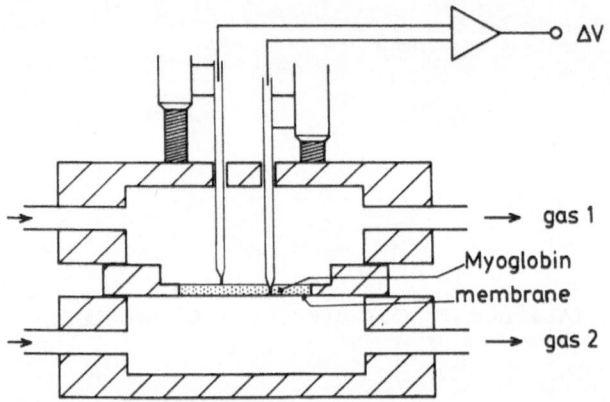

Fig. 1. Cross section of diffusion chamber. A layer of myoglobin
solution, supported by a microporous membrane, divides the
chamber into a bottom and a top part, which can be flushed
with gas mixtures independently. Microelectrodes can be
placed at any vertical position in the layer by micrometers
attached on top of the chamber. Microelectrode signals are
fed into a high-impedance differential amplifier for the
voltage difference output.

cisely known depth in the layer, where the top of the layer (zero
depth) is considered to be that depth where contact with the electrode is made. Electrode signals were fed into a high-impedance
($10^{13}\Omega$) differential amplifier and the resulting signals were written
on a strip-chart recorder.

Microelectrodes were constructed from glass micropipettes
stretched out under local heat to yield tip diameters of between
8 μm and 15 μm. These tips were polished under an angle of 30° and
the electrodes were filled with a mixture of 1 mg/l $AgNO_3$ and 2.5
mol/l KCl in warm Agar solution. When the tip was filled completely,
a chlorinated silver wire was inserted. After cooling, and before
its use in an experiment, the electrode was stabilized in a 2.5
mmol/l KCl solution overnight until the electrode signal became
steady.

Myoglobin solutions were prepared by dissolving purchased myoglobin (Horse, type II, Sigma Co.) in distilled water. The myoglobin
was present in the met- (ferri) form; its concentration was determined spectrophotometrically as 1.5 mmol/l (Perkin Elmer 124 spectrophotometer). $NaHCO_3$ was added, if necessary, up to the correct concentration of $[Na^+]$; note that any excess of HCO_3^- will disappear as
CO_2 so that only the $[Na^+]$ concentration is known or, in fact, its
mean value over the whole layer. Prior to its use, the solution was
filtered through a Millipore GS filter (0.22 μm pore size) and a
few crystals of carbonic anhydrase were added to speed up the hydra-

tion reaction of CO_2 so that chemical equilibrium between CO_2, H_2O and H_2CO_3 could be assumed.

Gas mixtures were humidified and preheated to about $27°$ C before they were flushed through the chambers. In all cases, the low P_{CO_2} gas was flushed through the bottom chamber; in this chamber, a wet filter paper was present to prevent evaporation of the layer. Layers were applied on the membrane within a holder of 9.8 mm diameter and a thickness of either 0.5 or 1 mm. The layer was inserted with a microsyringe such that the layer surface appeared flat as seen from the reflection of a rectangular grid image, to yield layers of about the same thickness as the holder. Layer thickness was measured and checked during the experiment as the difference between top and bottom position of the electrode (when the electrode touches the bottom this is clearly visible as an abrupt change in stability of the electrode signal). During the experiment, both layer and electrodes were visible from outside and could be inspected with a looking glass.

THEORY

The theoretical treatment is based on the Nernst-Planck equation that describes diffusional transport of charged species (Meldon et al., 1978);

$$ J = D \left\{ \frac{d[C]}{dx} + z[C] \frac{F}{RT} \frac{dV}{dx} \right\} \tag{1} $$

where J is the flux of species C, D is its mobility (diffusion coefficient), [C] is its concentration, z is its charge, x is the distance in the layer, V is the electric potential, F is the Faraday constant, R is the universal gas constant and T is the absolute temperature. Chemical equilibrium is assumed between all forms of CO_2 in the layer:

$$ CO_2 \rightleftharpoons H_2CO_3 \rightleftharpoons HCO_3^- \rightleftharpoons CO_3^= \tag{2} $$

where the possibility of CO_2 binding to myoglobin, as carbamate, is neglected. The further constraints are that there is local electro-neutrality (no net charge at any place), zero electric current (net charge transport is zero) and no net myoglobin or Na^+ flux (since these species cannot leave the layer). Under these circumstances, an electric field will be set up in the layer due to differences in the mobilities of the different ionic species. This field can be expressed in the form (Stroeve et al., 1985):

$$ \frac{dV}{dx} = - \frac{RT}{F} \ln(10) \frac{dpH}{dx} \frac{\sum_i (D_c - D_i) [c_i]}{\sum_j D''_j z_j^2 [c_j]} \tag{3} $$

where D_C is an "effective bicarbonate diffusion coefficient", D_i is the diffusion coefficient of species i, with concentration $[C_i]$ and charge z_i, and D_i^u is a modified value for Mb and Na^+; z_j^2 is the (mean) squared charge of species j. The exact form is given in the reference. Equation 3 clearly shows the mechanism. A potential difference exists if there is a difference in mobility between species involved in ionic reactions (D_C-D_i; where species i is mainly Mb) together with a gradient in pH; a gradient in pH accompanies the gradient in HCO_3^- which in turn is due to the gradient in CO_2. The potential difference is decreased by addition of Na^+ because of a term $D_C [Na^+]$ present in the denominator (Stroeve et al., 1985); this term will become dominating and increase the denominator so that dV/dx is decreased. Note, however, that for larger amounts of $[Na^+]$ also pH increases and thus the gradient dpH/dx might increase; in this case, the electric field no longer will decrease when more $NaHCO_3$ is added.

For the evaluation of eq.3, also the charge of the myoglobin has to be known. We assumed the charge to be about linearly dependent on pH (buffer line):

$$z_{Mb} = \beta(pH_I - pH) \tag{4}$$

where β is the slope of the line (buffer capacity) and pH_I is the pH where the myoglobin in the solution has zero net charge.

Table I. Parameter values used in the calculations.

P_{CO_2}	$5.56 \quad 10^{-10}$	$mol \cdot m^{-1} \cdot kPa^{-1} \cdot sec^{-1}$
$D_{HCO_3^-}$	$1.06 \quad 10^{-9}$	m^2/sec
$D_{CO_3^=}$	$8.20 \quad 10^{-10}$	m^2/sec
D_{Mb}	$1.0 \quad 10^{-10}$	m^2/sec
$\dfrac{[H^+][HCO_3^-]}{P_{CO_2}}$	$1.390 \quad 10^{-10}$	$(mol/l)^2/kPa$
$\dfrac{[H^+][CO_3^=]}{[HCO_3^-]}$	$5.623 \quad 10^{-11}$	mol/l
β	2.8	pH units^{-1}
pH_I	7.61	pH units
RT/F	25.7	mV

Electric potentials in and across the layer were calculated from this theory using parameter values determined independently as listed in Table I. The values of P_{CO_2}, $D_{HCO_3^-}$, $D_{CO_3^=}$, RT/F and of the reaction equilibria were taken from the 25° C data compiled by Stroeve et al. (1985), where the decrease due to myoglobin concentration was taken to be identical to that of albumin if expressed in g%. D_{Mb} was taken from Riveros-Moreno and Wittenberg (1972); for the data of the buffer line see below.

RESULTS

Calculation of layer potentials requires the charge dependency of Mb on pH (buffer line) to be known under conditions of the experiments. Since data of buffer lines were available only in myoglobin solutions containing other ions too (salts), and since our measurements were in layers either salt-free or containing Na^+ only, we first checked the buffer line for these solutions, using a commercially available titration apparatus (Metrohm 655 Dorimat operated by a HP μP Controller). Mb charge data, for 3 μmol/l Mb, were obtained by titrating with NaOH in solutions either salt-free or with an initial addition of HCl to decrease the starting pH (pH≥5). For the pH range between 5.3 and 9.0, all data closely followed the straight line of equation (4), where β = 2.8 and pH_I = 7.61, with a maximum deviation of 0.04.

In Figure 2, the results are shown of measurements of potential difference ΔV across the layer as a function of sodium concentration added as $NaHCO_3$. The upper chamber was flushed with 5 % CO_2 in N_2, leading to a P_{CO_2} of 5 kPa, the lower chamber with 100 % N_2 so that P_{CO_2} should be close to zero. The Celgard membrane is assumed to offer only a negligible resistance to CO_2 (permeability is about 10^3 higher than that of the liquid layer). Each point represents a mean value with its standard deviation (bar).

The lines in the figure were calculated from the parameter values of Table I for a top P_{CO_2} of 5 kPa and bottom P_{CO_2}'s of 0.02, 0.2 and 1 kPa respectively. Calculated values appear to be much higher than the values actually measured; for a bottom P_{CO_2} of 0.02 kPa and $[Na^+]$ = 0 even a value as high as 46 mV was calculated. If the decrease in electric potential were due to a back pressure of CO_2, even a value as high as 1 kPa would be insufficient, although the calculations at this back pressure come quite close to the measurements. Nevertheless, the measured data follow the theoretical considerations qualitatively: a sharp decrease for increasing sodium concentration from $[Na^+]$ = 0 levelling off (maybe even a small increase) for higher concentrations ($[Na^+]$ around 100 mmol/l).

In Figure 3, the measured values of the electric potential V in the layer are shown (V = 0 taken at depth = 0). Again, the data points represent mean values with standard deviations as bars. Meas-

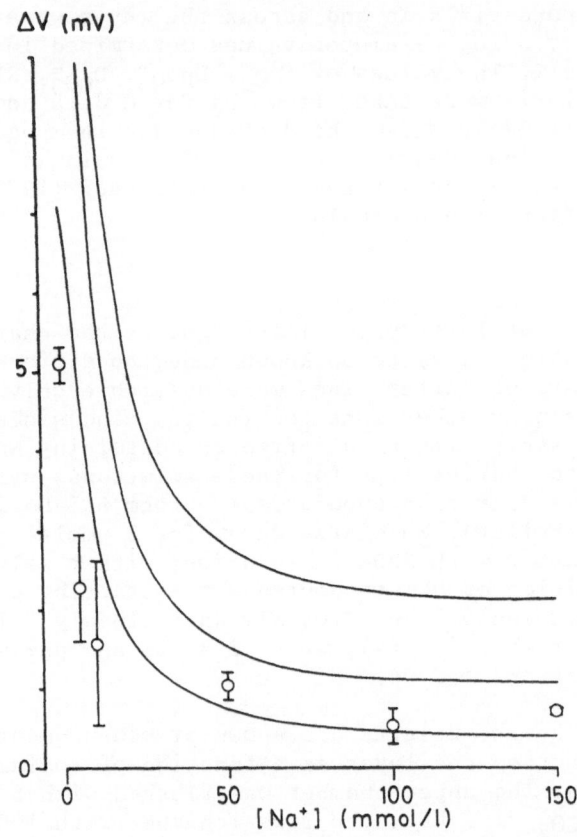

Fig. 2. Potential difference ΔV across layers containing 1.5 mmol/l
(met)myoglobin and different amounts of [Na^+], added as
$NaHCO_3$, in the presence of carbonic anhydrase, and for a
CO_2 partial pressure of 5 kPa above against no CO_2 below
the layer. Each data point represents a mean value with its
standard deviation as a vertical bar. Lines calculated are
for CO_2 back pressures of, from top to bottom, 0.02, 0.2
and 1 kPa respectively.

urements shown are for mean Na^+ concentrations of 0, 5 and 50 mmol/l,
as indicated in the figure. The lines in the figure were calculated
for P_{CO_2} = 5 kPa at depth 0 (top of the layer) against a back pressure of P_{CO_2} = 1 kPa at relative depth 1 (bottom of the layer).
These lines quite reasonably fit the data for 0 and 50 mmol/l [Na^+],
but poorly for 5 mmol/l [Na^+].

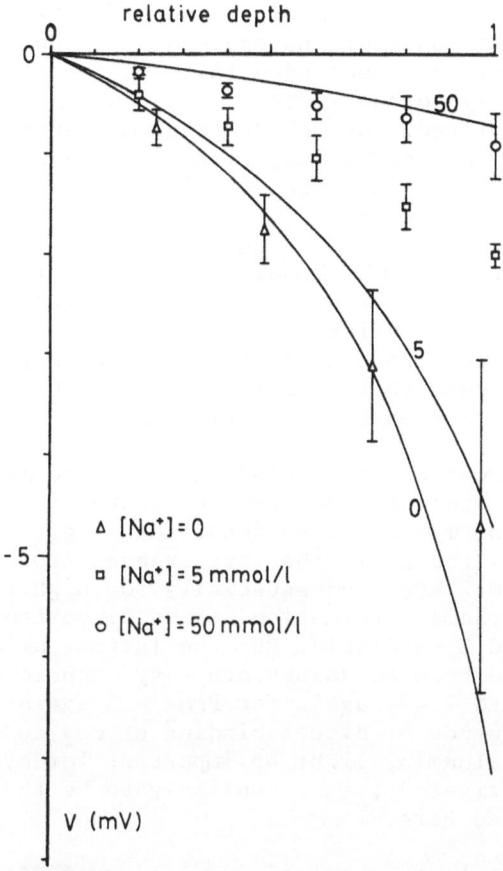

Fig. 3. Electric potential V in layers containing 1.5 mmol/l (met) myoglobin at various depths in the layer for three different mean concentrations of $[Na^+]$, added as $NaHCO_3$. Each point represents a mean value with its standard deviation as a vertical bar. Depth 0 is top of the layer (where the electric potential is taken as zero), depth 1 is the bottom. Top P_{CO_2} was 5 kPa; bottom P_{CO_2} was 1 kPa for the calculated lines; the experimental P_{CO_2} was (close to) zero.

DISCUSSION

The values of the diffusion potential as measured here are much lower than those predicted by theory. Although in the literature occasional discrepancies were found for the proteins hemoglobin and albumin these never were of the order found here. Stroeve et al. (1985) discussed the possible causes originating from insufficiencies in the modelling of the system or of the parameter values, where the fundamental idea of ionic diffusion leading to potential differences was left unchanged. They concluded that the theoretical treatment led to qualitatively correct results whereas quantitative agreement was not always achieved. But such a large difference as found here, e.g., for zero Na^+ concentration, with a calculated potential difference of 46 mV against a measured value of about 7 mV, calls for a more rigorous explanation.

The parameters of Table I, used in the calculations, were all obtained from independent sources. Another choice of a parameter set would lead to different values of the electric potential calculated, but these differences are not significant. There is no "critical" parameter in the sense that a small change in that parameter leads to a large change in electric potential.

Carbamate formation, i.e. binding of CO_2 to myoglobin, is not considered in the present theories. For increasing Na^+ concentrations, carbamate formation might become important. E.g., if $[Na^+]$ = 50 mmol/l, the calculated pH in the layer ranges from 7.83 to 9.15 for P_{CO_2} = 5 against 0.2 kPa, and especially for higher pH values of above 8 to 8.5 carbamate formation becomes important (Morrow et al., 1974; Wittmann and Gros, 1981). But the largest discrepancy is found for $[Na^+]$ = 0, and here pH values are very much lower: the calculated values were 6.63 to 7.49, again for P_{CO_2} = 5 against 0.2 kPa. So, although the influence of direct binding of CO_2 to protein, contrary to hemoglobin or albumin, might be important for myoglobin and remains to be investigated , it is unlikely to be the cause of the discrepancies detected here.

Another point is the hydration velocity of CO_2. Carbonic anhydrase was added to speed up the hydration so that chemical equilibrium between CO_2 and H_2CO_3 or HCO_3^- can be assumed. If there were no chemical equilibrium, the electric potential would be depressed and become layer thickness dependent (Stroeve et al., 1985). In the experiments, neither the addition of more carbonic anhydrase nor an increase in layer thickness from 0.5 to 1 mm led to an increase in electric potential, indicating that there was no such nonequilibrium. As a check, two measurements were performed without addition of carbonic anhydrase; in these cases, there was no measurable electric potential across the layer.

Both the finite permeability of the Celgard membrane and the transport of CO_2 by diffusion to the lower chamber will lead to an increase in P_{CO_2} at the bottom of the layer. We calculated CO_2 fluxes of between 2.5 and 90 $\mu mol \cdot m^{-2} sec^{-1}$. Across the Celgard membrane, with a permeability of 5.6 10^{-7} $mol \cdot m^{-1} \cdot kPa^{-1} \cdot sec^{-1}$ and a thickness of 25 μm (1 mil) this will lead to a pressure drop of between 0.1 and 4.0 Pa. Over the diffusion layer area of 0.75 cm^2, the CO_2 fluxes are calculated to range from 0.0046 to 0.165 $\mu l/sec$; gas flow in the lower chamber was about 50 μl/sec so that the P_{CO_2} build up in this chamber is between 0.1 and 3.3 Pa. These considerations result in CO_2 back pressures of between 0.2 and 7.3 Pa, or even smaller than the lowest value of 0.02 kPa chosen in the calculations. Also, the low CO_2 fluxes and thus low back pressures hold for those cases where the potentials are high.

It is interesting to note that the effect of nonequilibrium also resembles a "virtual" back pressure (Kreuzer and Hoofd, 1985). For an explanation of the measurements, such a back pressure has to be around 1 kPa. But even then there remain discrepancies, as clearly shown in Fig. 3 for the 5 mmol/l [Na^+] case. We must conclude that the present theoretical treatment offers no satisfactory explanation for the measurements presented here.

REFERENCES

Kreuzer, F., and Hoofd, L. J. C., 1985, Facilitated diffusion of O_2 and CO_2, in: "Handbook of Physiology: Respiration", in press.
Meldon, J. H., de Koning, J., and Stroeve, P., 1978, Electric potentials induced by CO_2 gradients in protein solutions and their role in CO_2 transport. Bioelectrochem. Bioenergetics, 5:77-87.
Morrow, J. S., Keim, P., and Gurd, F. R. N., 1974, CO_2 adducts of certain amino acids, peptides, and sperm whale myoglobin studied by carbon 13 and proton nuclear magnetic resonance. J. Biol. Chem., 249:7484-7494.
Riveros-Moreno, V., and Wittenberg, J. B., 1972, The self-diffusion coefficients of myoglobin and hemoglobin in concentrated solutions. J. Biol. Chem., 247:895-901.
Stroeve, P., Hoofd, L. J. C., and Kreuzer, F., 1985, Carbon dioxide facilitated transport in bovine albumin solutions. Ann. Biomed. Engng., in press.
Wittmann, B., and Gros, G., 1981, The carbamate kinetics of α-and ε-amino groups of myoglobin. J. Biol. Chem., 256:8332-8340.

BLOOD

OXYGEN SUPPLY AND MICROCIRCULATION OF THE BEATING DOG HEART AFTER HAEMODILUTION WITH FLUOSOL DA20%

D.K. Harrison, H.Günther, H.Vogel*, R.Eller-
mann, M.Brunner, J.Höper and M.Kessler

Institut für Physiologie und Kardiologie der
Universität Erlangen-Nürnberg
Waldstr. 6, D-8520 Erlangen, FRG
* Institut für Anaesthesiologie der
Universität München, FRG

INTRODUCTION

Previous studies on local tissue oxygen supply after haemodilution with the colloidal perfluorocarbon Fluosol DA20% (FDA20%) carried out in the liver (Höper et al.,1982), pancreas, kidney and skeletal muscle (Kessler et al.,1982), and the heart (Vogel et al.,1983; Kessler et al.,1983) have demonstrated that an improvement in local tissue oxygen supply was observed which was greater than could be explained simply in terms of the increased quantity of oxygen delivered by the fluorocarbon. It was evident that changes in flow occured (Höper et ai.,1982), probably at the microcirculation level.

In order to investigate this property of FDA20% experiments were carried out to investigate the changes in local myocardial pO_2 and microflow on the beating heart in 7 anaesthetised (Fentanyl/Diazepam) relaxed (Pancuronium bromide) artificially ventilated open chest mongrel dogs.

METHODS

Tissue pO2

Local tissue pO2 was measured polarographically by means of the multiwire surface electrode of Kessler and Lübbers (Kessler et al.,1976).

Microflow

Capillary blood flow was measured by means of the hydrogen clearance technique also using a multiwire surface electrode. The method, as applied to skeletal muscle, is described in detail elsewhere in this volume (Harrison et al.,1985). The technique used for measuring myocardial microflow was almost identical (Harrison et al.,1984).

The electrodes were held in place on the beating heart, within the region of the myocardium supplied by the left anterior descending coronary artery (LAD), by means of a special silicone rubber disc incorporating an "O"-ring holder (Kessler et al.,1984).

Regional and Global Parameters

The blood flow in the LAD was recorded by means of a Statham electromagnetic flowmeter. Left ventricular and aortic pressures were recorded using tip manometers (Miller), and central venous pressure by means of a Statham pressure transducer via a catheter located in the abdominal vena cava. These parameters, together with ECG were recorded semi-continuously using a Digital Equipments PDP11/34 computer (Ellermann et al.,1984). In addition, haematocrit, haemoglobin concentration and Fluocrit were measured at regular intervals.

Experimental Procedure

The various experimental stages of the investigation are illustrated in Figs.1-3. Following initial control measurements of all parameters, the dogs were isovolumetrically haemodiluted with Hydroxyethylstarch (HES) to Hct 14. By prediluting with HES the pronounced drop in blood pressure, which can occur during dilution with Fluosol, can be avoided (Pohl et al.,1981).

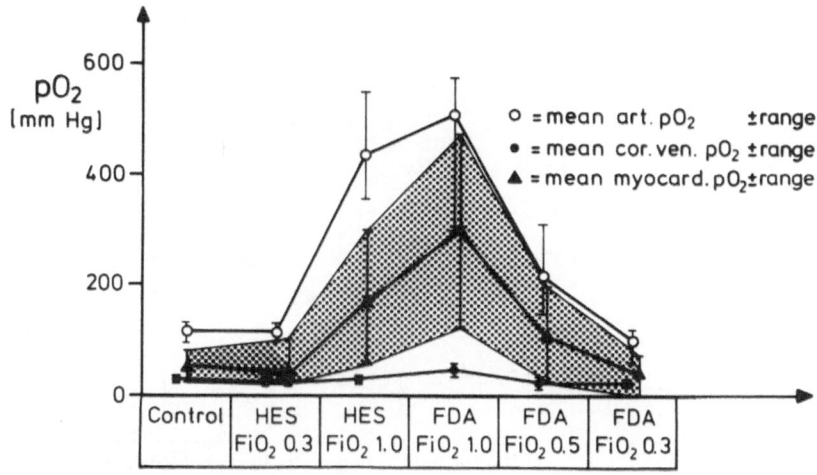

Fig.1 Arterial, coronary venous and myocardial pO2 values during haemodilution with HES and FDA.

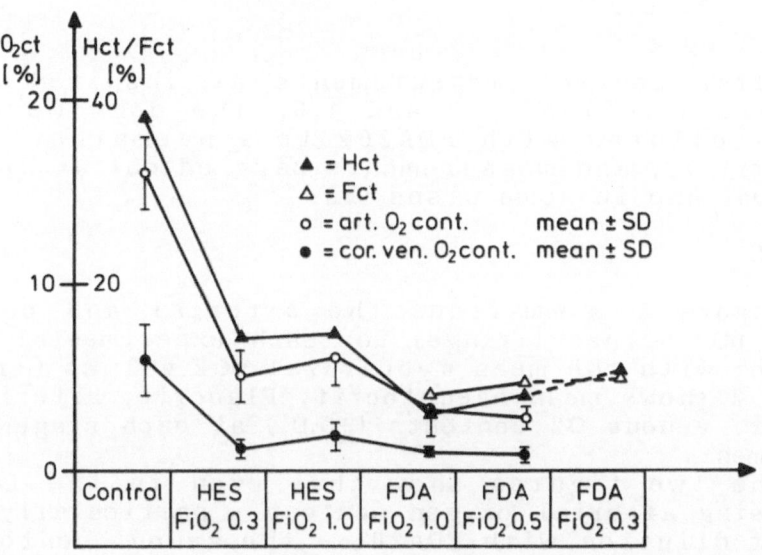

Fig.2 Mean haematocrit, Fluocrit, and arterial and coronary venous O2 contents at the various experimental stages.

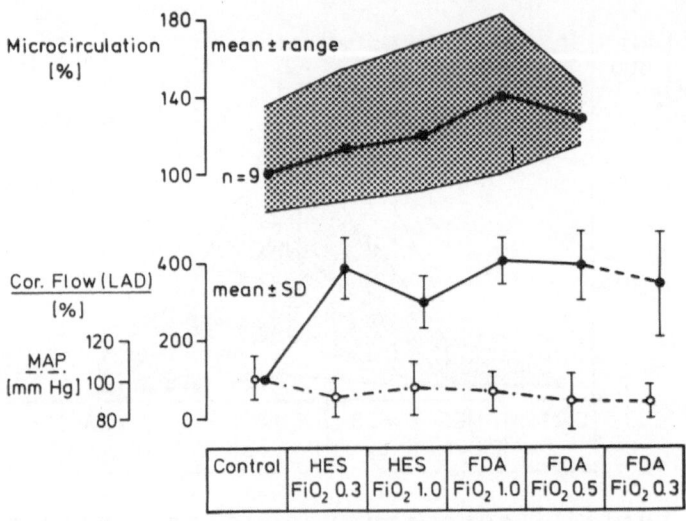

Fig.3 Changes in mean arterial blood pressure, coronary blood flow and microflow due to haemodilution with HES and FDA.

After control measurements at inspired oxygen fractions (FiO2) of 0.3 and 1.0, the dogs were then further diluted with FDA20% to a haematocrit of 8 (Fluocrit 7), and measurements carried out at FiO2s of 1.0, 0.5, and in some cases 0.3.

RESULTS

Figure 1 summarises the arterial and coronary venous pO2 values (+range) for each experimental stage, together with the mean myocardial pO2 values (+range). Figure 2 shows mean haematocrit, Fluocrit, arterial and coronary venous O2 contents (+S.D.) at each stage of the experiment.

The two figures show that even in the face of decreasing arterial oxygen content - particularly after further dilution with FDA20% - the venous content remained constant, and the arterial and tissue pO2 values increased. Most significant was the increase in the lowest pO2 values to above the dangerous, potentially anoxic level. Also worth noting is that the mean increase in tissue pO2 was even greater than that in the arterial pO2.

Mean arterial blood pressure and LAD flow values
(+S.D.) and microflow values (+range) are summarised in
Fig.3. It is remarkable that, in the myocardium, the
large increase in coronary blood flow induced by iso-
volumetric haemodilution with HES (to Hct 14) is not
accompanied by a proportional increase in microflow at
the surface of the myocardium. The mean ratio of the
increase in LAD flow to the increase in microflow was
23:1 indicating that a considerable amount of the flow

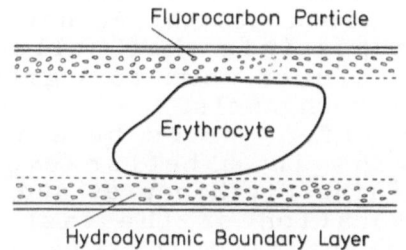

Fig.4 Schematic representation of an erythrocyte within
a capillary after dilution with FDA.

was being shunted through fast channels less effective
for exchange of oxygen. Further halving of the haematocrit by dilution with Fluosol, however, produced an
improvement of this ratio to 1.7:1 indicating a more
efficient flow pattern.

DISCUSSION

Haemodilution with FDA20% from Hct 14 to Hct 8 (Fct 7) induced a slight increase in viscosity of around 10%. It might therefore be expected that a decrease in flow would be observed. This was not the case, though, partly due to the inhibiting effect of Fluosol on the alpha receptors of the vascular smooth muscle (Suyama et al., 1979).However, in order to explain the fact that an improved myocardial pO2 was observed despite a further reduction in arterial O2 content, a redistribution of microflow must be postulated, and the following hypothesis is proposed as a possible explanation.

Figure 4 is a schematic representation of an erythrocyte within a capillary. Around it, and between it and the capillary wall, at the hydrodynamic boundary layer, are fluorocarbon particles (of the order of 0.1 microns in diameter) representing a source of friction to the movement of the red blood cell along the capillary. This friction is proportional to the velocity of the erythrocyte, it is thus possible that cells in faster shunt channels could be slowed down to a greater degree than those in the slower channels.

The overall effect would be a redistribution of microflow resulting in a better exchange of oxygen between the remaining erythrocytes and the tissue.

The exact location of the fast, shunt channels could not been identified in this study, but it is probable that large changes in capillary flow distribution occur deeper within the myocardium. The existence of such channels is indicated by our studies in skeletal muscle and is discussed elsewhere in this volume (Harrison et al.,1985).

Our studies suggest that the microrheological properties of the flourocarbon particles themselves may play a major role in improving the conditions for oxygen exchange between red blood cells and myocardial tissue by inducing a redistribution of capillary blood flow.

ACKNOWLEDGEMENTS

The authors are indebted to Miss A.Brehm and Mr. G.Kerl for their valuable technical assistance, and to Mrs. G.Schuster for the preparation of illustrations.

450

REFERENCES

Ellermann, R., Brunner, M., Kessler, M, Höper, J., Frank, K.H. and Harrison, D.K., 1984, Microcomputers for intraoperative and bedside monitoring. Measuring methods, data acquisition, processing, display, Proc. 6th Int. Symp. on Computers in Critical Care and Pulmonary Medicine, Heidelberg, June 1984, in press.

Harrison, D.K., Vogel, H., Günther, H. and Kessler, M., 1984, Hydrogen clearance applied to the measurement of capillary blood flow on the beating dog heart during haemodilution with Fluosol DA20%, Int. J. Microcirc. Clin. and Exp., 3:440.

Harrison, D.K., Knauf, S.K., Vogel, H., Günther, H. and Kessler, M., 1985, Redistribution of microcirculation in skeletal muscle during hypoxaemia, in: this volume.

Höper, J., Ji, S., and Kessler, M., 1982, Tissue oxygen supply of the isolated rat liver perfused with fluorocarbon, in:"Oxygen Carrying Colloidal Blood Substitutes," R. Frey, H. Beisbarth, K. Stosseck, ed., Zuckschwerdt, Munich.

Kessler, M., Höper, J. and Krumme, B.A., 1976, Monitoring of tissue perfusion and cellular function, Anesthesiology, 45:184.

Kessler, M., Höper, J. and Pohl, U., 1982, Tissue oxygen supply of liver, pancreas, kidney and skeletal muscle, in: "Oxygen Carrying Colloidal Blood Substitutes," R. Frey, H. Beisbarth, K. Stosseck, ed., Zuckschwerdt, Munich.

Kessler, M., Vogel, H., Günther, H., Harrison, D.K. and Höper, J., 1983, Local oxygen supply of the myocardium after extreme hemodilution with Fluosol DA, in: Advances in Blood Substitute Research, R.B. Bolin, R.P. Geyer and G.J. Nemo, ed., Alan R Liss, New York.

Kessler, M., Klövekorn, W.P., Höper, J., Sebening, F., Brunner, M., Frank, K.H., Harrison, D.K., Kernbach, C., Anderer, W., Richter, H. and Ellermann, R., 1984, Local oxygen supply and regional wall motion of the dog's heart during critical stenosis of the LAD, in: " Oxygen Transport to Tissue (V), D.W. Lübbers, H. Acker, E. Leniger-Follert and T.K. Goldstick, ed., Adv. Exp. Med. Biol., 169, Plenum, New York and London.

Pohl, U., Güggi, M., Höper, J. and Kessler, M., 1981, Oxygen supply of skeletal muscle after extreme hemodilution with fluosol, Biblthca. anat., 20:399.

Suyama, T., Watanabe, M., Hanada, S., Yano, K., Yokoyamo, K. and Naito, R., 1979, Pharmacological analysis of the mode of transient hypotensive action of Fluosol-DA found in dog, in: Proc. 4th Int. Symp. of Perfluorocarbon Blood Substitutes, Excerpta Medica, Amsterdam.

Vogel, H., Günther, H., Harrison, D.K, Höper, J., Frank, K.H. and Kessler, M., 1983, Oxygen tension and microflow of the myocardium following hemodilution with Fluosol DA 20%, Intensive Care Medicine, 9:231.

O_2 AND CO_2 SOLUBILITY OF THE FLUOROCARBON EMULSION FLUOSOL-DA 20% AND O_2 AND CO_2 DISSOCIATION CURVES OF BLOOD - FLUOSOL-DA 20% MIXTURES

J. Grote, K. Steuer, R. Müller, C. Söntgerath, and K. Zimmer

Institute of Physiology, University of Bonn
5300 Bonn, FRG

Since perfluorochemicals are characterized by a high solubility for gases, emulsions of perfluorinated compounds have been proposed as artificial blood substitutes (Clark and Gollan, 1966; Naito and Yokoyama, 1978; Beisbarth and Suyama, 1982; Geyer, 1982, 1983). Among the different perfluorochemicals investigated, Fluosol-DA 20% (FDA20) has been used successfully as an O_2 transport medium and plasma expander for different experimental animals and for humans. Our knowledge of respiratory gas transport of FDA20 and blood-FDA20 mixtures is, however, mainly based on theoretical investigations and calculations, which have been derived from separate data for blood and FDA20, and presumes that the fluorocarbon emulsion does not affect the O_2-affinity of hemoglobin or the acid-base status of blood. In addition, calculations and measurements of the O_2 solubility in the two Fluosol emulsions (FDA20 and FDA35) have resulted in disagreement (Naito and Yokoyama, 1978; Zander and Makowski, 1982). The aim of the present study was to determine the O_2 and CO_2 solubility coefficients of the perfluorochemical FDA20 as well as the O_2 and CO_2 dissociation curves and the pH-log PCO_2 equilibration lines of blood-FDA20 mixtures with a hemoglobin concentration of 7 $g \cdot dl^{-1}$.

MATERIAL AND METHODS

Fluosol-DA 20% (The Green Cross Corporation, Osaka) was prepared as described by Naito and Yokoyama (1978) and immediately used for measuring the C_{O_2}-P_{O_2} and the C_{CO_2}-P_{CO_2} dependence of FDA20. The O_2 and the CO_2 solubility coefficients were calculated from the O_2 and CO_2 dissociation curves. To produce blood-FDA20 mixtures, freshly drawn heparinized blood was obtained by venipuncture from eleven female and thirteen male volunteers. The blood was diluted with FDA20 in a volume ratio of about 1:1 to reach a hemoglobin concentration of 7 $g \cdot dl^{-1}$. Samples of the fluorocarbon emulsion as well as of the blood-FDA20 mixtures were equilibrated at 37°C with various water vapor saturated O_2-CO_2-N_2 mixtures of known composition, in the Radiometer Blood Microsystem (BMS 2 Mk 2, Radiometer, Copenhagen). The gas mixtures were supplied by a Corning Gas Mixing Apparatus 192 (Corning Medical GmbH, Giessen). The accuracy of the mixing system was checked by measuring the composition of the gas mixtures in a Scholander apparatus (Scholander, 1947) or by determining the O_2 and the CO_2 concentrations of the equilibrating gases in the same manner as in samples under investigation. Following complete equilibration the O_2 and the CO_2 content of FDA20 and the blood-FDA20 mixtures was measured with the Lex-O_2-CON TL (Lexington Instruments, Waltham, USA) and the Corning Carbon Dioxide Analyzer 965 D (Corning Medical GmbH, Giessen), respectively. The O_2 and CO_2 concentrations and the corresponding P_{O_2} and P_{CO_2} values were used to draw the O_2 or CO_2-dissociation curves. The pH-log P_{CO_2} equilibration lines of the blood-FDA20 mixtures were obtained at S_{O_2} = 100% and 0% by the Astrup micromethod using the pH meter PHM 84 (Radiometer, Copenhagen). The hemoglobin concentration of the blood and of the blood-FDA20 mixtures was determined photometrically after conversion to cyanmethemoglobin.

RESULTS AND DISCUSSION

The mean C_{O_2}-P_{O_2} dependence in Fluosol-DA 20% determined at 37°C and a P_{CO_2} of 40 mmHg is given in Fig 1. The measurements provided an O_2 solubility coefficient of 0.055 $\pm$0.004 $mlO_2 \cdot ml^{-1} \cdot atm^{-1}$. A decrease in P_{CO_2} had no significant effect on O_2 solubility in the fluorocarbon emulsion. At P_{CO_2} = 0 mmHg a coefficient of 0.057 $\pm$0.003 $mlO_2 \cdot ml^{-1} \cdot atm^{-1}$ was determined. Both values agree with the O_2 solubility measurements in FDA20 of Zander and Makowski (1982), however, they are below the value of 0.076 $mlO_2 \cdot ml^{-1} \cdot atm^{-1}$ calculated by Naito and Yokoyama (1978). According to the above results the O_2 solubility of FDA20 is about 2 to 2.5 times higher than in whole blood and water (Sendroy et al., 1934; Gertz and

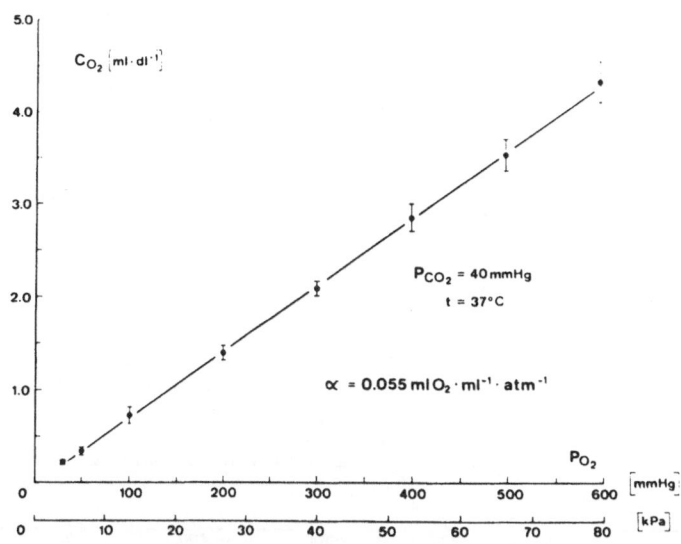

Fig. 1. C_{O_2}-P_{O_2} dependence in FDA20 at 37°C and P_{CO_2} = 40 mmHg. Given are mean values ±SD, n=7.

Loeschcke, 1954; Grote, 1967; Power, 1968; Zander, 1969).

CO_2 solubility in FDA20 was determined in non-acidified as well as in acidified samples of the perfluorocarbon emulsion. Small amounts of lactic acid (van Slyke et al., 1928) were added to about 50% of the samples to give a final lactic acid concentration of 2 ml·dl^{-1}. The addition of lactic acid to the perfluorochemical reduces the pH to below 4. Under these conditions only negligible amounts of bicarbonate can be formed and all the CO_2 measured can be looked upon as being dissolved (Siesjö; 1962; Austin et al., 1963). In the non-acidified FDA20 samples, however, the increase of C_{CO_2} with increasing P_{CO_2} is greater due to the additional formation of bicarbonate. Though the addition of acids will slightly influence the solubility of gases, there is sufficient evidence that the addition of small amounts of lactic acid to the fluorocarbon emulsion as described above does not produce any significant change in the O_2 solubility coefficient (Austin et al., 1963). The results of both series of CO_2-concentration measurements are summarized in Fig. 2. The C_{CO_2}-P_{CO_2} dependence of the non-acidified emulsion is given by curve A, while curve B shows the inter-relation of both parameters of the acidified FDA20

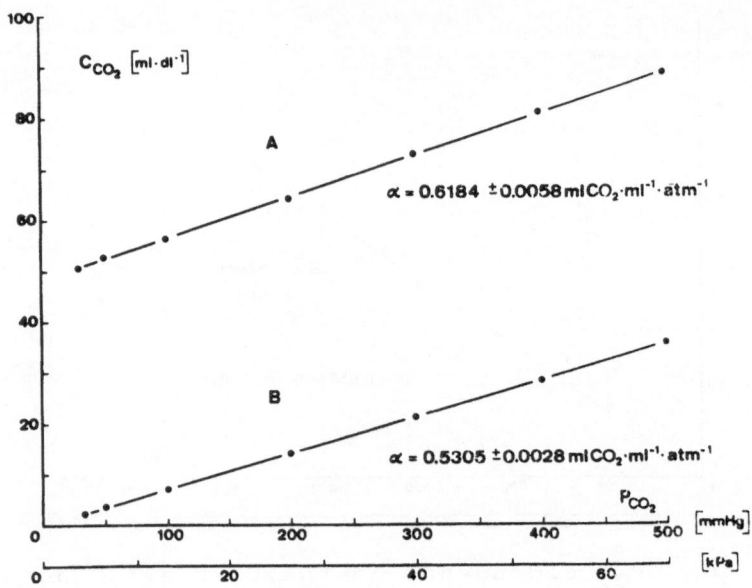

Fig. 2. C_{CO_2}-P_{CO_2} dependence in non-acidified (A) and in
          acidified FDA20 (B) at 37°C. Given are mean
          values, n=10.

samples. As expected, the mean CO_2 solubility coefficient
of the acidified perfluorocarbon emulsion ($0.531\,mlCO_2 \cdot ml^{-1} \cdot atm^{-1}$) was smaller than the coefficient of the untreated emulsion ($0.618\ mlCO_2 \cdot ml^{-1} \cdot atm^{-1}$)and is comparable
to the CO_2 solubility coefficients of water, serum, plasma
and whole blood (van Slyke, 1928; Bartels and Wrbitzky,
1960; Siesjö, 1962; Austin et al., 1963), but is below
the value calculated for FDA20 by Naito and Yokoyama
(1978).

Fig. 3 shows the mean O_2 dissociation curve of the blood-FDA20 mixture (upper curve), determined at 37°C and a
P_{CO_2} of 40 mmHg. The mean hemoglobin concentration of
the thirteen samples investigated was $7.06\ g \cdot dl^{-1}$. From
the linear part of the O_2 dissociation curve of each
individual sample the corresponding O_2 solubility
coefficient was determined. The mean value for the O_2
solubility constant of the blood-FDA20 mixture was
$0.044 \pm 0.003\ mlO_2 \cdot ml^{-1} \cdot atm^{-1}$ which is in close agreement
with the value ($0.041\ mlO_2 \cdot ml^{-1} \cdot atm^{-1}$) which can be
calculated from the ratio of whole blood and FDA20 in the
samples and the O_2 solubility coefficients of both

456

components. Using the measured O_2 solubility coefficients of the blood-FDA20 mixtures the amount of chemically bound oxygen per 100 ml was calculated for the different P_{O_2} levels. The results are given by the lower curve in Fig. 3. The mean O_2 capacity of the investigated samples was 9.5 $mlO_2 \cdot dl^{-1}$. Taking into account a Hüfner's number of 1.34 $mlO_2 \cdot gHb^{-1}$ a corresponding hemoglobin concentration of 7.065 $g \cdot dl^{-1}$ was determined. This value coin-

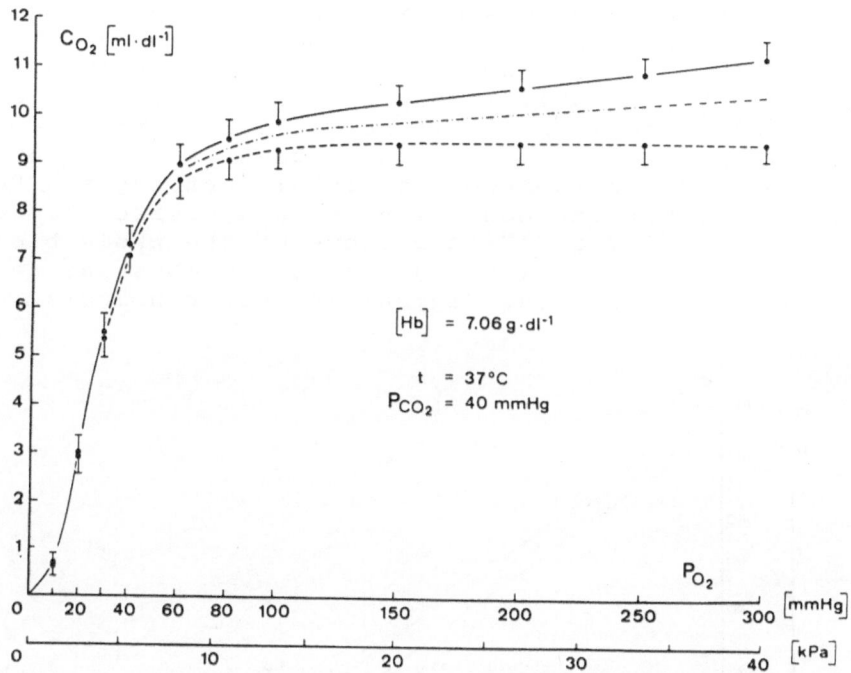

Fig. 3. Mean O_2 dissociation curve of blood-FDA20 mixtures (Hb = 7.06 $g \cdot dl^{-1}$) at 37°C and P_{CO_2} = 40 mmHg (upper curve). The amount of chemically bound oxygen is given by the lower curve.

cides with the measured hemoglobin concentration. The P_{50} read at the mean O_2 dissociation curve is 26.0 mmHg. A P_{50} of about 25 mmHg is to be expected from the pH of the blood-FDA20 mixtures evaluated for the condition S_{O_2} = 50% from the determined pH-log P_{CO_2} equilibration lines (Severinghaus, 1966, 1979; Grote, 1971).
Using the above results together with the O_2 solubility coefficient of whole blood the O_2 dissociation curve can

be computed for the conditions Hb = 7.0 g·dl^{-1}, P_{CO_2} = 40 mmHg and t = 37°C. The O_2 dissociation curve so derived is indicated in Fig. 3 by the dot-dash curve. The influence of the fluorocarbon emulsion on the O_2 concentration of the blood-FDA20 mixtures is given at each P_{O_2} level by the c_{O_2}-difference between the calculated O_2 dissociation curve and the directly determined O_2 dissociation curve of the samples investigated.

The addition of the fluorocarbon emulsion to the blood samples induced a decrease in the slope as well as a slight shift to the right of the pH-log P_{CO_2} equilibration lines as can be seen in Fig. 4, which gives a typical example. The slope of the mean pH-log P_{CO_2} equilibration line of the blood-FDA20 mixture (Fig. 5) is -1.27 at S_{O_2} = 100%. In oxygenated normal blood comparable values between -1.57 and -1.73 have been reported by different investigators (von Mengden et al., 1969; Grote, 1971; Siggaard-Andersen, 1974; Castaing and Pocidalo, 1979). For the conditions of a decreased hemoglobin concentration of 7 g·dl^{-1} the slope of the whole blood pH-log P_{CO_2} equilibration line for S_{O_2} = 100% was calculated as -1.37 using the Siggaard-Andersen nomogram.

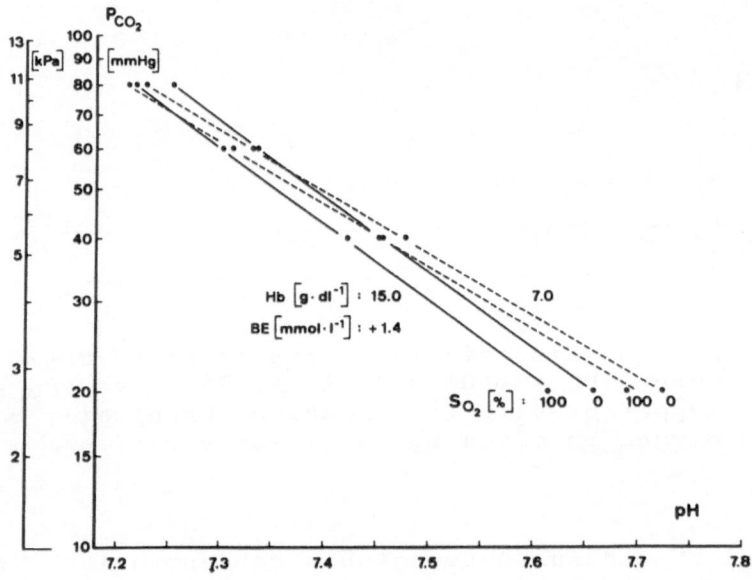

Fig. 4.   pH-log P_{CO_2} equilibration lines of normal blood and of a blood-FDA20 mixture with Hb = 7.0 g·dl^{-1} determined at 37°C and S_{O_2} = 100% and 0%.

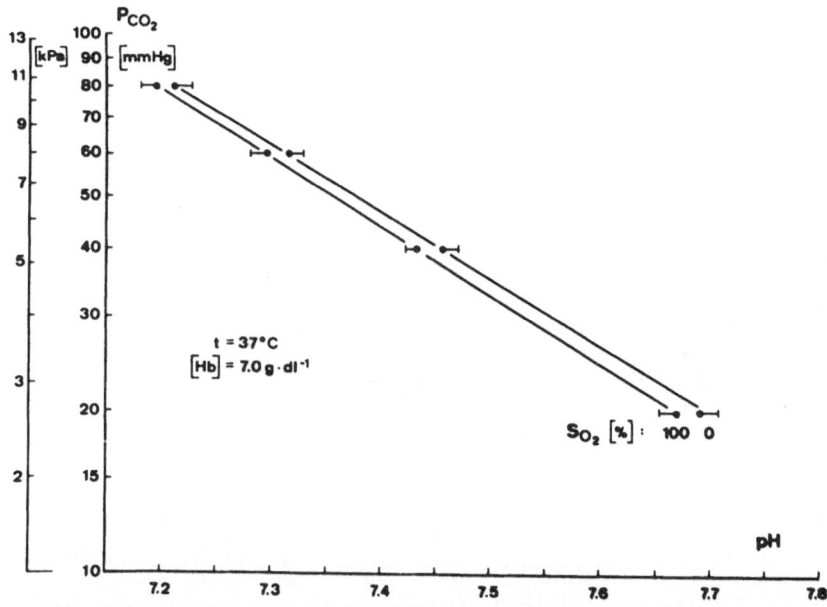

Fig. 5. Mean pH-log P_{CO_2} equilibration lines of blood-
FDA20 mixtures (Hb = 7.0 g·dl^{-1}), determined at
37°C and S_{O_2} = 100% and 0%.

In anemic blood samples with hemoglobin concentrations
between 6.7 and 10 g·dl^{-1} a mean slope of -1.41 was
determined (Grote and Söndgen, 1976). At a P_{CO_2} of
40 mmHg the mean pH of the oxygenated blood-FDA20 mixtures was 7.434 indicating a small shift to the right
of the pH-log P_{CO_2} equilibration lines. Since according
to Astrup (1956) an increase in the plasma protein concentration induces a left shift of the equilibration
lines, a shift to the right would be expected in the
samples under investigation because the blood was diluted. In addition, the right shift of the pH-log P_{CO_2}
equilibration lines of the blood-FDA20 mixtures may be
caused by the buffer content of FDA20 (HCO_3^--concentra-
tion = 25 mmol·l^{-1}).

The mean CO_2 dissociation curves of the blood-FDA20
mixtures determined at S_{O_2} = 100% and 0% are given in
Fig. 6. Both dissociation curves are comparable to those
of normal blood (Harms and Bartels, 1961; Rispens et al.,
1973; Mochizuki et al., 1982; Loeppky et al., 1983),
however, they are below the CO_2 dissociation curve calculated for the conditions Hb = 7 g·dl^{-1} and S_{O_2} = 100%
using the Siggaard-Andersen nomogram and the modified

459

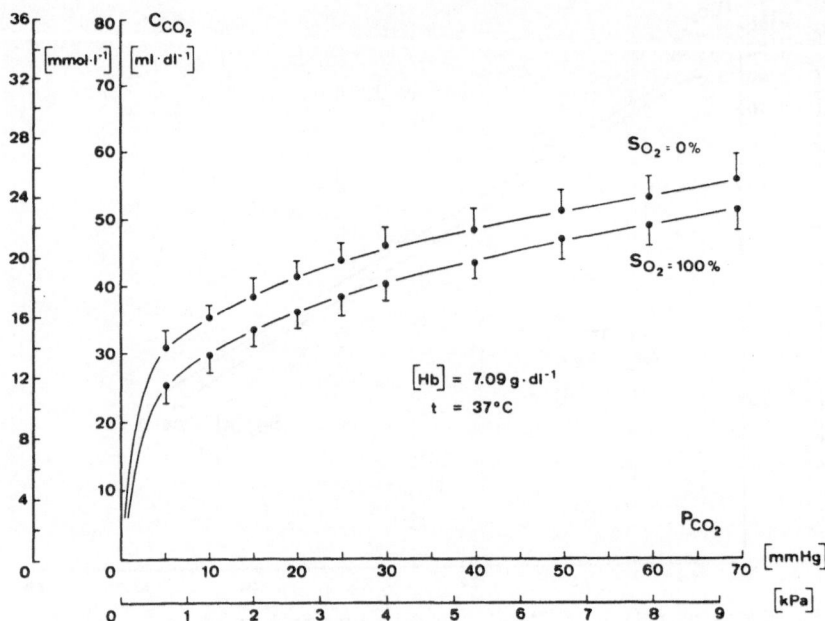

Fig. 6.   Mean CO_2 dissociation curve of blood-FDA20 mix-
          tures (Hb = 7.09 g·dl^{-1}), determined at 37°C
          and S_{O_2} = 100% and 0%.

Singer-Hastings nomogram of Rispens and coworkers (1973).
The mean CO_2 concentration of the samples was at
P_{CO_2} = 40 mmHg and S_{O_2} = 100% 19.5 mmol·l^{-1}.

REFERENCES

Astrup, P., 1956, Scand.J.clin.Lab.Invest.,8: 33-43
Austin, W.H., Lacombe, E., Rand, P.W., and Chatterjee, M.,
        1963, J.Appl.Physiol.,18: 301-304
Bartels, H., and Wrbitzky, R., 1960, Pflügers Arch.,271:
        162-168
Beisbarth, H., and Suyama, T., 1982, in: Frey, R., Beis-
        barth, H., Stosseck, K.(eds.) Oxygen carrying
        colloidal blood substitutes. Zuckschwerdt,
        München, pp. 3-12
Castaing, M., and Pocidalo, J.J., 1979, Respir.Physiol.,
        38: 243-256
Clark, L.C., and Gollan, F., 1966, Science, 152: 1755-1756

Gertz, K.H., and Loeschcke,H.H., 1954, Z. Naturforsch.,
      9b: 1-9
Geyer, R.P., 1982, in: Frey, R., Beisbarth, H., Stosseck,
      K.(eds.) Oxygen carrying colloidal blood substi-
      tutes. Zuckschwerdt, München, pp. 19-29
Geyer, R.P., 1983, in: Bolin, R.B., Geyer, R.P., Nemo,
      G.J.(eds.) Advances in blood substitute research.
      Progr.Clin.Biol.Res., vol. 122. Liss, New York,
      pp. 157-168
Grote, J., 1967, Pflügers Arch., 296: 202-211
Grote, J., 1971, in: Thews, G.(ed.) Nomogramme zum Säure-
      Basen-Status des Blutes und zum Atemgastransport,
      Anaesthesiology and Resuscitation, vol. 53.
      Springer, Berlin, Heidelberg, New York, pp. 47-83
Grote, J., and Söndgen, W., 1976, Pflügers Arch.,365: R22
Harms, H., and Bartels, H., 1961, Pflügers Arch.,272: 384-
      392
Loeppky, J.A., Luft,U.C., and Fletcher, E.R., 1983, Respir.
      Physiol., 51: 167-181
von Mengden, H.-J., Schultehinrichs, D., and Thews, G.,
      1969, Respir.Physiol., 6: 151-159
Mochizuki, M., Tazawa, H., and Tamura, M., 1982, Jpn.J.
      Physiol., 32: 231-244
Naito, R., and Yokoyama, K., 1978, Perfluorochemical blood
      substitutes. Techn.Inform.Series No.5, Green Cross
      Corporation, Osaka
Power, G.G., 1968, J.Appl.Physiol., 24: 468-474
Rispens, P., Brunsting, J.R., Zock, J.P., and Zijlstra,
      W.G., 1973, J.Appl.Physiol., 34: 377-382
Scholander, P.F., 1947, J.Biol.Chem., 167: 235-250
Sendroy, J., Dillon, R.T., and van Slyke, D.D., 1934,
      J.Biol.Chem., 105: 597-632
Severinghaus, J.W., 1966, J.Appl.Physiol., 21: 1108-1116
Severinghaus, J.W., 1979, J.Appl.Physiol., 46: 599-602
Siesjö, B.K., 1962, Acta physiol.scand., 55: 325-341
Siggaard-Andersen, O., 1974, The acid-base status of the
      blood. Munksgaard, Copenhagen, 4.th.ed.
van Slyke, D.D., Sendroy, J., Hastings, A.B., and Neill,
      J.M., 1928, J.Biol.Chem., 78: 765-799
Zander, R., 1969, Pflügers Arch., 308: 127-136
Zander, R., and Makowski, H.V., 1982, in: Frey, R.,
      Beisbarth, H., Stossek, K.(eds.) Oxygen carrying
      colloidal substitutes. Zuckschwerdt, München,
      pp. 131-141

GAS EXCHANGE DURING PERITONEAL PERFUSION WITH PERFLUOROCARBON

EMULSIONS

N.S. Faithfull*, P.J. Salt**, J. Klein*,
H.T. van der Zee***, H. Soini**, and W. Erdmann*

Departments of Anaesthesia, Erasmus University
Rotterdam, The Netherlands*, Addenbrookes Hospital
Cambridge, UK** and Albany Medical College, New York
State, USA***

The fact that fluorocarbons have a very high solubility for oxygen was very dramatically demonstrated by Clark and Gollan (1966), when they were able to show survival of mice completely immersed in these liquids for extended periods of time. The animals were able to obtain sufficient oxygen by respiring the liquid. After removal from the fluorocarbons the animals showed no apparent ill effects from the experience.

Pure fluorocarbons at 37°C can contain 40 or more volumes percent of oxygen (Geyer, 1975). These substances are however immiscible with blood and, if introduced into the circulation in an unmodified form, would cause embolic phenomena. In order to be of use as oxygen carrying blood substitutes they must therefore be used in an emulsified form. Such a blood substitute, containing either 20 or 35 percent fluorocarbons by weight, is produced commercially under the trade name of Fluosol-DA (Green Cross Corporation, Osaka, Japan). The compositions of Fluosol-DA 20% and 35% are shown in Fig. 1. Pluronic F68 and egg yolk phosphatides are used as emulsifying agents and the resulting very fine emulsion has a mean particle size of approximately 0.1 micron, with more than 90 percent of particles being smaller than 0.2 micron in diameter (Naito and Yokoyama, 1978).

The oxygen content of perfluorocarbon emulsions is directly dependent on the partial pressure of oxygen and, unlike haemoglobin, the amount of oxygen that can be taken up is directly proportional to the oxygen tension. At full saturation, blood with a haematocrit of 45 percent will contain something in the region of 20 ml of oxygen per 100 ml of blood and this will be achieved at a PO_2 of about 120 mm Hg. At this PO_2, Fluosol-DA 20% will contain approximately 1.2 ml of oxygen per 100 ml of emulsion. This amount, though small, is nevertheless more than three times as much as can be carried by plasma alone. The above figures from Naito and Yokoyama (1978) have recently been drawn into question by work of Grote et al. (this volume).

| | *Fluosol* | |
	−DA 20%	−DA 35%
Perfluoro-		
tripropylamine (FTPA)	6·0	10·5
decalin (FDC)	14·0	24·5
Pluronic F-68 (%)	2·7	
Egg yolk phosphatide	0·4	
Glycerol	0·8	
HES	3·0	
Glucose (mmol/l)	10	9·1
Na^+	128	117
K^+	4·6	4·2
Mg^{++}	2·1	1·9
Ca^{++}	2·5	2·3
Cl^-	112	102·5
HCO_3^-	25	23
HPO_4^{--}		
SO_4^{--}		
Osmotic pressure (mosm/l)	410 (320)	
Oncotic pressure (mmH$_2$O)	380–395	

Fig. 1 Composition of Fluosol-DA 20% and 35% emulsions.

As the oxygen content of Fluosol depends on the PO_2, it was postulated that oxygenated fluorocarbons might release useful amounts of oxygen when perfused through the peritoneal cavity, the mean PO_2 of which (in rabbits) was found by Klossner et al. (1974) to be 42 mm Hg. It should also be possible to decrease carbon dioxide by the same methods though, as will be later apparent, other plasma substitutes can equally well be substituted for fluorocarbon emulsions. This paper reports results obtained during perfusion using fluorocarbon emulsions in both spontaneously breathing rats and artificially ventilated rabbits.

EXPERIMENTS USING MECHANICALLY VENTILATED RABBITS

Methods

A group of six New Zealand white rabbits were anaesthetised with nitrous oxide, oxygen and halothane and, after endotracheal intubation, were artificially ventilated with mixtures of nitrous oxide and oxygen. Muscular relaxation was obtained by using a continuous intramuscular infusion of pancuronium bromide at a rate of 5.5 microgram per kg per hour. The arterial pressure in the femoral artery was monitored, using a Gould Statham P23 ID transducer, on a Grass 7D polygraph and inkwriting oscillograph. Expired carbon dioxide was continuously monitored using a Gould Godart capnograph Mark III and recorded on the Grass polygraph.

Via a small midline upper abdominal laparotomy, catheters were introduced for inflow and outflow of Fluosol-DA 20% which was oxygenated using a homemade bubble oxygenator, through which pure oxygen was bubbled. Sufficient oxygenation of the Fluosol, which was warmed to 37°C, was checked at regular intervals using a Radiometer ABL 1 acid/base laboratory. Before Fluosol perfusion was commenced, baseline values for arterial partial pressure of oxygen (PaO_2) and arterial carbon dioxide tension ($PaCO_2$) were obtained while the FIO_2 was progressively lowered in a stepwise fashion (allowing time for equilibration at each step) from an initial value of 0.5. At no time in this control procedure did the arterial oxygen saturation fall below 80 percent. The FIO_2 of the inspired gas mixture was measured using an Instrumentation Laboratory oxygen monitor 404.

After the controls had been performed at various FIO_2's, Fluosol perfusion was commenced using a Driessen roller pump at a rate of 25 ml min^{-1} and the FIO_2 was set to 0.5. The first measurements of arterial blood gases were performed after perfusing for at least 30 minutes. The FIO_2 was again progressively lowered and blood gas measurements were regularly performed. At the end of the experiments, arterial blood was taken and centrifuged to ascertain if measurable quantities of fluorocarbon emulsion had entered the circulation. On no occasion was a measurable fluorocrit obtained.

Results

A pair of measurements in the context of these experiments is taken to mean two measurements obtained at the same FIO_2, one before and one in the presence of intraperitoneal perfusion. The mean rise in the partial pressure of oxygen in the arterial blood amounted to 23.1 mm Hg ($\pm$ 2.9 SEM). This was highly significant as assessed by the Student paired t test ($p < 0.001$). The changes in PaO_2 following intraperitoneal Fluosol at different FIO_2's are given in Table I, and it can be seen that these changes were significant in every case as assessed on the paired t test, or in the case of the FIO_2 of 0.16 (at which there were only three measurements), the standard Student t test.

TABLE I.   Changes in PaO_2 ($\pm$ 1 SEM) following intraperitoneal perfusion of Fluosol-DA 20% (25 ml/min) at various FIO_2's. The figures are given in mm Hg and the numbers in each group are given in parenthesis. Statistical significance is indicated by asterisks :   * = $p < 0.05$ ** = $p < 0.01$

FIO_2	0.5	0.4	0.3	0.2	0.16
Change	23.0 *	25.1 **	25.7 **	15.8 **	22.0 *
in	$\pm$ 9.42	$\pm$ 6.46	$\pm$ 5.47	$\pm$ 3.19	$\pm$ 8.28
PaO_2	(6)	(6)	(6)	(6)	(3)

The PaO_2 values were plotted against the FIO_2 values in regression diagrams as shown in Fig. 2. The correlation coefficients were good for both control animals ($r=0.96$) and Fluosol perfused animals ($r=0.97$). It will be noticed that the two regression lines tend to converge at lower levels of FIO_2. This may be due to oxygen being taken up in the peritoneal cavity and then passing from the pulmonary capillaries into the alveoli and hence "excreted". This process would only occur if the PO_2 of the mixed venous blood was higher than the alveolar PO_2.

The mean decrease in arterial carbon dioxide tensions was less marked and amounted to only 2.2 mm Hg ($\pm$ 2.4 SEM). These changes were not significant on a paired t test. However, if all measurements were excluded where the pre-Fluosol PaO_2 was less than 75 mm Hg, these mean changes amounted to 1.5 mm Hg ($\pm$ 0.3

SEM). These changes, though small, were significant on a paired t test ($p < 0.05$). It should be noted that changes occurring if the PaO_2 was less than 75 mm Hg were insignificant; in many cases rises in $PaCO_2$ occurred when hypoxia was relieved. This was probably a reflection of increased CO_2 production in the face of improved oxygenation. A statistically significant correlation was found between the control level of PCO_2 (in non-hypoxic animals) and the decrease in PCO_2 during perfluorocarbon perfusion.

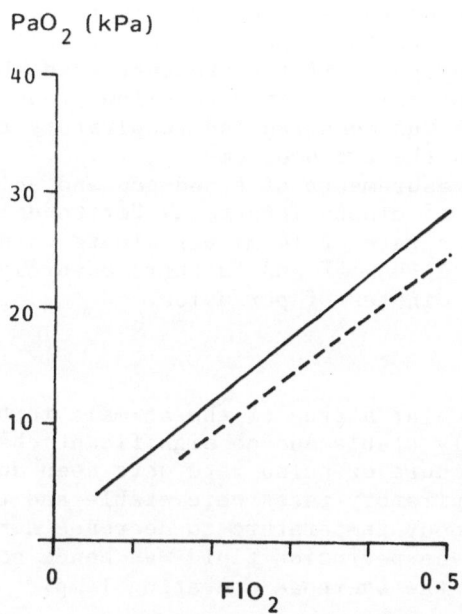

Fig. 2 Regression lines for oxygen tension (PaO_2) against inspired oxygen concentration (FIO_2) for both control measurements (----) and those obtained during intraperitoneal Fluosol perfusion (——).

EXPERIMENTS USING SPONTANEOUSLY BREATHING RATS

Methods

This study was carried out using male Wistar rats, ranging in weight from 200 to 300 grams. Anaesthesia was induced with 0.15 ml

of Hypnorm (Duphar BV, Amsterdam) per 100 gm body weight. This preparation contains 10 mg fluanisone and 0.2 mg of fentanyl per ml and was administered by intramuscular injection. Anaesthesia was maintained by continuous infusion of Althesin (5 ug per 100 gm per hour) into the tail vein. Tracheostomy was performed to ensure an open airway. The left femoral artery was cannulated with a 1 mm external diameter polythene cannula and systemic arterial pressure was monitored using a Gould Statham P23ID pressure transducer and Grass 7D polygraph and ink writing oscillograph. The in and outgoing lines for Fluosol perfusion consisted of a 7 French gauge Argyle oxygen catheter and a 16 gauge Salem gastric tube in the left and right iliac fossae respectively.
Fluosol, or Haemaccel, was oxygenated in a homemade bubble oxygenator and circulated using a self-constructed roller pump. Intra-abdominal pressure was monitored by a 1 mm internal diameter catheter inserted into the upper abdomen, a P23ID Transducer and the Grass 7D polygraph. If the pressure rose above 10 mm Hg, perfusion was temporarily stopped to allow pressure to normalise. Rectal temperature was measured and respiratory rate was monitored by a thermistor in the tracheostomy.

   Three control measurements of blood gas and acid/base status were performed at 15 minute intervals. Peritoneal perfusion was then performed at a rate of 14 ml per minute using either Haemaccel or Fluosol-DA 35% and further measurements were continued till 90 minutes of perfusion.

Results

   The cardiovascular status of the animals in both groups remained reasonably stable and no significant changes in either mean arterial pressure or pulse rate were seen during the course of perfusion. Respiratory rates were stable and there was no tendency for the body temperature to decrease during perfusion. Any heat loss to the perfusion fluid was hence compensated for by radiant heat from the overhead operating lamp.

   Changes in PaO_2, PCO_2 and hydrogen ion concentration for both control periods (C0, C15, and C30) and during prolonged peritoneal perfusion (P15 to P90) are shown in fig 3. The changes are illustrated as mean percentage changes with respect to the values obtained at the 30 minute control point (C30). It can be seen that no significant changes in PaO_2 occurred in the Haemaccel perfused animals, whereas a significant increase in PaO_2 was to be observed in the Fluosol perfused group after 45 minutes of treatment. This continued to rise until the termination of the experiment after 90 minutes of perfusion.

   When the graphs for changes in $PaCO_2$ are examined, it can be seen that intraperitoneal perfusion with both Haemaccel and

468

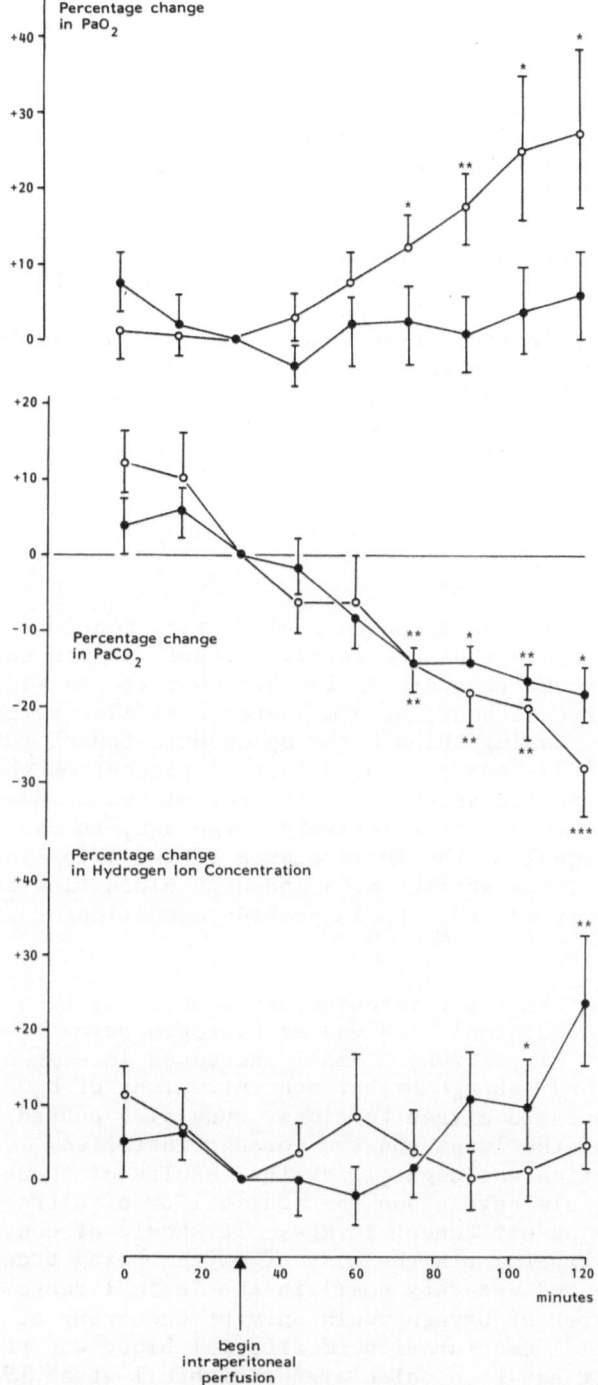

Figure 3. Percentage changes in PaO_2, $PaCO_2$ and hydrogen ion concentration during intraperitoneal perfusion of rats with Fluosol-DA 35% at a rate of 14 ml per minute. Asterisks indicate statistical significance as in fig. 1.

Fluosol results in progressive decreases in $PaCO_2$ and, after 45 minutes of perfusion, these changes achieve statistical significance. During the control periods (C0 to C30) the $PaCO_2$ also decreased - significantly so in the case of the Fluosol group. These effects can be attributed to recovery of the animals from the respiratory depressant effects of fentanyl (in the Hypnorm) used during the induction of anaesthesia.

The above mentioned improvement in respiratory exchange is reflected by falling hydrogen ion concetration in the arterial blood during this period. Prolonged intraperitoneal perfusion with Fluosol caused no further significant changes in acid/base balance but hydrogen ion concentration rose progressively in the Haemaccel group and after 60 and 90 minutes of perfusion these changes were significant ($p < 0.05$ and < 0.01 respectively). Base excess (not shown) was considerably lower in the Haemaccel group during this period ($p < 0.01$).

DISCUSSION

In most mammals the splanchnic blood flow accounts for a substantial percentage of the cardiac output. In man this amounts to about 25 percent (Cooperman, 1972). McDivitt and Niess, 1976, using microsphere methods, have measured a similar percentage of cardiac output passing through the splanchnic bed of rats and White et al.(1967) have estimated that 17 percent of the cardiac output of the rabbit passes along the portal vein. The surface area of the peritoneum is relatively large and, in man, is approximately equal to the surface area of the skin. This combination of large surface area and high blood flow in an area with a relatively low PO_2 should provide conditions suitable for gas exchange.

Oxygenation via the peritoneum has previously been attempted using oxygen (Awad et al., 1970a) or hydrogen peroxide solutions (H_2O_2) (Awad et al., 1970b). Small increases in oxygen tension were observed and, though higher concentrations of H_2O_2 caused greater increases in oxygen tensions, they also caused embolization of the lungs and the coronary arteries. Carbon dioxide extraction was negligible. The results of these preliminary trials have shown the feasibility of extra-pulmonary oxygenation using peritoneal lavage. It should of course be noted that in these experiments the mass of oxygen being transfered to the splanchnic bed was very small in the "normal range" of pO_2's and mass transfer of oxygen would only be occurring at pO_2's in which substantial desaturation of arterial blood was present. Nevertheless it has been calculated (Faithfull et al.,1984) that something in the order of 50 percent of the body's oxygen could theoretically be supplied by intraperitoneal oxygenation.

It might be argued that, in the rabbit studies, exclusion of $PaCO_2$ measurements, where control values of PaO_2 were less than 75 mm Hg, was unjustifiable. The mean PaO_2 in these animals was 57.8 mm Hg ($\pm$ 3.3 SEM) and there is evidence that this degree of hypoxia may be sufficient to cause decreases in oxygen consumption (Harzbecker et al., 1979; Levitan and Bungo, 1982). In the rat experiments, carbon dioxide clearance apppears to be equally effective with both Haemaccel and Fluosol. This is not surprising in view of the high solubility of carbon dioxide in aqueous media.

In view of the decreases in $PaCO_2$ that were seen, it might be expected that the arterial pH would rise in both the Haemaccel and Fluosol groups. These anomalous results can be explained on the basis of the occurrence of critical decreases in cardiac output during perfusion and subsequent impairment of tissue oxygenation. Improved oxygen supply in the fluorocarbon perfused animals prevented significant increases in hydrogen ion concentration in this group as opposed to the Haemaccel group.

The results of this preliminary trial have shown the feasibility of extra-pulmonary oxygenation using peritoneal lavage. It is possible that this technique may find application in the treatment of some forms of respiratory failure. It would be particularly indicated in cases of pulmonary damage by oxygen radical formation in paraquat poisoning.

REFERENCES

Awad, J.A., Brassard, A. and Caron, W.M., 1970a. Intraperitoneal Oxygenation. An Experimental Study in Dogs. Int. Surg., 53:162.

Awad, J.A., Brassard, A., Caron, W.M. and Cadrin, C., 1970b. Intraperitoneal oxygenation with hydrogen peroxide. Int. Surg. 54:276

Clark, L. C., and Gollan, F., 1966. Survival of mammals breathing organic liquids equilibrated with oxygen at atmospheric pressure. Science, 152:1755.

Cooperman, L. H., 1972. Effects of anaesthetics on splanchnic circulation. Brit. J. Anaesth., 44:967.

Faithfull, N. S., Klein, J., van der Zee, H. and Salt, P. J., 1984. Intraperitoneal oxygenation using perfluorocarbon substitutes. Brit. J. Anaesth., 56:867.

Geyer, R. P., 1975. Review of perfluorochemical-type blood substitutes. Proc. Xth Intern Cong Nutrition Symposium on PFC Artificial Blood, Kyoto, Japan: p.3.

Grote, J., Steuer, K., Müller, R., Söntgerath, C. and Zimmer, K, 1984. O_2 and CO_2 transport properties of fluorocarbon emulsions (Fluosol-DA) and Blood-Fluosol-DA mixtures. Abstracts of the Intern. Soc. on Oxygen Tranport to Tissue, Nijmegen, The Netherlands : p 38.

Harzbecker, K., Krause, M., Krämer, U. and Müller, H-R., 1979. Der Einfluss von Hypoxie auf den pulmonalen Gaswechsel und die Hämodynamik. Z. Ges. Inn. Med., 34;:330.

Klossner, J., Kivisaari, J. and Niinikosi, J., 1974. Oxygen and Carbon Dioxide Tensions in the Abdominal Cavity of the Rabbit. Am. J. Surg., 127:711.

Levitan, B. M. and Bungo M. W., 1982. Measurement of cardio pulmonary performance during acute exposure to a 2440-m equivalent atmosphere. Aviat. Space Environ. Med. , 53:639.

McDivitt D. G. and Nies A. S., 1976. Simultaneous measurement of cardiac output and its distribution with microspheres in the rat. Cardiovasc. Res., 10:494.

Naito R. and Yokoyama K., 1978. In: Perfluorochemical blood substitutes. Green Cross Corporation Technical Information Service No.5, Osaka, Japan.

White, S. W., Chalmers, J. P., Hilder, R., and Korner, P. I., 1967. Local thermodilution methods for measuring blood flow in the portal and renal veins of the unaesthetized rabbit. Aust. J. exp. Biol. med. Sci., 45:453-468.

This work was supported in part by a grant from the East Anglian Regional Health Authority.

OXYGEN AFFINITY OF HEMOGLOBIN SOLUTIONS MODIFIED BY COUPLING WITH
NFPLP AND THE EFFECTS ON TISSUE OXYGENATION IN THE ISOLATED
PERFUSED RAT LIVER

J. van der Plas, W.K. Bleeker, A. de Vries-van Rossen,
A. van Hamersveld, G. Rigter, J.A. Loos, and J.C. Bakker

Central Laboratory of the Netherlands Red Cross Blood
Transfusion Service, Plesmanlaan 125, Amsterdam
The Netherlands

INTRODUCTION

The use of a stroma-free hemoglobin solution as a plasma
expander with oxygen transport capacity is limited due to two
unfavourable properties: 1. An increased oxygen affinity, which is
mainly caused by the loss of 2,3-diphosphoglycerate (2,3-DPG) from
the central cavity of the hemoglobin tetramer, and 2. A shortened
vascular retention time, which is mainly due to excretion of the
dimeric form of hemoglobin through the kidneys (Bunn et al., 1969).
The goal of our research project is to modify the hemoglobin molecule so that a normal oxygen affinity and vascular retention time
are obtained. In order to change these intrinsic properties, organic
phosphate molecules were coupled covalently in the central cavity.
The binding of pyridoxal 5'-phosphate was the first modification
that has been studied (Benesch et al., 1972; Bakker et al., 1983, in
press). It was observed that this derivative has a decreased oxygen
affinity, but the main product cannot be produced in yields higher
than 25%, because the phosphate-containing β chain redistributes due
to dissociation of the tetramer. The binding of another phosphate,
2-nor-2-formylpyridoxal 5'-phosphate (NFPLP) could solve this
problem, because it couples between both β chains (Benesch et al.,
1975). It appeared that the main coupled product of NFPLP with hemoglobin (HbNFPLP) could be obtained reproducibly in yields of 60-70%
(Bakker et al., 1983, in press). The present paper describes the
effects of the covalent coupling of NFPLP to hemoglobin on tissue
oxygenation in the isolated perfused rat liver.

METHODS

Preparation of hemoglobin solutions

Packed erythrocytes, which had been made leukocyte free by filtration via special columns (Diepenhorst et al., 1972), were washed
three times with a physiological saline solution to remove the
traces of plasma proteins and thrombocytes. The erythrocytes were
lysed by adding two volumes of cold distilled water. The effective
removal of membrane fragments was established by tangential filtration (0.45 μm) and subsequent filtration through sterile 0.22 μm
membrane filters. This solution was dialysed against either 0.1 M
Tris-HCl (pH 7.0) or against a perfusion medium (see below) and
stored at 4°C as solutions of 7 g% stroma-free hemoglobin (7 g
SFH/100 ml).

Coupling of NFPLP to hemoglobin (Hb)

The coupling of NFPLP to Hb is essentially the same as that of
PLP (pyridoxal-phosphate) to Hb as described by Benesch et al.
(1972). A 7 g% stroma-free hemoglobin solution in 0.1 M Tris-HCl
(pH 7) was deoxygenated in a rotating flask under a stream of nitrogen. NFPLP was added in a molar ratio of 1:1 to hemoglobin. After 3
hours of rotating under nitrogen, a 40-fold excess of sodium borohy-
dride in 1 mM KOH was added, and the rotating was continued for
another 30 minutes. Thereafter, the solution was oxygenated by a
stream of air during 15 min. After filtration via 0.22 μm membrane
filters and dialysis against an electrolyte medium, the solution was
stored at 4°C.

Synthesis of 2-nor-2-formylpyridoxal 5'-phosphate (NFPLP)

NFPLP was synthesized in a five-step procedure, starting from
pyridoxal hydrochloride, as described by Pocker (1973) and Benesch
and Benesch (1981) with some modifications necessary for synthesis
on a gram scale (van der Plas et al., in preparation).

Perfusion medium

The composition of the perfusion medium was as follows:
NaCl, 115 mM; KCl, 4.7 mM; $MgCl_2$, 1.1 mM; $CaCl_2$, 2.6 mM; NaH_2PO_4,
1.2 mM; $NaHCO_3$, 25 mM; D-glucose, 50 mM; pyruvate, 0.1-3 mM;
lactate, 3-10 mM; hemoglobin 7 g%, pH 7.4.

Perfusion system

In Figure 1 a schematic drawing of the system is shown. It was
designed to be used with constant flow rates of the perfusates
through the liver. The system contained two recirculation circuits.
In one of these the perfusate was equilibrated with O_2 and CO_2 to
obtain the desired pH, PCO_2 and PO_2. A membrane oxygenator was used
to obtain a proper gas exchange. Via the other circuit the liver was

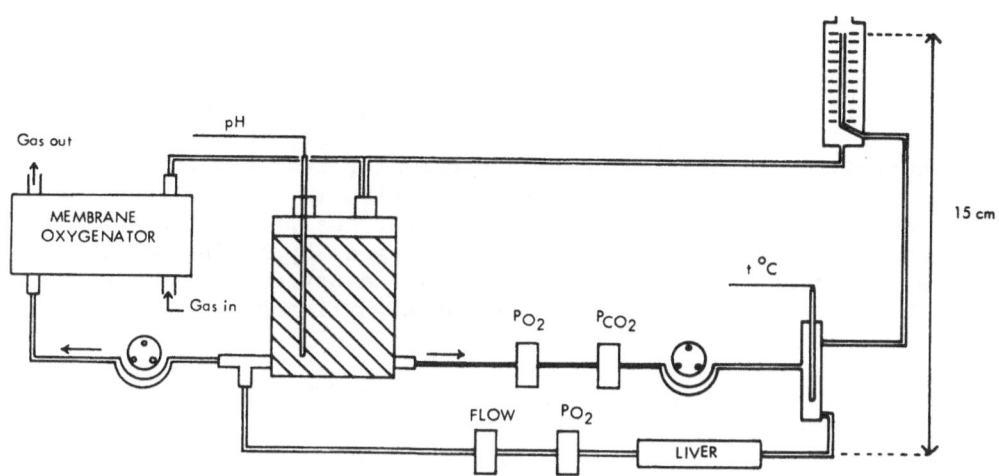

Fig. 1. Recirculation flow perfusion system

perfused with a flow rate of 18 ml/min or less. An overflow system limited the perfusion pressure to 15 cm H_2O maximally. A peristaltic pump was used to circulate the perfusate. The system was placed in a thermostatically controlled cabinet (37°C).

Analytical methods

P_{50} values were derived from the oxyhemoglobin dissociation curves recorded with the DCA-1 (Radiometer, Copenhagen) in diluted hemoglobin samples (Duvelleroy et al., 1970; Teisseire et al., 1975) under standard conditions (pH 7.4, PCO_2 = 40 mm Hg, temp.=37°C).

O_2 content of the perfusate was measured with the Lex-O_2-Con (Lexington Instruments Corp., Waltham, Mass.) in 20 µl samples taken from the portal vein and from the hepatic vein.

The bile production was determined by marking the progression of the bile front on the tubing inserted in the bile duct every 5 min and from these values the bile flow rate was estimated.

Hemoglobin concentrations were measured at 540 nm as cyano-methemoglobin.

Perfusion experiments

The aim of this liver perfusion study was the evaluation of the oxygen transport and release capacity of the modified hemoglobin solution. The criteria were the following oxygen sensitive para-meters:
-Venous PO_2
-Oxygen consumption/extraction
-Bile flow rate
-Lactate/pyruvate (L/P) ratio, as a reflection of the redox level in the cytoplasm
-β-Hydroxybutyrate/acetoacetate (βOH/Acac) ratio, as a reflection of the redox level in the mitochondria

475

RESULTS AND DISCUSSION

Figure 2 shows the mean data of oxygen supply and oxygen consumption of two series of rat liver perfusions with the indicated solutions. The P50 values of these solutions were 16 and 26 mm Hg respectively. For both series of experiments, the same hemoglobin concentration (7 g/100 ml), the same PO_2 (100 mm Hg) and the same flow rate (18 ml/min) were used; therefore, the perfusates had about the same oxygen transport capacity and oxygen supply in the two series. The differences in oxygen supply and oxygen consumption between the two series (Fig. 2) are not significant.

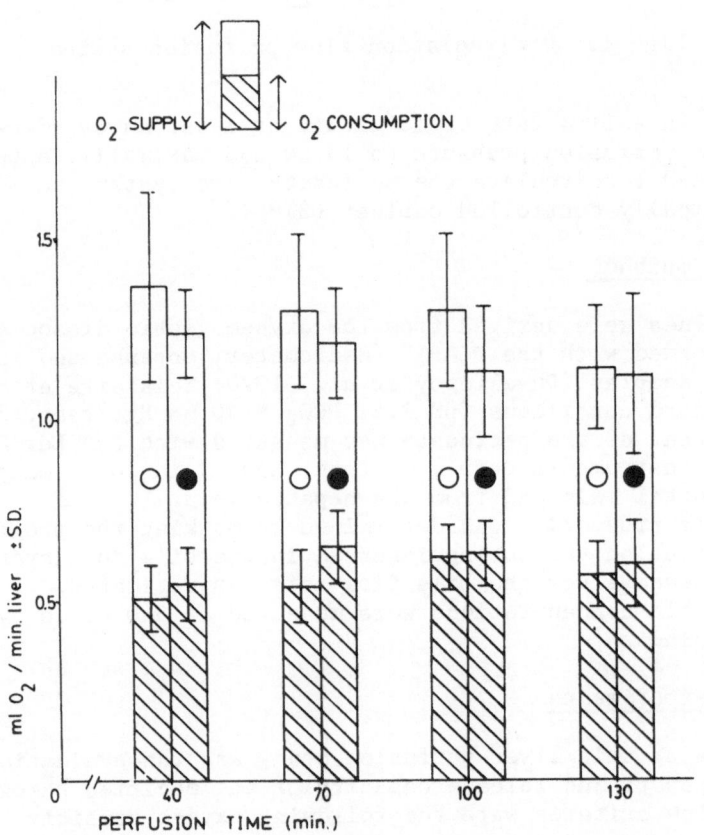

Fig. 2. Oxygen supply and oxygen consumption by the isolated perfused rat livers at different perfusion times. Values are means ± S.D. of perfusions with Hb (O, n=5) and a mixture of 45% unmodified hemoglobin and 55% coupled hemoglobin (Hb/HbNFPLP = 45/55; ●, n=5).

476

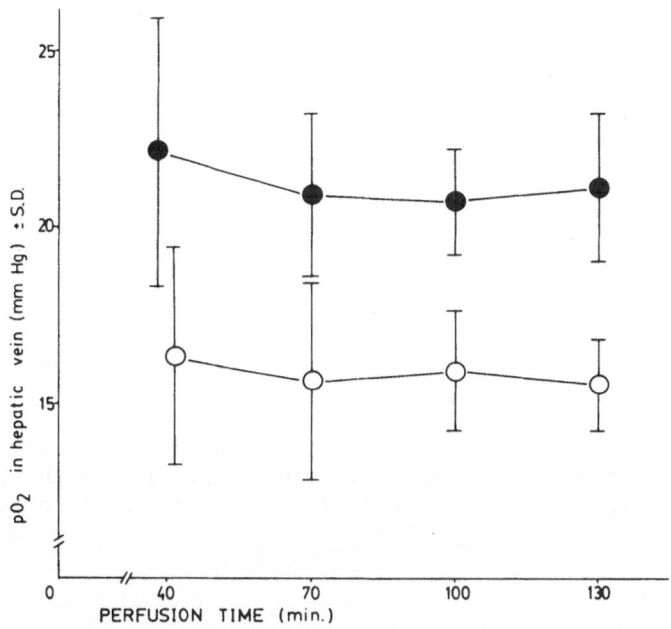

Fig. 3. Venous PO$_2$ in hepatic vein at different perfusion
times. Values are means ± S.D. of perfusions with
Hb (0, n=5) and Hb/HbNFPLP (45/55; ●, n=5) solutions

In Figure 3 the influence of the coupling of NFPLP to hemoglobin
on the venous PO$_2$ is shown. The figure shows a significantly higher
venous PO$_2$ in the case of the perfusions with the modified hemoglobin solutions, with p values between 0.02 and 0.001. These data
were in accordance with the different oxygen dissociation curves of
the perfusates (P$_{50}$ values 16 and 26 mmHg for the Hb and Hb/HbNFPLP
solutions, respectively) because the oxygen supply and consumption
data were equal.

Figure 4 shows the perfusion pressure of the inflowing perfusates. At t = 40 min the pressure of the Hb solutions is slightly
lower than that of the coupling mixture (p = 0.05). However, from
t = 70 min to t = 135 min no significant differences were observed.
During all perfusions the flow rate could be kept constant at 18 ml/
min. These data indicate that the modification of the hemoglobin
molecule introduced by coupling to the NFPLP does not result in a
change in rheological properties of the hemoglobin solution during
the perfusions.

In Figure 5 the observed bile flow rates have been plotted for
both series of liver perfusions. At time 40 min a slightly higher
bile flow rate was observed for the Hb solutions (p = 0.038). At the
other times no significant differences were found.

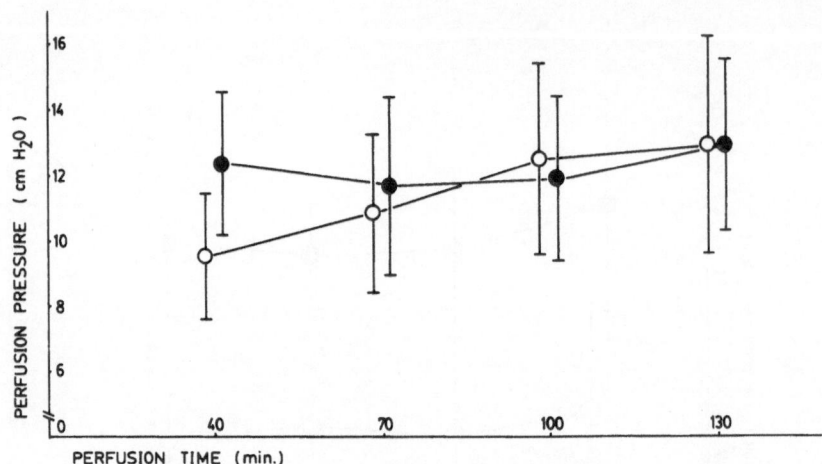

Fig. 4. Perfusion pressure of the inflowing perfusates.
Values are means ± S.D. of perfusions with Hb
(O, n=5) and Hb/HbNFPLP (45/55; ●, n=5) solutions

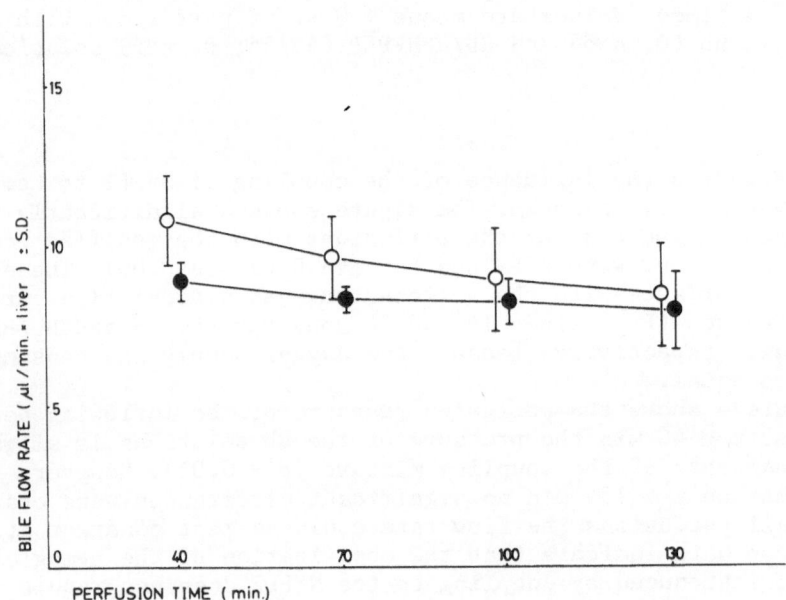

Fig. 5. Bile flow rate of the isolated rat liver.
Values are means ± S.D. of perfusions with Hb
(O, n=5) and Hb/HbNFPLP (45/55; ●, n=5) solutions

Because the oxygen supply was about twice as high as the oxygen consumption, the experimental conditions may not have been discriminent enough to show any differences in oxygen release between the two perfusates. In order to create a more critical situation, another series of perfusions was performed under conditions of hypoxia achieved by a decrease in perfusion flow rate. At time 75 and 105 min, the flow rate was adjusted to 9 ml/min and 6 ml/min, respectively. The degree of coupling of the modified hemoglobin solution used in these series was 66% which resulted in a P_{50} value of 34 mmHg.

Before the decrease in perfusion flow rate, a situation similar to that of the previous series was established (Fig. 6). Again, a difference in oxygen supply was noticed between the two perfusates, although all known parameters that determine oxygen supply were equal (hemoglobin concentration, methemoglobin concentration, PO_2 of the inflowing perfusate and perfusion flow rate). This time however, the difference was significant throughout the perfusion. P values

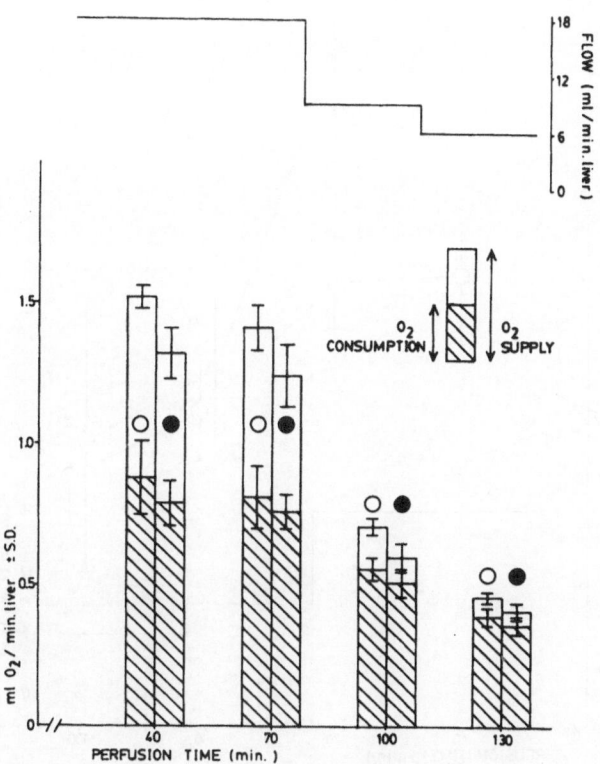

Fig. 6. Oxygen supply and oxygen consumption by the isolated perfused rat liver at different perfusion times. Values are means + S.D. of perfusions with Hb (0, n=8) and Hb/HbNFPLP (34/66; ●, n=8) solutions

less than 0.00003, 0.002, 0.00005 and 0.001 were found at the indicated perfusion times. It is well possible that this significance is caused by the higher degree of coupling in this Hb/HbNFPLP solution (66%) in comparison with the degree of coupling in the previous series (55%). This could mean that the HbNFPLP exhibits other oxygen binding properties than unmodified Hb. From the recent data of Benesch et al. (1984) a similar change in oxygen binding capacity at a PO_2 level of 160 mm Hg could be derived. However, in this heart model an enhanced unloading of oxygen by the modified hemoglobin was observed, although very low hemoglobin concentrations were used. For the liver perfusions the differences in oxygen consumption were significant at time 100 and 130 min (p = 0.013 and p = 0.018). Oxygen extraction was slightly different at time 100 min (p = 0.083).

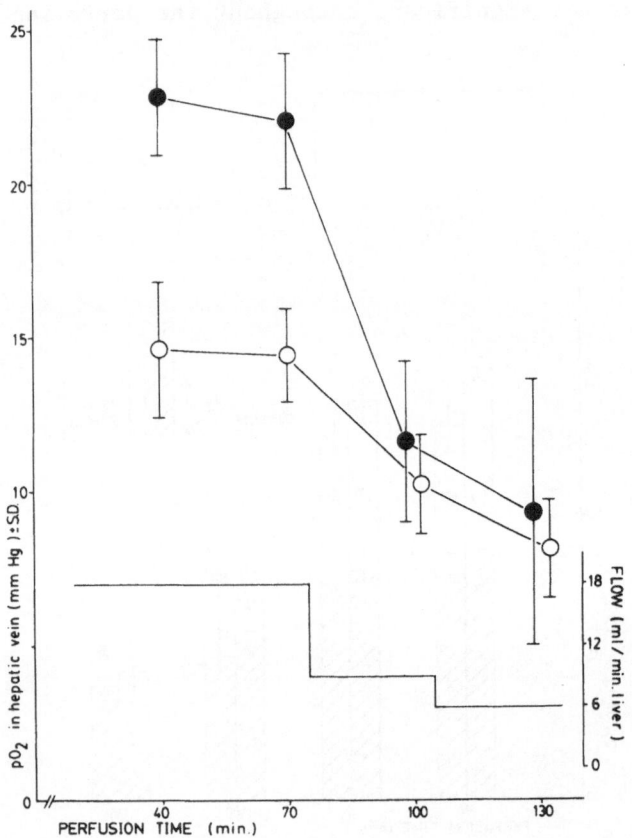

Fig. 7. Venous PO_2 in hepatic vein at different perfusion times. Values are means + S.D. of perfusions with Hb (0, n=8) and Hb/HbNFPLP (34/66; ●, n=8) solutions

For the venous PO$_2$ at times 40 and 70 min again a significantly higher value was found for the modified solution with p values of 8×10^{-7} and 5×10^{-7}, respectively. After the decrease in perfusion flow from 18 ml/min to 9 ml/min, this difference between both solutions disappeared.

Apparently, the oxygen-consuming processes require so much oxygen that the PO$_2$ has to drop to about 10-12 mmHg. At these pressures the oxygen dissociation curves of both perfusates do not differ very much. Therefore, it can not be expected that the oxygen consumption/extraction data differ significantly, which is in agreement with what was observed.

In Figure 8 the mean values of the bile flow rate have been plotted for both series of liver perfusions. As can be seen from the figure, the bile flow rate responds directly to the drop in perfusion flow from 18 to 9 ml/min. The same holds for the second drop to 6ml/min. No significant differences were observed between both perfusates.

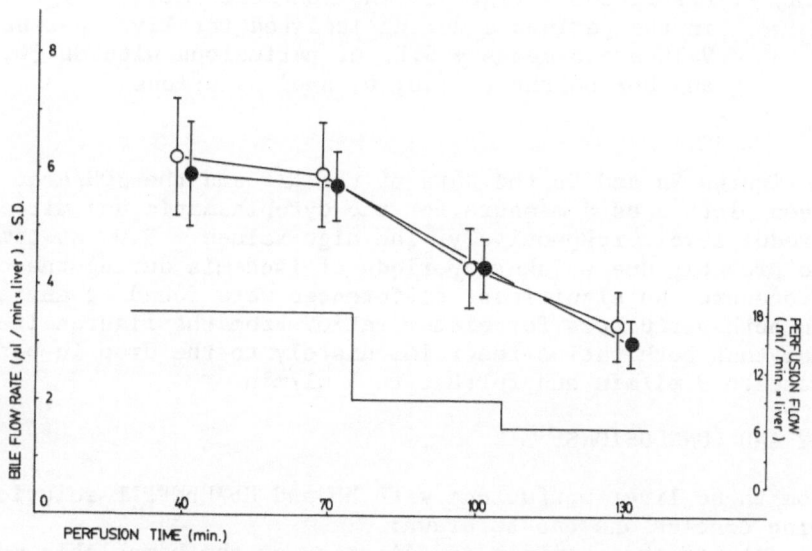

Fig. 8. Bile flow rate of the isolated rat liver. Values are means + S.D. of perfusions with Hb solutions (0, n=8) and Hb/HbNFPLP (34/66; ●, n=8) solutions

481

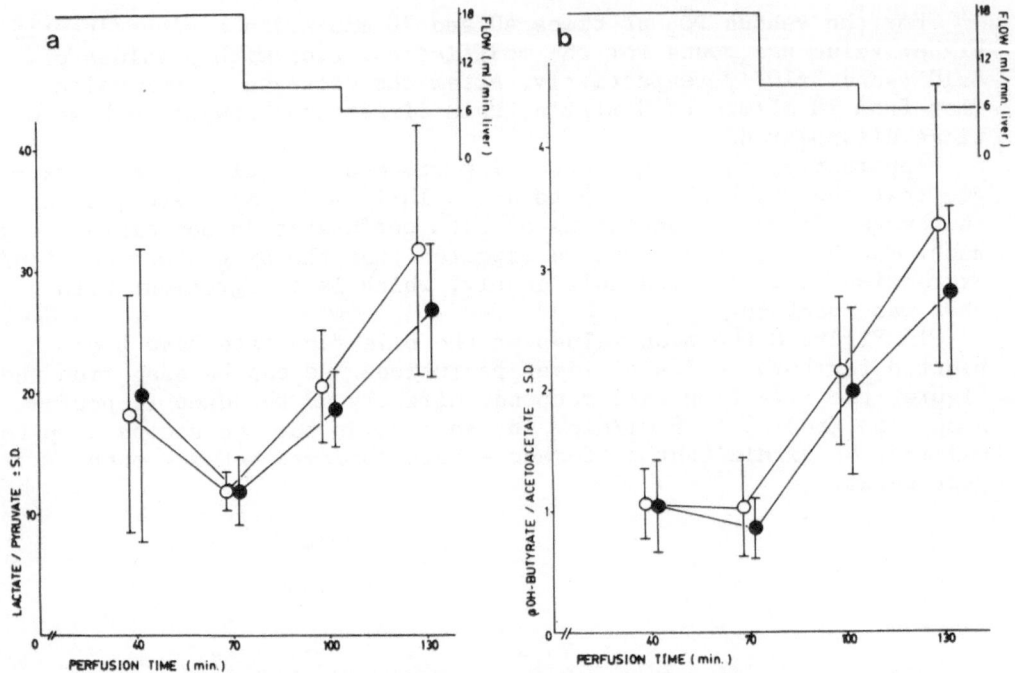

Fig. 9a, b. L/P ratios (Fig. 9a) and βOH/Acac ratios (Fig. 9b)
in the perfusate during isolated rat liver perfusions.
Values are means ± S.D. of perfusions with Hb (O, n=8)
and Hb/HbNFPLP (34/66; ●, n=8) solutions

In figures 9a and 9b the data of the L/P and the βOH/Acac ratios
have been plotted as a measure for the cytoplasmatic and mitochondrial redox level, respectively. The high values ± S.D. at time 40
min are probably due to short periods of ischemia during the operation procedure. No significant differences were found at any time
between both perfusates for either ratio. From the figures it should
be clear that both ratios react immediately to the drop in perfusion
flow rate to 9 ml/min and further to 6 ml/min.

SUMMARY AND CONCLUSIONS

From these liver perfusions with Hb and Hb/HbNFPLP solutions the
following conclusions can be drawn:
1. In spite of the chemical modification of the hemoglobin mole-
    cule, no rheological differences are seen.
2. All parameters measured were sensitive to hypoxia induced by a
    decrease in perfusion flow rate.
3. The NFPLP-induced decrease in oxygen affinity was reflected in a
    higher venous PO_2. These in-vivo observations are in agreement
    with the in-vitro measured oxygen dissociation curves. The dif-
    ference in PO_2 did not result in a change in the other oxygen-
    sensitive parameters in this model under the chosen conditions.

482

Possible causes for these observations are:
  i. the level of hypoxia was too low
  ii. the oxygen supply in the perfusions with the modified hemo-
      globin solutions was lower than the oxygen supply in the
      perfusions with normal hemoglobin. Whether or not this
      observation is due to an intrinsic property of the modified
      hemoglobin molecule remains to be established.

REFERENCES

Bakker, J. C., van der Plas, J., Bleeker, W. K., de Vries-van
    Rossen, A., Schoester, M., Brummelhuis, H. G. J., and Loos, J.
    A., 1983, Oxygen affinity of hemoglobin solutions modified by
    coupling to PLP or NFPLP and the effects on tissue oxygenation,
    in: "Oxygen transport to tissue - VI", Plenum Press, New York,
    in press.
Benesch, R. E., Benesch, R., Renthal, R. D., and Maeda, N., 1972,
    Affinity labeling of the polyphosphate binding site of hemo-
    globin, Biochemistry, 11:3576-3582.
Benesch, R., Benesch, R. E., Yung, S., and Edalji, R., 1975, Hemo-
    globin covalently bridged across the polyphosphate binding site,
    Biochem. Biophys. Res. Commun. 4, 63:1123-1129.
Benesch, R., and Benesch, R. E., 1981, Preparation and properties of
    hemoglobin modified with derivatives of pyridoxal, in: "Methods
    in Enzymology", Vol. 76, p 147-159, Academic Press, New York.
Benesch, R., Triner, L., Benesch, R. E., Kwong, S., and Verosky, M.,
    1984, Enhanced oxygen unloading by an interdimerically cross-
    linked hemoglobin in an isolated perfused rabbit heart, Proc.
    Natl. Acad. Sci. USA, 81:2941-2943.
Bunn, H. F., Esham, W. T., and Bull, R. W., 1969, The renal handling
    of hemoglobin. I. Glomerular filtration, J. Exp. Med.,129:909-924.
Diepenhorst, P., Sprokholt, R., and Prins, H. K., 1972, Removal of
    leucocytes from whole blood and erythrocytes suspension by fil-
    tration through cotton wool, Vox sang., 23:308-320.
Duvelleroy, M. A., Buckles, R. G., Rosenkaimer, S., Tung, S., and
    Laver, M. B., 1970, An oxyhemoglobin dissociation analyzer. J.
    Appl. Physiol., 28:227-233.
Pocker, A., 1973, Synthesis of 2-nor-2-formylpyridoxal 5'-phosphate,
    a bifunctional reagens specific for the cofactor site in pro-
    teins, J. Org. Chem., 38:4295-4299.
Teisseire, B., Lousance, D., Soulard, C., Herigault, R., Teisseire,
    L., and Laurent, D., 1975, A method of continuous recording on
    micro-samples of the Hb-O_2 association curve. I. Technique and
    direct registration of standard results, Bull. Europ. Physio-
    path. Resp., 11:837-851.

The investigations were supported (in part) by the Foundation for
Medical Research (FUNGO) (grant no. 13-36-38).

OXYGEN BINDING PROPERTIES OF EARLY DEFINITIVE RED CELLS FROM NORMOXIC AND HYPOXIC CHICK EMBRYOS

Rosemarie Baumann and Jens Fischer

Zentrum Physiologie Medizinische Hochschule
3000 Hannover, FRG

INTRODUCTION

During vertebrate ontogeny one observes large changes of the oxygen binding properties of the blood,reflecting the transition from the specific embryonic hemoglobins to fetal and/or adult hemoglobin as well as changes in the concentration of those metabolites of the red cell that act as allosteric regulators of hemoglobin function. While these changes have been extensively investigated for later stages of development in mammals and birds,there exist only few data on the functional properties of embryonic blood (1,2,3),and control of hemoglobin function at this stage is not well understood.

In the chick embryo,the specific embryonic hemoglobins are synthezised by the first erythrocyte population, the primitive red cells originating in the yolk sac (4).These cells are unable to produce adult hemoglobin and from the sixth day of incubation onwards there appears a new red cell line, the definitive red cells, which produce the two adult hemoglobins A and D.By day nine of incubation about 60% of the circulating hemoglobin is already of the adult type. The life-span of the first definitive red cells is low i.e. about 5 days (5) and there are also distinct morphological differences between the various transient red cell populations (5).
However it is not known to which extent the first generations of definitive red cells also show differences in their functional pro-perties.Since the embryonic and adult hemoglobins are contained in different cell populations measurements of whole blood oxygen affinity give no information about the behaviour of the individual population.

The aim of the present study was to investigate the oxygen bin-ding properties of definitive red cells,prepared from the blood

of chicken embryos between 7 to 14 days of incubation, which covers
the period of transition from embryonic to adult hemoglobin almost
completely. Further experiments were carried out on hypoxic embryos
between 7 to 9 days of development, where definitive red cells appear
in the circulation at an earlier time (6), and where oxygen affinity
of the blood is increased compared to normoxic embryos.

The results suggest, that the increase of embryonic blood oxygen
affinity observed during the second week of incubation is caused in
part through a programmed release of definitive red cell populations
with intrinsically different oxygen affinities.Moreover within a cell
population the oxygen affinity seems to increase as the red cell
matures.

MATERIALS and METHODS

Fertilized eggs from white-leghorn chicken were incubated at
37.5°C and 60% relative humidity in air or in 13.5% oxygen.Timing of
the eggs started when they were put in the incubator.Blood was taken
from the embryos between 7 to 14 days of development by venipuncture
of a large extra-embryonic blood vessel.Packed red cells were washed
3 times in buffer (10 mmol/ L Tris pH 7.4; 5 mmol/L glucose; 4 mmol/L
KCl and 140 mmol/ L NaCl) and finally resuspended in the same buffer
to give a hematocrit of about 20%.Definitive and primitive red cells
were separated by density gradient centrifugation on a linear gradient
of Ficoll 400, prepared from solutions of 10g% and 20g% Ficoll (7).
The red cells were centrifuged for 8 minutes at 1700 rpm and 4°C.After
centrifugation the gradient was divided in 9 subfractions.The top
fraction of lowest density contained the most immature definitive
red cells .This fraction was called Fl. Fraction 5, which was also
 analysed contained a mixture of primitive red cells and more mature
definitive red cells between day 7 to 9,from day 10 onwards it was
essentially free of primitive red cells.

Oxygen equilibrium curves of red cell suspensions from Fl and
F5 were recorded with a stepwise photometric method as described
elsewhere (2).The hemoglobin pattern of the separated fractions was
examined by isoelectric focusing on polyacrylamide gels and quanti-
tated by densitometry.ATP was measured with a test-kit (Boehringer
Co. Mannheim). The adult hemoglobins A and D were prepared from
adult chicken blood by column chromatography (2). Oxygen equilibrium
curves of concentrated solutions (200 g/L) of the two adult hemoglobins were determined with the Lex-O_2 -Con.The pH of the solutions
was adjusted to 6.9, the chloride concentration to 100 mmol/L and
ATP was added to give a stoechiometric ratio of ATP/Hb of 3:1.The
pH and ATP concentration correspond to the values measured in unfractionated red cells from 9 day old chick embryo.

486

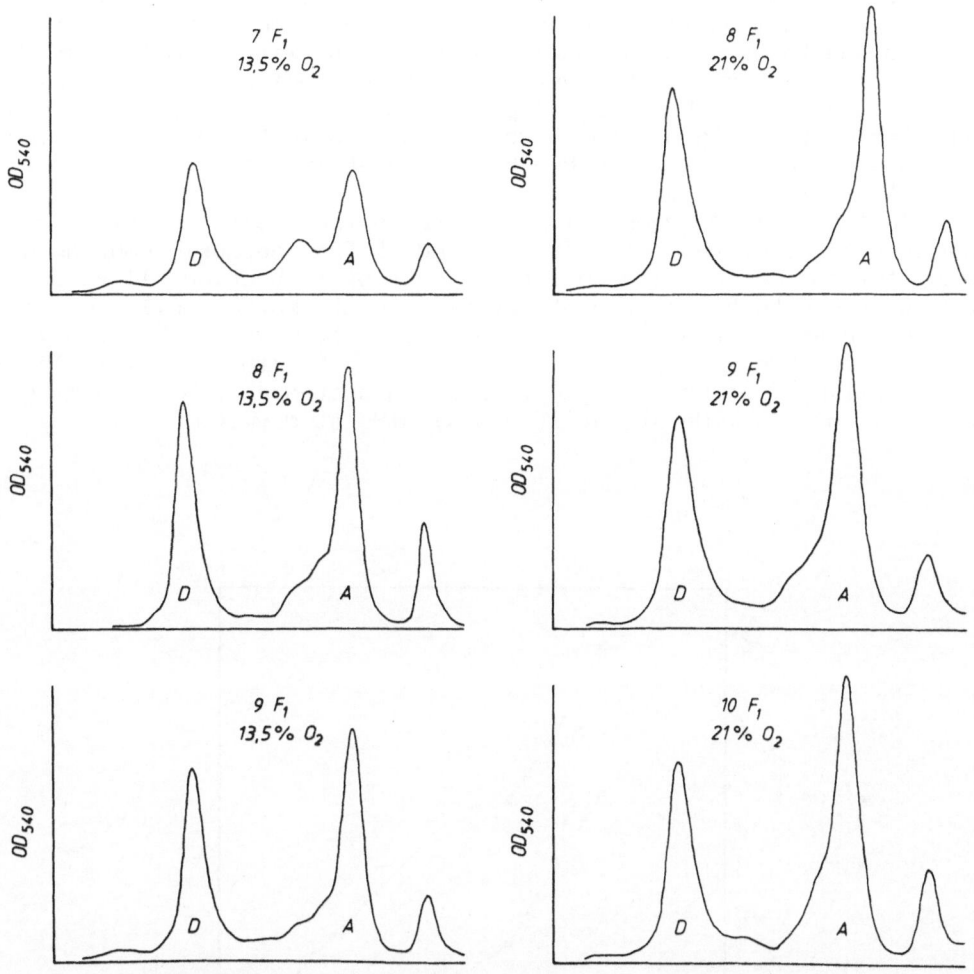

Fig. 1. Hemoglobin pattern of definitive red cells from fraction 1
(Fl) prepared from the blood of normoxic and hypoxic chick
embryos. Letters A and D denote the two adult hemoglobin
fractions.

RESULTS

Fig.1 shows the hemoglobin pattern of fraction 1 from the blood of 7 to 9 day old hypoxic embryos and 8 to 10 day old normoxic embryos. In all preparations minor amounts of embryonic hemoglobin were found. This is due to some unavoidable contamination with primitive cells; of equal importance is however the fact that definitive red cells of 7 to 9 day old embryos still produce minor quantities of embryonic hemoglobin (8). Between 7 to 10 days of development the adult hemoglobins are present in a ratio HbA/HbD of about 1:1; in adult red cells the ratio is about 2.5:1.

In figure 2 the mean values for the oxygen halfsaturation pressure (P_{50}) of red cells from F1 and F5 from normoxic embryos are shown for the period between 7 to 14 days of incubation. All values derive from 4 to 5 measurements at each point. For F1 cells the P_{50} related to an external pH of 7.4 decreases from 90.5 mmHg at day 7 to about 70 mmHg at day 10 and further on to 53 mmHg at day 14. The oxygen affinity of F5 is higher; here P_{50} decreases from 73.5 mmHg at day 7 to 54.5 mmHg at day 10 and 47 mmHg at day 14.

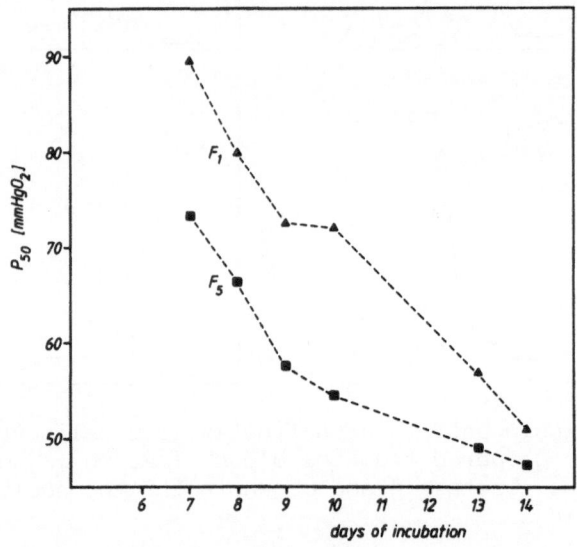

Fig. 2.   Oxygen half saturation pressure (P_{50}) of cells from F1 compared to cells from F5 between 7 to 14 days of incubation. Measurements were carried out at 37° C and external pH 7.4.

In table 1 we compare the P_{50} values obtained in the blood of norm-oxic embryos with results obtained for hypoxic embryos. It can be seen that the oxygen affinity of F1 cells from hypoxic embryos is always higher.The difference in P_{50} amounts to about 12 mmHg. Excepting day 7 the same can also be said for cells from F5, however the difference in P_{50} is only 6 to 7 mmHg.

Table 1. P_{50} in $mmHgO_2$ for F1 and F5 cells from normoxic and hypoxic chick embryos. 37°C,pH 7.4.

	13.5% O_2				21% O_2			
day	$\overline{x}$ F1	S.D.	$\overline{x}$ F5	S.D.	$\overline{x}$ F1	S.D.	$\overline{x}$ F5	S.D.
7	78.8	10.4	74.6	8.4	90.5	6.4	73.5	7.6
8	67.9	14.7	59.8	9.1	80.1	6.2	66.6	2.8
9	60.6	6.1	50.8	5.8	72.5	7.2	57.5	10.2

Aside from the pronounced changes of the oxygen affinity of cells from F1,we also noted that the shape of the oxygen equilibrium curve is altered substantially, indicating changes in the cooperativity of oxygen binding (fig.3). When one compares the oxygen binding curves for F1 cells from day 9,10 and 14 it is obvious that the steepness of the curve in the upper saturation range decreases with increasing age.

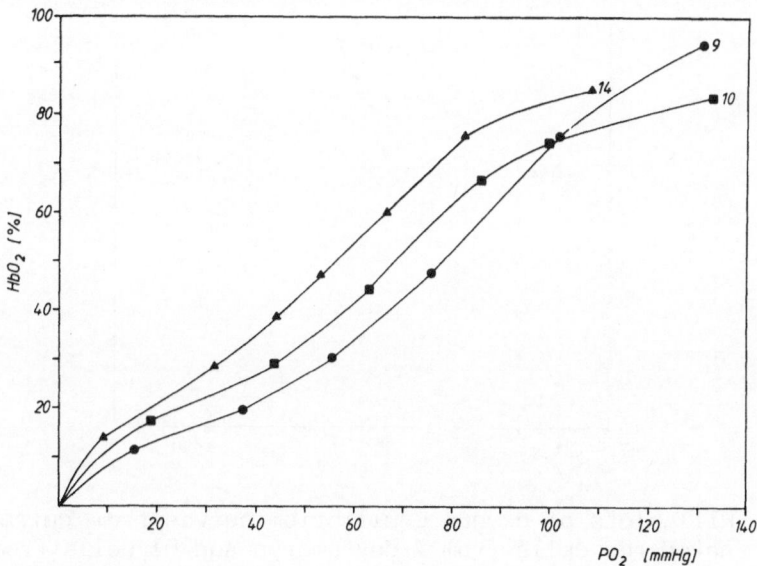

Fig. 3 . Oxygen binding curves of red cells from F1 for day 9,10 and 14. pH 7.4 ,37°C.

We found that for F1 cells harvested between day 7 to 9 the n-value always exceeded 4 in the saturation range between 60% to about 90%. After day 10 the n-value was always below 4.Moreover the cooperativity of oxygen binding for F1 cells between day 7 to 9 is very dependent on oxygen saturation.In fig. 4 the Hill-plots of the oxygen equilibrium curve of unfractionated red cells from day 7 and F1 cells from day 7 are compared .It is evident that cooperativity increases with rising oxygen saturation.Another striking fact is that both curves are nearly identical,despite the fact that the unfractionated red cells consist mainly of primitive red cells and the concentration of embryonic hemoglobin is about 70%. When we tried to simulate the oxygen binding curve of 9 day F1 cells by measuring the oxygen binding to concentrated solutions of hemoglobin A and D which were adjusted to physiological concentrations of ATP and pH (fig.5) we found that neither HbA nor HbD showed n-values above 4.For HbA n= 2 was measured and for HbD n=3.This finding indicates that the elevated cooperativity must depend on other factors present in the early definitive red cells.

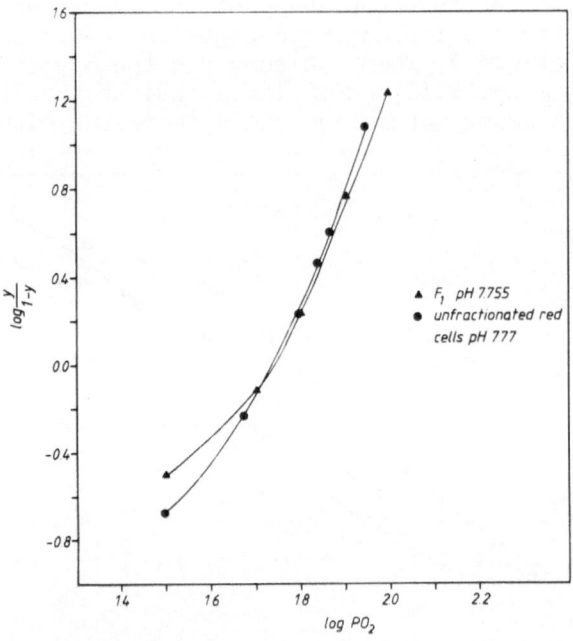

Fig. 4.   Hill-plots of oxygen equilibrium curves from unfractionated red cells from 7 day embryo and F1 cells from day 7. 37°C.

490

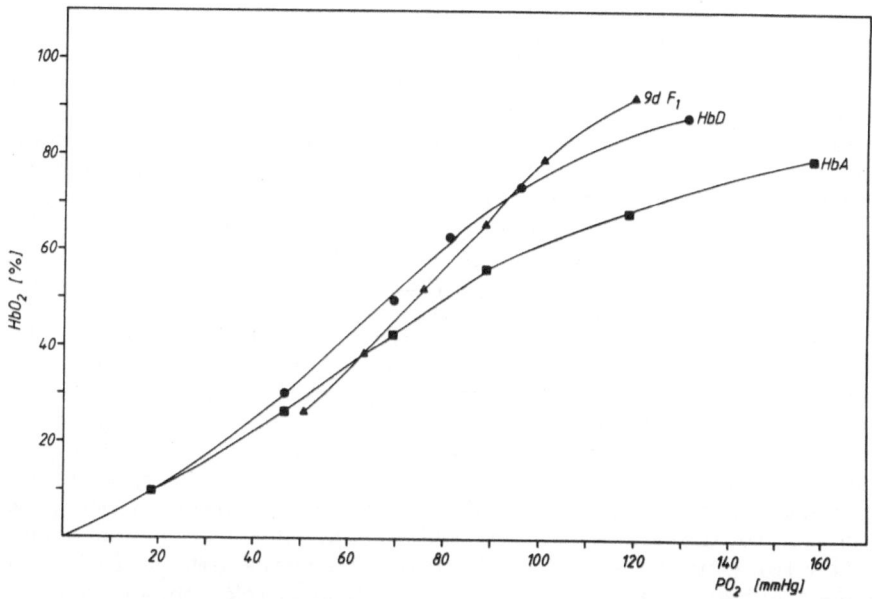

Fig. 5.Comparison of oxygen binding curves for 9 day Fl cells and
concentrated solutions of HbA and HbD respectively. The pH
for Fl cell suspensions was 7.4, that of the Hb solutions
6.9. ATP was 3mol/mol Hb,total Chloride 0.1mol/L. 37°.

Since the embryonic red cells contain high concentrations of ATP (9)
we were interested to see if the separation procedure had an effect
on the ATP concentrations.Measurements of fractions 1,5 and 9 from
the blood of 8 day hypoxic embryos gave the following values (mean
of at least 3 determinations) : 2.6molATP/ molHb in Fl;2.2molATP/Hb
in F5; 2.4molATP/molHb in F9,compared to a value of 3.1molATP/Hb for
whole blood (6).Similar results were obtained for day 9 and normoxic
cell fractions also had between 0.5 to 1molATP/molHb less ATP than
the controls. The results indicate that there is some loss of ATP
during the preparation of the cells.

DISCUSSION
        The present study shows that the oxygen affinity and cooperati-
vity of oxygen binding of definitive red cells is subject to drastic
changes between day 7 to 14.The fall of the P_{50} of the Fl cells
from about 90 mmHg at day 7 to 53 mmHg at day 14 parallels the change
in whole blood, where P_{50} falls from about 88 mmHg at pH 7.4 and day
7 (6) to 46 mmHg at day 14 (10). A major cause for the rapid
increase of the oxygen affinity during the second week of incubation
is the changing function of the definitive red cells.Since the total
red cell volume increases about tenfold between day 7 to 14 (11) and
primitive red cell production stops at day 6 to 7 ,it is reasonable

to assume that the cells of F1 represent definitive red cells that have entered the circulation during the last 24 h. Our data indicate that there are distinct differences in the various subpopulations of definitive red cells. Not only are the immature F1 cells characterized by different oxygen affinities and different cooperativity of oxygen binding, there is also some indication that within a population the oxygen affinity increases as the cells mature, since the definitive red cells found in F5 at day 10 must of necessity have been F1 cells at the preceeding stages. However their P_{50} has decreased by about 20 mmHg during maturation.

The mechanisms that are responsible for the increase of the oxygen affinity are not completely understood. While the decrease of the red cell ATP concentration measured in whole blood certainly contributes to the rise in oxygen affinity , other mechanisms also play a role. Thus red cell pH increases during development (12). However, neither of the known cofactors can be made responsible for the observed changes in cooperativity. n-values higher than 4, which is the theoretical limit for a fully cooperative tetramer have been reported for primitive red cells from the chick embryo (2) and have been measured in whole blood from the chick embryo up to day 10 (3).

We have shown, that the principal embryonic hemoglobin HbP forms stable aggregates of at least two tetramers under physiological conditions (13). However, concentrated solutions of HbP do not show elevated cooperativity. High n-values are apparently induced through the interaction of HbP with cellular cofactors that have yet to be identified. The same reasoning can be applied to the data obtained for F1 cells between day 7 to 9. In these cells hemoglobin D is present in a much higher concentration than during later stages of development. Like hemoglobin P hemoglobin D forms stable aggregates(13) of at least two tetramers under physiological conditions and the aggregation is independent of oxygenation . The oxygen binding curve of the concentrated HbD solution displays normal cooperativity, hence we conclude, that the first generations of definitive red cells must contain a factor influencing the cooperativity of the HbD molecule in the same way as HbP; perhaps the factor is identical for both primitive and definitive red cells.

The finding that the oxygen affinity changes drastically within the definitive cell population explains our previous data obtained for embryos incubated in hypoxia (6). Here we observed that definitive cells entered the circulation at an earlier time , we were however unable to correlate the observed increase of hemoglobin oxygen affinity with the amount of circulating adult hemoglobin. The results from the present study show that because of earlier start definitive populations that have a higher oxygen affinity are released at an earlier time than in the normoxic controls. Finally it seems as if within the definitive cell population the factor responsible for the increased cooperativity is not produced in cells that emerge between 9 to 10 days and later. An equally sharp transition in cellular function was observed by Chapman and Tobin (8) who found that up to day nine all circulating definitive red cells contained minor quantities of embryonic hemoglobin,and that cells from later stages apparently had lost the capacity for embryonic hemoglobin synthesis.Thus the morphologically different transient definitive cell populations described by Lemez (5),may also show distinct functional properties.Since the ontogenetic changes in red cell populations and hemoglobin types are very similar for avian species, the results of the present study , especially as regards the function of hemoglobin D, may apply in principle to far more species than the chicken.

REFERENCES

1. J.G. Gilman. Rat embryonic and fetal erythrocytes.High 2,3 - bisphosphoglycerate and low oxygen affinity in vitro for nucleated embryonic red cells.Biochem. J. 192: 335, 1980
2. R. Baumann, S.Padeken and E.A. Haller. Functional properties of embryonic chicken hemoglobins. J. Appl. Physiol. 53: 1439,1982
3. G.N. Lapennas and R. B. Reeves. Oxygen affinity and equilibrium curve shape in blood of chicken embryos. Respir. Physiol. 52: 13, 1983
4. G.A. Bruns and V.M. Ingram. The erythroid cells and hemoglobins of the chick embryo. Philos. Trans. R. Soc. London Ser. B. 266: 225, 1973
5. L. Lemez. Quantitative Studie der fünf Typen der definitiven Erythrozyten (E II) beim Hühnerembryo.Verh. Anat. Ges. 71: 235, 1977
6. R. Baumann, S. Padeken, E.A. Haller and Th. Brilmayer. Effect of hypoxia on oxygen affinity ,hemoglobin pattern and blood volume of early chicken embryos. Am. J. Physiol.244: R 733, 1983
7. L.Cirotto, A. Scotto di Tella and G. Geraci. The hemoglobin of the developing chicken embryos.Fractionation and globin composition of the individual component of total erythrocytes and a single erythrocyte type. Cell Differ. 4: 87, 1975
8. B.S. Chapman and A. J. Tobin. Distribution of developmentally regulated hemoglobin in embryonic erythroid populations .Dev.Biol. 69: 375,1979
9. G.R. Bartlett and T.A. Borgese. Phosphate compounds in red cells of the chicken and duck embryo and hatchling.Comp. Biochem.Physiol. A. 55: 207, 1976
10.H. Tazawa , T. Ono and M. Mochizuki.Oxygen dissociation curve for chorioallantoic blood for chicken embryo.J.Appl. Physiol. 40:393 1976

11. A.L. Romanoff." Biochemistry of the avian embryo. A quantitative analysis of prenatal development",Interscience,New York,1969
12. R.Baumann. Regulation of oxygen affinity of embryonic chicken blood during hypoxia. In press.
13. R. Baumann and G. Gros.A comparative study of the aggregation of avian embryonic and adult hemoglobin.in: " Hemoglobin ". A.G. Schnek and C. Paul eds. Editions de l'Université de Bruxelles, Brussels,1984

RED CELL O_2 TRANSPORT AT ALTITUDE AND ALTITUDE TRAINING

Heimo Mairbäurl and Wolfgang Schobersberger

Department of Physiology
University of Innsbruck
A - 6020 Innsbruck
Austria

INTRODUCTION

Ascent to altitude brings people, who are adapted to low elevations, into a more or less hypoxic environment. The degreé of hypoxia depends on the altitude. It has to be distinguished between moderate altitude, which we understand to be between 1600 m and 3500 m above sea level, and high altitude, which are elevations higher than 3500 m. This distinction is necessary from a physiological point of view, since different mechanisms are involved in the adaptation of oxygen transport by the erythrocyte to moderate altitude or high altitude.

At high altitude the oxygen content of the alveolar gas is reduced to an extent which diminishes dramatically blood oxygenation in the lungs. Oxygen saturation of hemoglobin is far from complete. Among other mechanisms an increase in the oxygen binding capacity by stimulating erythropoiesis helps to maintain oxygen delivery to the tissues (10). Besides, an increase in the hemoglobin oxygen affinity occurs to improve the oxygen extraction in the lungs (5). The latter might impair the unloading of oxygen from hemoglobin in the blood capillaries, since oxygen is bound more tightly. This might result in a decrease in the exercise performance capacity at high altitude.

The situation at moderate altitude is different. The oxygen tension is reduced slightly, but only to an extent which does not impair blood oxygenation in the lungs very much. In fact, normally the hemoglobin oxygen saturation does not decrease below 90%. The oxygen supply to tissue should therefore not be impaired.

Nevertheless the organism responds to the slightly hypoxic environment with immediate hyperventilation, which lasts for a short period of time until the respiratory system adapts. In the meanwhile a second mechanism is induced. It concerns the oxygen transport by the erythrocyte: The concentration of 2,3-DPG in the erythrocyte increases within a few hours after the ascent to altitude (8) or after exposure to air with low oxygen content (14). 2,3-DPG remains then elevated during the whole period of staying at moderate altitude. Parallel to the increase in the concentration of 2,3-DPG the oxygen affinity of hemoglobin is lowered, which means that the oxygen unloading from hemoglobin is improved.

The situation is peculiar: On one hand the oxygen uptake is not impaired, so that tissue oxygenation should be normal, on the other hand mechanisms are induced which improve tissue oxygenation, which is not necessary as the oxygen demand is about the same at this elevation as compared to sea level.

Both the reason for the above described effects of moderate altitude on hemoglobin oxygen transport, and the mechanisms which cause 2,3-DPG to increase and therefore decrease the hemoglobin oxygen affinity, are yet unknown. The present study should provide further information on the mechanisms involved in the increase in red cell 2,3-DPG, and should evaluate the contribution of exercise performance at altitude to altitude adaptation.

MATERIALS AND METHODS

Twelve healthy males (mean age 21 years) participated in an altitude study which was performed in a mountain lodge at an elevation of 2300 m above sea level in midwinter. The study at altitude lasted 13 days. Six of the subjects behaved passively during the stay (controls), the remaining ones performed a bicycle ergometer training at 75% of their maximal exercise performance capacity for 45 min daily, except on days before a test. The training was controlled by monitoring the heart rate.

Incremental bicycle ergometer tests were performed before, within 48 hours after the ascent, at the end of the stay at altitude, as well as after the descent to record exercise performance during the study. In the tests the beginning work load was 50 W and was increased by 50 W every 2 min until subjective exhaustion. Heart rates at each work load, maximal work capacity (W/kg) and the concentration of lactate in cubital venous blood in exhaustion were determined in the exercise tests performed during the stay at altitude. In pre- and post-altitude tests the maximal oxygen uptake ($\dot{V}_{O_2}$, mlO_2/min.kg) and the anaerobic treshold (at 4 mmol/l lactate, expressed in % of max. work capacity) were determined in addition to the other exercise parameters.

Blood samples were collected from antecubital veins before each exercise test (rest). The blood was immediately heparinized (10 IU/ml). Hemoglobin (Hb), hematocrit (Hct), red cell count (RBC) and reticulocyte counts were determined by standard hematological methods. The metabolic substrates glucose, lactate, ATP and 2,3-DPG were determined from 1:7 extracts of blood in perchloric acid using test kits from Böhringer (FRG) and Sigma Chemicals (USA).

As a measure for the hemoglobin oxygen affinity the P-50 value was determined (oxygen tension at 50% oxygen saturation of hemoglobin). The Hill coefficient was calculated for the middle part of the oxygen dissociation curve. Therefore blood samples were equilibrated to gas mixtures, which were prepared from pure O_2, CO_2 and N_2 to achieve an oxygen saturation of hemoglobin in the range of a) 40 to 50% and b) between 50 and 60%. CO_2 was kept constant at 40 mmHg. The oxygen saturation was determined in the equilibrated samples using an OSM 2a (Radiometer, Denmark). The pH was measured in the equilibrated samples for pH-correction of the P-50 value.

RESULTS

Red Cell Parameters

In blood samples collected at rest the hemoglobin concentration decreased slightly during the stay in both groups (-4.5±7 g/l, p< 0.8),and no change in hematocrit and red cell counts was measured. Reticulocytes were already increased significantly within 2 days after the ascent and continued to increase during the stay at altitude. This increase was more pronounced in training subjects as compared to controls (p<0.1). After the descent the reticulocyte counts decreased but were still above pre-altitude values (figure 1a).

The concentration of 2,3-DPG increased after the ascent to altitude (figure 1b). At the start of the stay at altitude this elevation was about 0.7 μmol/gHb in controls, but about 1.9 μmol/gHb in training subjects as compared to pre-altitude values. Towards the end of the stay at altitude an additional increase in red cell 2,3-DPG was found in both control and training subjects. After the descent 2,3-DPG concentration decreased slightly below pre-altitude values in controls. A decrease was also found in training subjects, but the values remained significantly above pre-altitude 2,3-DPG. The concentration of ATP was 627±31 μmol/l blood in both groups initially and did not change significantly in neither group during the stay at altitude or after the descent.

Figure 2 shows the actual P-50 values and the actual Hill coefficients during this altitude study. It can be seen that in both groups the P-50 value increased from 25.8 mmHg to about 28.4 mmHg right after the ascent to altitude. This high value was maintained during the stay in training subjects. In contrast in control subjects the P-50 value decreased significantly during the first half of the stay at altitude by about 1 mmHg as compared to early altitude values and remained at this lower level. After the descent the P-50 values decreased as compared to altitude values but remained still about 1 mmHg higher than pre-altitude values.

The Hill coefficients did not change within 2 days after the

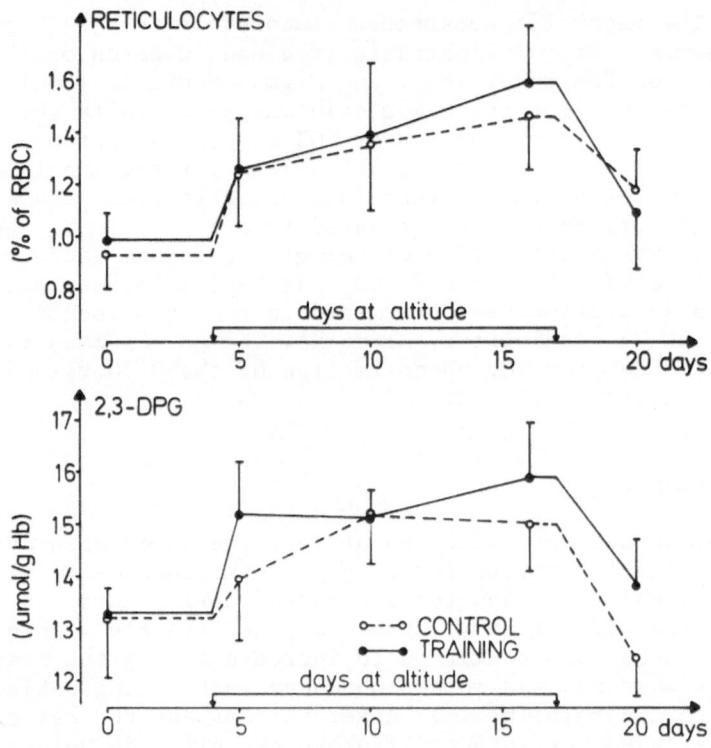

Figure 1: Reticulocyte counts and red cell concentration of 2,3-DPG (means ± S.Dev.) during the altitude study.

ascent to altitude, neither in controls nor in training subjects (figure 2). But with prolonged stay at altitude the Hill coefficient decreased consistently in controls, but increased significantly in training subjects. After the descent the Hill coefficient normalized in controls, but remained increased in the training group. No changes in arterial pH and P_{CO_2} were found in the study.

Exercise Parameters

The maximal work capacity decreased significantly after the arrival at altitude (-10%), but normalized during the stay at altitude (table 1). After the descent the maximal work capacity was unchanged in controls, but was elevated significantly by about 8% in training individuals as compared to pre-altitude values. No change in the maximal oxygen uptake was found during the study. The anaerobic treshold was unchanged in controls, but increased significantly in training subjects by about 12.5% after the stay at altitude as compared to pre-altitude.

The maximal heart rate (in exhaustion) was significantly lower at altitude (table 1) as compared to pre- or post-altitude values. This effect was significantly higher in training subjects than in controls. Not only in exhaustion, but also during the exercise tests

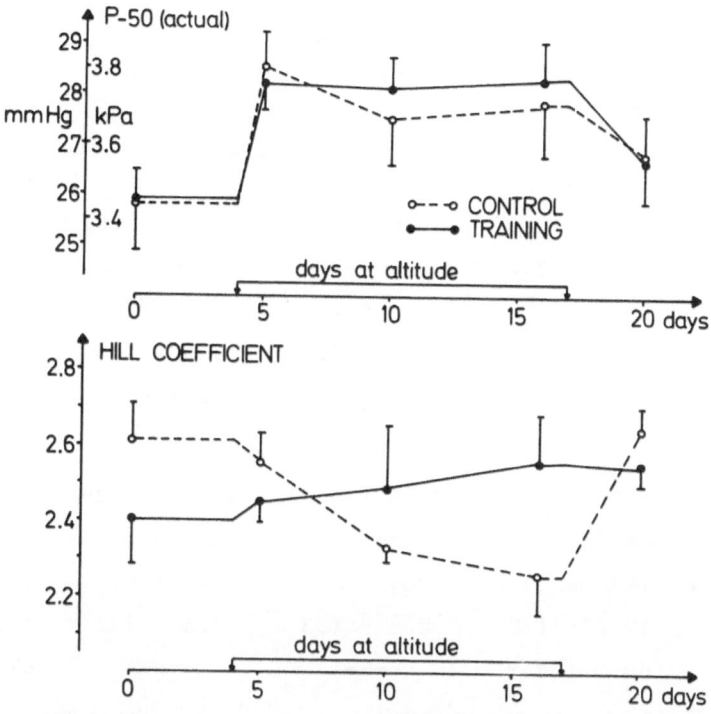

Figure 2: Actual P-50 values and Hill coefficients (means ± S.Dev)
before, during and after a 13-day stay at altitude.

at all work loads the heart rates were lower, in controls by
about 10 to 13/min after the ascent to altitude. This lowered value
was maintained during the stay at altitude and shifted towards normal after the descent. It remained then still lower than during the
pre-altitude exercise tests. In training subjects the heart rates
during the exercise tests were lowered by about the same as in controls. But there was an additional decrease in the heart rates during the exercise tests found at the end of the stay at altitude
(- 15 to - 20/min as compared to pre-altitude values). These lower
heart rates were maintained also after descent in the training group.

The concentration of lactate in venous blood collected in exhaustion was significantly lower during the stay at altitude as
compared to pre- or post-altitude values, significantly more pronounced in training subjects as compared to controls (table 1).

DISCUSSION

Red Cell Metabolism

A decrease in the hemoglobin oxygen affinity as an effective
mechanism for the adaptation to moderate altitude or any hypoxic
environment has been described earlier (11). In many reports as

Table 1: Exercise parameters (determined in exhaustion) before, during and after staying at altitude (2300 m). Mean values ± S.D.

CONTROL:	before	altitude beginning	end	
Work load	4.21 ± 0.37	3.90 ± 0.45	4.09 ± 0.67	4.37 ± 0.39
$\dot{V}_{O_2}$	49.6 ± 3.4	----	----	47.5 ± 3.2
Heart rate	200 ± 8	192 ± 7	186 ± 7	197 ± 7
Lactate	11.9 ± 1.3	8.5 ± 2.0	9.5 ± 1.4	12.0 ± 1.1
AT	58.3 ± 7.5	----	----	61.8 ± 7.1
TRAINING:				
Work load	4.02 ± 0.32	3.58 ± 0.38	4.01 ± 0.29	4.32 ± 0.22
$\dot{V}_{O_2}$	45.9 ± 1.1	----	----	44.5 ± 1.9
Heart rate	197 ± 11	190 ± 6	179 ± 7	191 ± 8
Lactate	12.6 ± 1.0	8.2 ± 1.3	7.6 ± 1.1	11.2 ± 0.9
AT	60.2 ± 4.8	----	----	67.8 ± 2.4

Work load (W/kg); $\dot{V}_{O_2}$ (maximal O_2 uptake, ml/min.kg); heart rate (beats/min); lactate (mmol/l); AT (anaerobic treshold, % of maximal work load).

well as in this one the decrease in Hb-O_2-affinity (increase in P-50 value) was paralleled by an elevation of red cell 2,3-DPG concentration. The attempt of explaining the increased P-50 value found within 2 days after the ascent to altitude quantitatively by the increase in 2,3-DPG fails in control subjects: The measured increase in 2,3-DPG accounts for only about 60% of the decrease in the Hb-O_2-affinity, when using a factor of $\Delta \log P_{O_2}/\Delta DPG = 0.01$ for the calculations of the DPG-effect on P-50 value.[2] There have to be other factors influencing the oxygen affinity of hemoglobin acutely after an ascent to altitude, which are yet unknown. After prolonged stay (more than one week) at altitude the concentration of 2,3-DPG continues to increase and reaches values high enough to explain the increase in the P-50 value quantitatively in both controls and training subjects.

Unknown, besides factors inducing the decrease in Hb-O_2-affinity shortly after ascent to altitude, is furthermore the mechanism which induces the increase in 2,3-DPG concentration in the red cell at altitude. Several factors can be discussed as possible explanations:

One might be alkalosis, which stimulates the red cell metabolism under certain conditions and thereby causes an increase in erythrocyte 2,3-DPG. A respiratory alkalosis was not found in this study throughout the whole period of staying at altitude. Mild alkalosis has been described to occur within a few hours after transfer into an hypoxic environment (8) like altitude or the low pressure chamber. But this alkalosis was not high enough to be able to explain the high increase in 2,3-DPG, as can be seen from the experiments of Rapoport et al. (13). In addition, all studies published on adaptation to moderate altitude showed that alkalosis was compensated within a few days after the ascent, but the concentration of 2,3-DPG remained still high or even tended to increase further (7).

A stimulation of glycolysis in order to increase red cell 2,3-DPG concentration might be caused by other factors than alkalosis. It might be induced by hormones like catecholamines and/or corticosteroids. Both hormones have been shown to decrease the hemoglobin oxygen affinity by increasing red cell 2,3-DPG concentration (2,9,12). So hormonal stimulation of red cell metabolism after acute exposure to altitude may cause the increase in 2,3-DPG.

Also a stimulation of erythropoiesis can lead to an increase in the concentration of 2,3-DPG. Young erythrocytes have a higher metabolic activity (6) and therefore produce more 2,3-DPG as compared to old ones. So an increasing number of young erythrocytes circulating in the blood may cause an overall increase in 2,3-DPG concentration. It can be seen in figure 1 that the number of reticulocytes increases after the ascent to altitude, indicating a stimulated erythropoiesis. This decrease in the mean age of circulating erythrocytes might be another factor contributing to the elevation of 2,3-DPG after prolonged stay at moderate altitude, but not after acute exposure to this environment. Although erythropoiesis seems to be stimulated, the hemoglobin concentration did not change significantly. This might be explained by an increased sequestration of older red cells at altitude or altitude training.

It was found in this study that all parameters of red cell metabolism are changed more in training subjects as compared to control ones during the stay at altitude. Therefore it can be concluded that the adaptation to moderate altitude occurs independently of performing exercise at altitude. Exercise seems to act as a separate stimulus for changing red cell function and decreasing the hemoglobin oxygen affinity, thus adding to the mechanism of passive adaptation to altitude.

Exercise performance

Exercise performance capacity is reduced after the ascent to altitude as has been shown in this study as well as by others (15), but normalizes after about two weeks of staying at altitude. The reason is not quite clear. The heart rate during rest and exercise, even in exhaustion, is significantly lower at altitude as compared to pre- or post-altitude values. This indicates that the cardiac output is decreased at rest and during exercise performance at altitude. This might, of course, impair the exercise performance capacity at altitude. But after prolonged stay at altitude the exercise performance capacity is restored and heart rates during exercise are still low or lowered even more, indicating a still decreased cardiac output. Other studies support this finding, describing a decreased stroke volume and a slightly decreased heart rate at rest and during exercise during a ten-day stay at altitude (1). So the argument of a decreased work capacity due to a decreased cardiac output does not hold. There is no sign of tissue hypoxia due to a decreased cardiovascular activity.

Another factor indicating that there is no hypoxia during performance of exercise at altitude is the decreased lactate concentration in exhaustion, which was found in this study as well as by others (3). This would even imply that there is more oxygen available during exercise at altitude as compared to lower elevations, and that anaerobic energy production is not required to the same extent.

But how can the organism perform exercise at altitude comparable in strength to that performed at lower elevations having a decreased cardiac output and a diminished anaerobic energy production? The answer to this question is speculative. The reason for the more efficient performance at altitude may be found in the change in red cell oxygen transport at moderate altitude. As described above the oxygen affinity of hemoglobin decreases shortly after the ascent to altitude and remains lowered during prolonged stay. A right shift of the oxygen dissociation curve, as indicated by the increased P-50 values, indicates that the arterio-venous oxygen difference ($AVDO_2$) is higher to maintain a certain tissue oxygen tension, as oxygen is unloaded more easily from hemoglobin. In fact, using the data on $AVDO_2$ during exercise at altitude (1), an increase in P-50 value to about the same extent as described in this study can be calculated.

Doing these estimations the other way round by using the P-50 values and Hill coefficients determined in the present study, oxygen dissociation curves (ODC) can be calculated from the Hill plot. Using data on the oxygen tension in femoral-venous blood during rest (45 mmHg) and exercise (21 mmHg) (4), at constant blood hemoglobin concentration of 160 g/l, the $AVDO_2$ can be calculated. These values are listed in table 2. It can be seen that there is an increase in the $AVDO_2$ at altitude as compared to pre- and post-altitude values in both controls and training individuals. At rest the $AVDO_2$ is increased more at altitude in controls as compared to training subjects. In contrast, at exercise, at a low PO_2, the change in the $AVDO_2$ is higher in the training subjects than in controls. This can be explained by the changes in the position and the shape of the ODC during altitude adaptation: In controls altitude adaptation induces a right shift of the ODC by a flattening of the curve. In training subjects the ODC is shifted towards the right and the slope is increased. This combination results in an improved release of oxygen from hemoglobin at low oxygen tensions and is therefore an advantage during exercise performance.

Table 2: Calculated arterio-venous oxygen differences (ml O_2/100 ml of blood) before, during and after a 13-day stay at an altitude of 2300 m above sea level.

	femoral-venous blood at[*]:	
	rest	exercise
CONTROL:		
pre-altitude	2.43	12.04
begin-altitude	3.38	13.00
end-altitude	3.67	12.41
post-altitude	2.92	12.77
TRAINING:		
pre-altitude	2.81	11.83
begin-altitude	3.05	12.74
end-altitude	3.25	13.20
post-altitude	3.16	12.80

[*] For oxygen tensions see text. The calculations are based on actually measured arterial O_2 saturations, and venous O_2 saturations calculated from the Hill plot.

It can be summarized that adaptation to moderate altitude of red cell oxygen transport occurs independently of performing exercise at altitude. Altitude training provides an additional positive effect resulting in an improved tissue oxygenation as compared to people who adapt passively. Since the effects induced are maintained for a certain periode of time even after descent, a higher exercise performance capacity in healthy subjects, or a significant improvement of patients with cardio-vascular disease might result.

REFERENCES

1) ALEXANDER,J.K., L.H.HARTLEY, M.MODELSKI and R.F.GROVER (1967). Reduction of stroke volume during exercise in man following ascent to 3100 m altitude. J.Appl.Physiol. 23:849-858.
2) BAUER,C. and A.M. RATHSCHLAG-SCHÄFER (1968). The influence of aldosterone and cortisol on oxygen affinity and cation concentration of the blood. Respir.Physiol. 5:360-370.
3) CUNNINGHAM,D.A. and J.R.MAGEL (1970). The effect of moderate altitude on post-exercise lactate. Int.Z.angew.Physiol. 29:94-100.
4) DOLL,E., J.KEUL and C.MAIWALD (1968). Oxygen tension and acid base equilibria in venous blood of working muscle. Am.J.Physiol. 215:23-29.

5) EATON,J., T.D.SELTON and E.BERGER (1974). Survival at extreme altitude: Protective effect of increased hemoglobin-oxygen affinity. Science 183:743-744.

6) FORNAINI,G., M.MAGNANI, M.DACHA and V.STICCHI (1978). Relationship between glucose phosphorylating activities and erythrocyte age. Mech.Aging Develop. 8:249-256.

7) HUMPELER,E., K.INAMA and P.DEETJEN (1979). Improvement of tissue oxygenation during a 20 day's stay at moderate altitude in connection with mild exercise. Klin.Wschr. 57:267-272.

8) HUMPELER,E., K.INAMA and H.JUNGMANN (1980). Die Sauerstoffaffinität des Hämoglobins 3 Stunden nach passivem Höhenwechsel von 400 auf 1800 m. Wiener Klin.Wschr. 92:326-332.

9) HUMPELER,E., F.SKRABAL and G.BARTSCH (1980). Influence of exposure to moderate altitude on plasma concentrations of cortisol, aldosterone, renin, testosterone and gonadotropins. Eur.J.Appl.Physiol. 45:167-176.

10) HURTADO,A., C.F.MERINO and D.DEGADO (1945). Influence of anoxemia on the hematopoetic activity. Arch.Intern.Med. 75:284-323.

11) LENFANT,C., J.D.TORRANCE, R.WOODSON and C.A.FINCH (1970). Adaptation to hypoxia. In: Red Cell Metabolism and Function, G.BREwer, ed. p. 203-212. New York, Plenum Press.

12) MAIRBÄURL,H., and E.HUMPELER (1981). In vitro influences of adrenaline on erythrocyte metabolism and on oxygen affinity of hemoglobin. In: The Red Cell: Fifth Ann Arbor Conference, G. BREWER,ed. p.311-319. New York, A.R. Liss.

13) RAPOPORT,I., T.A.RAPOPORT and S.M.RAPOPORT (1978). Analysis of pH-induced changes of glycolysis of human erythrocytes. Acta Biol.Med.Germ. 37:393-401.

14) RÖRTH,M., F.NYGAARD and H.H.PARVING (1972). Effect of exposure to simulated high altitude on human red cell phosphates and oxygen affinity of Hb. Influence of exercise. Scand.J.clin.Lab.Invest. 29:329-333.

15) TURKMENOW,M.T. and J.J.IMANKULOV (1975). Human work capacity at high altitude. Xogm.Biol.Aviakosm.Med. 9:70.

504

MODELLING WHOLE BLOOD OXYGEN EQUILIBRIUM: COMPARISON

OF NINE DIFFERENT MODELS FITTED TO NORMAL HUMAN DATA

J.F. O'Riordan,[1] T.K. Goldstick,[1] L.N. Vida,[2]
G.R. Honig,[2] and J.T. Ernest[3]

[1]Department of Chemical Engineering, Northwestern
University, Evanston, IL 60201
[2]Department of Pediatrics, University of Illinois,
Chicago, IL 60612
[3]Department of Ophthalmology, University of Illinois Eye
and Ear Infirmary, Chicago, IL 60612

ABSTRACT

The ability of nine different models, prominent in the literature, to meaningfully characterize the oxygen-hemoglobin equilibrium
curve (OHEC) of normal individuals was examined. Previously reported
data (N=33), obtained using the DCA-1 (Radiometer, Copenhagen), and
new data (N=8), obtained using the Hemox-Analyzer (TCS, Southampton,
PA), from blood samples of normal, non-smoking volunteers were used
and these devices were found to give statistically similar results.
The OHECs were digitized and fitted to the models using least-squares
techniques developed in this laboratory. The "goodness-of-fit" was
determined by the root-mean-squared (RMS) error, the number of parameters, and the parameter redundancy, i.e., correlation between the
parameters. The best RMS error did not necessarily indicate the best
model. Most literature models consist of ratios of similar-order
polynomials. These showed considerable parameter redundancy which
made the curve fitting difficult. The best fits gave RMS errors as
low as 0.2% saturation. The Hill model gave a good characterization
over the saturation range 20%-98% with RMS errors of about 0.6% saturation. On the other hand, good characterizations over the entire
range were given by several other models. The relative advantages
and disadvantages of each model have been compared as well as the
difficulties in fitting several of the models. No single model is
best under all circumstances. The best model depends upon the particular circumstances for which it is to be utilized.

INTRODUCTION

The oxygen-hemoglobin equilibrium curve (OHEC) is used widely in clinical and basic research to determine hemoglobin abnormalities and identify oxygen transport deficiences. It is helpful to have a mathematical description of the OHEC in order to make comparisons among the OHECs of different individuals. By far the most commonly used characterization of the OHEC is the Hill model (1910) which unfortunately applies over only a limited saturation range (20% to 98%). This, however, is the range of major physiological interest. Numerous other models have appeared in the literature. It is possible that one or more of these might better describe the OHEC and be capable of covering the complete saturation range as well as having parameters which are of greater theoretical significance than the Hill parameters P_{50} and n. Nevertheless, no systematic, comparative study of the many reported models has been previously attempted using a large, accurate pool of normal human data.

We applied the nine models shown in Table I to 41 sets of OHEC data from 36 normal, non-smoking, sedentary adults to determine model parameters. These models were tested for accuracy of fit, quality of fit (RMS error), singularities and local minima in the sum-of-squares (SOS) function, redundancy of parameters (parameter correlation) and physical significance of the parameters.

One of the earliest models, that of Haldane (Douglas et al., 1912), has been historically overshadowed by the earlier Hill model. Haldane, like Hill, believed that the fundamental Hb subunit existed in an aggregated state. But Haldane theorized that the aggregation was a function of saturation whereas Hill had previously proposed that it consisted of a constant number of Hb subunits. Although today it is known that neither model is theoretically correct, the Hill model is still widely used for empirical characterization of the OHEC. Unlike all of the other models discussed here, the Haldane model predicts PO_2 from saturation and the complexity of the equation prevents a simple transformation that would allow prediction of saturation. This prevented us from making a complete comparison of it with the other models of Table I.

Adair's stepwise hypothesis of 1925 paved the way for the modern conception of the hemoglobin molecule. Adair proposed that four oxygen molecules bind to a single Hb molecule sequentially, giving four equilibrium constants, one for each sequential reaction. This was the first of several models in which the equation for saturation consisted of a ratio of closely ordered polynomials. This type of equation is difficult to fit because the parameters are rather closely correlated (i.e., the parameters are redundant). The Pauling (1935) model has only two parameters which arise from an energy analysis of a proposed hemoglobin reaction mechanism. One (K) describes the energy of the $Hb-O_2$ reaction while the other (alpha) is a measure

Table I. Models describing the Oxygen-Hemoglobin Equilibrium Curve.

MODEL NAME	EQUATION

Hill (1910)

$$Y = \frac{(P/P_{50})^n}{1 + (P/P_{50})^n}$$

$P \equiv PO_2$, torr

$Y \equiv$ fractional sat.

Haldane (1912)

$$P = \frac{KY(1 - b(1-Y))}{(1-y)(1+aY)}$$

Adair (1925)

$$Y = \frac{a_1 P + 2a_2 P^2 + 3a_3 P^3 + 4a_4 P^4}{4(1 + a_1 P + a_2 P^2 + a_3 P^3 + a_4 P^4)}$$

Pauling (1935)

$$Y = \frac{KP + (2\alpha+1)K^2 P^2 + 3\alpha^2 K^3 P^3 + \alpha^4 K^4 P^4}{1 + 4KP + (4\alpha+2)K^2 P^2 + 4\alpha^2 K^3 P^3 + \alpha^4 K^4 P^4}$$

Margaria (1963)

$$Y = \frac{\left[\frac{1 + KP}{KP}\right]^3 + m - 1}{\left[\frac{1 + KP}{KP}\right]^4 + m - 1}$$

MWC (1965)

$$Y = \frac{LcX(1 + cX)^3 + X(1+ X)^3}{L(1 + cX)^4 + (1 + X)^4}$$

$X \equiv K_R P$

Kelman (1966)

$$Y = \frac{a_1 P + a_2 P^2 + a_3 P^3 + P^4}{a_4 + a_5 P + a_6 P^2 + a_7 P^3 + P^4}$$

Severinghaus (1979)

$$Y = \left[\frac{a}{P^3 + bP} + 1\right]^{-1}$$

Easton (1979)

$$Y = (Y_m - Y_a)\left[\frac{-Y_a}{Y_m - Y_a}\right]^{e^{-KP}} + Y_a$$

of the energy of interaction between Hb subunits. Another model
(Wyman, 1948) fitted the OHEC to the Hill model but used the Hill parameters P_{50} and n to further predict other parameters based on an
assumed, theoretical Hb structure. Since Wyman's mathematical description of the OHEC is identical to the Hill equation, the results
with his model would simply repeat the Hill results and so were
omitted. Margaria (1963) simplified the Adair model by equating the
first three equilibrium constants because they were of similar magnitude while the fourth was much higher. Criticism of Adair's assumptions has also led to other hypotheses such as the recent Monod-
Wyman-Changeux (MWC) model (Monod et al., 1965). The MWC model is
the only theoretical approach supported by experimental observation
(Perutz, 1978). As will later be shown, the MWC model is equivalent
to the Margaria model. Recently there have been attempts to develop
even more complex models (Perutz, 1978) in order to take into account
some deficiencies in the above models. These, however, were beyond
the scope of this study. Being the most theoretically correct equation, the MWC model was expected to give the best results.

Empirical models include the Kelman (1966) model. Kelman completely generalized the Adair equation parameters, thus allowing
greater flexibility. Unfortunately, this also caused the parameter
redundancy to reach unacceptable levels. The Severinghaus (1979)
model is also a purely empirical model with completely arbitrary parameters. But since it arises from the Hill equation, it is a much
different type of model than the polynomial ratios. Actuarial mathematics provided Easton (1979) with an equation that fitted the OHEC
surprisingly well. Furthermore, unlike some other models this equation gives a non-zero derivative at zero PO_2, as found experimentally. The model must be used in its most general form to obtain a good
fit. This, however, increases parameter redundancy. Easton includes
the parameter B, which describes the leftward or rightward shift of
the OHEC, in his model, much like the Hill parameter P_{50}. The Easton
parameter B is simply a grouping of his parameters Y_a and Y_m, such
that: $B = \ln ((Y_a - Y_m)/Y_a)$. Also, his parameter K is supposed to
determine the slope of the OHEC, like the Hill parameter n.

Other models are certainly possible and modifications of literature models have been considered by us. However, it was the purpose
of our study to examine only the models that have been previously reported in the literature.

METHODS

A set of 33 OHECs previously reported (O'Riordan et al., 1983),
in addition to eight OHECs (for three individuals) obtained using the
Hemox-Analyzer (TCS Medical Products Div., Southampton, PA, USA) were
individually fitted to all nine models. The continuous curves from
the Hemox-Analyzer were digitized every 2.5 torr on the PO_2 axis

using a graphics tablet (Tektronix model 4954, Tektronix, Beaverton, OR, USA). All OHECs were either determined at or corrected to pH 7.40 and 37.0°C.

A nonlinear regression and graphics routine, reported previously by us (O'Riordan et al., 1983), was used to fit each model to each set of OHEC data. Most OHECs were fitted using the Gauss method (Robinson, 1981) to search for the minimum sum-of-squares (SOS). The Marquardt method (Robinson 1981) usually gives faster convergence but could rarely be employed here because of the problems of parameter redundancy and scaling. All equations were fitted to unweighted data sets. The points from each OHEC data set were distributed evenly

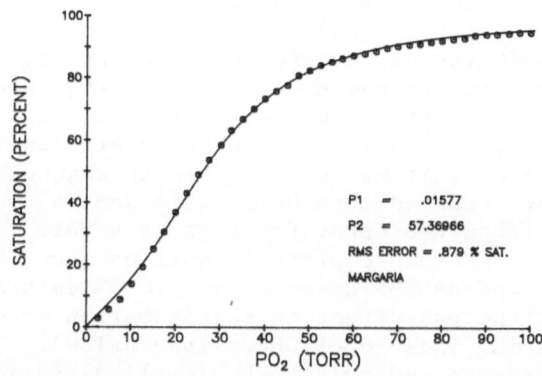

Figure 1. Typical fit of the oxygen-hemoglobin equilibrium curve.

over the PO_2 range from 0 to approximately 100 torr. Initial estimates of the parameters in each model were obtained either from the literature or found by trial and error. No parameters were fixed or limited even though physical interpretation may have suggested some bounds. This was done in order to obtain the best possible fit. The convergence criteria for the SOS minimization routine was a relative change of less than 1.5×10^{-8} for all parameters on two succesive iterations. The residuals of each fit were examined to determine the quality of the fit. RMS errors and parameter values were compared between models. Linear regression was performed between some model parameters and the Hill P_{50} and n to evaluate the physical significance of the model parameters.

RESULTS

A typical fit is shown in Figure 1, in this case for an OHEC obtained with the Hemox Analyzer (12/2/82 12:40). The residuals resulting from fitting this typical OHEC to eight of the models are shown in Figure 2 as functions of saturation (Figure 2A) and PO_2 (Figure 2B). The Haldane model was not included here because it cannot predict saturation. Because the OHECs were digitized at equal intervals of PO_2, there is a cluster of points at high saturation in Figure 2A. One measure of the quality of a fit is the number of times the residuals change sign. The Hill model residuals cross zero seven times, somewhat more than usual. Of course there are large residuals at saturations below 20% because these data were not included in the fit. Although the Margaria and MWC model residuals each cross zero only four times below 90% saturation, these models appear to follow the data just as closely as the Hill model. On the other hand, the Severinghaus model residuals, which also cross zero four times, exhibits marked deviations from the data which result in an unusually high RMS error (1.6% saturation). Figure 2 also demonstrates for this particular OHEC (as we have found for every other OHEC we have studied) that the Margaria and MWC models fit the data almost identically. Adair's model, with nine zero crossings, fits the data very well but the parameter a_3 was found to be indeterminate, tending towards zero. Therefore, it was set to zero throughout. The residuals for Pauling's model crossed zero only twice and, as would be expected, gave a very large RMS error for this data set. Also, as expected, the 7-parameter Kelman empirical equation gave the best fit with 12 zero crossings and an RMS error of only 0.3% saturation. However, the redundancy of the parameters in this equation makes it almost useless for comparing individual OHECs (see below). The Easton model gave six zero crossings and only rather small deviations in the residuals compared to other models. It rivals the Adair model in its fit without the problem of having an indeterminate parameter.

Aggregate parameter values, RMS error and parameter correlation (redundancy), all with their coefficient of variation, were obtained for the 33 OHECs determined using the DCA-1 (Table II) and the averages for each of the three individuals determined using the Hemox-Analyzer (Table III). Coefficients of variation $(SD/\overline{x})$ were given rather than standard errors to provide a better measure of the spread of parameter values. Only the highest parameter correlation for each model is included. No significant differences were found in any parameter values or RMS errors between the DCA-1 and Hemox-Analyzer data using a two-tailed t-test with $p < .05$. Results from the two different devices could therefore have been lumped together although this was not done here.

Reich and Zinke (1974) first pointed out the redundancy in the parameters in several models for the OHEC. This redundancy is clearly seen in the inter-parameter correlation (normalized covariance)

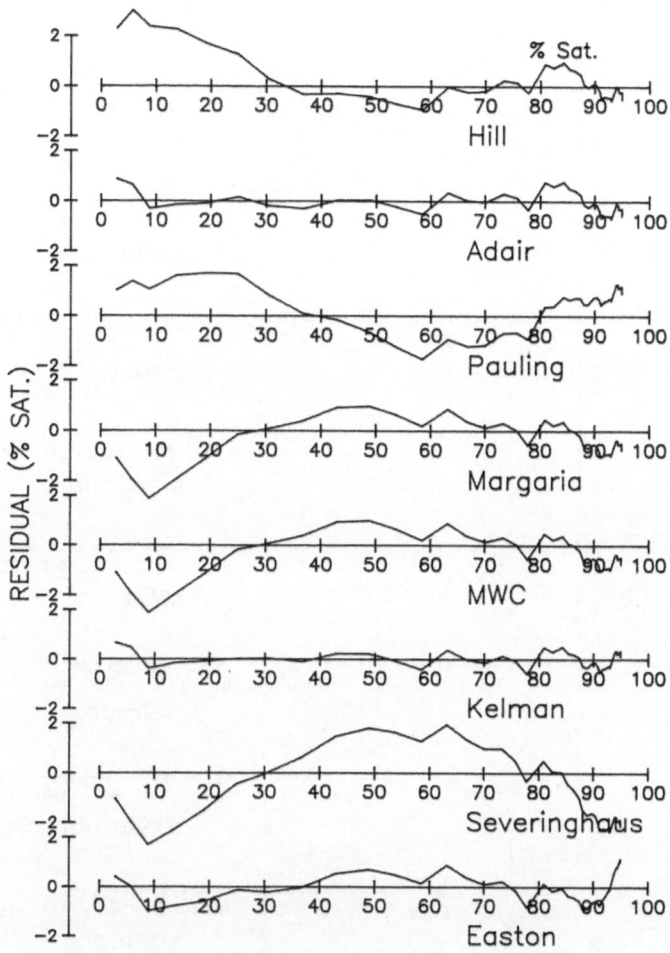

Figure 2A. Residuals for typical fits for one OHEC vs. saturation

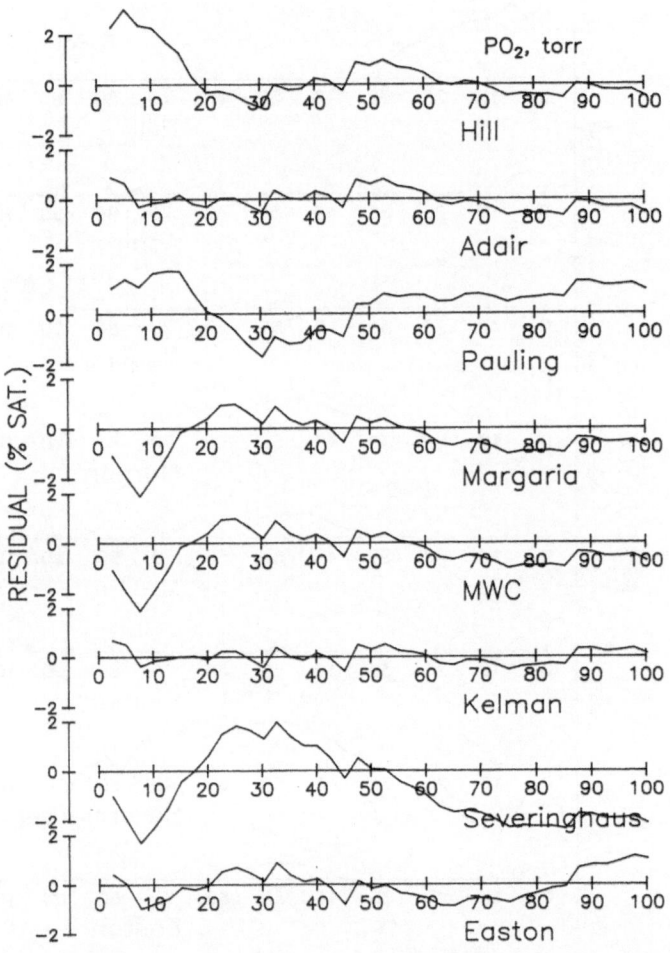

Figure 2B. Residuals for typical fits for one OHEC vs. PO_2.

Table II. Parameter values, RMS errors, and parameter correlation for DCA-1 data fit to each model.

MODEL	SAT. RANGE FITTED	PARAMETERS ± COEFFICIENT OF VARIATION	RMS ERROR (% sat.)	PARAMETER CORRELATION
Hill	20 – 98	$26.2 \pm 3.1\%$ P_{50} $2.50 \pm 2.7\%$ n	$0.488 \pm 25\%$	$0.505 \pm 3.0\%$
Haldane	0 – 100	$3.08 \pm 4.7\%$ K $0.350 \pm 83\%$ a $-22.0 \pm 32\%$ b	$1.767 \pm 14\%$ *torr	$0.982 \pm 0.6\%$ K vs. a
Adair	0 – 100	$0.0181 \pm 37\%$ a_1 $0.00147 \pm 14\%$ a_2 $2.56 \times 10^{-6} \pm 15\%$ a_4	$0.409 \pm 24\%$	$0.805 \pm 18\%$ a_1 vs. a_4
Pauling	0 – 100	$9.12 \pm 8.0\%$ alpha $0.00422 \pm 8.3\%$ K	$1.133 \pm 20\%$	$-0.990 \pm 0\%$
Margaria	0 – 100	$0.0120 \pm 6.6\%$ K $153 \pm 22\%$ m	$0.922 \pm 20\%$	$-0.989 \pm 0.2\%$
MWC	0 – 100	$7.54 \times 10^{-7} \pm 2.9\%$ K_R $9.03 \times 10^{-9} \pm 5.5\%$ c $1.02 \times 10^{30} \pm 3.0\%$ L	$0.931 \pm 20\%$	$-1.000 \pm 0\%$ K_R, c vs. L
Kelman	0 – 100	$-6.33 \times 10^{6} \pm 620\%$ a_1 $5.22 \times 10^{5} \pm 680\%$ a_2 $-1.12 \times 10^{5} \pm 1000\%$ a_3 $-8.04 \times 10^{8} \pm 550\%$ a_4 $-7.84 \times 10^{7} \pm 1130\%$ a_5 $9.72 \times 10^{5} \pm 1240\%$ a_6 $-1.14 \times 10^{5} \pm 1020\%$ a_7	$0.237 \pm 87\%$	See text.
Severinghaus	0 – 100	$2.63 \times 10^{4} \pm 10\%$ a $252 \pm 17\%$ b	$0.941 \pm 33\%$	$0.842 \pm 1.2\%$
Easton	0 – 100	$0.0691 \pm 2.7\%$ K $-0.0177 \pm 19\%$ Y_a $0.958 \pm 0.8\%$ Y_m	$0.595 \pm 15\%$	$0.932 \pm 0.4\%$ K vs. Y_a

513

Table III. Parameter values, RMS errors, and parameter correlation for Hemo-Analyzer data fit to each model.

MODEL	SAT. RANGE FITTED	PARAMETERS ± COEFFICIENT OF VARIATION			RMS ERROR (% sat.)	PARAMETER CORRELATION
Hill	20 - 98	$24.6 \pm 11\%$ P_{50}	$2.57 \pm 8.1\%$ n		$0.671 \pm 24\%$	$0.469 \pm 7.2\%$
Haldane	0 - 100	$1.53 \pm 65\%$ K	$-0.0567 \pm 549\%$ a	$-43.8 \pm 69\%$ b	$3.163 \pm 73\%$ * torr *	$0.816 \pm 14\%$ K vs. b
Adair	0 - 100	$0.0372 \pm 17\%$ a_1	$0.00149 \pm 51\%$ a_2	$4.12 \times 10^{-6} \pm 43\%$ a_4	$0.380 \pm 27\%$	$0.824 \pm 1.8\%$ a_1 vs. a_4
Pauling	0 - 100	$10.2 \pm 28\%$ alpha	$0.00435 \pm 32\%$ K		$1.515 \pm 9.8\%$	$-0.556 \pm 34\%$
Margaria	0 - 100	$0.0128 \pm 25\%$ K	$201 \pm 73\%$ m		$0.521 \pm 35\%$	$-0.986 \pm 0.5\%$
MWC	0 - 100	$7.11 \times 10^{-7} \pm 12\%$ K_R	$8.95 \times 10^{-9} \pm 16\%$ c	$1.00 \times 10^{30} \pm 3.1\%$ L	$0.529 \pm 35\%$	$-0.981 \pm 0.5\%$ K_R vs. L
Kelman	0 - 100	$8.44 \times 10^{7} \pm 206\%$ a_1 $-3.50 \times 10^{9} \pm 222\%$ a_4 $1.42 \times 10^{6} \pm 170\%$ a_7	$-2.59 \times 10^{6} \pm 142\%$ a_2 $9.97 \times 10^{8} \pm 147\%$ a_5	$1.34 \times 10^{6} \pm 170\%$ a_3 $-1.61 \times 10^{7} \pm 122\%$ a_6	$0.330 \pm 51\%$	See text.
Severinghaus	0 - 100	$1.37 \times 10^{4} \pm 9.2\%$ a	$233 \pm 37\%$ b		$0.628 \pm 43\%$	$0.806 \pm 6.0\%$
Easton	0 - 100	$0.0710 \pm 6.1\%$ K	$-0.0244 \pm 41\%$ Y_a	$0.971 \pm 1.1\%$ Y_m	$0.539 \pm 25\%$	$-0.601 \pm 23\%$ K vs. Y_m

shown in Tables II and III. This value can be looked at as a normalized measure of the dependence between pairs of parameters. As this value approaches one, a large change in one parameter of the pair gives a large change in the other parameter but results in an insignificant change in the SOS. An example of this is seen in the SOS surface for the MWC model, depicted in Figure 3. Increasing the parameter L while simultaneously decreasing c over a wide range has only a slight effect on the SOS. Another indication of this is shown in Figure 4 where K_R and c are clearly functions of L and, at large L, the RMS error was constant independent of L. These points were determined by fitting the MWC model to one OHEC repeatedly using different initial parameter estimates. In Figure 5, the SOS surface is shown for the Hill equation. A clearcut minimum is seen and the independence of the parameters is evident because there are no diagonal valleys. Perhaps the worst redundancy is found with the Kelman model. Its seven parameters were all intricately interconnected. The parameter a_3-a_7 correlation was nearly always 1.00 with most other values greater than 0.75. Models with high redundancy give parameters with little practical or theoretical value, nor are they useful in comparing individual OHECs.

Figure 6 shows the RMS error (means ± SD) for each model while Figure 7 compares RMS errors for different models for several representative OHECs. The Kelman and Adair models generally gave the lowest RMS errors for most OHECs while the Pauling model generally gave the highest. The results for the MWC model almost exactly mimicked the results of the Margaria model in every case, while the

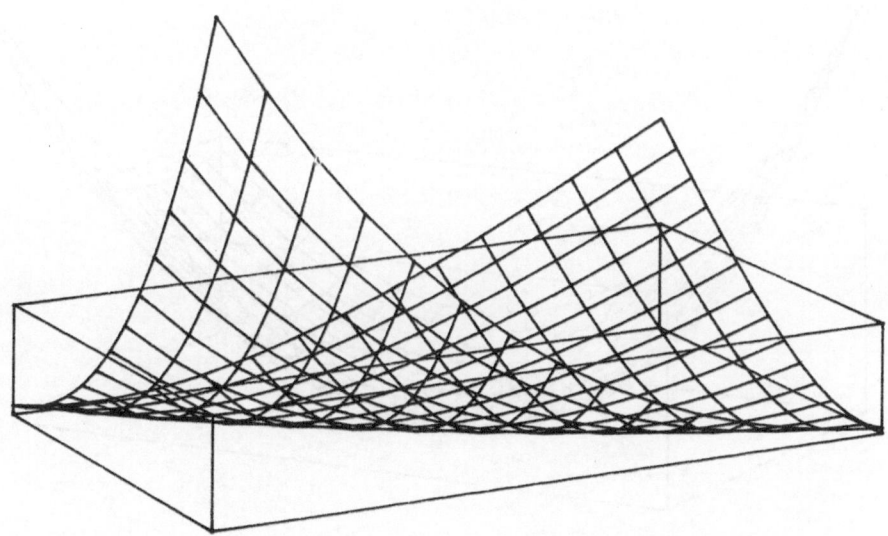

Figure 3. Sum of squares surface for typical MWC model fit.

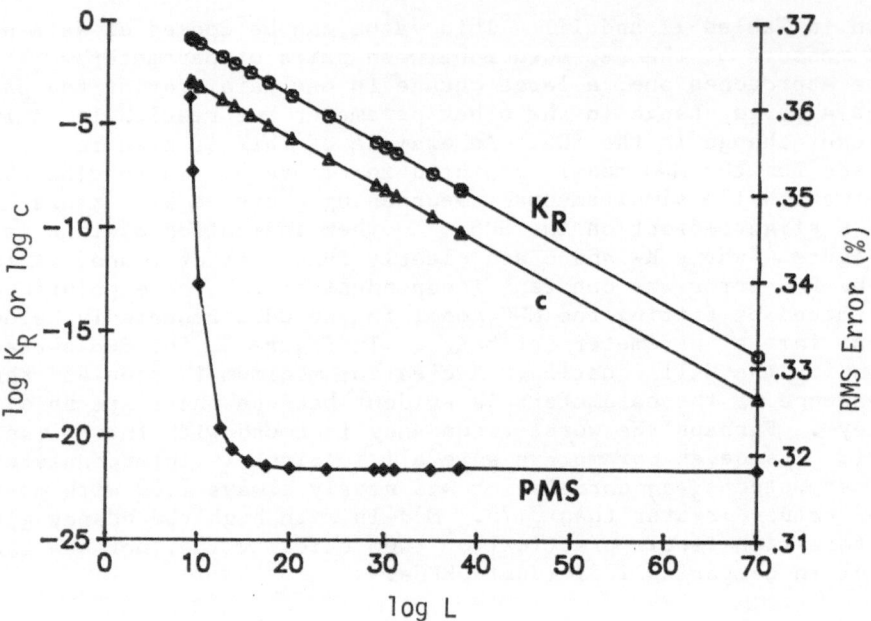

Figure 4. Relationship between the MWC parameters and the RMS error for a typical fit.

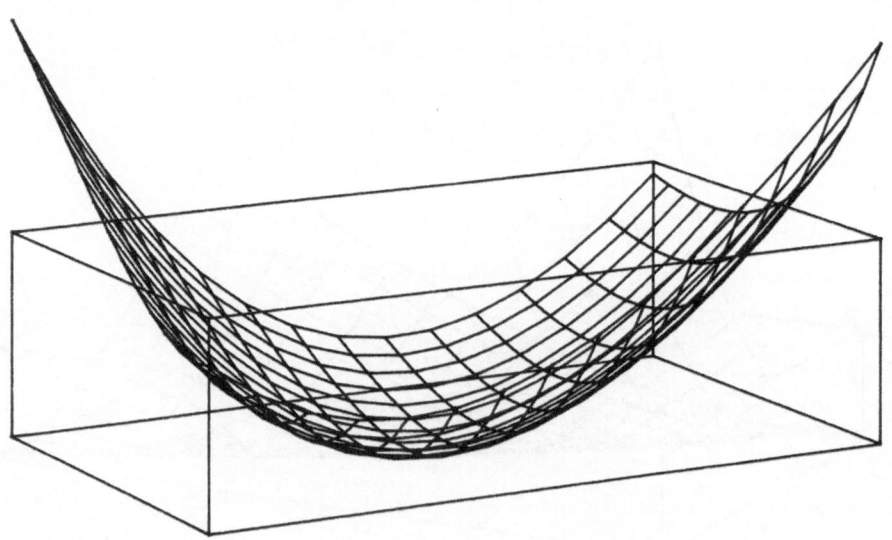

Figure 5. Sum of squares surface for a typical Hill model fit.

Severinghaus model usually provided RMS errors higher than the MWC and Hill values. The Pauling model seems to have completely opposite fitting characteristics than that of the Margaria model. Whenever there was a good fit to the Margaria model by a particular OHEC, there was invariably a poor fit to the Pauling model and vice-versa. This is evident in Figure 2 where the Pauling residuals appear to mirror the Margaria residuals. The Pauling model RMS errors were

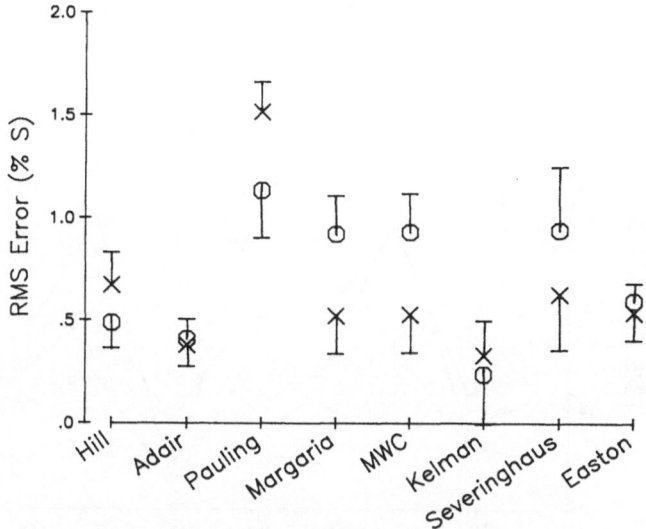

Figure 6. RMS error means and standard deviations for each model. DCA-1 data is represented by o and Hemox-Analyzer data is shown as x. Error bars associated with each data point represent standard deviation.

consistent with, although not as good as, the Adair values. In turn, the Adair model consistently fitted better than the Hill model, but the results reported here could only be obtained with a_3 set equal to zero. The Kelman seven parameter equation, of course, fitted the data extremely well but the parameter values exhibited wide variation and redundancy as discussed above. Easton's model consistently fitted the data better than the Severinghaus model.

Excluding the Adair model because by setting $a_3 = 0$ it is no longer theoretically consistent and the Kelman model because of redundancy, the Hill and Easton models provided the best fits. The average RMS error was a bit higher for the Easton model but the standard deviation was much smaller (i.e., the parameters were more consistent). In addition, the Easton model describes the complete OHEC while the Hill model covers only 20% to 98% saturation. The two-parameter Hill model, however, exhibited the least redundancy. A sig-

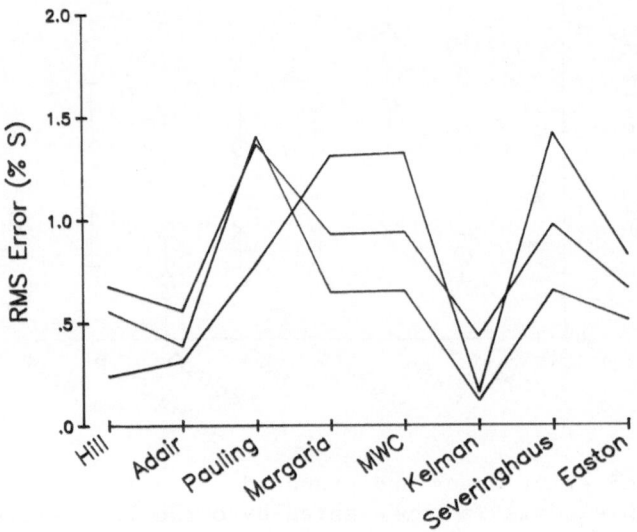

Figure 7.   RMS error relationship between models for several typical OHECs.

nificant advantage of this model would seem to be that the parameters are quite independent. The independence of the Severinghaus parameters was consistently intermediate between that for the Hill equation and that for the other models. Although its underlying thesis is supported by observation, the MWC model is extremely difficult to fit because of the redundancy (covariance) between all three parameters (Figure 4).

DISCUSSION

The 1978 study of Winslow et al. gives aggregate results for the Adair fits of OHECs from 48 adults. Their Adair parameters ($a_1 = 0.0157$ +65%, -36%; $a_2 = 0.00117$ + 11%, -45%; $a_3 = 0$; $a_4 = 2.45 \times 10^{-6}$ +7%, -6%) are practically the same as our values (Tables II and III). They also found a_3 particularly difficult to fit. Their subject group included smokers, although the P_{50} range of their OHECs was 22.5 to 29.9 torr which agrees well with our range of 21.9 to 28.0 torr. It is important to note that Winslow et al. used a much different experimental method to determine their OHECs and very different fitting techniques. Nevertheless their Adair parameters are indistinguishable from ours. Although not shown here, it is clear from our results that the redundancy in the Adair model can be significantly reduced by setting a_3 to zero and that this does not affect the quality of the fit.

The residual plots for the Margaria and MWC models are remarkably similar, suggesting the models are also very similar. This may be explained by examining the models themselves. When both models are fully expanded as ratios of polynomials in PO_2, a relationship between the two appears (Table IV). Each of the expressions multiplies one of the terms of the PO_2 polynomial in the appropriate model. If, as we have found, L is very large (10^{30} for our OHECs), the MWC expressions approach the limits shown at the right side of the table. The (c/K_R) expression is almost identical to the Margaria parameter K explaining the similarity between the Margaria and MWC model results. Because of parameter redundancy, the MWC parameters will remain difficult to obtain and imprecise. The difficulty of fitting the MWC model may be circumvented by finding one or more parameters by some independent means (i.e., reducing the number of parameters). The fit would then be obtained using a smaller number of parameters, in the manner of Imai (1983). It would be necessary, however, to find these fixed parameter values for the particular blood under study. One cannot use a "standard" value for all blood.

The fit of the Severinghaus model was fair for some curves and poor for others. On average the RMS error was high as was its coefficient of variation. Because of this, in addition to the completely empirical nature of the model, compared to the other models, the Severinghaus model was not ranked among the best choices for characterizing the OHEC.

The Margaria model with its two parameters is certainly easier to fit than the four-parameter Adair model from whence it was derived but it does not supply us with as much information as does the Adair equation nor does it fit as well. Nevertheless, based on its similarity to the MWC equation, it may lead to an entirely new model.

For most applications, the Hill equation still appears to give

Table IV. Similarity of terms in Margaria and MWC Equations

Margaria Expression	MWC Expression	MWC Limit
K^4_m	$\dfrac{Lc^4 + 1}{K_R^4(L+1)}$	$\left(\dfrac{c}{K_R}\right)^4$
K^3	$\dfrac{Lc^3 + 1}{K_R^3(L+1)}$	$\left(\dfrac{c}{K_R}\right)^3$
K^2	$\dfrac{Lc^2 + 1}{K_R^2(L+1)}$	$\left(\dfrac{c}{K_R}\right)^2$
K	$\dfrac{Lc + 1}{K_R(L+1)}$	$\dfrac{c}{K_R}$

an adequate fit over the physiologically important part of the OHEC. In the present study the Hill model generally gave RMS errors which were at the low end but showed less randomness in the residuals than the other models possibly indicating that it is less accurate. As expected, when compared with the Hill model, an increase in accuracy was obtained with the Margaria, MWC, and Severinghaus models. Although these three models are also applicable over the complete range of saturation, this extra information is of little physiological interest. In summary, for most applications the Hill equation is a sufficiently accurate model for description of OHEC data. The significance of the Hill parameters is well-known and the parameters are easy to determine using nonlinear regression.

When the most accurate description of the OHEC is required, as when looking for small changes in the OHEC, the Easton model would appear to be the best choice. The three parameters are relatively easy to determine although the high parameter redundancy necessitates good initial parameter estimates. Linear regression of the Hill P_{50} with Easton's B ($r^2 = 0.22$) and the Hill n with Easton's K ($r^2 = 0.06$) did not support Easton's hypothesis that B indicated curve shift and K indicated curve slope.

Using nonlinear regression to fit multi-parameter models to OHEC data is of limited value when the parameters exhibit redundancy. More robust estimation techniques such as maximum likelihood which do not assume a normal distribution of residuals and are less sensitive to outliers may be required. Independent evaluation of some of the parameters in order to reduce their total number, however, appears to be the most promising method for complex parameter estimation problems.

ACKNOWLEDGEMENTS

We are grateful for the technical assistance of Louise Ellis, Cheryl Evans, Beverly Glover and Steve Neumann. This work was supported in part by National Eye Institute Grant EY-04085.

REFERENCES

Adair, G.S., 1925, The hemoglobin system VI. The oxygen dissociation curve of hemoglobin, J. Biol. Chem. 63:529-545.

Douglas, C.G., Haldane, J.S., and Haldane, J.B.S., 1912, The laws of combination of haemoglobin with carbon monoxide and oxygen, J. Physiol., 44:275-304.

Easton, D.M., 1979, Oxyhemoglobin dissociation curve as expo-exponential paradigm of asymmetric sigmoid function, J. Theor. Biol., 76:335-349.

Hill, A.V., 1910, The possible effects of the aggregation of the molecules of hemoglobin on its dissociation curves, J. Physiol., London, 40:(Proceedings), iv.

Imai, K., 1983, The Monod-Wyman-Changeux allosteric model describes haemoglobin oxygenation with only one adjustable parameter, J. Mol. Biol., 167:741-749.

Kelman, G.R., 1966, Digital computer subroutine for the conversion of oxygen tension into saturation, J. Appl. Physiol.,21:1375-1376.

Margaria, R., 1963, A mathematical treatment of the blood dissociation curve for oxygen, Clin. Chem., 9:745-762.

Monod, J., Wyman, J., Changeux, J., 1965, On the nature of allosteric transitions: a plausible model, J. Mol. Biol., 12:88-118.

O'Riordan, J.F., Goldstick, T.K., Ditzel, J., Ernest, J.T., 1983, Characterization of oxygen-hemoglobin equilibrium curves using nonlinear regression of the Hill equation: parameter values for normal adults, Adv. Exp. Med. Biol., 159:435-444.

Pauling, L., 1935, The oxygen equilibrium of hemoglobin and its structural interpretation, Proc. Nat. Acad. Sci., Wash., 21:186-191.

Perutz, M.F., 1978, Hemoglobin structure and respiratory transport, Sci. Amer., 239:92-125.

Reich, J.G., Zinke, I., 1974, Analysis of kinetic and binding

measurements IV. Redundancy of model parameters, <u>Studia
Biophysica,</u> 43:91-107.
Robinson, B., 1981, NLREG-Nonlinear regression subroutine package,
Vogelback Computing Center document no. 328, Northwestern
University, Evanston, IL.
Severinghaus, J.W., 1979, Simple, accurate expressions for human
blood oxygen dissociation computations, <u>J. Appl. Physiol.:
Respirat. Environ. Exercise Physiol.</u>, 46:599-602.
Winslow, R.M., Morrissey, J.M., Berger, R.L., Smith, P.D., Gibson,
C.C., 1978, Variability of oxygen affinity of normal blood:
an automated method of measurement, <u>J. Appl. Physiol.: Respira-
tion Environ. Exercise Physiol.</u>, 45:289-297.
Wyman, J., 1948, Heme proteins, <u>in</u>: "Advances in Protein Chemistry,"
M.L. Anson and J.T. Edsall, eds., Academic Press, New York.

RHEOLOGICAL FACTORS INFLUENCING OXYGEN TRANSFER

IN HEART AND BRAIN

Hideyuki Niimi and Takashi Yamakawa

National Cardiovascular Center Research Institute
Suita, Osaka, 565 Japan

INTRODUCTION

Among numbers of factors affecting the oxygen transport to tissue from capillaries, capillary rheology and its distribution are most important in regulating the oxygen transport so as to comply with the metabolic requirement of organs such as heart and brain. To date, a number of studies have been performed to examine the role of the capillary topology (geometry and distribution) in the oxygen supply to tissue, but rheological factors have not yet received much attention (Niimi et al, 1983). The purpose of this research is to clarify the significance of the rheological factors in regulation of the oxygen transport to tissue from capillaries. Especially, we will emphasize how variable capillary hematocrits possibly affect the transcapillary oxygen transport. After describing some direct observations related to microcirculatory heterogeneity, such as the preferential flow in capillaries of heart and brain, we will numerically investigate the transcapillary oxygen transport phenomena by generating the flow conditions based on a "two-fluid model".

INTRAVITAL OBSERVATION

We made a direct observation of blood cells flowing through capillaries in the heart and brain of cats using a transilluminator-microscope-cine system. The method used was reported in detail elsewhere (Yamakawa and Niimi, 1983; Niimi et al., 1984). We here show the results relevant to the phenomena of oxygen transport (Yamakawa and Niimi, 1983; Niimi et al., 1984; Yamakawa et al., 1984).

Coronary Microcirculation

Most capillaries observed in the left atrium of cats were asymmetric without tortuosity. The red blood cells (RBC's) flowing through capillaries were uniformly distributed and therefore the inter-RBC distance, i.e. distance between two adjacent RBC's, was almost constant. The capillary hematocrit (Hcap) was 31% ± 5.2% (SD) when the systemic Ht was 40%. The Hcap of the heart was higher than those of other organs (Lipowsky et al., 1980).

During acute ischemia, RBC's flowrate through capillaries was reduced. Immediately following the induction of ischemia, the Hcap increased in most capillaries, but after several minutes it decreased in some capillaries. White blood cells (WBC's) also appeared in the capillary networks and several of them stopped or plugged at the capillary branching. Due to them, RBC's accumulated upstream but were almost absent downstream (plasma-WBC-accumulated RBC flow), and their distribution was not uniform along the capillary. The calculated inter-RBC distance scattered more widely compared to the normal one though their mean values were almost equal. Another surprising phenomenon was the appearance of heterogeneous RBC flow without WBC in some capillaries. This is probably due to the increased variation in the RBC transit time through capillaries at the lowered arterial-to-venous pressure difference.

In our experiments, no capillary recruitment was observed under normal and acute ischemic conditions.

Cerebral Microcirculation

Most capillaries observed in the cerebral cortex showed asymmetric distribution with high tortuosity. Based on 5-sec observation, the capillary blood flow could be classified into three patterns: perfused, unperfused and intermittently perfused capillary. The unperfused capillary occupied approximately one third of the total and contained very few RBC's. In the perfused capillary, the Hcap increased linearly with the RBC velocity until it approached about 30%.

In hemorrhagic shock, the RBC velocity in capillaries was decreased. During the shock, WBC's appeared in the microvascular networks, several of which stopped or plugged at the capillary branching. The same flow patterns as those in the coronary capillaries were observed. Especially, the RBC distribution also became heterogeneous along the capillary under the hemorrhagic shock. These phenomena are probably induced by rheological and morphological differences between WBC and RBC.

MODEL AND ANALYSIS

In order to theoretically examine the transcapillary oxygen transport, we simulated capillary blood flow using a "two-fluid flow" in which the blood was assumed to consist of the two fluids: RBC and plasma. The properties of the two fluids, such as velocity and oxygen pressure (PO_2), represented the quantities averaged over a segment of the capillary smaller than the capillary length but larger than the cell size, and also a time period longer than the passage time of RBC through the inter-RBC distance (see APPENDIX). The relative motion between RBC and plasma was included to describe the variation in the capillary hematocrit, and also the mass exchange of oxygen between RBC and plasma was included to describe a non-equilibrium state in which mean values of RBC and plasma PO_2 are not equal.

Two-Fluid Model

Considering a single capillary with a length L between an arteriole and a venule, we take the z-axis along the capillary. Here, the capillary is not necessarily straight in the z-axis. If the hematocrit in the capillary is denoted by H_c, the volume fraction of plasma becomes $1 - H_c$. If we represent the mean velocities of RBC and plasma fluid by V_r and V_p, respectively, the RBC and plasma flowrates, Q_r and Q_p, can be described as

$$Q_r = H_c V_r S_c, \qquad Q_p = (1 - H_c) V_p S_c \qquad (1)$$

where S_c is the cross-sectional area of the capillary. In quasi-steady flow, both Q_r and Q_p are constant along the capillary so that they are prescribed at the capillary end. If the ratio of RBC to total flowrate is denoted by H_s, we obtain

$$V_r = H_s Q / H_c S_c, \quad V_p = (1 - H_s) Q / (1 - H_c) S_c \qquad (2)$$

where Q is the total flowrate. If H_s is taken to be the systemic hematocrit, V_r and V_p can be expressed as functions of Q and H_c. Note that when H_c is smaller than H_s, V_r is larger than V_p.

Mass Balance of Oxygen in Flow

Considering both oxygen dissolved in the plasma and that bound to hemoglobin and also dissolved in the RBC, the mass balance describing the mass flux from RBC to plasma and from plasma into tissue across the capillary wall can be written as

$$(\alpha_r + N \, d\psi/dP_r) \, Q_r \, dP_r/dz = -qH_c S_c , \qquad (3)$$

$$\alpha_p Q_p \, dP_p/dz = qH_c S_c - J. \qquad (4)$$

where P_r, P_p are mean PO_2 in RBC and plasma, respectively; α_r and α_p are coefficients of oxygen solubility in RBC and plasma, respectively; N is the oxygen capacity per unit volume of RBC; $\psi(p)$ represents the fractional saturation of hemoglobin with oxygen, and q and J are the mean rate of oxygen transfer from RBC to plasma and from plasma to tissue, respectively. In order to solve eqs.(3) and (4) for P_r and P_p, q and J must be defined.

Since P_r and P_p average the corresponding PO_2 values over the segment, they are not always equal. We here assume, for simplicity, that the rate of oxygen transfer q is proportional to the difference between RBC and plasma PO_2 levels, namely,

$$q = \kappa \, (\, P_r - P_p \,) \tag{5}$$

where κ is the proportionality constant (see DISCUSSION).

As for J, considering that the total oxygen transported across the capillary wall is consumed in the whole region of tissue surrounding it, we obtain the relation : $\langle J \rangle = A_t \, (V/L)$ where $\langle J \rangle$ represents the mean value of J over a total volume, V, of the tissue and A_t corresponds to the rate of oxygen consumption per unit volume of tissue. Since J, in general, depends upon the distribution of PO_2 at the boundary between the capillary wall and the tissue, it cannot be determined rigorously without solving the diffusion equation of oxygen within the tissue. In the present analysis, however, we simply approximate J as

$$J = A_t \, S_t \tag{6}$$

where S_t corresponds to the cross-sectional area of the local tissue. This approximation may be valid for the case when the axial diffusion of oxygen in tissue is very small in comparison with the radial diffusion.

Capillary-Tissue Unit and Calculation Procedure

A simple Krogh type model based on a capillary-tissue unit was utilized to model a complex organ that contains counter-current capillary networks (see APPENDIX). In the modified Krogh model, the maximal diffusional distance was assumed to vary along a single capillary, and the geometry of tissue was characterized by the mean outer radius R_0 and the taper index β as $R_0 = (R_a + R_v)/\,2$, $\beta = (R_a - R_v)/\,R_a$ where R_a and R_v represent the radii of the tissue at the arterial and venous end of capillary, respectively.

Using the finite difference method, we numerically solved a set of non-linear differential equations (1)-(6). To examine effects of rheological parameters on the transcapillary oxygen transport, the actual values of blood and tissue physical variables, and of geometrical and dynamical parameters as follows were used:

α_r (ml O_2 / ml.mmHg) = 3.4 x 10^{-5}, α_p (ml O_2 / ml.mmHg) = 3.4 x 10^{-5}, N (ml O_2 /ml)= 0.45, κ (ml O_2 / ml sec mmHg) = 3.6 x 10^{-2}, α_t(ml O_2 / ml.mmHg) = 3.2 x 10^{-5}, D_t (cm^2/sec)=1.7 x 10^{-5}, A_t* (ml O_2 / ml.sec) = 3.3 x 10^{-3}, R_c (μm) = 2.1, R_t** (μm)= 9.5, L (μm)= 600, P_a**(mmHg)= 87 (* values at rest, ** standard values)

NUMERICAL RESULTS

To examine the potential role of H_c associated with the oxygen transport to tissue, we calculated the RBC and plasma PO_2 values along the capillary of the cylinder model (β=0) for several values of H_c, and then evaluated the PO_2 drops (ΔPO_2) between the arterial and venous ends (Fig.1). When H_s and Q (and thus Q_r) were kept constant, the H_c did not affect the RBC PO_2 but plasma PO_2; the plasma PO_2 increased with decrease in H_c, but approached the RBC PO_2 as H_c increased. Particularly for H_c exceeding 0.4, the plasma could be considered to be in an oxygen-equilibrium state with the RBC. As for PO_2 at the capillary venous end, we could demonstrate that the venous PO_2 levels in RBC and plasma decreased (or increased) with increase (or decrease) in the arterial PO_2.

We changed the taper index β to examine the effect of the tissue geometry on the oxygen transfer. Fig. 2 shows an example

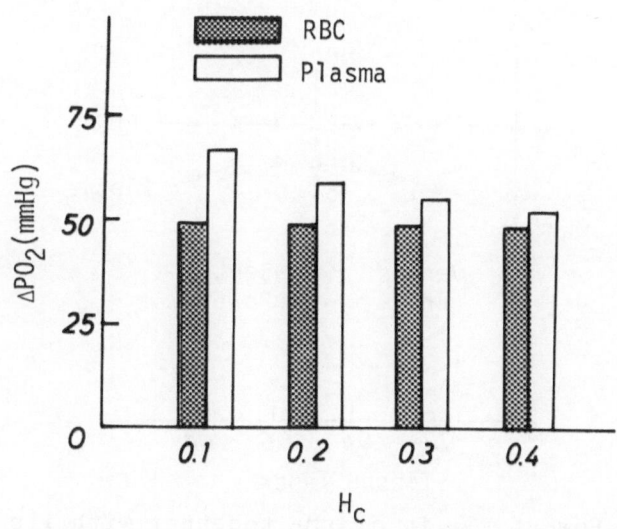

Fig. 1 Arertio-venous PO_2 drop against capillary hematocrit for H_s = 0.45 and V_r = 2mm/sec.

527

of RBC and plasma PO_2 distributions along the capillary for β = 0.8. The PO_2 in plasma became the lowest at the central portion of the capillary, differently from that in RBC. Fig. 3 shows the lowest plasma PO_2 values and its location against the taper index. As compared with the cylinder model, a novel feature appears in plasma, the venous PO_2 level being higher than that in the cylinder model.

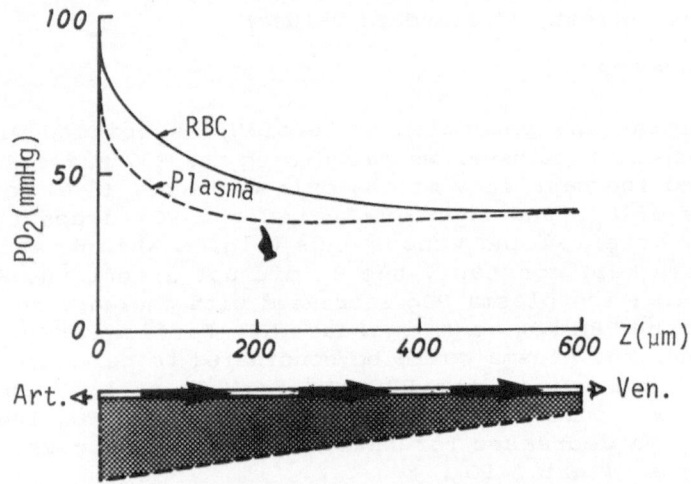

Fig. 2. Distributions of RBC and plasma PO_2 along the capillary for β = 0.8 . The minimum in plasma appears at the location represented by a finger.

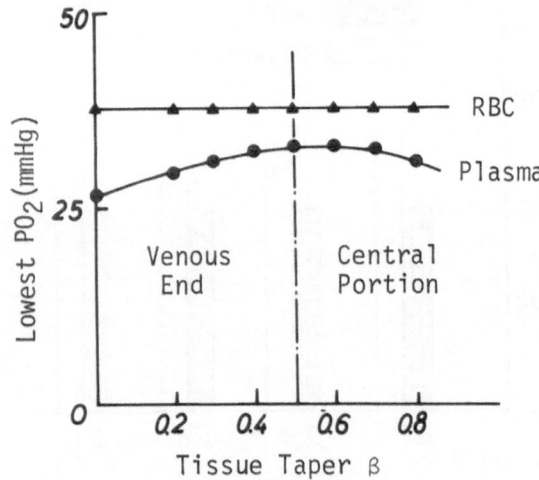

Fig. 3. The lowest PO_2 in plasma together with its location against the tissue taper for H_s= 0.45 and V_r= 2mm/sec.

DISCUSSION

It has been widely accepted that the capillary blood flow is the most important factor related to the oxygen supply to tissue. If the blood flow corresponds to the RBC flowrate, i.e. the product of RBC velocity and hematocrit, equal rates of oxygen supply can be achieved by either a low hematocrit and a high RBC velocity or by a high hematocrit and a low RBC velocity (Klitzman and Duling, 1979). According to our simulation, this concept is true so far as the plasma and RBC are in an oxygen-equilibrium state, but it becomes invalid in non-equilibrium states.

One important factor attributable to such non-equilibrium conditions is the low hematocrit in capillaries. If the capillary hematocrit is reduced with the RBC flux being held constant, the number of RBC's and consequently the total surface area of RBC's in contact with plasma in unit capillary length will be reduced. This will, in turn, restrict the capacity of oxygen exchange between RBC's and plasma, so that the capillary hematocrit may contribute appreciably to the oxygen transport process. Another factor is the parameter κ in eq.(5) where smaller κ values require larger PO_2 gradients between RBC and plasma in order to assure a fixed amount of oxygen transport. The present κ includes the combined effect of both cell membrane oxygen transfer and convective (or "bolus") flow inside and outside the moving cell (see Fig. A).

The current microscopic observations clearly proved that local hematocrits in coronary and cerebral microvasculatures are lower compared with the systemic hematocrit. Under some patho- and physiological conditions, dilute and/or accumulated blood cells appeared in the capillary networks. Such low and high hematocrits probably reflect individual behaviors of RBC's and plasma in capillaries (Gaehtgens, 1984). Actually, using eq.(2) in our two-fluid model, we could generate variable capillary hematocrits by changing RBC and plasma velocities.

Under conditions where capillary hematocrit is extremely reduced, the plasma PO_2 may be significantly different from the RBC PO_2 even if the flowrate is kept constant. In fact, Fig. 1 showed how the arterio-venous PO_2 drop of RBC does not depend upon the capillary hematocrit, while the plasma PO_2 drop is increased with decreasing hematocrit. Although little oxygen is dissolved in plasma , the plasma PO_2 level may affect the PO_2 distribution within tissue via the capillary wall. Particularly when capillary RBC and plasma PO_2 are not in an equilibrium state, the plasma may play an essential role in the transcapillary oxygen transport. A measure of such non-equilibrium conditions will be the PO_2 difference between RBC and plasma. As shown in Fig. 3, the location of the largest PO_2 difference may be affected by the variation in the tissue taper. It must be emphasized here that the lowest PO_2 in plasma may occur at a central portion between the arterial and venous ends in the tapered tissue unit.

Finally, let us briefly mention the significance of capillary tortuosity in the oxygen supply to tissue. By numerically calculating the distribution of the PO_2 in tissue, we can predict that the lowest PO_2 may appear at a point of the outer border of tissue between arterial and venous ends under non-equilibrium conditions, but that the capillary with tortuosity may possibly decrease the volume of the lowest PO_2 in the tissue (Niimi and Sugihara, 1984). In view of oxygen supply economy, the smaller low PO_2 region may be favorable. Therefore, the capillary tortuosity may play an important role in the tissue oxygenation.

The authors thank M. Sugihara and I. Sugiyama for their numerical calculation and S. Takatani for a critical reading of the manuscript.

REFERENCES

Gaehtgens, P., 1984, Regulation of capillary haematocrit, Int J Microcirc: Clin Exp 3, 3: 147-160.

Lipowsky, H.H., Usami,S., and Chien, S., 1980, In vivo measurement of microvessel hematocrit, red cell flux, velocity, and transit time, Am. J. Physiol., 243: H1018-H1026.

Klitzman, B., and Duling, B.R., 1979, Microvascular hematocrit and red cell flow in resting and contracting striated muscle, Am. J. Physiol., 237: H481-H490.

Niimi,H, Sugihara,M., and Yamakawa, T., 1983, Hemorheological factors of oxygen transfer in capillary tissue unit, Biorheology, 20: 603-614.

Niimi, H, Sugihara, M., and Yamakawa,T., 1984, Microvascular topology and blood flow in microvessel, in: "Proc. 1st China Japan USA Conf. Biomechanics", Beijing, Science Press.

Niimi, H., and Sugihara, M., 1984, Hemorheological approach to oxygen transport between blood and tissue, Biorheology, 21: 445-461.

Yamakawa,T., and Niimi,H., 1983, Intravital microscopic study of coronary microcirculation during acute ischemia, in: "Intravital Observation of Organmicrocirculation", M. Tsuchiya, H. Wayland et al, eds, Amsterdam, Excerpta Medica, pp. 205-219.

Yamakawa,T., Sugiyama, I., and Niimi, H., 1984, A direct observation method of brain microcirculatory flow using transilluminator-intravital microscope system (in Japanese), in: "Proc. 23rd Conf. Japan Soc. ME & BE", pp106-107.

APPENDIX

Conservation Laws of Capillary Flow

Physical properties of RBC and plasma flowing in a capillary are functions of the position. The mean quantities over a cross-section of the capillary also fluctuate in time. Here, by averaging a mean quantity Q over a time period T longer than the passage time of RBC through one inter-RBC distance, we express it in terms of the average ($\langle Q \rangle$) and fluctuation (Q') as follows:

$$Q = \langle Q \rangle + Q' , \qquad \langle Q \rangle = \frac{1}{T}\int_T Q \, dt$$

Note that $\langle Q' \rangle = 0$, and as for two quantities Q_1 and Q_2, $\langle Q_1 \cdot Q_2 \rangle = (1 + e_{12}) \langle Q_1 \rangle \langle Q_2 \rangle$ where $e_{12} = \langle Q'_1 \cdot Q'_2 \rangle / \langle Q_1 \cdot Q_2 \rangle$. In the present formulation, the e_{12} value is assumed to be negligibly small.

Here we consider conservation laws associated with capillary blood flow in a small segment between z_j and z_{j+1} shown in Fig. A, in which the segmental length is longer than the cell size. Then, the mass conservations of RBC and plasma can be expressed in the forms:

$$[\, Q_r \,]_j = 0 , \qquad [\, Q_p \,]_j = 0$$

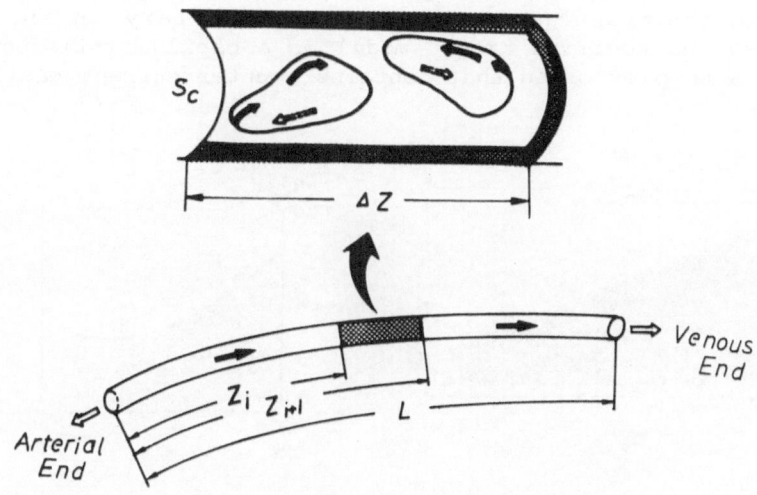

Fig. A. Schematic representation of a small segment of a single
capillary and asymmetric motion of cells.

where Q_r and Q_p are the flowrates defined in the text and the symbol $[\Psi]_j$ represents the difference of a quantity between the two cross-sections. The above equations can be easily integrated along the capillary to give the corresponding relationships in the text.

Considering the net convective flux of dissolved and hemo-globin-bound oxygen across the two cross-sections, the mass flux of oxygen from RBC into plasma and also from plasma into tissue across the capillary wall, we can describe the mass conservation equations of oxygen as follows:

$$[(\alpha_r + N\,\psi(p))\,Q_r]_j = -\,q_j\,H_c\,S_c\,\Delta z$$

$$[\,\alpha_p\,q_p\,]_j = q_j\,H_c\,S_c\,\Delta z - J_j\,\Delta z$$

where q_j and J_j represent the rate of oxygen transfer from RBC to plasma and the rate of oxygen transfer from plasma to tissue, respectively, in the segment.

Modified Krogh Model

Here we consider a couple of counter-current capillaries shown in Fig.B where Ca and Cv are symmetric but have anti-parallel input and output. At a cross-section (s-s'), blood PO_2 of Ca is different from that of Cv. Since the blood PO_2 level depends upon the capillary site, the maximal distance of oxygen diffusion from Ca may not be equal to that from Cv, and also the PO_2 distribution in the tissue may be asymmetric with respect to Ca and Cv. Hence, when we consider one of the two capillaries alone like the Krogh tissue cylinder, we must regard the cross-section of the tissue to vary along the capillary. In the text, we adopted the modified Krogh model as a capillary-tissue unit to model a complex organ that contains counter-current capillary networks.

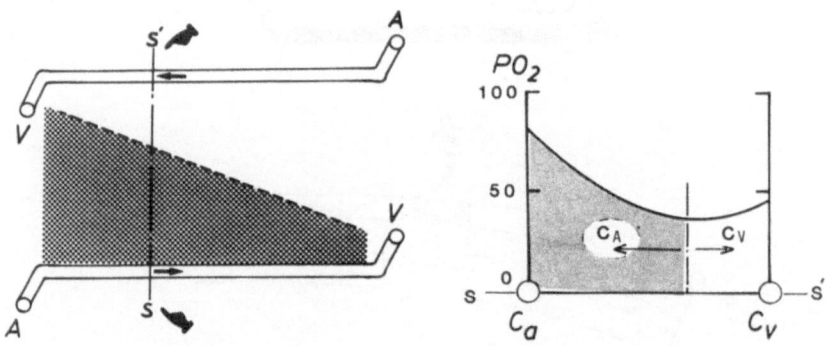

Fig. B. Schematic representation of a couple of counter-current capillaries, and PO_2 in capillary blood and tissue.

CARBOXYHEMOGLOBIN: DETERMINATION AND SIGNIFICANCE IN OXYGEN TRANSPORT

W.G. Zijlstra, A. Buursma, G. Kwant, B. Oeseburg and
A. Zwart

Department of Physiology, University of Groningen, and
Clinical Chemical Laboratory, Diakonessenhuis Groningen
Groningen, The Netherlands

Apart from being the direct cause of quite a few cases of near-fatal poisoning, carbon monoxide is a very common noxious agent functioning as an additional factor in human disease. The extent of the possible role of carbon monoxide in human pathology is demonstrated by the following data from the Diakonessenhuis Groningen, a 400-bed private hospital[1]. During a five-month period the carboxyhemoglobin fraction (FHbCO) was measured in the blood of all pre-operative patients. In 64.4% of the 1358 cases FHbCO was < 1.5%, in 26.8% it was between 1.5 and 5.0%, in 8.5% between 5.0 and 10.0% and in 0.4% it was > 10%. The highest value measured in this series was 15.5%. Thus it appears that in a considerable number of patients HbCO fractions are present that are of possible pathophysiological significance. This shows the practical importance of the pathophysiology of carboxyhemoglobin and the need for easy and reliable methods for the determination of FHbCO in blood.

For the determination of FHbCO in human blood spectrophotometric methods are well suited. Some thirty years ago a joint investigation in our two laboratories[2] resulted in two spectrophotometric methods which, with only minor modifications, have been in use till the present day. In both methods a two-component system is analyzed through absorbance measurement at two wavelengths of which one is at an isobestic point of the two components. The fraction of component 2 (F_2) follows from the absorbance ratio according to the following equation:

$$F_2 = c_2/c = a(A^{\lambda_1}/A^{\lambda_2}) + b \tag{1}$$

where c_2 is the concentration of component 2; c is the sum of the concentration of components 1 and 2; A^{λ_1} and A^{λ_2} are the absorbances at wavelength λ_1 and λ_2, respectively, λ_2 being at an isobestic point; a and b are constants[3].

In one method the mixture Hb/HbCO is used and measurements are made at λ = 540 and 578 nm after a 200-fold dilution of the blood with 0.1% ammonia solution, using a lightpath length of 1.00 cm. At λ = 540 nm there is a considerable difference in absorbance between Hb and HbCO, whereas at the isobestic point at λ = 578 nm the difference is by definition zero (Fig. 1). A small amount of sodium dithionite ($Na_2S_2O_4$) is added to the diluted blood to ensure that all hemoglobin other than HbCO is in the form of Hb.

In the other method, the mixture HbO_2/HbCO is used and measurements are made at λ = 562 and 540 nm in almost undiluted blood – only a very small amount of a non-ionic detergent is added for hemolysis – using a lightpath length of 0.01 cm. At λ = 562 nm there is a considerable difference in absorptivity between HbO_2 and HbCO, while 540 nm is the isobestic wavelength (Fig. 1).

The constants a and b in the two equations of the type of Eq. 1 used in the two methods have been determined by measuring the absorbance ratios of solutions containing the pure components separately, for the 540/578 method Hb and HbCO, for the 562/540 method HbO_2 and HbCO. The methods thus were originally based on the unproven assumption that Lambert-Beer's law, from which Eq. 1

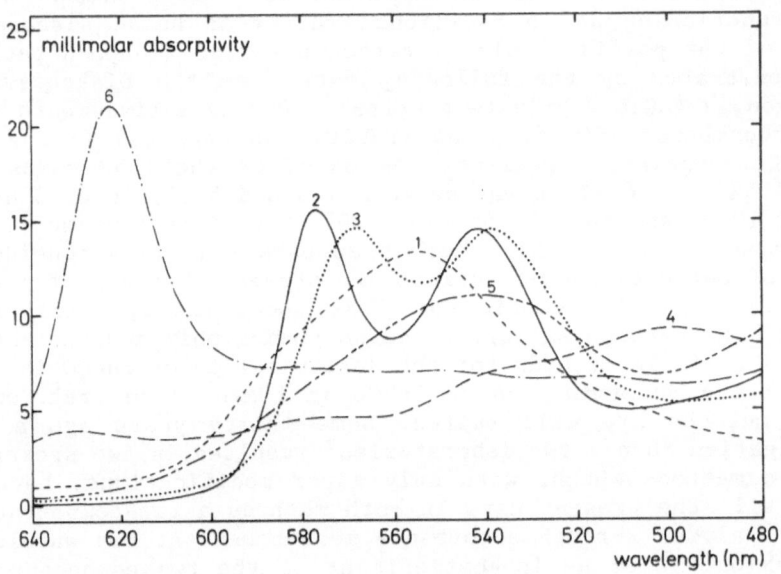

Fig. 1. Absorption spectra of (1) de-oxyhemoglobin (Hb), (2) oxyhemoglobin (HbO_2), (3) carboxyhemoglobin (HbCO), (4) hemiglobin = methemoglobin (Hi) at pH 7.0–7.4, (5) hemiglobincyanide (HiCN) and (6) sulfhemoglobin (SHb). The millimolar absorptivity is expressed in $l \cdot mmol^{-1} \cdot cm^{-1}$.

is derived, is valid for the components to be measured in the mixtures and that the samples used for the determination of the two constants of each equation really contained no light-absorbing substances except HbCO, Hb or HbO_2.

Putting these assumptions to the test in order to prove the validity of the spectrophotometric methods requires a reference method for measuring CO in blood with a high accuracy over a wide range. Van Slyke's manometric method does not meet the requirements of a reference method for CO in blood, because it measures CO as a residual gas pressure after elimination of N_2, O_2 and CO_2 from the measuring chamber. The titrimetric method described by Dijkhuizen et al.[4] on the other hand, which is specific for CO and has a coefficient of variation of about 1% as calculated from duplicate determinations, is very suitable for this purpose. In this method the blood sample is hemolyzed and the CO bound to hemoglobin is set free by converting HbCO into Hi with the help of $K_3Fe(CN)_6$; CO is oxidized to CO_2 in a furnace containing CuO at 400 °C and the CO_2 is subsequently bubbled through a solution of $BaCl_2$ in a water/tert.butanol mixture at pH = 10; the H^+ ions formed are titrated with a NaOH solution of known strength. The reactions involved are the following:

$$CO + CuO \longrightarrow CO_2 + Cu$$
$$CO_2 + H_2O + Ba^{2+} \longrightarrow BaCO_3\downarrow + 2\ H^+$$
$$2\ H^+ + 2\ OH^- \longrightarrow 2\ H_2O$$

Fig. 2 shows the instrumental set-up for carrying out this procedure.

The reference method was used to test the validity of the 562/540 spectrophotometric method. To this end 46 blood samples were prepared containing 0-90% HbCO, using blood from 22 healthy donors. Of each sample FHbCO was determined at least in duplicate with the titrimetric method, and the absorbance ratio A^{562}/A^{540} measured. The result, shown in Fig. 3, proves that an equation of the type of Eq. 1 correctly represents the relationship between FHbCO and A^{562}/A^{540}, and allows the constants a and b to be calculated from it. This yields:

$$FHbCO = 3.215\ (A^{562}/A^{540}) - 1.923 \tag{2}$$

All two-wavelength spectrophotometric methods depend on the presence of only two hemoglobin derivatives in the solution of which the absorbance is measured. This condition cannot always be fulfilled and therefore it is important to choose the wavelengths in such a manner that any possible error introduced by other common hemoglobin derivatives is minimal. Because of a proper choice of the wavelengths the 562/540 method for the determination of FHbCO is almost insensitive to the presence of hemiglobin. A more fundamental solution of course is multicomponent analysis by absorbance measurements at many wavelengths. It has for long been

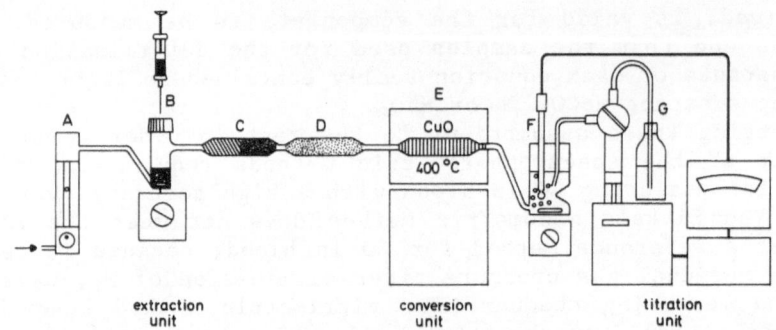

extraction
unit

conversion
unit

titration
unit

Fig. 2.   Measuring system for CO in blood[4]. A = supply of carrier
gas (N_2) with flowmeter; B = extraction vessel with
stirrer in which the blood is hemolyzed and the CO bound
to hemoglobin is set free; C, D = filter units filled
with activated charcoal (a liquid nitrogen trap can be
used instead) and with soda asbestos and magnesium per-
chlorate; E = furnace for converting CO into CO_2; F =
titration vessel with stirrer; G = automatic titrator
keeping the pH in the titration vessel at 10 by adding a
0.1 mol/l NaOH solution.

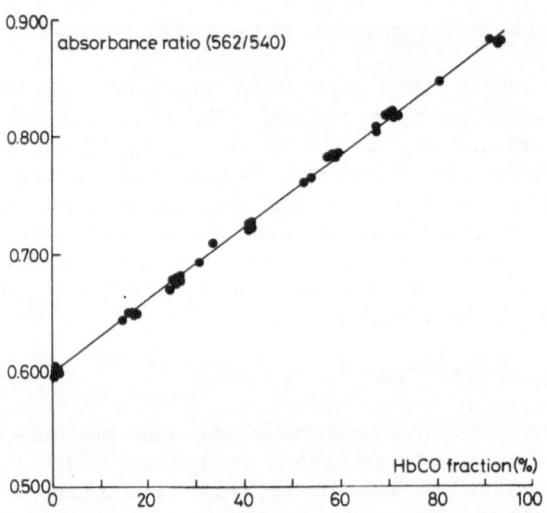

Fig. 3.   Absorbance ratio A^{562}/A^{540} plotted against FHbCO
determined with the titrimetric method of Dijkhuizen et
al.[4] The equation of the regression line is A^{562}/A^{540} =
0.3118 FHbCO + 0.5976. The correlation coefficient r =
0.999.

appreciated that, given sufficiently different absorption spectra, any number of components in a mixture can be analyzed by absorbance measurements at at least as many wavelengths as there are components in the mixture. For various technical reasons, multicomponent analysis of hemoglobin derivatives has developed only slowly, however.

Practical multicomponent methods for the determination of hemoglobin derivatives are the five-wavelength method of Zwart et al.[5] and the method implemented in the IL282 CO-Oximeter[6,7]. Recently, we developed a new multiwavelength method for the simultaneous determination of Hb, HbO_2, HbCO, Hi and SHb, to be carried out by means of a Hewlett-Packard HP 8450 or 8451 diode array spectrophotometer[8]. The calculations, made by the built-in microcomputer, are based on the absorption spectra 1, 2, 3, 4 and 6 shown in Fig. 1. To check the accuracy of the determination of HbCO by this technique, we again used the titrimetric CO determination as a reference method. Fig. 4 shows the result of 42 comparative measurements. The difference of the multicomponent analysis with respect to the chemical method was +0.53% ± 1.31% FHbCO (SD).

By combining this spectrophotometric technique with our method for recording oxygen dissociation curves of whole blood[9,10], we were able to study the influence of HbCO on the oxygen affinity of

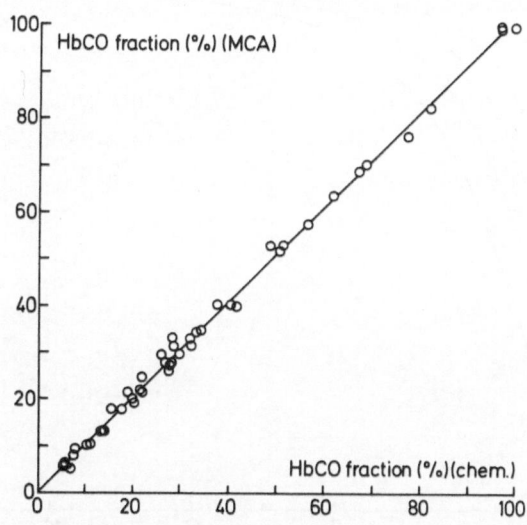

Fig. 4.   FHbCO measured by multicomponent analysis (MCA) plotted against FHbCO measured by the titrimetric method (chem.)[8]. The equation of the regression line is FHbCO (MCA) = 1.02 FHbCO (chem.) − 0.01. The correlation coefficient r = 0.999.

hemoglobin accurately . The reason for restudying the effect of CO on the oxygen dissociation curve (ODC) of human blood was the scarcity of the available literature data, which, moreover, are not in full mutual agreement[11]. Fig. 5 shows, for blood from a single donor, four ODC's recorded in the presence of four different HbCO fractions, under otherwise standard conditions. There is a considerable shift of the ODC to the left when FHbCO is increased. The position of an ODC can be expressed as P_{50}, i.e. the oxygen tension (pO_2) corresponding to an oxygen saturation (sO_2) of 50%. A fall in P_{50} reflects a shift of the ODC to the left. Fig. 6 shows the P_{50} of the remaining (i.e. the non-HbCO) hemoglobin as a function of FHbCO for 26 blood samples from seven healthy donors. The slope of the regression line ($\Delta P_{50}/\Delta FHbCO$) is -3.6 kPa, which is in excellent agreement with the values which can be calculated from the data of Roughton and Darling[12] and Hlastala et al.[13], -3.7 kPa and -3.6 kPa, respectively. Fig. 5 also shows that in the presence of HbCO the ODC of the remaining hemoglobin becomes less S-shaped. This is also reflected in the corresponding n values of the Hill equation, which decrease from 2.56 to 1.63 when FHbCO increases from < 1% to 52% [11].

In order to illustrate the dual effect of CO on the O_2 transport capability of the blood more clearly, Fig. 7 is presented in which, instead of sO_2, the O_2 content of the blood is plotted

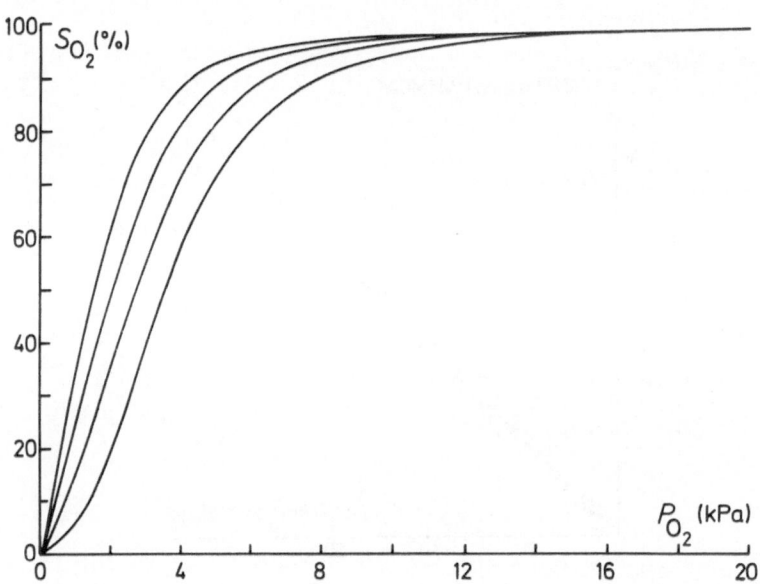

Fig. 5.   Oxygen dissociation curves (pH = 7.4, pCO_2 = 5.33 kPa, temperature = 37 °C) in the presence of four different HbCO fractions, blood from a single donor[11]. From left to right: FHbCO = 50.8, 32.5, 14.4 and < 1%.

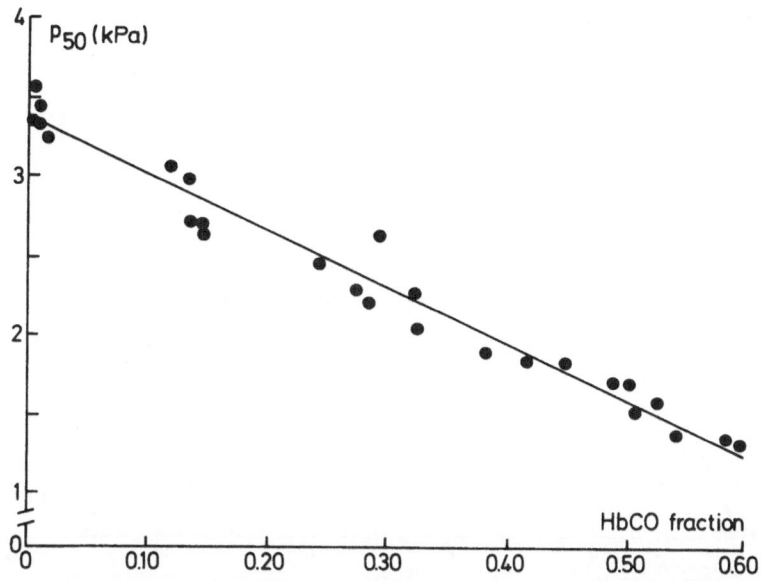

Fig. 6.   Standard P_{50} (pH = 7.4, pCO_2 = 5.33 kPa, temperature 37
°C) plotted against FHbCO for 26 blood samples from
seven donors[11]. The equation of the regression line is
P_{50} = -3.6 FHbCO + 3.4. The correlation coefficient r =
0.98.

against pO_2. The O_2 content was calculated on the basis of the
total hemoglobin concentration (cHb* = 9.43 mmol/l), according to
the following equation:

$$O_2 \text{ content} = cHb* \cdot \beta O_2 \cdot sO_2 \qquad\qquad (3)$$

where βO_2 is the oxygen binding capacity: 1 mol O_2 per 1 mol Fe.
The normal O_2 content vs. pO_2 curve is shown, together with two
other curves, one representing blood of which cHb* is reduced by
50.8%, and the other representing blood with FHbCO = 50.8%. It can
clearly be seen that a certain amount of HbCO in the blood impedes
O_2 transport more than anemia of a corresponding degree, because
of the concomitant shift to the left of the ODC.

A comparison has been made between the ODC's recorded in the
presence of various amounts of HbCO and those calculated from the
standard ODC[9] for the same values of FHbCO by means of the procedure described by Roughton and Darling[12]. This calculation is
based on two assumptions, already made by Haldane[14] in 1912: (1)
the concentration of unliganded hemoglobin in blood with a certain
pO_2 and pCO is the same as in blood without CO with an oxygen
tension equal to pO_2 + M·pCO, where M is the relative affinity
factor for CO in relation to O_2 for the binding site in hemo-

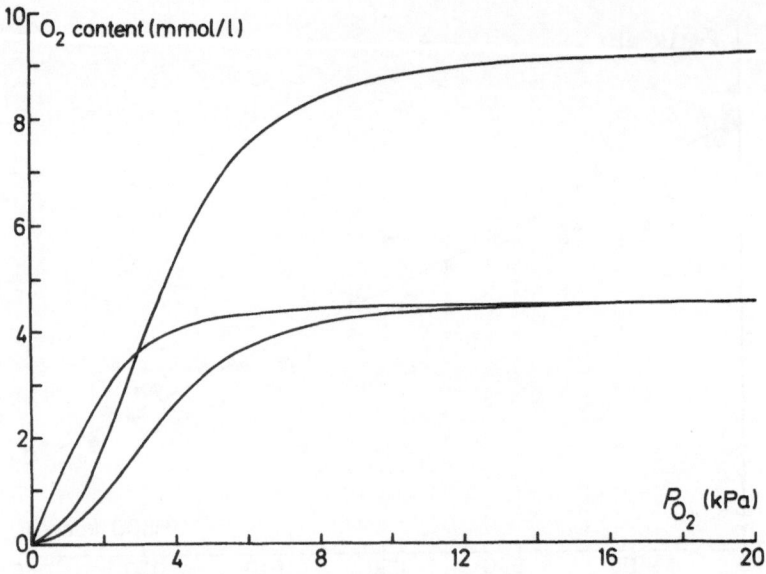

Fig. 7. O_2 content plotted against pO_2 (pH = 7.40, pCO_2 = 5.33 kPa, temperature = 37 °C), based on the data of Fig. 5. The upper line represents blood without HbCO; the lower right line relates to blood without HbCO after reduction of cHb* by 50.8%; the lower left line relates to blood with FHbCO = 50.8%.

globin; (2) hemoglobin combined with either CO or O_2 is partition-ed between HbCO and HbO_2 according to

$$\frac{cHbCO}{cHbO_2} = M \cdot \frac{pCO}{pO_2} \qquad (4)$$

where cHbCO and $cHbO_2$ are the concentrations of HbCO and HbO_2 in the blood and pCO and pO_2 the corresponding partial pressures; $M \approx 230$[15].

An appreciable difference between measured and calculated ODC's in the range of sO_2 = 20–80% proved to be present only when FHbCO was > 50%; the measured ODC was then situated to the left of the calculated one[11]. At lower values of FHbCO there was only a slight difference at low sO_2. Thus it may be concluded that for FHbCO < 50% there is hardly any difference as regards heme–heme interaction between the reactions of hemoglobin with CO and O_2, except at very low sO_2. However, at higher values of FHbCO, CO has a somewhat larger effect on heme–heme interaction than O_2. This is compatible with Roughton's finding that the carbon monoxide dis-sociation curve is somewhat steeper than the ODC[15].

Since in the reaction of hemoglobin with CO as compared to O_2 an appreciably stronger heme–heme interaction is only present at

very high FHbCO or at very low sO_2, this factor hardly contributes to the toxicity of CO. The very strong effect of CO on O_2 transport can be explained by the two factors already distinguished by Haldane[14] and more clearly described by Roughton and Darling[12].
(1) The presence of HbCO in the blood diminishes the oxygen capacity, i.e. the amount of oxygen that can be bound per unit of blood; in this respect the effect of HbCO is analogous to anemia.
(2) The gas pressure at which O_2 is released in the tissue capillaries is $pO_2 + M \cdot pCO$. Because M is large (ca. 230), $M \cdot pCO$ is a considerable part of the releasing pressure. This leaves only a low pO_2 available for actually driving the O_2 diffusion to the tissue cells.

REFERENCES

1. A. Zwart, Unpublished data (1984).
2. E.J. van Kampen, H.C. Volger, and W.G. Zijlstra, Spectrophotometric determination of carboxyhaemoglobin in human blood and the application of this method to the estimation of carbon monoxide in gasmixtures, Proc.Kon.Ned.Akad. Wet. C57: 320 (1954).
3. E.J. van Kampen and W.G. Zijlstra, Spectrophotometry of hemoglobin and hemoglobin derivatives, Adv.Clin.Chem. 23: 199 (1983).
4. P. Dijkhuizen, A. Buursma, A.M. Gerding, E.J. van Kampen, and W.G. Zijlstra, Carboxyhaemoglobin. Spectrophotometric determination tested and calibrated using a new reference method for measuring carbon monoxide in blood, Clin.Chem.Acta 80: 95 (1977).
5. A. Zwart, A. Buursma, E.J. van Kampen, B. Oeseburg, P.H.W. van der Ploeg, and W.G. Zijlstra, A multiwavelength spectrophotometric method for the simultaneous determination of five haemoglobin derivatives, J.Clin.Chem.Clin.Biochem. 19: 459 (1981).
6. L.J.A. Brown, A new instrument for the simultaneous measurement of total hemoglobin, % oxyhemoglobin, % carboxyhemoglobin, % methemoglobin, and oxygen content in whole blood, I.E.E.E. Trans.Bio-Med.Electron. 27: 132 (1980).
7. A. Zwart, A. Buursma, B. Oeseburg, and W.G. Zijlstra, Determination of hemoglobin derivatives with the IL282 CO-Oximeter as compared with a manual spectrophotometric five-wavelength method, Clin.Chem. 27: 1903 (1981).
8. A. Zwart, A. Buursma, E.J. van Kampen, and W.G. Zijlstra, Multicomponent analysis of hemoglobin derivatives with a reversed-optics spectrophotometer, Clin.Chem. 30: 373 (1984).
9. A. Zwart, G. Kwant, B. Oeseburg, and W.G. Zijlstra, Oxygen dissociation curves for whole blood, recorded with an instrument that continuously measures pO_2 and sO_2 independently at constant t, pCO_2 and pH, Clin.Chem. 28: 1287 (1982).

10. W.G. Zijlstra, G. Kwant, B. Oeseburg, and A. Zwart, Oxygen affinity of human whole blood investigated by means of a new analytic set-up, in: "Hemoglobin", A.G. Schneck and C. Paul, eds. Editions de l'Université de Bruxelles, Brussels (1984).

11. A. Zwart, G. Kwant, B. Oeseburg, and W.G. Zijlstra, Human whole-blood oxygen affinity: effect of carbon monoxide, J. Appl.Physiol.: Respirat.Environ.Exercise Physiol. 57: 14 (1984).

12. F.J.W. Roughton and R.C. Darling, The effect of carbon monoxide on the oxyhemoglobin dissociation curve, Am.J.Physiol. 141: 17 (1944).

13. M.P. Hlastala, H.P. McKenna, R.L. Franada, and J.C. Detter, Influence of carbon monoxide on hemoglobin-oxygen binding, J.Appl.Physiol. 41: 893 (1976).

14. J.B.S. Haldane, The dissociation curve of oxyhaemoglobin in human blood during partial CO-poisoning, J.Physiol.London 45: XXII (1912).

15. F.J.W. Roughton, The equilibrium of carbon monoxide with human hemoglobin in whole blood, Annals N.Y.Acad.Sci 174: 177 (1970)

CONTRIBUTION OF THE HALDANE EFFECT TO THE INCREASE IN ARTERIAL CARBON DIOXIDE TENSION IN HYPOXAEMIC SUBJECTS TREATED WITH OXYGEN

J. Kraan and P. Rispens

Departments of Pulmonary Diseases and Physiology
University of Groningen, Groningen, The Netherlands

INTRODUCTION

Carbon dioxide retention is a well-known risk of oxygen administration to hypoxaemic patients. The classic explanation for this retention is that oxygen cuts off the hypoxic drive for ventilation leading to a decreased ventilation in patients in whom the ventilatory response to carbon dioxide is diminished. However, Aubier et al.[1] found only a slight decrease in steady state minute ventilation ($\dot{V}E$) in patients with chronic obstructive pulmonary disease (COPD) in whom hypoxaemia had been relieved by oxygen administration. Nevertheless, the mean rise in arterial oxygen tension ($pO_2(a)$) of 38 to 225 mmHg and in arterial oxygen saturation ($sO_2(a)$) of 65% to 100% in their patients was attended by a mean rise in arterial carbon dioxide tension ($pCO_2(a)$) of 65 to 88 mmHg. The greater part of this rise is explained by an increased inhomogeneity of the ventilation/perfusion ($\dot{V}/\dot{Q}$) distribution within the lungs, which may be due to the relief by oxygen of hypoxic vasoconstriction in poorly ventilated lung units. In addition a substantial part of the rise in $pCO_2(a)$ is ascribed to the Haldane effect. Aubier et al. calculate that in their series the Haldane effect caused a rise in $pCO_2(a)$ of 7 mmHg. This value was derived from changes in pCO_2 seen when in blood in vitro some of the CO_2 bound as bicarbonate and carbamate is set free by oxygenation and converted into dissolved CO_2. In their calculations the CO_2 set free by oxygenation was handled as if it did not escape from the blood. However, in vivo CO_2 set free by oxygen administration escapes to the alveolar space and is eliminated with the expiratory gas. Hence the Haldane effect can only be held responsible for a transient increase in $pCO_2(a)$ lasting until the CO_2 set free by oxygenation is expired.

Steady state $pCO_2(a)$ in vivo is mainly governed by metabolic CO_2 production ($\dot{V}CO_2$) and alveolar ventilation ($\dot{V}A$). In an ideal lung, with equal $\dot{V}/\dot{Q}$ ratios in all compartments, $pCO_2(a)$ may be assumed to be equal to the alveolar pCO_2 ($pCO_2(A)$):

$$pCO_2(a) = pCO_2(A) = \frac{\dot{V}CO_2}{K \cdot \dot{V}A} \qquad (1)$$

where $K = 1/(pB-pH_2O)$. Therefore, steady state pCO_2 cannot change in an ideal lung when $\dot{V}CO_2$ and $\dot{V}A$ remain constant. However, in patients with chronic obstructive pulmonary disease (COPD) the situation is more complex. Most hypoxaemic COPD patients to whom O_2 is administered have lungs with abnormal $\dot{V}/\dot{Q}$ distribution, which may cause large alveolo-arterial differences in pCO_2. Hence Eq. (1) cannot be applied without restriction in these patients. We therefore calculated the effect of oxygen administration on steady state $pCO_2(a)$ both at hypoxaemia with normal $\dot{V}/\dot{Q}$ distribution and at hypoxaemia with abnormal $\dot{V}/\dot{Q}$ distribution. For the calculations, we used the computer program for the ten-compartment lung model of West and Wagner[2]. A case of normal $\dot{V}/\dot{Q}$ distribution was used to demonstrate that O_2 administration as such has no influence on $pCO_2(a)$ through the Haldane effect in healthy conditions. A case of abnormal $\dot{V}/\dot{Q}$ distribution was used to obtain the contribution of the Haldane effect per se to the increase in $pCO_2(a)$, found by Aubier et al. in their patients.

CALCULATIONS

The computer program of West and Wagner allows the calculation of steady state gas tensions and concentrations of mixed venous blood, blood equilibrated in different lung compartments and arterial blood in subjects with given oxygen consumption ($\dot{V}O_2$), carbon dioxide production ($\dot{V}CO_2$), alveolar ventilation ($\dot{V}A$) and cardiac output ($\dot{Q}$). Calculations are made at given body temperature, haemoglobin concentration, haematocrit, inspiratory volume fractions of O_2 and CO_2 ($FO_2(I)$ and $FCO_2(I)$) and barometric pressure (pB). Different degrees of inhomogeneous $\dot{V}/\dot{Q}$ distribution can be introduced by assigning different values for the log standard deviation of ventilation and blood flow in the ten lung compartments. In addition a percentage of true shunt circulation can be introduced.

In our calculations, administration of O_2 in a case of hypercapnia and hypoxaemia at normal $\dot{V}/\dot{Q}$ distribution and at abnormal $\dot{V}/\dot{Q}$ distribution was simulated. Input values are shown in table 1. The input values were so chosen that before O_2 administration degrees of hypercapnia and hypoxaemia comparable to those found in Aubier's patients before the O_2 treatment were obtained. In the case of normal $\dot{V}/\dot{Q}$ distribution $\dot{V}A$ had to be decreased to obtain the desired degree of hypercapnia ($pCO_2(a) = 59.6$ mmHg) and $FO_2(I)$

Table 1. Input values for studying the influence of $FO_2(I)$ on $pCO_2(a)$ at normal and abnormal $\dot{V}/\dot{Q}$ distributions

	normal case	abnormal case
$\dot{V}O_2$ (ml·min^{-1})	300	300
$\dot{V}CO_2$ (ml·min^{-1})	240	240
$\dot{Q}p$ (l·min^{-1})	6	5.5
$\dot{V}A$ (l·min^{-1})	3.5	4.4
cHb (g·l^{-1})	148	148
pB (mmHg)	760	760
log SD ($\dot{V}A$)	0.25	1.15
log SD ($\dot{Q}$)	0.001	0.001
true shunt (%)	–	20
$FO_2(I)$	0.15 →1	0.21 →1

had to be decreased to obtain the desired degree of hypoxaemia ($pO_2(a)$ = 40.0 mmHg, $sO_2(a)$ = 68%). In the case of abnormal $\dot{V}/\dot{Q}$ distribution a true shunt of 20% was added to the $\dot{V}/\dot{Q}$ inequality. This was done because otherwise during administration of pure O_2, $pO_2(a)$ would rise to values much higher than those found in Aubier's patients. At the values chosen for the abnormal case, degrees of hypercapnia ($pCO_2(a)$ = 61.1 mmHg) and hypoxaemia (pO_2 (a) = 40.6 mmHg, $sO_2(a)$ = 69%) obtained during air breathing were comparable with those seen in Aubier's patients, and during administration of pure O_2 the same increase in $pO_2(a)$ as seen in Aubier's patients was obtained.

RESULTS

The effects of increasing $FO_2(I)$ on pO_2, sO_2, pCO_2 and total CO_2 concentration (cCO_2) in arterial blood, mixed venous blood and blood equilibrated in a lung compartment with high $\dot{V}/\dot{Q}$ ratio and with low $\dot{V}/\dot{Q}$ ratio is shown in figs. 1A through 4A in the case of normal $\dot{V}/\dot{Q}$ distribution and in figs. 1B through 4B in the case of abnormal $\dot{V}/\dot{Q}$ distribution with true shunt. It should be noted that in the case of normal $\dot{V}/\dot{Q}$ distribution the top (nr. 1) and bottom (nr. 10) compartments with the highest $\dot{V}/\dot{Q}$ and the lowest $\dot{V}/\dot{Q}$ ratio, respectively, have been chosen, whereas in the case of abnormal $\dot{V}/\dot{Q}$ distribution two less extreme compartments (nr. 3 and 7) were chosen.

Both at normal and at abnormal $\dot{V}/\dot{Q}$ distribution breathing of pure oxygen results in improved oxygenation of arterial blood. $pO_2(a)$ and $sO_2(a)$ rise to 645 mmHg and 100% at normal $\dot{V}/\dot{Q}$ distribution and to 230 mmHg and 99.5% at abnormal $\dot{V}/\dot{Q}$ distribution and shunt circulation. Both in the compartments with a high $\dot{V}/\dot{Q}$ and those with a low $\dot{V}/\dot{Q}$ ratio, pO_2 increases to values around 650 mmHg and sO_2 to 100%. This is the case both at normal and abnormal

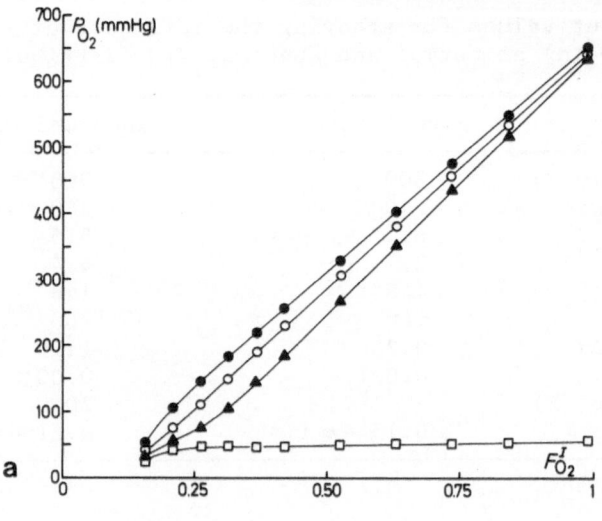

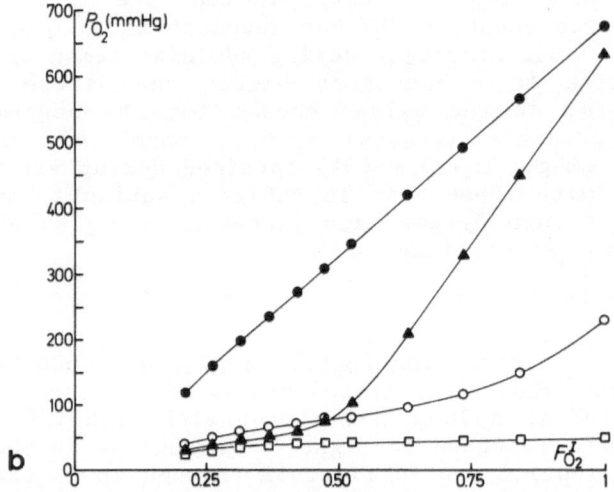

Fig. 1.   Effect of $FO_2(I)$ on pO_2 in mixed venous blood (▭),
arterial blood (○), blood equilibrated in a high $\dot{V}/\dot{Q}$
compartment (●) and blood equilibrated in a low $\dot{V}/\dot{Q}$
compartment (▲).
A: normal case; B: abnormal case. In the normal case the
top compartment (nr. 1, $\dot{V}$ = 0.021 $l \cdot min^{-1}$; $\dot{Q}$ = 0.018 $l \cdot
min^{-1}$) and the bottom compartment (nr. 10, $\dot{V}$ = 0.005
$l \cdot min^{-1}$, $\dot{Q}$ = 0.018 $l \cdot min^{-1}$) are shown. In the abnormal
case compartment nr. 3 ($\dot{V}$ = 1.195 $l\ min^{-1}$; $\dot{Q}$ = 0.341 $l \cdot
min^{-1}$) and nr. 7 ($\dot{V}$ = 0.047 $l \cdot min^{-1}$; $\dot{Q}$ = 0.480 $l \cdot min^{-1}$)
are shown.

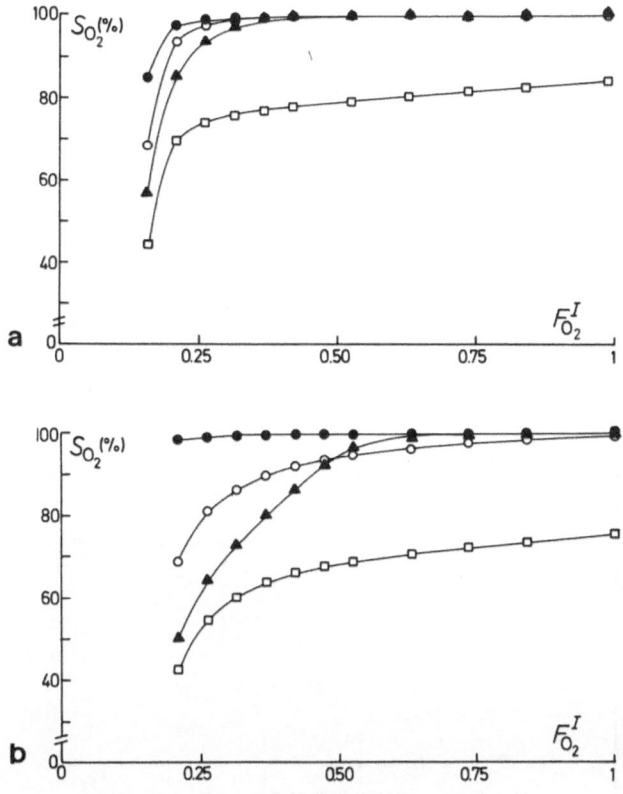

Fig. 2.   Effect of $FO_2(I)$ on sO_2. Details in Fig. 1.

$\dot{V}/\dot{Q}$ distribution.

Both at normal and at abnormal $\dot{V}/\dot{Q}$ distribution, correction of hypoxaemia is attended by an increase in $pCO_2(\bar{v})$, an increase in pCO_2 in the lung compartments with a low $\dot{V}/\dot{Q}$ ratio, a decrease in pCO_2 in the lung compartment with a high $\dot{V}/\dot{Q}$ ratio, and an increase in veno-arterial difference in pCO_2. At normal $\dot{V}/\dot{Q}$ distribution these changes go along with hardly any increase in $pCO_2(a)$ (0.2 mmHg). However, at abnormal $\dot{V}/\dot{Q}$ distribution and true shunt circulation a substantial increase in $pCO_2(a)$ (3.7 mmHg) is found.

DISCUSSION

In the calculations presented here the contribution of the Haldane effect per se to the increase in steady state $pCO_2(a)$ found when hypoxaemic subjects are treated with O_2 is obtained; the possible effects of O_2 on ventilation and $\dot{V}/\dot{Q}$ distribution are excluded by keeping these quantities constant when oxygen is

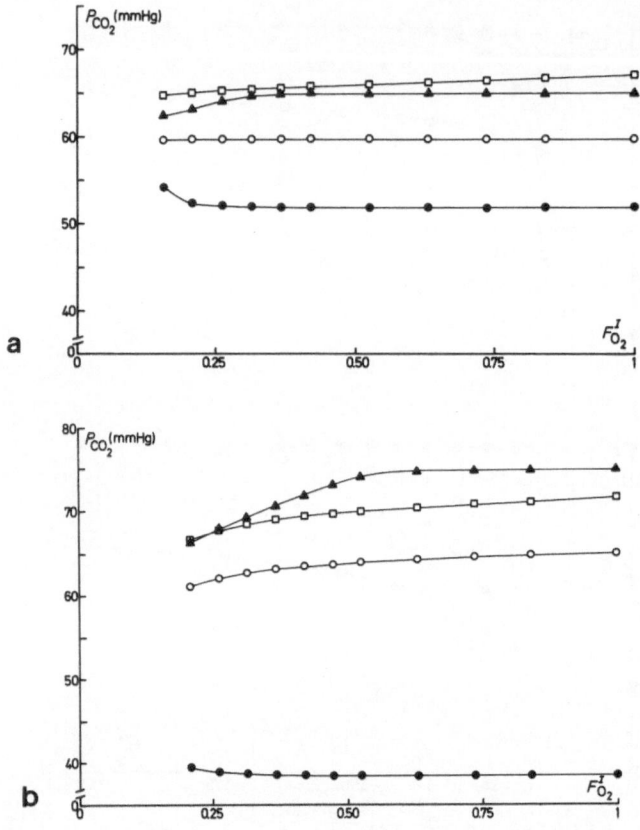

Fig. 3.   Effect of $FO_2(I)$ on pCO_2. Details in Fig. 1.

administered. The calculations were carried out because, in our opinion, the contribution of the Haldane effect is overestimated in the literature[1,3,4].

In an ideal lung, steady state $pCO_2(a)$ solely depends upon $\dot{V}CO_2$ and $\dot{V}A$ and is not influenced by $FO_2(I)$ (Eq.(1)). Normal $\dot{V}/\dot{Q}$ distribution comes close to the ideal lung situation.
Using Eq. (1) a $pCO_2(a)$ = 59.2 mmHg is calculated from $\dot{V}CO_2$ = 240 ml (stpd)·min^{-1} and $\dot{V}A$ = 3500 ml (btps)·min^{-1}, while the ten compartment lung model used here yields $pCO_2(a)$ = 59.6 mmHg at $FO_2(I)$ = 0.15 and $pCO_2(a)$ = 59.8 mmHg at $FO_2(I)$ = 1 at normal $\dot{V}/\dot{Q}$ distribution. Hence, at normal $\dot{V}/\dot{Q}$ distribution, steady state $pCO_2(a)$ is virtually uninfluenced by $FO_2(I)$. At abnormal $\dot{V}/\dot{Q}$ distribution and shunt circulation, a notable increase in $pCO_2(a)$ is found: from 61.1 mmHg at $FO_2(I)$ = 0.2 to 64.8 mmHg at $FO_2(I)$ = 1. These changes correspond well with the data of Grant[5] who calculated the effect of <u>complete</u> elimination of the Haldane effect on $pCO_2(a)$. At normal $\dot{V}/\dot{Q}$ distribution no increase in $pCO_2(a)$

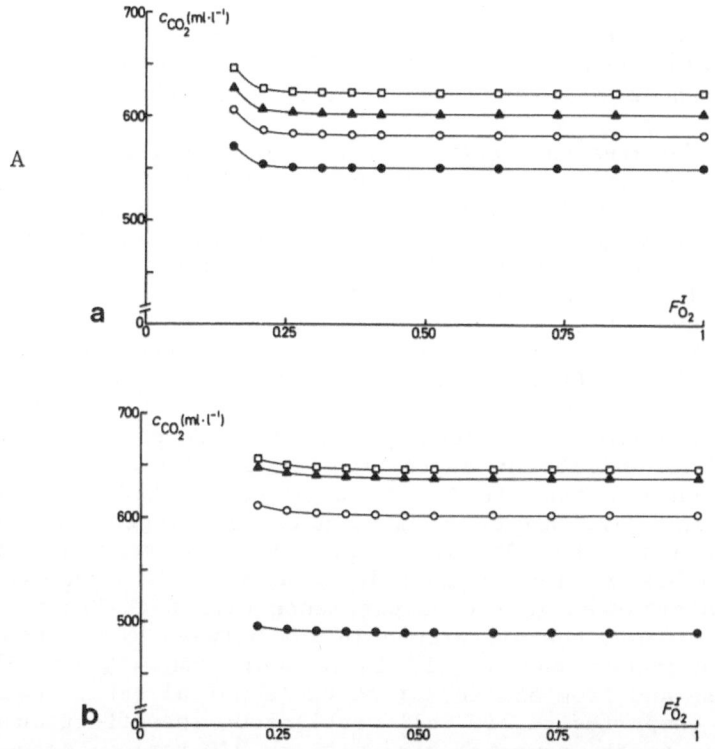

Fig. 4.   Effect of $FO_2(I)$ on cCO_2. Details in Fig. 1.

was found, but at abnormal $\dot{V}/\dot{Q}$ distribution increases in $pCO_2(a)$ of up to 10 mmHg were calculated. In our calculations only part of the Haldane effect is eliminated by increasing $FO_2(I)$. Therefore only part of the maximum increase in $pCO_2(a)$ can be expected.

To understand why $pCO_2(a)$ does increase at abnormal $\dot{V}/\dot{Q}$ distribution and shunt circulation and not at normal $\dot{V}/\dot{Q}$ distribution, the effect of increasing $FO_2(I)$ on gas values in mixed venous blood and blood in lung compartments with high and low $\dot{V}/\dot{Q}$ ratios has to be considered. Both at normal and at abnormal $\dot{V}/\dot{Q}$ distribution increase in $FO_2(I)$ is accompanied by an increase in $pCO_2(\bar{v})$. The increase in $pCO_2(\bar{v})$ is attended by an increase in the arterio-venous difference in pCO_2: from 5.1 to 7.3 mmHg at normal $\dot{V}/\dot{Q}$ distribution and from 5.5 to 6.7 mmHg at abnormal $\dot{V}/\dot{Q}$ distribution and shunt circulation. The increase in arterio-venous difference in pCO_2 is due to a reduction of the (reversed) Haldane effect: at $pO_2(a) = 645$ and 231 mmHg, a substantial part of the O_2 delivered to the tissues is transported by the blood as dissolved O_2. This part of the O_2 delivery does not contribute to the buffering of CO_2 by the Haldane effect. At normal $\dot{V}/\dot{Q}$ distribution the increase in $pCO_2(\bar{v})$ cannot influence $pCO_2(a)$ (Eq. (1)), but at abnormal $\dot{V}/\dot{Q}$ distribution with shunt circulation, part of the increased $pCO_2(\bar{v})$ can be transmitted directly to the arterial blood by the shunt and can thus contribute to the increase in $pCO_2(a)$.

However, the greatest contribution comes from the increase in pCO_2 in the lung compartments with low $\dot{V}/\dot{Q}$ ratios. This increase is seen both at normal $\dot{V}/\dot{Q}$ distribution (fig. 3A) and at abnormal $\dot{V}/\dot{Q}$ distribution (fig. 3B). In the latter case, pCO_2 in the low $\dot{V}/\dot{Q}$ compartment rises above $pCO_2(\bar{v})$. Nevertheless, some CO_2 is released from blood even in this compartment: cCO_2 in the blood leaving this compartment is less than $cCO_2(\bar{v})$ at all values of $FO_2(I)$ (fig. 4B). The rise in pCO_2 is due to the increase in oxygenation with $FO_2(I)$ of blood entering the low $\dot{V}/\dot{Q}$ compartments. The difference in sO_2 between mixed venous blood entering the low $\dot{V}/\dot{Q}$ compartment and blood leaving this compartment is 13% at $FO_2(I) = 0.15$ and 16% at $FO_2(I) = 1$ in the normal case (fig. 2A); in the abnormal case it is 7% at $FCO_2(I) = 0.2$ and 24% at $FO_2(I) = 1$ (fig. 2B). Owing to this increased oxygenation, more CO_2 is released to the alveolar space. Because ventilation in these compartments is low, a notable rise in pCO_2 results. Opposite changes are seen in the compartments with high $\dot{V}/\dot{Q}$ ratios. In these compartments the difference in sO_2 between blood entering and leaving decreases when $FO_2(I)$ increases: from 41% to 16% in the normal case and from 55% to 24% in the abnormal case. However, because these compartments are well ventilated, the effect on pCO_2 is smaller than in the compartments with low $\dot{V}/\dot{Q}$ ratios, especially in the abnormal case. At normal $\dot{V}/\dot{Q}$ distribution, the changes in pCO_2 in the different lung compartments hardly influence the value of $pCO_2(a)$: the increase in the low $\dot{V}/\dot{Q}$ compartments is balanced by the decrease in the high $\dot{V}/\dot{Q}$ compartments. At abnormal $\dot{V}/\dot{Q}$ distribution, however, the increase in pCO_2 in the low $\dot{V}/\dot{Q}$ compartments does result in an increase in $pCO_2(a)$: first because the increase in pCO_2 in the low $\dot{V}/\dot{Q}$ compartments is much larger than the decrease in the high $\dot{V}/\dot{Q}$ compartments; and second because, owing to the substantial blood flow in the low $\dot{V}/\dot{Q}$ compartments, these compartments contribute significantly to the composition of arterial blood.

Although in the case of abnormal $\dot{V}/\dot{Q}$ distribution and shunt circulation approximately the same changes in $pO_2(a)$ and $sO_2(a)$ were obtained by us as those seen in Aubier's patients, the increase in $pCO_2(a)$ in our calculation (3.7 mmHg) was less than that derived by Aubier et al. for the contribution of the Haldane effect (7 mmHg). Even smaller increases in $pCO_2(a)$ were calculated when Aubier's changes in $pCO_2(a)$ and $sO_2(a)$ were simulated by manipulating $\dot{V}/\dot{Q}$ distribution inequality without shunt or by manipulating the skewness of the distribution of $\dot{V}$ and $\dot{Q}$.

It has been pointed out above that the contribution of the Haldane effect as estimated by Aubier et al. was based on the erroneous assumption that all CO_2 set free by oxygenation remains in the blood. It can be seen in figs. 4A and 4B that cCO_2 decreases at increasing $FO_2(I)$ in mixed venous and arterial blood and in blood in the various lung compartments. Thus CO_2 set free by oxygenation is eliminated. Hence, Aubier's value of 7 mmHg is an overestimation of the contribution of the Haldane effect to the increase in $pCO_2(a)$ seen when hypoxaemic COPD patients are treated with O_2.

REFERENCES

1. M. Aubier, D. Murciano, J. Milic-Emily, E. Touaty, J. Dagfous, R. Pariente, and J.P. Derenne, Effects of the administration of O_2 on ventilation and blood gases in patients with chronic obstructive pulmonary disease during acute respiratory failure, Am.Rev.Respir.Dis. 122: 747 (1980).
2. J.B. West, and P.D. Wagner, Pulmonary gas exchange, in: Bio-engineering aspects of the lung, J.B. West, ed., M. Dekker, New York, (1977).
3. N.R. Anthonisen, Hypoxemia and O_2 therapy. Am.Rev.Respir.Dis. 126: 729 (1982).
4. U.C. Luft, E.M. Mostyn, J.A. Loeppky, and M.D. Venters, Contribution of the Haldane effect to the rise of arterial pCO_2 in hypoxic patients breathing oxygen. Crit.Care Med. 9: 32 (1981).
5. B.J.B. Grant, Influence of Bohr-Haldane effect on steady-state gas exchange, J.Appl.Physiol. 52: 1330 (1982).

CHANGES IN ARTERIAL CARBON DIOXIDE TENSION AND ARTERIO-VENOUS

DIFFERENCE IN OXYGEN CONTENT WITH pH DURING METABOLIC ACIDOSIS

A.J.M. Langbroek, P. Rispens and W.G. Zijlstra

Department of Physiology, University of Groningen
Groningen, The Netherlands

INTRODUCTION

The decrease in arterial pH (pH(a)) during metabolic acidosis stimulates ventilation. Knowledge of the magnitude and time course of this response is important for the assessment of acid-base disturbances from pH, pCO_2 and $cHCO_3^-$ [1,2] and for the treatment of these disturbances. However, the time course is still a matter of controversy. Owing to the poor permeability of the blood brain barrier to H^+ and HCO_3^- it has been generally assumed that there is a time lag in the ventilatory response to metabolic acidosis [3]. Some authors [4,5] have indeed found a further decrease in arterial pCO_2 (pCO_2(a)) when after induction of metabolic acidosis by means of intravenously administered HCl, pH(a) was kept low by additional administration of HCl. However, in recent years it has been demonstrated that in dogs and cats a fast exchange of HCO_3^- across the blood brain barrier is possible [6,7]. In agreement with this fast exchange, Kaehny and Jackson found no time lag in the ventilatory response to metabolic acidosis in an investigation in dogs about the role of the peripheral chemoreceptors [8].

Another effect of the decrease in pH(a) during metabolic acidosis is a decreased O_2 affinity of the blood. It is usually supposed that the decreased O_2 affinity favours O_2 delivery to the tissues. However, to our knowledge it has not been investigated whether the decreased O_2 affinity during metabolic acidosis actually results in an increase in mixed venous pO_2 ($pO_2(\bar{v})$) or an increase in the arterio-venous difference in O_2 concentration ($cO_2(a)-cO_2(\bar{v})$).

In this investigation the controversy of the time dependence of the ventilatory response to metabolic acidosis was studied in conscious dogs in which an acidosis was induced by intravenous or oral administration of HCl or NH_4Cl. In some of the experiments, the effect of acidosis on O_2 delivery to the tissues was also studied.

MATERIAL AND METHODS

Experiments were carried out in mongrel dogs of either sex weighing 18-43 kg. The dogs were equipped with permanent catheters in the aorta and pulmonary artery[9]. The catheter in the aorta was used for sampling, that in the pulmonary artery both for sampling and administration of acid.

Time course of the ventilatory response. Four series of six experiments each were carried out to study the time course of the ventilatory response as indicated by $pCO_2(a)$ to a metabolic acidosis: intravenous administration of HCl, intravenous administration of NH_4Cl, oral administration of HCl and oral administration of NH_4Cl.

Before the start of an experiment the dogs were fasted for 16 h except for the use of water. During the experiment the animals lay quietly in a basket for 16 h under continuous supervision. This 16 h period was divided in a control phase of 1 h, an induction phase of 3 h and a maintenance phase of 12 h. Thereafter the dog was brought to its cage where it was kept acidotic for another 16 h. The total maintenance phase thus lasted 28 h. In the presentation of the results, this period is divided into a first part of 6 h (maintenance phase I), a second part of 6 h (maintenance phase II) and a third part of 16 h (maintenance phase III). After the maintenance phase pH was allowed to return to normal (recovery phase). The whole procedure is shown in fig. 1.

In the experiments with intravenous administration of HCl or NH_4Cl, pH was decreased to approximately 7.2 in about 3 h with the help of a 500 $mmol·l^{-1}$ HCl or NH_4Cl in 0.9% NaCl solution. The initial infusion rate was 0.04 mmol acid per kg per min. During the induction phase the infusion rate was adjusted on the basis of the measured pH(a) values. During maintenance phases I and II pH(a) was kept low with 200 or 100 $mmol·l^{-1}$ acid in 5% glucose solution. In maintenance phase III, pH was kept low by feeding the dogs a semi-synthetic protein-rich, electrolyte-free diet (URL, Vlaardingen). Thereafter pH was allowed to return to normal by feeding normal dog food.

In the experiments with oral administration, HCl or NH_4Cl dissolved in the semi-synthetic food was given via a gastric tube. A total amount of 10 mmol per kg was given in one to three doses. Within 3 h pH(a) decreased to about 7.2. This period was taken as the induction phase. In the following maintenance phases I and II the dogs were only allowed to drink distilled water. During maintenance phase III the animals were given semi-synthetic food. In the recovery phase normal dog food was given.

O_2 delivery to the tissues. The effect of acidosis on O_2

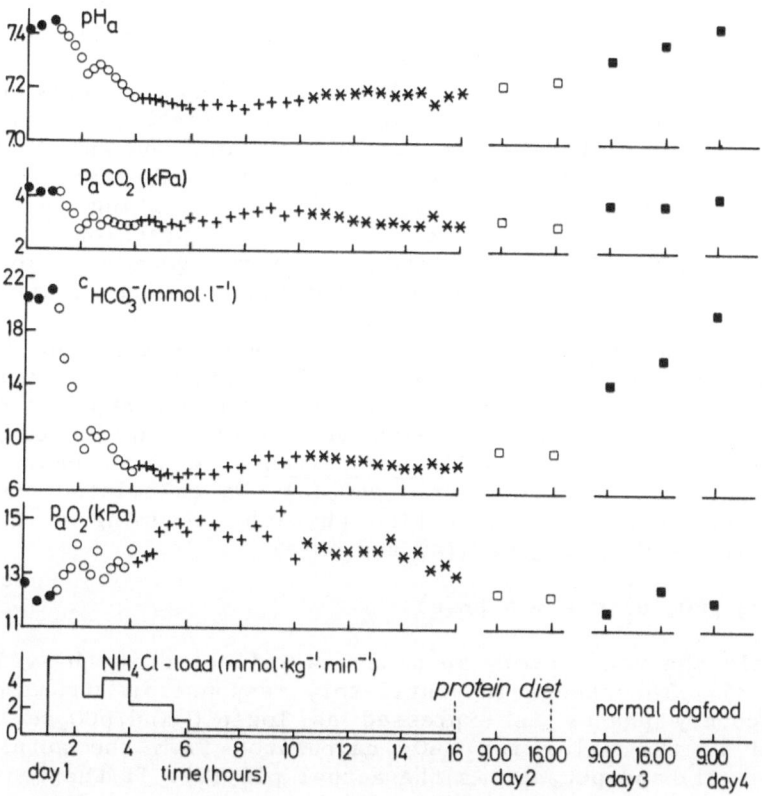

Fig. 1.   The course of pH(a), pCO_2(a), $cHCO_3^-$ and pO_2(a) in one
acidosis experiment. ● = control phase; o = induction
phase; + = maintenance phase I; * = maintenance phase
II; □ = maintenance phase III; ■ = recovery phase.

delivery to the tissues was studied in four of the experiments. In
this study each dog was used for an acidosis experiment (v.s.) and
a control experiment. In the acidosis experiments pH was decreased
to about 7.2 by oral administration of HCl (n=1) or NH_4Cl (n=3).
O_2 delivery was studied in maintenance phases I and II. $pO_2(\bar{v})$ and
$(cO_2(a)-cO_2(\bar{v}))$ in this period were compared with those in the
corresponding period of the control experiment. In the control
experiment, a 4 h period of habituation was followed by a 12 h
period of studying O_2 delivery.

Sampling. In the control phase three arterial blood samples
were drawn at 30 min intervals. In the induction phase samples
were taken every 15 min. In the maintenance phases I and II
samples were taken every 30 min. In maintenance phase III two samples were taken at an interval of 8 h. During the recovery phase
two samples were taken every day, one at 8 a.m. and one at 4 p.m.
In the experiments on O_2 delivery the arterial and mixed venous
samples were taken simultaneously.

Habituation to the sampling procedure. During the first 16 h of the experiments the dogs were in the experimental room. Sampling took place while the animals were lying quietly in their basket in continuous presence of the investigator. In maintenance phase III and in the recovery phase, however, the animals were in their cages. Meeting the investigator again the next morning may have caused excitement in some animals, resulting in an extra stimulation of the ventilation. To get an impression of this effect the course of $pCO_2(a)$ during the first 90 min following the renewed meeting with the investigator was studied in six dogs by taking arterial samples every 15 min.

Analytical techniques. pH, pO_2 and pCO_2 were measured with an automatic blood gas analyzer (ABL-2, Radiometer, Copenhagen). Plasma $cHCO_3^-$ was calculated from pH and pCO_2. sO_2 and cHb were measured with the help of a hemoxymeter (OSM-2, Radiometer).

Calculation. The ventilatory response to a decrease in pH(a) is manifested in a decrease in $pCO_2(a)$. We calculated the ventilatory response in the induction phase by assuming a linear relationship between $\log pCO_2(a)$ and pH(a).

$$\log pCO_2(a) = a + b\ pH(a) \tag{1}$$

Obviously the ventilatory response is reflected in the value of b in Eq. (1). The change in ventilatory response in the maintenance and recovery phases is expressed as $\log(pCO_2ind/pCO_2act)$, where pCO_2ind is the value for pCO_2 calculated from the actual pH(a) with Eq. (1) and pCO_2act is the actual $pCO_2(a)$. If the ventilatory response is increased $\log(pCO_2ind/pCO_2act)$ is positive; if it is decreased $\log(pCO_2ind/pCO_2act)$ is negative. The induction line as calculated with the help of Eq. (1) is plotted in a $pH/cHCO_3^-$ diagram together with all individual values measured during the experiments (figs. 2 and 3). If the ventilatory response is increased during the maintenance phase points of this phase are found right from the induction line (fig. 3), if it is decreased, points fall to the left of the induction line (fig. 2).

Arterio-venous differences in cO_2 were calculated with the help of Eq. (2).

$$cO_2(a)-cO_2(\bar{v}) = cHb \cdot \beta O_2 \cdot (sO_2(a)-sO_2(\bar{v})) \tag{2}$$

cO_2 is expressed in $ml \cdot l^{-1}$, cHb in $g \cdot l^{-1}$. For βO_2, 1.36 ml O_2 per g Hb was used.

Statistical analysis of differences was carried out using the Student T test: ns = $P > 0.05$, * = $0.05 > P > 0.01$, ** = $0.01 > P > 0.001$ and *** = $0.001 > P$.

RESULTS

Ventilatory response in the induction phase. In all experiments a decrease in $pCO_2(a)$ with pH(a) was observed in the induc-

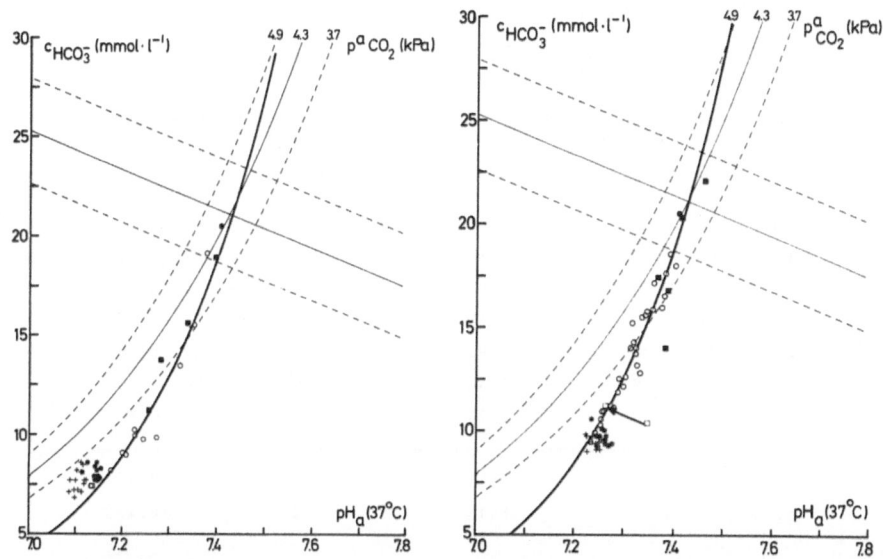

Fig. 2.   pH-cHCO₃⁻-plot of the experiment of fig. 1. The
(left)   induction line is given by $\log pCO_2(a) = -3.91 + 0.61$
           $pH(a)$. A decreased ventilatory response is seen during
           the maintenance phases I and II relative to the induc-
           tion phase. Symbols as in fig. 1.

Fig. 3.   pH-cHCO₃⁻-plot of another experiment. The induction line
(right)   is given by $\log pCO_2(a) = -4.90 + 0.74 pH(a)$. An in-
           creased ventilatory response is seen during the main-
           tenance phases I and II relative to the induction phase.
           Arrow indicates the change in ventilatory response
           during a habituation experiment in maintenance phase III.

tion phase. The ventilatory stimulation $b (= \Delta\log pCO_2/\Delta pH$, cf. Eq.
(1)) found in the experiments is shown in table 1, together with
the intercepts a. For the intravenous HCl and NH₄Cl experiments,
$b = 0.52 \pm 0.20$ and $b = 0.51 \pm 0.15$, respectively. In the oral HCl
and NH₄Cl experiments, the stimulation was somewhat smaller
($b = 0.28 \pm 0.27$ and $b = 0.36 \pm 0.19$, respectively). No
significant differences in ventilatory response between the four
series were revealed by the Student T-test.

 Ventilatory response during maintenance phases I and II.
Figs. 2 and 3 show different ventilatory responses in two
experiments. In fig. 2 a decrease in ventilatory response in
comparison with the induction phase is indicated; in fig. 3 an
increase is indicated. Table 2 presents mean values and s.d. of
$\log(pCO_2ind/pCO_2act)$ found in the maintenance phases I and II in
each experiment. From this table large dog-to-dog differences in

Table 1. Intercepts (a) and slopes (b) of the
four series of metabolic acidosis
experiments.

| | Intravenous | | | | Oral | | | |
| | HCl | | NH_4Cl | | HCl | | NH_4Cl | |
no	a	b	a	b	a	b	a	b
1	-2.36	0.41	-3.40	0.55	-0.22	0.11	-1.27	0.26
2	-4.08	0.64	-3.91	0.61	-3.85	0.61	-2.24	0.39
3	-2.02	0.36	-2.16	0.38	-0.68	0.18	-4.32	0.67
4	-1.31	0.26	-2.57	0.44	-4.03	0.63	-1.27	0.26
5	-4.42	0.69	-1.91	0.34	+0.55	0.01	-2.56	0.43
6	-4.81	0.74	-4.90	0.74	-0.41	0.14	-0.25	0.12
Mean		0.52		0.51		0.28		0.36
s.d.		0.20		0.15		0.27		0.19

the time course of the ventilatory response to metabolic acidosis
become apparent. In eight experiments a significant increase in
the ventilatory response is to be found in maintenance phase I in
comparison to the induction phase; in six experiments there is a
significant decrease and in 10 experiments no significant changes
in response can be observed. In maintenance phase II, ventilatory
response can be seen to be larger in comparison to the induction
phase in 11 experiments, in three experiments a significant decrease is to be found and in 10 experiments there are no significant changes. In nine experiments the ventilatory response in
maintenance phase II is larger than in maintenance phase I, in
four experiments it is smaller and in 11 experiments there is no
significant difference to be seen.

Ventilatory response during maintenance phase III and during
the recovery phase. Role of habituation in the sampling. In the
experiment represented in fig. 2, ventilation in maintenance phase
III and recovery phase shows no increase in comparison with the
induction phase: the measured values are found scattered around
the induction line. In the experiments represented in fig. 3,
values measured in maintenance phase III and in the recovery phase
fall clearly to the right of the induction line. However, if
during the 90 min after the first sample in maintenance phase III
new samples are taken every 15 min while the dog was lying quietly
in its basket, the measured values return to those corresponding
to the induction curve (indicated by the arrow). This was found in
all habituation experiments in which ventilation seemed to have
been stimulated in maintenance phase III (table 3).

O_2 delivery to the tissues. Fig. 4 shows $pO_2(\bar{v})$ and
$(cO_2(a)-cO_2(\bar{v}))$ as found in one dog in the presence of acidosis
and in a control experiment. Mean values and s.d. of $(cO_2(a)-cO_2(\bar{v}))$

and $pO_2(\bar{v})$ as found in four dogs during acidosis and in control experiments are presented in table 4. In each dog $(cO_2(a)-cO_2(\bar{v}))$ is significantly higher in the presence of acidosis while no significant change is to be seen in $pO_2(\bar{v})$.

Table 2. Ventilatory stimulation (log pCO_2ind/pCO_2act) during maintenance phase I (3-9 h) and maintenance phase II (9-15 h) compared to the induction phase.

Intravenous HCl		Oral HCl	
3-9 h	9-15 h	3-9 h	9-15 h
0.101 ± 0.018 ***	0.060 ± 0.027 ***	0.012 ± 0.023 n.s.	0.022 ± 0.018 **
-0.025 ± 0.035 *	-0.063 ± 0.023 ***	-0.032 ± 0.030 *	0.006 ± 0.041 n.s.
0.007 ± 0.023 n.s.	-0.013 ± 0.031 n.s.	0.048 ± 0.022 ***	0.017 ± 0.020 *
0.010 ± 0.022 n.s.	0.019 ± 0.039 n.s.	-0.042 ± 0.045 **	-0.009 ± 0.030 n.s.
0.046 ± 0.048 *	-0.001 ± 0.022 n.s.	0.047 ± 0.035 ***	0.026 ± 0.023 **
-0.043 ± 0.035 *	-0.080 ± 0.009 ***	0.019 ± 0.033 n.s.	0.023 ± 0.013 n.s.

Intravenous NH_4Cl		Oral NH_4Cl	
3-9 h	9-15 h	3-9 h	9-15 h
-0.046 ± 0.010 ***	0.010 ± 0.018 n.s.	0.051 ± 0.040 ***	0.077 ± 0.029 ***
-0.083 ± 0.033 ***	-0.049 ± 0.029 ***	-0.001 ± 0.023 n.s.	0.022 ± 0.020 *
0.017 ± 0.046 n.s.	0.048 ± 0.028 **	0.013 ± 0.020 n.s.	0.032 ± 0.048 *
-0.004 ± 0.029 n.s.	-0.009 ± 0.023 n.s.	0.000 ± 0.029 n.s.	-0.002 ± 0.036 n.s.
0.000 ± 0.019 n.s.	0.013 ± 0.019 n.s.	0.019 ± 0.021 *	0.044 ± 0.022 ***
0.026 ± 0.025 ***	0.046 ± 0.036 ***	0.053 ± 0.026 **	0.097 ± 0.035 ***

Table 3. Ventilatory stimulation (log pCO_2ind/pCO_2act) in six habituation experiments in maintenance phase III.

Dog	time (min)						
	0	15	30	45	60	75	90
1	0.084	0.033	0.005	0.057	-0.040	0.020	0.014
2	0.039	0.031	0.007	0.003	-0.009	-0.011	-0.013
3	-0.040	-0.015	-0.022	0.015	0.015	-0.012	-0.032
4	0.167	-0.037	0.074	0.040	0.072	0.046	0.066
5	0.021	0.005	-0.008	0.010	0.012	-0.041	0.007
6	0.075	-0.008	-0.003	0.044	0.022	0.034	-0.023
mean	0.058	0.002	0.009	0.028	0.012	0.006	0.003
s.d.	0.070	0.027	0.034	0.022	0.037	0.033	0.035

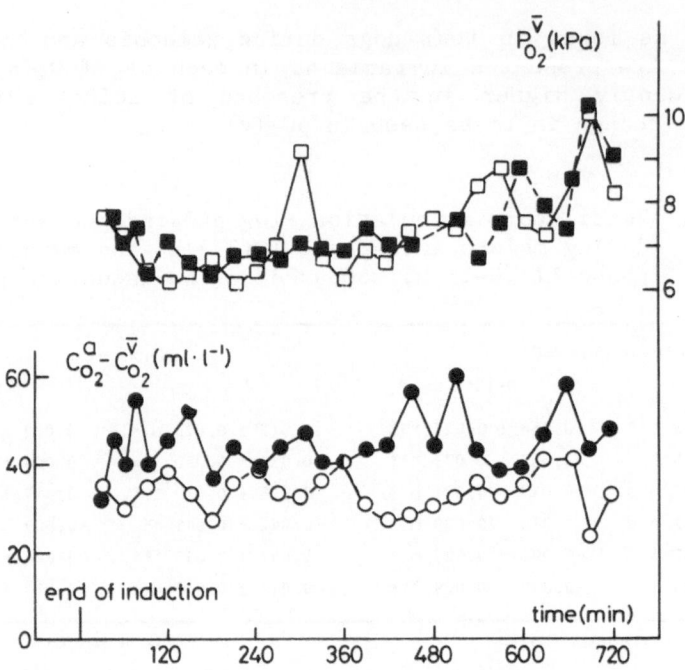

Fig. 4. $(cO_2(a)-cO_2(\bar{v}))$ (●) and $pO_2(\bar{v})$ (■) during 720 min after
induction of acidosis and in a control experiment
(o and □).

DISCUSSION

  Ventilatory response in the induction phase. In this study
changes in $pCO_2(a)$ are considered to be a measure of ventilatory
stimulation. The changes in $pCO_2(a)$ with $pH(a)$ in the induction
phase are seen as the acute response of ventilation to metabolic
acidosis. In all four series of experiments an acute increase in
ventilation was observed upon induction of the acidosis. The response is of about the same magnitude as reported for dogs in other
studies[4,8]. No signs of depression of the ventilation by NH_4Cl, as
mentioned by Winterstein et al.[10] and Loeschcke and Sugioka[11],
were observed. In the experiments with intravenous administration,
no difference was observed between the responses to HCl and NH_4Cl,
neither in magnitude nor in time course. The same holds for the
experiments with oral administration of HCl and NH_4Cl. In comparison to intravenous administration, the mean acute response to
oral administration was somewhat smaller, but in view of the large
dog-to-dog variations, these differences are not significant.
  Ventilatory response in the maintenance phase. Contrary to
Asch et al.[4] and Bureau et al.[5] but in accordance with Kaehny and
Jackson [8], no systematic further increase in ventilatory response

Table 4. $(cO_2(a)-cO_2(\bar{v}))$ and $pO_2(\bar{v})$ and standard deviations as found in four acidosis and control experiments.

Exp	$c^a_{O2}-c^{\bar{v}}_{O2}$ control ml·l^{-1}	$c^a_{O2}-c^{\bar{v}}_{O2}$ acidosis ml·l^{-1}	$P^{\bar{v}}_{O2}$ control kPa	$P^{\bar{v}}_{O2}$ acidosis kPa
1	34.3 ± 4.0	51.6 ± 10.6 ***	5.37 ± 0.52	5.78 ± 0.53 *
2	40.1 ± 8.7	45.4 ± 6.9 *	5.63 ± 0.38	5.72 ± 0.48 n.s.
3	48.1 ± 6.7	53.9 ± 7.4 *	5.46 ± 0.27	5.40 ± 0.27 n.s.
4	33.8 ± 4.1	44.3 ± 7.5 ***	7.08 ± 1.73	7.42 ± 0.89 n.s.

was observed in the maintenance phases I and II. Some of the dogs indeed showed a further increase in ventilation, but in most of the experiments either no change or a decrease was found. One explanation of the discrepancy between our results and those of Asch et al. and Bureau et al. may be that the sampling procedure has influenced the results obtained by the latter. We sampled three to six times more frequently than Asch et al. and Bureau et al. during the maintenance phases I and II, while our animals were continuously in the company of the investigator. It may therefore be assumed that in the maintenance phases I and II the animals were accustomed to the sampling procedure. In the experiments of Bureau et al., however, the animals were in their cages between samplings. Asch et al. do not report where their animals spent the time between samplings, but it is clear from their paper that during the maintenance phase samples were taken at intervals of at least 2 h. Table 3 demonstrates that meeting the investigator again, can cause a temporary extra stimulation of ventilation in sensitive animals.

The ventilatory response is easily overestimated if no time is allowed for habituation of the animals to the sampling procedure. Because for practical reasons it was impossible to allow in all our experiments enough time for habituation to the sampling procedure in the maintenance phase III and during the recovery phase, the values obtained should be considered with caution. The general impression that in many animals no further stimulation of ventilation occurs during sustained acidosis is, however, confirmed by the results of the maintenance phase III and the recovery phase.

The absence of a further increase in ventilation during the maintenance phase is in agreement with the fast exchange of HCO_3^- across the blood brain barrier found in dogs and cats in recent investigations[6,7]. If this fast exchange also takes place in man, the reluctance in treating metabolic acidosis with rapid restoration to normal blood pH by means of intravenous administration of $NaHCO_3$ should be reconsidered. The frequently reported transient respiratory alkalosis in the course of treatment with $NaHCO_3$ and the transient decrease in pH in cerebrospinal fluid would be difficult to understand. The classic explanation that the central drive for ventilation through chemosensitive areas in the medulla oblongata would remain operative and even be increased for some time during $NaHCO_3$ therapy[3] is incompatible with a fast HCO_3^- exchange across the blood brain barrier.

O_2 delivery during metabolic acidosis. The values found for $(cO_2(a)-cO_2(\bar{v}))$ and $pO_2(\bar{v})$ indicate that in the four dogs studied, O_2 transport indeed profits from the decreased O_2 affinity of the blood during metabolic acidosis: more O_2 per 1 cardiac output is delivered to the tissues at an unchanged or increased $pO_2(\bar{v})$ level. This shows that during metabolic acidosis the O_2 supply to the tissues can be accomplished with a lower cardiac output. This is of course an advantage, because in this condition the low pH may decrease the contractility of the heart. To our knowledge this is the first study in intact, conscious animals in which an indication of such a compensatory effect has been obtained. To prove the existence of this effect, the experiments described here will have to be extended with simultaneous measurements of O_2 consumption and cardiac output.

REFERENCES

1. P. Rispens, W.G. Zijlstra, and E.J. van Kampen, Significance of bicarbonate for the evaluation of non-respiratory disturbances of acid-base balance. Clin.Chim.Acta 54:335 (1974).
2. O. Siggaard-Andersen, The acid-base status of the blood, Munksgaard, Copenhagen (1976).
3. R.A. Mitchell, C.T. Carman, J.W. Severinghaus, B.W. Richardson, M.M. Singer, and S. Shnider, Stability of cerebrospinal fluid pH in chronic acid-base disturbances in blood. J.Appl.Physiol. 20: 443 (1965).
4. M.J. Asch, R.B. Dell, G.S. Williams, M. Cohen, and R.W. Winters, Time course for development of respiratory compensation in metabolic acidosis. J.Lab.Clin.Med. 73: 610 (1969).
5. M.A. Bureau, G. Ouellet, R. Begin, N. Gagnon, L. Geoffroy, and Y. Berthiaume, Dynamics of the control of ventilation during metabolic acidosis and its correction. Am.Rev.Resp.Dis. 119: 933 (1979).
6. H.R. Ahmad, and H.H. Loeschcke, Fast bicarbonate-chloride exchange between plasma and brain extracellular fluid at maintained pCO_2. Pflügers Arch. 395: 300 (1982).
7. J. Weyne, J.B. Nshimyumuremyi, G. Demeester, and I. Leusen, Correction of CSF HCO_3 after its experimental increase in normocapnia: inhibition by acetazolamide. Pflügers Arch. 396: 66 (1983).

8. W.D. Kaehny, and J.T. Jackson, Respiratory response to HCl acidosis in dogs after carotid body denervation. J.Appl.Physiol. 46: 1138 (1979).

9. J. Zweens, and P. Schiphof, Permanent catheterization of aorta and pulmonary artery in the dog. Pflügers Arch. 362: 201 (1976).

10. H. Winterstein, and N. Gökhan, Ammoniumchlorid-Acidose und Reactionstheorie der Atmungsregulation. Arch.Intern.Pharmacodyn.Thér. 93: 212 (1953).

11. H.H. Loeschcke, and K. Sugioka, pH of cerebrospinal fluid in the cisterna magna and on the surface of the choroid plexus of the 4th ventricle and its effect on ventilation in experimental disturbances of acid balance transients and steady states. Pflügers Arch. 312: 161 (1969).

OXYGEN PERMEABILITY OF METHEMOGLOBIN SOLUTIONS SOAKED IN MILLIPORE

FILTERS

L. Hoofd and A. Lamboo

Department of Physiology, University of Nijmegen
6525 EZ Nijmegen, The Netherlands

SUMMARY

For the measurement of gas diffusion through liquids, Millipore filters are an interesting and easy tool. They keep the fluid in place, and layer thickness can be determined precisely and easily. We soaked Millipore type SM filters with solutions containing 1.66 mmol/l methemoglobin to measure the oxygen permeability at 25° C, and compared the results with former measurements in liquid layers. Data scattered between 1.0 and 1.5 10^{-11} mol$\cdot$m$^{-1}\cdot$kPa$^{-1}\cdot$sec^{-1} and a decrease with increasing KCl concentration, as found for liquid layers, could neither be confirmed nor rejected. Nitrogen/oxygen permeability ratio of 0.465 $\pm$ 0.016 SE was in agreement with literature data.

METHODS

Methemoglobin solutions were prepared as described by Breepoel et al. (1982). Concentration determined spectrophotometrically (Perkin Elmer 124 spectrophotometer) was 1.66 mmol/l. Millipore filters type SM were soaked with solutions containing different amounts of KCl by placing the filters on top of the solution until they were evenly filled. Filters then were wiped with a clean tissue and mounted into a stainless steel diffusion chamber (Fig. 1).

Gas phases above and below the layer were flushed with wetted gases of known composition supplied by a gas mixing pump (Wösthoff M300/a-f). With these gases, the polarographic oxygen electrodes (Kimmich and Kreuzer, 1969) in both chambers were calibrated. After reaching steady state, the valves were closed, and oxygen partial pressure in each chamber was recorded by the oxygen electrodes.

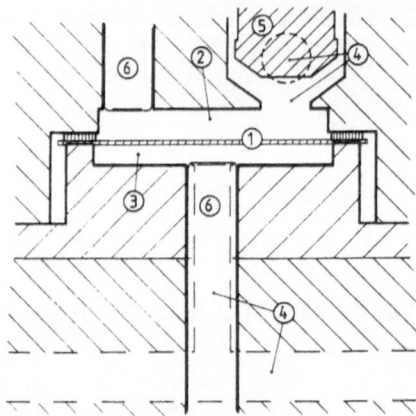

Fig. 1. Cross section of diffusion chamber. Millipore filter (1) is
clamped between upper (2) and lower (3) gas chamber. Gas
inlets (4) can be closed by valves (5); valve of lower
chamber, perpendicular to the cross section, is not shown.
Oxygen partial pressure in both chambers is measured by
oxygen electrodes (6). The whole chamber is thermostated in
a water bath at 25°C.

Oxygen pressures change due to a difference in partial pressures of
top and bottom chamber, resulting in gas fluxes through the layer;
from the oxygen electrode recordings, oxygen fluxes into or out of
the gas chambers were derived (see section THEORY). Mixtures of O_2
and N_2 were used, with O_2 percentages chosen between 0 % and 70 %.
All measurements were performed in a water bath at constant temperature (25° C).

   Filter thickness was measured with a screw micrometer before
the methemoglobin was soaked in. The filter type was Millipore SM,
pore size 5.0 μm, porosity 84 %, filter thickness around 150 μm. As
a check, some of the filters were measured after the experiment too;
in no case a change in thickness could be detected.

THEORY

   From the change in oxygen partial pressure and the volumes of
the gas chambers, oxygen flux through the filter layer can be derived. Additionally, also the nitrogen/oxygen permeability ratio is
derived (Hoofd et al., in prep.); here a short outline of the method
is presented. Both oxygen and nitrogen diffuse through the layer so
that in each chamber the amount of each gas and consequently the
product of volume and partial pressure of the gas change. For oxygen,
in each chamber this yields:

$$RT\frac{dn}{dt} = \frac{dP}{dt} V + P\frac{dV}{dt} \tag{1}$$

566

where R = gas constant, T = absolute temperature, n = moles of O_2, P = O_2 partial pressure, V = chamber volume and t = time. The change in amount is due to a flux through the layer:

$$\frac{dn}{dt} = A\,J \tag{2}$$

where J = O_2 flux and A = area of diffusion. Similar relations hold for nitrogen, where nitrogen pressure and flux are denoted by P' and J' respectively. Furthermore, the changes in volume of top and bottom chamber are opposite and the sum is equal to the total chamber volume (0.208 cm^3 minus the volume of the Millipore layer). Considering also the fact that the total pressure (P_T = P+P' is unchanged (the quite flexible Millipore does not allow for a pressure build up), and thus $dP_T/dt=0$, we derive:

$$ART\,(J + J') = P_T\,\frac{dV}{dt} \tag{3}$$

Flux is due to a difference in partial pressure. For O_2:

$$J = \frac{P}{L}\,(P_b - P_t) \tag{4}$$

where P = oxygen permeability (Krogh's diffusion coefficient), L = layer thickness, and P_b and P_t are the partial pressures in the bottom and in the top chamber respectively. Note that the permeability P is equal to the product of diffusion coefficient D and solubility α. Equation (4) holds for steady state, with constant values of e.g. P_b and P_t. Although in the experimental set-up here, after closing the valves both P_b and P_t change and this change is utilized to calculate the flux J, these changes add up to at most 0.1 kPa and thus are negligibly small as compared with the actual pressures in the chamber where the experiment is run under atmospheric pressure. Consequently, also the volume changes are negligibly small; they only are important as compared with the equally small partial pressure changes. Therefore, the situation is one of quasi steady state.

For the other gas, nitrogen, the pressure difference is just the opposite of oxygen, so that:

$$J' = \frac{P'}{L}\,(P'_b - P'_t) = -\frac{P'}{L}\,(P_b - P_t) \tag{5}$$

If this set of equations is worked out for dP/dt, the following relationship can be derived:

$$\frac{dP}{dt} = \pm\frac{ART}{V}\,\frac{P}{L}\,(P_b - P_t)\left[1 - \frac{1-P'/P}{P_T}\,P\right] \tag{6}$$

where the + sign holds for the top chamber (P=P_t) and the − sign for the bottom chamber (P=P_b).

Both parameters P and P'/P occur in this equation. A least-square fitting procedure was applied to the measured data of dP/dt in both chambers to provide these parameters.

RESULTS

The results of the measurements are presented in Fig. 2. In the lower part, the measured values of P'/P are shown. The mean value of 0.465 ± 0.016 SE compares well with 0.56 ± 0.05 of Breepoel et al.

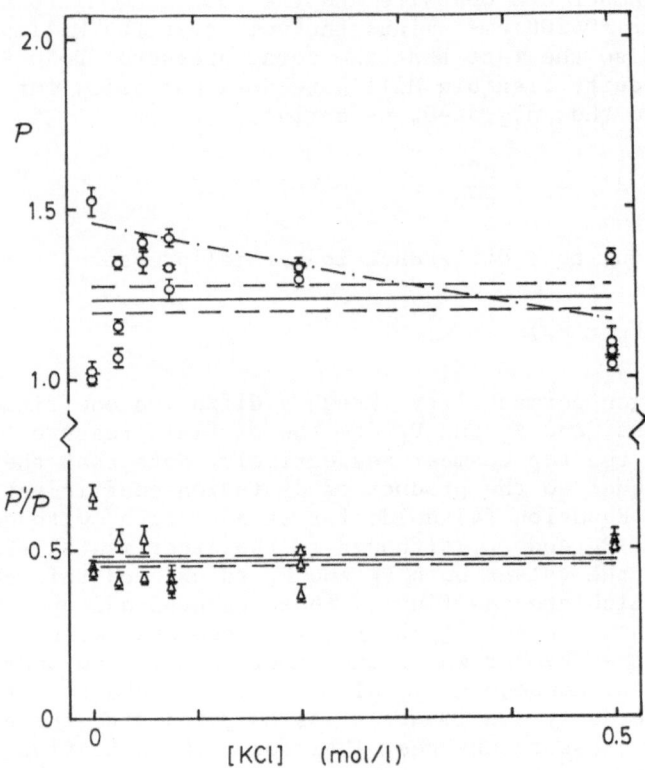

Fig. 2. Plots of P (upper part, in 10^{-11} mol·m^{-1}·kPa^{-1}·sec^{-1}) and of P'/P (lower part) at 25° C in SM Millipore filters containing 1.66 mmol/l methemoglobin solution with various amounts of KCl added. Bars indicate SE for each experiment as resulting from the fitting procedure. Solid lines are weighted mean values; broken lines indicate SE of the mean. Broken dotted line is calculated from literature data.

(1982) as well as with the permeability ratio of 0.476 ± 0.025 in filters soaked with water (Hoofd et al., in prep.). No dependency on [KCl] is observed. Oxygen permeability P, shown in the upper part of Fig. 2, shows a large scatter in the measurements. No significant dependency on [KCl] was visible either; the mean value of P for all measured data was 1.28 10^{-11} mol·m^{-1}·kPa^{-1}·sec^{-1} with a Standard Error of 0.04 in the same units. However, due to the scatter in the data, a dependency on [KCl] cannot be excluded. The dash-dotted line in the figure represents a possible dependency on [KCl] as interpolated from the data of Breepoel et al. (1982), constant values of P of 2.75 10^{-11} mol·m^{-1}·kPa^{-1}·sec^{-1} at zero Hb concentration in water and of 1.77 10^{-11} mol·m^{-1}·kPa^{-1}·sec^{-1} in SM filters (Hoofd et al., in prep.), and assuming a linear dependency of ln (P) on [Hb]:

$$P = 1.46 \ 10^{-11} \exp \{- 0.45[KCl]\} \tag{7}$$

This line is also not significantly different from the measured data: a least-square linear regression analysis of ln (P) against [KCl] yields a slope of 0.10 ± 0.17 SE, for the 19 data points, so that neither a value of zero (no dependency) nor the value of 0.45 of equation (7) can be excluded.

DISCUSSION

Measurements of oxygen permeability in solutions soaked in a Millipore filter are much easier than in liquid layers. Therefore, they are recommended for a quick determination of permeabilities (Cadman et al., 1981). Measurements of oxygen diffusion in hemoglobin solutions soaked in Millipore filters type HA were to initiate the interest in the facilitation of oxygen diffusion by hemoglobin (Scholander, 1960). However, at least for the filter type used here, the measurements appear to be subject to much more scatter than measurements in liquid layers; this is clearly seen from a comparison of the data presented here with those of Breepoel et al. (1982), where exactly the same experimental set-up was used for liquid layers confined between Teflon membranes.

Although the oxygen permeability is determined here with an accuracy of a few percent of the mean value, for more specific information like a possible decrease with increasing [KCl] the method proves inconclusive. The source of the scatter in the data is not clear, but it should be recalled that these filters in fact have not been developed as a tool for diffusion measurements. For SM filters, there is considerable scatter in pore size and porosity (Hoofd et al., in prep.).

Apart from this, the mean value of the oxygen permeability P could be determined with sufficient accuracy, and in good agreement with literature data. For confirmation or rejection of the KCl effect on P, however, these measurements must be considered as insufficient.

REFERENCES

Breepoel, P. M., de Koning, J., and Hoofd, L., 1982, Diffusion of oxygen in methemoglobin solutions. Dependence on salt concentration. Biochem. Biophys. Res. Commun., 109: 848-850.

Cadman, A. D., Fleming, R., and Guy, R. H., 1981, Diffusion coefficient determination using a filter-paper diaphragm cell technique. J. Pharm. Pharmacol., 33: 121-123.

Hoofd, L., de Koning, J., Lamboo, A., and Kreuzer, F., Determination of permeabilities for two gases from recording the partial pressure of one gas, in preparation.

Kimmich, H. P., and Kreuzer, F., 1969, Telemetry of respiratory oxygen pressure in man at rest and during exercise, in: "Oxygen Pressure Recording in Gases, Fluids, and Tissues", Progr. Resp. Res., Vol. 3, F. Kreuzer, ed., Karger, Basel, pp 22-41.

Scholander, P. F., 1960, Oxygen transport through hemoglobin solutions. Science 131: 585-590.

RETICULOCYTOSIS AND BONE MARROW cAMP LEVEL IN RATS FOLLOWING PHYSICAL EXERCISES

Z. Szygula[1], Z. Dabrowski[2], R. Kubica[3], and H. Miszta[4]

[1] Department of Sport Medicine, Akademy of Physical
Education. Al. Planu 6-letniego 62a, 31-571 Krakow
Poland
[2,4] Laboratory of Animal Physiology and Toxicology
Department of Animal Physiology, Institute of Zoology
Jagiellonian University, ul. Karasia 6, 30-060 Krakow
Poland
[3] Department of Physiology and Biochemistry. Academy
of Physical Education, Al, Planu 6-letniego 62a
31-571 Krakow, Poland

INTRODUCTION

In the course of intensive physical exercises the blood serum
erythropoietin level becomes elevated [16,21]. Erythropoietin, being
a protein hormone of a big molecular weight, does not penetrate the
target cell, but is bound by a surface receptor[15] and affects the
processes occurring within the erythropoietin-sensitive cell according to the generally accepted theory of the "second messenger".
As it has been demonstrated[2,5,7], erythropoietin triggers an increase
of cAMP in the bone marrow cells. On the other hand, an elevation in
the intracellular cAMP concentration has been shown to stimulate
erythropoiesis in vitro.

The available literature on the subject has not yielded any information on the changes in the bone marrow cAMP level as induced by
physical exercises and training.

The present authors have aimed at the investigation of the bone
marrow erythropoietic activity as influenced by physical exercises,
accepting the peripheral blood reticulocyte count and the bone marrow
cAMP level as indicators of this activity.

MATERIAL AND METHODS

The investigations were carried out on 43 male Wistar rats at 3-4 months of age and with a mean body weight of 224.2 g. Throughout the experiment the animals were fed standard fodder and given tap water ad libitum, being kept under constant light conditions (N/D:12/12). The physical exercises consisted in running a speed of 1.47 km/h within an electric treadmill. The running tests were carried out between 9 a.m. and 1 p.m. under stable environmental conditions (at a temperature approximating 20-23°C, and relative humidity of 50-65%). The rats selected for the experiment were familiar with a training treadmill. The control group C animals (n=9) were kept resting at all times. Groups I (n=10) and II (n=9) were subjected to a single exercise till signs of fatigue developed. The Group III rats (n=7) were trained for 35 days; for the first five days they ran for one minute daily, on the sixth day for two minutes, and on the consecutive days the time of running was extended by two minutes daily to reach finally 60 minutes on the last experimental day. Group IV (n=8) was trained for one minute daily for the first six days, and starting from the seventh day the time was extended by one minute to reach 30 minutes on the final 35th day of the experiment.

Blood samples were collected from the tail vein and served as the material for reticulocyte count determinations done after routine methods. Four age groups of reticulocytes were distinguished while counting following the concept developed by Heilmeyer and Trachtenberg[1], and the percentage constituted by each particular age group was calculated.

Blood samples were collected for the first time prior to a single physical exercise in Groups I and II, as well as immediately after the exercise (Group I) and following a 24-hour rest (Group II). In the two training groups the first blood collection occurred prior to the training, and the second 24 hours after the final exercise. The control rats were also drawn blood twice in order to determine whether the amount of blood collected for the determinations might trigger significant changes in the reticulocyte count.

The bone marrow samples for the cAMP determinations wer collected from both femoral bones immediately after the exercise (Group I), 24 hours following a single exercise (Group II), and 24 hours following the last exercise of the series (Groups III and IV). Bone marrow samples collection was also performed in the control rats. The animals were etherized and exsanguinated by dissection of the bilaterally exposed femoral vessels. Subsequently the femurs were isolated and immediately frozen in liquid nitrogen. The time lapse between the etherization of the animal and the bone sample freezing did not exceed 3 minutes in each case. The procedures of bone sample collection were always carried out between 2 p.m. and 3 p.m.

The bone marrow extraction for cAMP level determinations was performed after the method developed by Tovey et al.[19]. The cAMP determinations in bone marrow extracts were done following the radio-competitive method developed by Gilman[9] and modified by Kolen and Channing[14]. The sample radioactivity was measured with the use of a liquid scintillation counter SL 30/200 Intertechnique. The results were expressed in pmols per 1 g of fresh bone marrow (1pmol/1 g of bone marrow).

The results were statistically worked out, using, apart from routine descriptive methods, the student t-test to evaluate the significance of differences between particular groups, having formerly tested the homogeneity of variances by means of the Fisher F-test.

RESULTS AND DISCUSSION

Peripheral Blood Reticulocytes.

The peripheral blood reticulocyte count and percentage are presented in Fig. 1.

A single blood collection in Group C did not evoke significant changes in the reticulocyte count and distribution into age groups. No youngest forms of reticulocytes (group 1) were found in the peripheral blood of the Group C rats. The group 2 and 3 reticulocytes were noted in scant amounts, and above 80% of all the reticulocytes were the oldest (group 4) forms. A similar reticulocyte count and distribution into particular age groups in the peripheral blood was observed at rest prior to physical exercises in Groups I and II and before training in Groups III and IV. Immediately after single physical exercises (Group I) the authors observed an increase in the peripheral blood reticulocytes by 83%, the appearance of the youngest reticulocyte forms (group 1) at the periphery, a more than threefold increase in the number of the group 2 reticulocytes, an increment in the number of the group 3 reticulocytes, and a drop in the number of the oldest forms (group 4) from 84% down to 65%. Following a 24-hour rest period and a subsequent single physical exercise, the reticulosis was still more pronounced, and the reticulocyte picture was shifted towards the youngest forms (group 2). An even more intensified reticulosis was apparent following training periods in the Group III and IV rats. The highest reticulosis value was encountered in Group III (573% of the value observed at rest) where the animals were subjected to very strenuous exercises during training periods. Both training groups revealed a very conspicuous shift of the reticulocyte picture towards the youngest forms with a simultaneous marked drop in the percentage of the oldest forms.

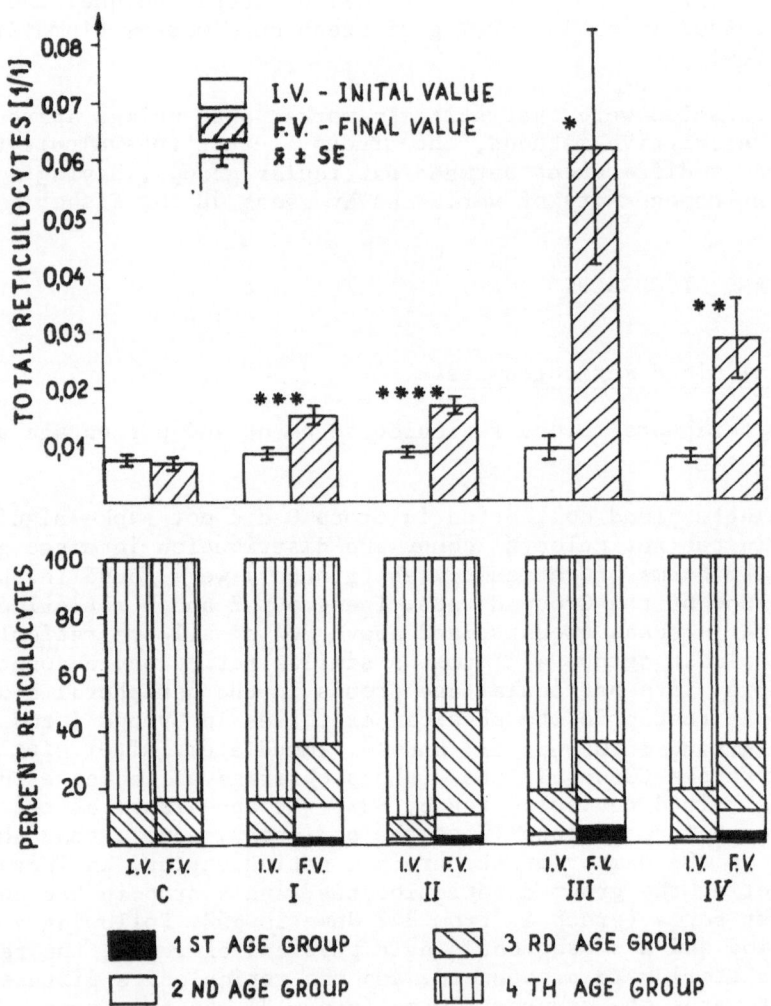

Fig. 1. The number of reticulocytes in peripheral blood – upper diagram and the percentages of their four age groups–lower diagram * p<0,03 **p<0,01 ***p<0,005 ****p<0,001

According to Hillmeyer and Trachtenberg, the group 1 reticulocytes are normally encountered solely in the bone marrow. Their appearance at the periphery testifies to an increased demand on the part of the organism for young red blood cells, as well as to an increased erythropoietic activity of the bone marrow. It seems that the elevation of the peripheral blood reticulocyte count following a single exercise in combination with the shift of the reticulocyte picture towards younger forms can be explained by an increased blood flow throught the bone marrow in the course of physical exercises[11], as well as by pressure changes in the marrow cavity during muscular contractions resulting from the vascular-muscular action and exerting a sucking effect upon the sinus walls, damaging the bone marrow barrier[6].

A pronounced reticulosis noted after training periods, especially in Group III, in conjunction with an apparent shift of the reticulocyte picture towards the youngest forms can testify to an intensified erythrocyte hemolysis in the course of exercises, an increased erythropoietic activity of the bone marrow, and to a "crossing" of the bone marrow barrier[18].

Bone Marrow cAMP Level.

Fig. 2 presents the bone marrow cAMP level in the controls C, in rats subjected to single exercises (Groups I and II) and to training (Groups III and IV). The cAMP level determined in rats immediately following their single physical exercises (Group I) was only slightly higher in comparison to the control group, the difference being statistically insignificant. The cAMP level measured after a 24-hour rest (Group II) surpassed the control result by 196.28 pmol/1 g of bone marrow, the difference reaching statistical significance ($p < 0.04$). The Group II animals subjected to training which induced a high reticulosis revealed a cAMP level that exceeded the control value by 326.57 pmol/1 g of bone marrow ($p < o.10$). The rats undergoing moderate training showed a post-training cAMP level higher than the control value by 330.72 pmol/1 g of bone marrow ($p < 0.006$).

The observed statistically significant increase of the bone marrow cAMP level following a single physical exercise maintained till signs of fatigue develop, which occurs after a 24-hour rest, can be the effect of erythropoietin. Similarly, an increment in the cAMP level noted after training periods can be the result of this hormone activity. A very interesting phenomenon which requires further studies seems to be a slight, statistically insignificant elevation of the bone marrow cAMP level immediately after a strenuous physical exercise. It is well known that in the course of physical exercises there occurs a rise in blood levels of such hormones as catecholamines, thyroid hormones, corticosteroids and

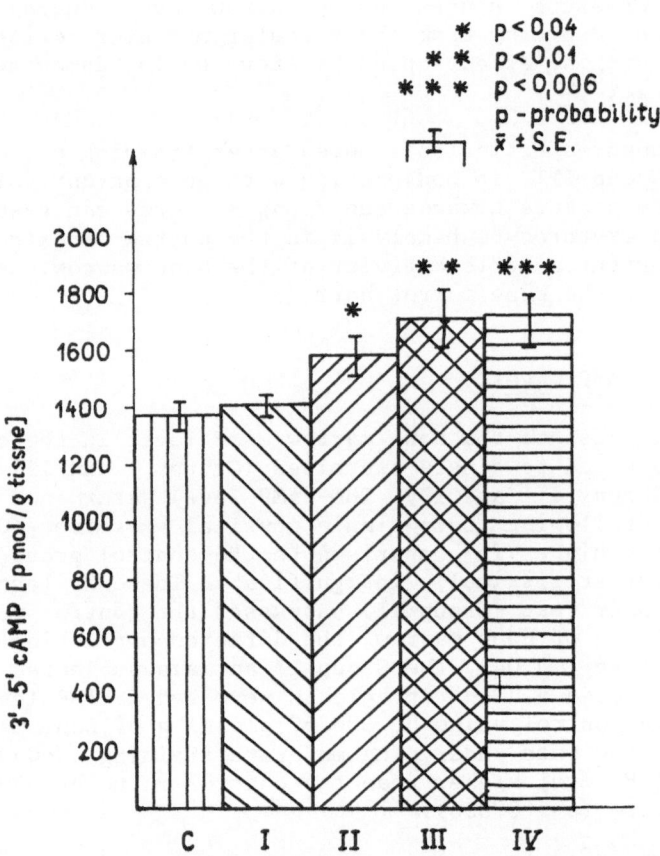

Fig. 2.   The level of cyclic AMP in bone – marrow.

androgens[3,12,13,20]. The generally accepted knowledge holds it that the above hormones stimulate the adenile cyclase system, resulting in an increase of the intracellular cAMP concentration[4,8,10,17].

CONCLUSIONS:

1. Both after single exercises and following training periods there occurs a gross increase in the peripheral blood reticulocyte count with a simultaneous shift of the reticulocyte picture towards youngest forms.

2. Twenty-four hours after strenuous physical exercises and trainings there is noted an elevation of the cAMP level.

3. The observed changes testify to a pronounced stimulation of the bone marrow erythropoietic activity, as well as to a "crossing" of the bone marrow barrier in the course of strenuous physical exercises employed during training.

REFERENCES

1. H. Gegemann and H.G. Harwerth, "Praktische Hämatologie", George Thieme Verlag, Stuttgart (1974).
2. J.E. Brown and J.W. Adamson, Studies of the influence of cyclic nucleotides on in vitro haemoglobin synthesis, Brit. J. Haematol., 35:193 (1977).
3. Z. Brzezinska, W. Kowalski and K. Nazar, Activity of the adrenergic system during prolonged running in dogs, Acta Physiol.Pol., 24:339 (1973).
4. J.W. Byron, Evidence for a β -adrenergic receptor initiating DNA synthesis in haemopoietic stem cells, Exptl.Cell.Res., 71:228 (1972).
5. F. Chiuini, G. Della Tore, G. Fano and A. Viti, Early increase of cyclic adenosine monophosphate level induced by erythropoietin on rabbit bone marrow cell suspensions, Acta Haematol., 61:251 (1979).
6. Z. Dabrowski, Z. Szygula and H. Miszta, Do changes in bone marrow pressure contribute to the egress of cells from bone marrow?, Acta Physiol.Pol., 32:729 (1981).
7. G. Della Tore, G. Fano and G. Menchetti, cAMP-cGMP ratio and Hb concentration in rabbit bone marrow cells stimulated by erythroproietin and NaF, IRCS Medical Sci., 9:344 (1981).
8. T. Ganchev, The influence of isoprenaline beta-adrenergic stimulation on erythropoiesis in white rats, Agressologie, 16:301 (1975).
9. A.G. Gilman, A protein binding assay for adenosine 3' : 5'-cyclic monophosphate, Proc.Natl.Acad.Sci.U.S., 67:305 (1970).

10. D. Gorshein, E.H. Reisner jr. and F.H. Graber, Tissue culture of bone marrow. V. Effect of 5 β /H/ steroids and cyclic AMP on heme synthesis, Am.J.Physiol., 228:1024 (1975).
11. P.M. Gross, D.D. Heistad and M.L. Marcus, Neurohumoral regulation of blood flow to bones and marrow, Am.J.Physiol., 237:H440 (1979).
12. W. Kindermann, A. Schnabel, W.M. Schmitt, G. Biro, J. Cassens and F. Weber, Catecholamines, growth hormone, cortisol, insulin and sex hormones in anaerobic and aerobic exercise, Eur.J.Appl. Physiol., 49:289 (1982).
13. V. Koivisto, R. Hendler, E. Nadel and Ph. Felig, Influence of physical training on the fuel - hormone response to prolonged low intensity exercise, Metabolism, 31:192 (1982).
14. J. Kolena and C.P. Channing, Stimulatory effects of LH, FSH, and Prostaglandins upon cyclic 3', 5' - AMP levels in porcine grandulosa cells, Endocrinology, 90:1543 (1972).
15. M.D. Lafferty, G.A. Ackerman, Ch.D.R. Dunn and R.D. Lange, Ultrastructural, immunocytochemical localisation of presumptive erythropoietin binding sites on developing erythrocytic cells of normal human bone marrow, J.Histochem.Cytochem., 29:49 (1981).
16. R. Lindemann, R. Ekanger, P.K. Opstad, M. Nummestad and R. Ljosland, Hematological changes in normal men during prolonged severe exercise, Amer.Corr.Ther.J., 37:107 (1978).
17. M. Pawlikowski and J. Lewandowski, Cyclic adenosine 3', 5' - -monophosphate as the intracellular mediator of hormonal action, Endokrynol. Polska, 24:105 (1973).
18. Z. Szygula, K. Spodaryk, Z. Dabrowski and H. Miszta, Post-effort anaemia and hemolytic phenomena during physical exercises, (in press).
19. K.C. Tovey, K.G. Oldham and J.A.M. Whelan, A simple direst assay for cyclic AMP in plasma and other biological samples using an improved competitive protein binding technique, Clinica Chemica Acta, 56:221 (1974).
20. J.E. Wilkerson, S.M. Horvath and B. Gutin, Plasma testosterone during treadmill exercise, J.Appl.Physiol.:Resp., Environ. Exercise Physiol., 49:249 (1980).
21. J. Zivny, J. Neuwirt and T. Travnicek, The effect of lactic acid on erythropoietin production and the rate of disappearance of erythropoietin from rat plasma during exercise, Life Sciences, 10:11 (1971).

POST-EXERCISE ANEMIA DURING EXAMINATION IN RATS

Zbigniew Szygula[1], Zbigniew Dabrowski[2], Tadeusz Krezel[3], and Helena Miszta[4]

[1,3] Department of Sport Medicine, Academy of Physical Education, Al. Planu 6-letniego 62a, 31-571 Krakow Poland
[2,4] Laboratory of Animal Physiology and Toxicology Department of Animal Physiology, Institute of Zoology Jagiellonian University, ul. Karasia 6, 30-060 Krakow Poland

INTRODUCTION

Numerous communications on the changes in the erythrocyte system as induced by physical exercises seem to be contradictory. Some authors point to an increase in hemoglobin concentration as well as erythrocyte and hematocrit count following single intensive physical exercises[3,4,5,10,18,24] and prolonged physical training periods[19,20]. Others report a drop below initial values in the above mentioned hematological indices after single intensive physical efforts[1,6,9,13,17] and also following training periods of various duration and intensity[5,7,12,15,22]. Moreover, cases of anemia have been described in athletes, and even in male and female members of the Olympic teams[21,23]. To stress the character of such anemia it has been called sports, athletes', or post-exercise anemia[11,12,16,22,25].

The present authors have aimed at tracing the changes in the basic erythrocyte system indices in the peripheral blood following single strenuous physical exercises and training periods of diversified intensity. Another objective has been to find out whether muscular effort results in an intensification of the erythrocyte hemolysis.

MATERIAL AND METHODS

Material

The experiments were carried out on 43 male Wistar rats at an age ranging from 3 to 5 months and with a mean body weight of 224.2 g. Throughout the experiment duration the animals were fed standard fodder and given tap water ad libitum, being kept in constant light conditions with a ratio of daytime to nighttime of 12/12.

Physical exercises

The rats ran with the speed of 1.47 km/h inside an electric treadmill. The physical exercises were carried out at constant time and under constant environmental conditions.

Experimental groups

Control group C (n=9). The rats were kept at rest all the time.
Group I (n=10) and Group II (n=9). The animals were subjected to single physical exercises till signs of fatigue developed.
Group III (n=7). The rats underwent a 35-day training. For the first five days they ran for one minute daily, on the sixth day for two minutes, and on each consecutive day the duration of the exercise was extended by two minutes to reach 60 minutes on the last training day.
Group IV (n=8). The animals were also trained for 35 days, but within the first six days the duration of the run was one minute daily, and subsequently it was increased by only one minute daily starting from the seventh day of the experiment to reach 30 minutes on its final day.

The studies included

The erythrocyte count, hemoglobin concentration and hematocrit value in the peripheral blood collected in Groups I and II for the first time prior to a single exercise, and for the second time immediately after the exercise (Group I) and following a 24-hour rest (Group II). The rats of the latter group rested in their regular cages given free access to water and fodder. The Group III and IV animals were subjected to blood collection prior to training and 24 hours after the last exercise.

580

In control group C blood samples were also drawn twice to serve as the material for the determination of the above mentioned indices. The results obtained at the first collection in Group C served as initial results for this group, whereas the second blood drawing results were to answer the question whether the amount of the collected blood might evoke significant changes in the blood picture.

The calculations included also the mean corpuscular volume (MCV), mean corpuscular hemoglobin concentration (MCHC) and mean corpuscular hemoglobin (MCH).

Blood samples were collected from the tail vein always at the same time of the day.

The determinations of hematological indices were done after routine methods[7].

In order to take into consideration the possible effect of exercise-evoked dehydration and rehydration at rest upon the hematological changes, the animals were weighed prior to the first and second blood collections.

To find out whether exercises induce hemolytic phenomena the authors determined the blood plasma hemoglobin level employing the O-toluidine method according to Beau[2] and using blood samples collected from the venous femoral vessels of the Group I rats directly following the exercise. Subsequently, the index of intravessel hemolysis level (IIHL) was calculated after the equation developed by Olearczyk and Krolak[14]:

$$IIHL = \frac{\text{blood plasma hemoglobin x value of venous blood plasma fraction}}{\text{total blood hemoglobin}}$$
$$= \frac{Hb_o \times (1 - Ht)}{\text{total blood Hb}}$$

The resultant values were compared to the values obtained according to the same method in Group C.

All the results were statistically worked out with the use of routine methods, presented in the form of an arithmetic average $\bar{x} \pm S.E.$, and verified from the statistical viewpoint employing the Student t-test.

RESULTS AND DISCUSSION

The changes evoked by a single blood collection in Group C were slight and statistically insignificant (Tab. 1).

Peripheral blood changes following single strenuous exercises

The Group I rats ran for 29 minutes, and the Group II animals for 25 minutes. It was determined that a single strenuous physical exercise triggered a statistically significant drop in the hemoglobin concentration, hematocrit value and erythrocyte count (Tab. 1) in the Group I animals. The alterations in the MCV, MCH and MCHC indices were minute and statistically insignificant (Tab. 2). The body weight (Tab. 3) was decreased, but the lack of significance of the changes pointed to the fact that in rats the loss of water during exercises does not play any decisive role (a limited role of dehydration).

After a 24-hour rest following a single exercise there was observed a still more intensified drop in the morphotic values of the erythrocyte system (Group II - Tab. 1), the changes being markedly significant from the statistical point of view. They were not triggered by an excessive hydration of the organism, since the body weight continued to be maintained at a level lower than the initial value (Tab. 3). The alterations in the MCV, MCH and MCHC indices were minute and statistically insignificant (Tab. 2).

Hemolytic phenomena in the course of physical exercises

The blood serum hemoglobin concentration determined in the Group I rats immediately after a single physical exercise was apparently elevated in comparison to the value obtained in the Group C animals kept at rest at all times (Fig. 1), the difference being markedly significant from the statistical viewpoint. Similarly, the value of IIHL was grossly increased in Group I in comparison to the controls, the difference reaching a high statistical significance level (Fig. 1). The above data testify to a strongly intensified erythrocyte intravessel hemolysis in the course of strenuous physical exercises.

Peripheral blood changes induced by training

Both training groups yielded a decrease of the hematological parameters in the peripheral blood erythrocyte system following training periods (Tab. 1). The intensity of the said changes reached its highest values in Group III, where the prescribed exercises were the most exhausting, thus leading to anemia development. Since the

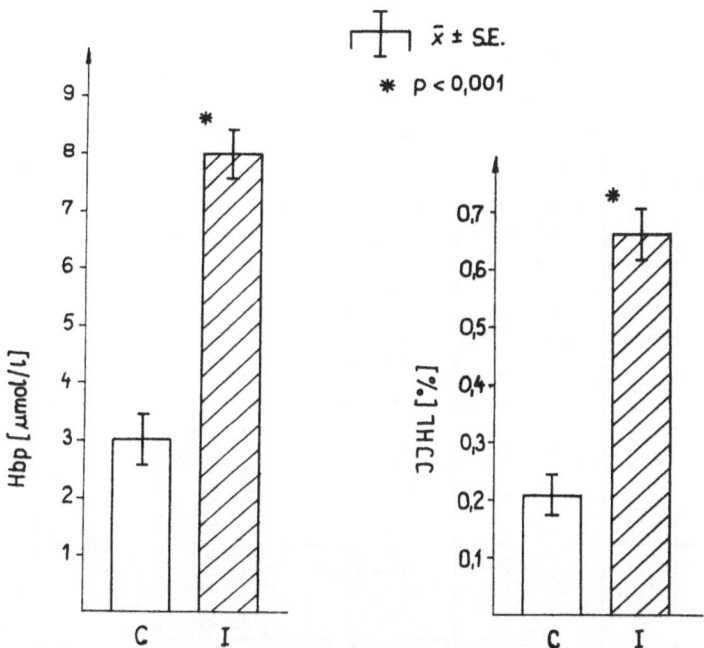

Fig. 1. Blood plasma hemoglobin (Hbp) - on the left, and the index of intravessel hemolysis level (IIHL) - on the right in control group (C) and in rats subjected to single exercises (I).

changes in the MCV, MCH and MCHC indices were slight and statistically insignificant (Tab. 2), the thus induced anemia might be termed normocytic and normochromic. The rats of this group also revealed a small body weight increment after a 35-day training period, what reflected the slowed-down development of those animals. (Tab. 3).

Group IV, consisting of rats subjected to moderate training, also showed a decrease in the hematological values, yet the drop was not so drastically expressed as in Group III (Tab. 1). The changes in the MCV, MCH and MCHC indices were also slight and insignificant from the statistical viewpoint (Tab. 2). The body weight increment in this group was bigger than in the Group IV animals (Tab. 3). The alterations in the hematological indices detected in this training group can be regarded as typical adaptative changes following pro-

Table 1. Values of peripheral blood morphotic indices in particular groups of animals

GROUPS	C			I			II			III			IV		
	I.V.	F.V.	Δ% Δp	I.V.	F.V.	Δ% Δp	I.V.	F.V.	Δ% Δp	I.V.	F.V.	Δ% Δp	I.V.	F.V.	Δ% Δp
Hb $\bar{x} \pm$ S.E. (mmol/1)	8,94 0,25	9,00 0,23	+0,06 0,67% St.I.	8,66 0,20	7,91 0,18	−0,75 8,66% <0,02	8,93 0,22	7,89 0,23	−1,04 11,65% <0,006	9,47 0,24	5,88 0,58	−3,59 34% <0,001	9,51 0,18	7,52 0,62	−1,99 21% <0,01
Ht $\bar{x} \pm$ S.E. (1/1)	0,393 0,006	0,39 0,005	−0,003 0,76% St.I.	0,39 0,005	0,35 0,004	−0,04 10,26% <0,001	0,37 0,005	0,34 0,008	−0,03 8,11% <0,005	0,40 0,007	0,31 0,02	−0,09 22,5% <0,005	0,40 0,01	0,36 0,02	−0,04 10% St.I.
E $\bar{x} \pm$ S.E. (T/1)	9,77 0,31	9,35 0,26	−0,42 4,3% St.I.	9,78 0,32	8,60 0,22	−1,18 12,07% <0,01	9,61 0,32	7,94 0,31	−1,67 17,38% <0,003	10,09 0,44	7,14 0,54	−2,94 29,2% <0,002	9,38 0,35	8,94 0,64	−0,44 4,73% St.I.

I.V. – initial value
F.V. – final value
Δ – F.V. – I.V.

St.I. – Statistically Insignificant

Hb – Hemoglobin
Ht – Hematocrit
E – Erythrocytes

Table 2. Values of MCV, MCH and MCHC in particular groups of animals

GROUPS	C			I			II			III			IV		
	I.V.	F.V.	Δp	I.V.	F.V.	Δp	I.V.	F.V.	Δp	I.V.	F.V.	Δp	I.V.	F.V.	Δp
MCV x̄ ± S.E. (fl)	40,47 1,45	42,05 1,30	+1,58 St.I.	39,91 1,39	40,63 1,15	+0,72 St.I.	38,91 1,38	43,16 1,97	+4,25 St.I.	39,73 1,87	43,71 4,75	+3,98 St.I.	42,30 1,92	40,20 4,02	-2,10 St.I.
MCH x̄ ± S.E. (fmol)	0,92 0,04	0,96 0,04	+0,04 St.I.	0,89 0,04	0,92 0,03	+0,03 St.I.	0,93 0,04	0,99 0,05	+0,06 St.I.	0,94 0,05	0,82 0,10	-0,12 St.I.	1,01 0,04	0,84 0,09	-0,17 St.I.
MCHC x̄ ± S.E. (mmol/1)	22,61 0,73	22,88 0,65	+0,27 St.I.	22,17 0,59	22,62 0,58	+0,45 St.I.	23,88 0,67	23,03 0,85	-0,86 St.I.	23,63 0,74	18,83 2,37	-4,8 St.I.	23,95 0,78	20,91 2,25	-3,04 St.I.

I.V. – initial value
F.V. – final value
Δ – F.V. – I.V.

St.I. – Statistically Insignificant

585

Table 3. Body weight in particular groups of rats

GROUPS	C	I	II	III	IV
I.V. $\overline{x}\pm$S.E.	223,56 7,13	243,15 4,54	239,9 5,49	201,00 3,66	210,13 10,60
F.V. $\overline{x}\pm$S.E.	223,11 7,25	240,45 4,55	238,44 5,9	206,57 2,21	219,50 11,48
F.V.–I.V.	-0,45	-2,7	-1,45	+5,57	+9,38
Δ%	0,20%	1,1%	0,6	2,77	4,46
p	St.I.	St.I.	St.I.	St.I.	St.I.

I.V. – initial value
F.V. – final value
St.I. – Statistically Insignificant

longed exercises, comparable to changes occurring in athletes engaged in high-endurance sport disciplines.

CONCLUSIONS

1. Strenuous single physical exercises result in a decrease in the peripheral blood hemoglobin concentration, hematocrit value and erythrocyte count.

2. In the course of strenuous physical exercises there occurs an intensification of the erythrocyte intravessel hemolysis.

3. The intensified erythrocyte hemolysis can provide an explanation for the drop in the hematological indices value of the erythrocyte system as triggered by single exercises.

4. Prolonged physical training leads to a decrease of the morphotic parameters in the peripheral blood erythrocyte system.

5. Should the exercises employed in the course of the training be very strenuous and the erythrocyte hemolysis transgress the hemopoietic processes in the bone marrow, post-exercise anemia can develop as a result.

REFERENCES

1. P.O. Astrand and B. Saltin, Plasma and red cell volume after prolonged severe exercise, J.Appl.Physiol., 19:829 (1964).
2. A.F.Beau, A Method for hemoglobin in serum and urine, Am.J.Clin. Pathology, 32:111 (1962).
3. W. van Beaumont, Red cell volume with changes in plasma osmolarity during maximal exercise, J.Appl.Physiol., 35:47 (1973).
4. W. van Beaumont, J.E. Greenleaf and L. Juhos, Disproportional changes in hematocrit, plasma volume, and proteins during exercise and bed rest, J.Appl.Physiol., 33:55 (1972).
5. D.L. Costill, A scientific aproach to distance running, Sport Wyczynowy, 14/8/:4 (1976).
6. A.J. Dalton and H. Selye, The blood picture during the alarm reaction, Fol.Haematol., 62:397 (1939).
7. D.B. Dill, F.G. Hall, K.D. Hall, C. Dawson and J.L. Newton, Blood, plasma, and red cell volumes: age, exercise, and environment, J.Appl.,Physiol., 21:597 (1966).
8. W.R. Faulkner and J.W. King, "Manual of Clinical Laboratory Procedures", Chem.Rub.CO, Cleveland (1970).
9. J. Karvonen and J. Saarela, Hemoglobin changes and decomposition of erythrocytes during 25 hours following a heavy exercise run, J.Sports Med.Phys.Fitness. 3:171 (1976).
10. M.A. Konstam, S. Tu'meh, J. Wynne, J.R. Beck, J. Kozlowski and B.L. Holman, Effect of exercise on erythrocyte count and blood

activity concentration after technetium-99m in vivo red blood cell lebeling, Circulation, 66:638 (1982).

11. E. Kvanta, Deficiency of iron and other metals in athlete's body, Sport Wyczynowy, 14/3-4/:36 (1976).

12. R. Lindemann, Low hematocrits during basic training: athletes anemia?, N.England J.Med., 21:1191 (1978).

13. J. Novosadova, The changes in hematocrit, hemoglobin, plasma volume and proteins during and after different types of exercise, Eur.J.Appl.Physiol., 36:223 (1977).

14. J. Olearczyk and M. Krolak, Investigations on postrainal intervascular haemolysis degree. I. Regular values of haemoglobin concentration in plasma and of intervascular haemolysis degree factor, in: Zeszyty Naukowe AWF we Wroclawiu, vol. 22, Wroclaw (1977).

15. J.L. Puhl and W.S. Runyan, Hematological variation during aerobic training of college women, Research Quarterly for Exercise and Sport, 51:533 (1980).

16. M.W. Radomski, B.H. Sabiston and P. Isoard, Development of "Sports Anemia" in physically fit men after daily sustained submaximal exercise, Aviat.Space Environ.Med., 51:41 (1980).

17. H.E. Refsum, G. Jordfald and S.B. Stromme, Hematological changes following prolonged heavy exercise, in: Medicine Sport. vol. 9, Advances in Exercise Physiology, Karger, Basel (1979).

18. R.J. Rose, Haematological changes associated with endurance exercise, Veterinary Record, 110:175 (1982).

19. R.J. Rose and D.R. Hodgson, Haematological and plasma biochemical parameters in endurance horses during training, Equine Veterinary J., 14:144 (1982).

20. G.A. Stewart, G.T. Clarkson and J.D. Steel, Hematology of the racehorse and factors affecting interpretation of the blood count, Proc.Am.Ass.Equine Pract., 17:35 (1970).

21. G.A. Stewart, J.E. Steel, A.H. Toyne and M.J. Stewart, Observations on the haematology and the iron and protein intake of Australian olympic athletes, Med.J.Australia, 2:1339 (1972).

22. D.E. Uddin, B. Puligandla, S.A. Strass and H.R. Schumacher, Low hematocrits during basic training: athlete's anemia?, N.Engl.J.Med., 21:1192 (1978).

23. J.F. de Wijn, J.L. Jongste, W. Mosterd and D. Willebrand, Hemoglobin, packed cell volume, serum iron binding capacity of selected athletes during training, Nutr.Metabol., 13:129 (1971).

24. J.E. Wilkerson, B. Gutin and S.M. Horvath, Exercise-induced changes in blood, red cell, and plasma volumes in men, Med. Scie.Sports, 9:155 (1977).

25. H. Yoshimura, Anemia during physical training (sports anemia). Nutrition Reviews, 28:251 (1970).

IN VIVO ARTERIAL PLATELET-VESSEL WALL INTERACTION AND THROMBOSIS:

INDUCTION, ON-LINE REGISTRATION AND ULTRASTRUCTURAL CONTROL

L. Maes, R. Andries, J.X. Wu[+], and R.H. Bourgain

Laboratory for Physiology and Physiopathology, V.U.B.
[+]Dept. of Pathology, Academic Hospital, V.U.B.
Laarbeeklaan 103, B-1090 Brussels, Belgium

ABSTRACT

A technique for induction and on-line quantification of local platelet thrombi in mesenteric arteries of small laboratory animals was developed and standardized in our laboratory.

In the past, this model was used to study the nature of platelet-vessel wall interaction in the living animal. The ultrastructure of the experimental intimal lesion and the vessel wall regeneration were assessed by transmission electron microscopy (TEM), both in normal and pathologic conditions.

Scanning electron microscopy (SEM) now shows the ultramorphology of platelet thrombi on the experimentally injured arterial segment following topical superfusion with ADP, mepacrine or platelet-activating factor (PAF). The application of these substances, each with proper bio-activity, leads to distinct types of platelet thrombi. Mepacrine or PAF superfusion causes large thrombotic masses, as compared to control, ADP induced thrombi, and seems toxic for the endothelial cells. Mepacrine thrombi differ significantly from PAF thrombi in their platelet density, degree of platelet activation and in their relation to the endothelium that surrounds the experimental lesion. Furthermore, PAF superfusion induces a phenomenon of spontaneous regeneration of the thrombus after its forced embolization. This is probably due to some unknown bio-action of PAF in the vessel wall.

(+) Dr. J.X. Wu is a visiting professor from the Department of Pathology, Bethune Medical College, The People's Republic of China.

INTRODUCTION

Experimental models for the study of in vivo platelet-vessel
wall interaction, as expressed by local platelet thrombosis on a
small endothelial lesion, ought to approximate normal physiologic
conditions. Several methods for the induction of a de-endothelializ-
ing arterial wall injury and for the generation of subsequent platelet thrombosis have been introduced (Begent and Born,1970; Hladovec,1971; Rosenblum,1978; Philp et al.,1978; Zimmerman et al.,1979;
Kovacs and Görög,1979; Ubatuba et al.,1979; Shishido and Katori,
1981; Van Der Byl et al.,1982; Takano and Suzuki,1982; Weichert et
al.,1983). All methods induce lesions with a large variety in localization. But the registration procedure, the "measurement" of the
actual thromboformation does not meet acceptable criteria for standardization and reproducibility.

A standardized technique for induction and reproducible, on-
line registration of platelet thrombi in small arteries of small
laboratory animals was developed in our laboratory (Bourgain and
Six,1974; Bourgain et al.,1984). Based on the desquamating properties of a well defined, standardized electric microcurrent, this
technique induces the immediate loss of 20 to 40 adjoining endothelial cells. Thrombus generation is performed by a time-limited topical superfusion of that injured arterial segment with a standard
ADP-solution. These ADP thrombi are considered as "normal", control
thrombi, and, providing similar experimental conditions, can be re-
induced in a reproducible way.

In the past, this model was used to investigate platelet-vessel
wall interaction in the living animal. The role of the prostaglandin
metabolism was assessed and commented in several publications (Bourgain,1978a and b,1979 and 1980; Bourgain et al.,1979,1981,1982 and
1983). The ultrastructure of the experimental intimal lesion and its
regeneration was studied by TEM, in normal and pathologic conditions,
in straight arterial segments and in bifurcation zones (Potvliege
and Bourgain,1976,1977,1979,1980 and 1982; Potvliege et al.,1984).

Recently, the overall topographic ultramorphology of this intimal lesion and the "normal" ADP thrombi were studied by SEM (Maes
et al.,1984).

To demonstrate the various possibilities of this thrombosis
model, we now present some examples of thrombotic phenomena induced
by superfusion of an injured arterial segment with ADP, mepacrine
and PAF.

MATERIALS AND METHODS

ADP and mepacrine platelet thrombosis was evaluated in normal, adult (250-350g), male Wistar rats. For the study of PAF thrombi we used normal, adult (600-800g), male guinea pigs. Both groups were fed on a standard pellet diet and received water ad libitum.

The preparation of the animals, the dissection of the mesenteric artery, the de-endothelialization, the thromboformation and its on-line registration were commented and documented in extenso in earlier publications (Bourgain and Six,1974; Bourgain et al.,1984) and will only be summarized in a few lines. After careful microdissection of an appropriate mesenteric artery (250-350 μm diameter), de-endothelialization is induced by a single, 1 minute electric current. The intensity of this current depends on the vessel diameter, its polarity is inversed every 5 seconds to minimize vasospasm. Then, a control thrombus is generated by a time-limited superfusion of that arterial segment with ADP (400 μM, 45s, 1ml/min, 37°C). Such an ADP thrombus embolizes spontaneously within 1 to 2 minutes after discontinuance of the ADP drip, but can be reproduced by its renewal after a suitable time interval, in casu 10 to 12 minutes. The quantification of the thromboformation is made possible by the microprojection of the vessel segment onto light sensitive electronic components. An appropriate optoelectronic transduction allows the on-line derivation of several discriminating parameters (duration, amplitude, density, surface,...).

For SEM the animals were total-body-perfusion-fixed at physiologic pressure with 2% glutaraldehyde in cacodylate buffer. The arteries were overnight immersion-fixed, post-fixed in osmium, dehydrated in ascending ethanol concentrations, critical-point-dried, opened lengthwise with the technique by Reidy and Schwartz (1982), coated with gold and examined with a Philips SEM 505. A detailled description of this procedure can be found in Maes et al.(1984a,b) and in Potvliege et al.(1984).

Mepacrine (quinacrine hydrochloride), an inhibitor of phospholipase activity, was superfused in a 5.10^{-5}M concentration. Platelet activating factor (PAF-acether, 1-O-alkyl-2-acetyl-sn-glycero-3-phosphorylcholine, (+)) was superfused in a 10^{-6}M concentration. In vivo, PAF is a toxic endogenous phospholipid. Its complex biochemistry and biology was summarized by O'Flaherty and Wykle(1983). Several publications treat its role in platelet aggregation (Chignard et al.,1979; Vargaftig et al.,1980; Benveniste,1981).

(+) PAF-acether was kindly provided by Dr. B.B. Vargaftig, Institut Pasteur, Paris, France.

RESULTS

The intimal lesion and the ADP induced control thrombus (figs. 1 and 2) were shown in detail in an earlier publication (Maes et al., 1984a). In general, the lesion is a circular or oval area with a central zone that is desquamated completely and covered by a multitude of activated platelets. Its periphery is often occupied by flaps of endothelial cell remnants. Mostly 20 to 40 adjoining endothelial cells get detached by the electric current. TEM equally reveals a restricted lesion of the medial smooth muscle cells under the intimal trauma (Potvliege and Bourgain,1976 and 1977). However, this deep injury did not influence the endothelial regeneration pattern, nor did it lead to scar formation with fibrous tissue deposition (Potvliege and Bourgain,1977 and 1980). Control thrombi are sponge-like platelet masses, anchored on the experimentally denuded subendothelium, plasma-permeable, with an irregular surface, very blood-streamlined. We never saw leukocytes in such thrombotic mass.

Mepacrine superfusion over an injured arterial segment is responsable for a significant initial decrease of the different thrombus parameters when one induces ADP thrombi during the mepacrine flow. But gradually, this decrease is reversed into a rather anarchic increase in thromboformation. In vivo light microscopy then shows a thrombotic mass that is spreading over the complete luminal circumference of that vessel segment. SEM (fig.3) confirms this impression. Instead of a single thrombotic mass, we see a multitude of small platelet clumps, interconnected by a monolayer of activated platelets, on a large denuded subintimal area. At this concentration, mepacrine superfusion seems toxic for the endothelial cells. As dying or dead endothelial cells detach very quickly, the denuded area gradually enlarges, leading to the characteristic thrombotic phenomena.

PAF-acether superfusion generates large thrombotic phenomena by itself, no subsequent ADP superfusion is needed. There is no spontaneous disappearance after discontinuance of the PAF application. To force its embolization one needs a PGE_1 superfusion ($10^{-5}M$). Moreover, such forced embolization is followed, a few minutes later, by the reappearance of a new, PAF-like, thrombus on the same spot, without having to renew the PAF superfusion. SEM (fig.4) reveals a large thrombus, based on a "normal" denuded subendothelium, but also spreading widely, both up-and downstream, over the adjoining, non-detached endothelium. A PAF thrombus is a densely packed platelet mass, always invaded by numerous leukocytes, mostly polymorphonuclears. The endothelium under the thrombus demonstrates large necrotic cytoplasmic vacuoles. A more detailled description of PAF induced thrombi can be found in Maes et al.(1984b).

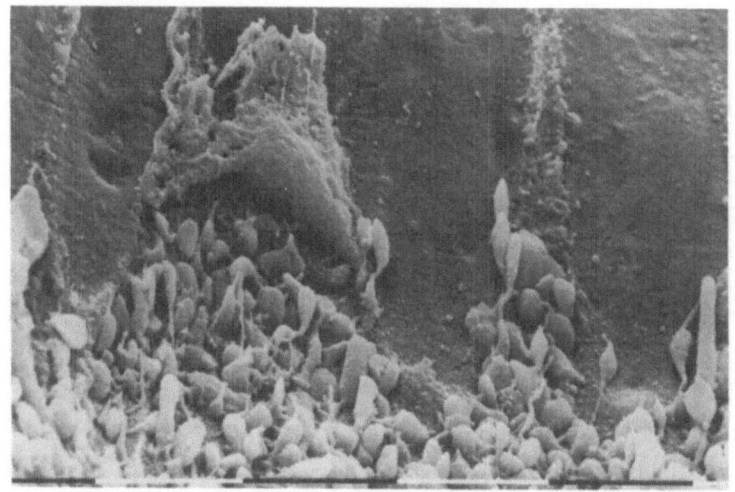

Fig.1 The edge of the lesion is occupied by flaps of
endothelial cell remnants. This specimen was
fixed a few seconds after the start of ADP superfusion. Platelets start forming a monolayer on
the denuded subendothelium (bar = 10μm).

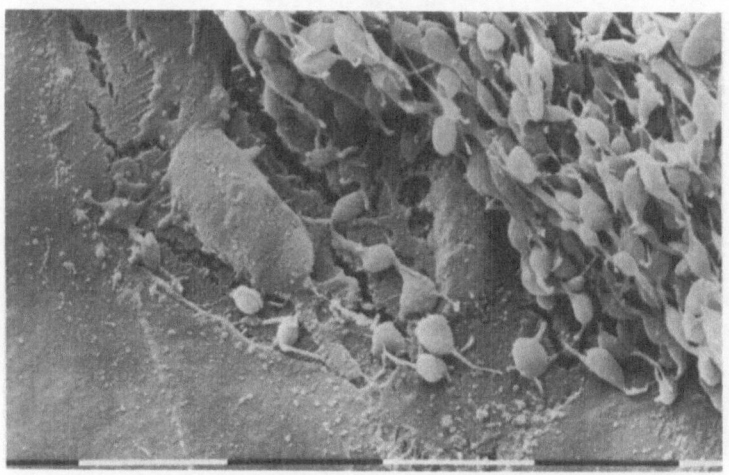

Fig.2 A part of the ADP thrombus. Platelets interconn-
ect by their pseudopods and form a porous mass.
The thrombus never extends beyond the sharp edge
of the lesion (bar = 10μm).

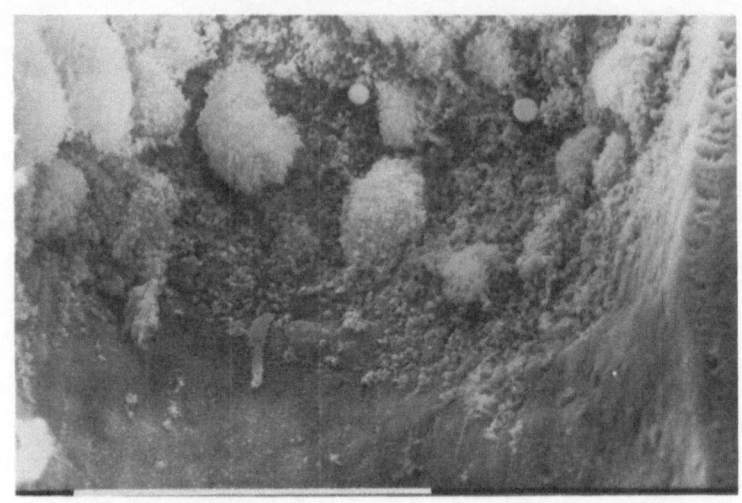

Fig.3 Thrombosis induced by ADP during continuous mepacrine superfusion. A multitude of small platelet
thrombi, interconnected by a platelet monolayer
cover the luminal vessel wall (bar = 0.1mm).

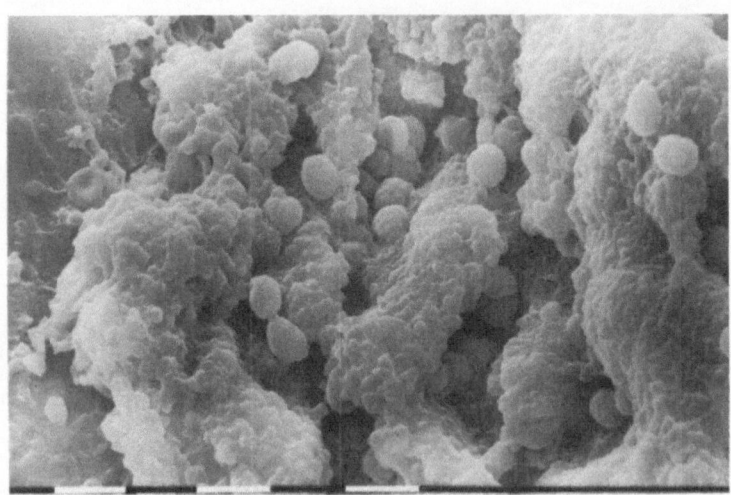

Fig.4 A PAF thrombus is a very dense platelet mass,
covering the denuded area and a part of the adjoining endothelium. Note the presence of numerous leukocytes (bar = 10μm).

DISCUSSION

Arterial platelet thrombosis is an expression of the complex interaction between platelets and the vessel wall. An experimental model should approximate the physiopathologic situation and provide for a standardized, reproducible and on-line registration of the transient, time-limited thromboformation.

An in vivo light microscopic evaluation of the experimental situation is not sufficient to elucidate all problems occuring during the experiment. On-line observations need complementation with ultra-morphologic data. This is clearly evidenced in the mepacrine or PAF experiments. In both situations thromboformation is augmented, giving rise to apparently similar light microscopic images. SEM and TEM show quite different structures. With mepacrine the enlargening is mainly due to a necrotic detachment of the endothelial cells, thereby exposing more subendothelium. In the PAF experiment the intoxicated cells do not detach. The platelets aggregate on the endothelium surrounding the experimental lesion, maybe due to a loss or partial destruction of their glycocalyx. Other significant differences with the mepacrine thrombi are a consequence of PAF's bioactivity: the powerful aggregating properties are reflected in the high density of the thrombus, the presence of leukocytes indicates its strong leukotaxic capacity. Autorepetition of PAF thrombi after a single PAF superfusion cannot be explained on the basis of an altered platelet function alone, but evidently necessitates some fundamental change in the endothelial metabolism as well. Recent experiments, combining PAF and mepacrine superfusion point to a possible autogeneration of PAF-like activity in the endothelial cell through a complex set of successive biochemical steps. This hypothesis, together with the possible influence of PAF on the endothelial glycocalyx, needs more experimental data.

REFERENCES

Begent, N. and Born, G.V.,1970, Growth rate in vivo of platelet thrombi, produced by iontophoresis of ADP, as a function of mean blood flow velocity, Nature, 227:926-930.

Benveniste, J.,1981, Platelet-activating factor (PAF-acether): present status, Agents Actions, 11:542-544.

Bourgain, R.H.,1978a, The effect of indomethacin and ASA on in vivo induced white platelet arterial thrombus formation, Thromb.Res., 12:1079-1086.

Bourgain, R.H.,1978b, Inhibition of PGI_2 (prostacyclin) synthesis in the arterial wall enhances the formation of white platelet thrombi in vivo, Haemostasis, 7:252-255.

Bourgain, R.H.,1979, The inhibitory effect of PGI_2 on white platelet arterial thrombus formation, Haemostasis, 8:117-119.

Bourgain, R.H.,1980, The inhibition of PGI_2 synthetase within the arterial wall by 15-hydroperoxyarachidonic acid enhances local white platelet thrombosis,Haemostasis, 9:345-351.

Bourgain, R.H. and Six, F.,1974, A continuous registration method in experimental arterial thrombosis in the rat, Thromb.Res., 4: 599-607.

Bourgain, R.H., Andries, R. and Finné, E.,1979, The role of prostaglandins in platelet-vessel wall interactions, Thér.,239:161-163.

Bourgain, R.H., Andries, R., Biagi, G. and Finné, E., 1981, The effect of arachidonic acid on platelet-vessel interaction, Arch.int.Pharmacodyn.Thér., 250:302-304.

Bourgain, R.H., Andries, R. and Six, F.,1982, Role of the prostaglandin biochemical pathway in platelet-vessel wall interaction and local thrombosis, Haemostasis, 11:133-138.

Bourgain, R.H., Andries, R. and Maes, L.,1983, Effect of cyclooxygenase inhibition on platelet-vassel wall interaction, Haemostasis, 13:102-108.

Bourgain, R.H., Vermarien, H., Andries, R.,Vereecke, F., Jacqueloot, J., Rennies, J., Blockeel, E. and Six, F.,1984(in press), A standardized "in vivo" model for the study of experimental arterial thrombosis. Description of a method., Proc.Int.Symp."Oxygen Transport to Tissue", U.S.A. 1983.

Chignard, M., Le Couedic, J.P., Tence, M., Vargaftig, B.B. and Benveniste, J.,1979, The role of Platelet-activating factor in platelet aggregation, Nature, 279:799-800.

Hladovec, J.,1971, Experimental arterial thrombosis in rats with continuous registration, Thrombos.Diathes.Haemorrh., 26:407-410.

Kovacs, I. and Görög, P.,1979, Laser induced thrombosis test suitable for pharmacological screening, Microvasc.Res., 18:403-412.

Maes, L., Andries, R. and Bourgain, R.H.,1984a(in press), Endothelial injury and platelet thrombosis in mesenteric arteries of rats. A scanning electron microscopic study., Microvasc.Res.

Maes, L., Bourgain, R.H., Andries, R. and Warson, F.,1984b(in press), the effect of PAF-acether on in vivo arterial platelet-vessel wall interaction in the guinea pig, Atherosclerosis.

O'Flaherty, J.T. and Wykle, R.L.,1983, Biology and biochemistry of platelet-activating factor, Clin.Rev.Allergy, 1:353-359.

Philp, R.B., Francey, I. and Warren, B.A.,1978, Comparision of antithrombotic activity of heparin, ASA, sulfinpyrazole and VK744 in a rat model of arterial thrombosis, Haemostasis, 7:282-293.

Potvliege, P.R. and Bourgain, R.H.,1976, Thrombosis induced in vivo in the mesenteric artery of rats. An electron microscopic study of the initial phases, Br.J.exp.Pathol., 57:722-732.

Potvliege, P.R. and Bourgain, R.H.,1977, Thrombosis induced in vivo in the mesenteric artery of normal and thrombocytopenic rats. An electron microscopic study of the early wall reaction, Br.J.exp. Pathol., 58:670-676.

Potvliege, P.R. and Bourgain, R.H.,1979, Inhibition by suloctidil of the early wall reaction induved by local thrombosis, Eur.J. Rheum.Inflamm., 2:204-207.

Potvliege, P.R. and Bourgain, R.H.,1980, The wall reaction to electric microinjury at branching sites of mesenteric arteries in the rat: an electron microscopic study of intimal cushions, Br.J.exp. Pathol., 61:324-331.

Potvliege, P.R. and Bourgain, R.H.,1982, The effect of a fat-rich diet on the ultrastructure of mesenteric arteries of the rat and their reaction to local desendothelialization, Br.J.exp.Pathol., 63:116-123.

Potvliege, P.R., Maes, L., Warson, F. and Bourgain, R.H.,1984(in press), The effect of the inhibition of platelet function on the development of the primary atherogenic lesion in rats on a fat-cholesterol rich diet, Br.J.exp.Pathol.

Reidy, M.A. and Schwartz, S.M.,1982, A technique to investigate surface morphology and endothelial cell replication of small arteries: a study in acute angiotensin-induced hypertensive rats, Microvasc. Res., 24:158-167.

Rosenblum, W.I.,1978, Fluorescence induced in platelet aggregates as a guide to luminal contours in the presence of platelet aggregation, Microvasc.Res., 15:103-106.

Shishido, M. and Katori, M.,1981, A quantitative method using continuous registration of platelet thrombus size in hamster cheek pouch, Microvasc.Res., 22:199-209.

Takano, S. and Suzuki, T.,1982, A study on in vivo production of thrombosis in rat mesenteric arterioles and action of prostaglandin (PG)I_2 on the thrombosis, Japan.J.Pharmacol., 32:439-444.

Ubatuba, F., Moncada, S. and Vane, J.R.,1979, The effect of prostacyclin on platelet behaviour, thrombus formation in vivo and bleeding time, Thromb.Haemostas.(Stuttg.), 41:425-435.

Van Der Byl, K.V., Honour, A.J. and Learry, W.P.P.,1982, A method for the study of platelet "white body" formation in the mesenteric arteries of the living animal, Life Sci., 31:2985-2989.

Vargaftig, B.B., Chignard, M., Le Couedic, J.P. and Benveniste, J., 1980, One, two, three or more pathways for platelet aggregation, Acta Med.Scand.(Suppl.), 642:23-29.

Weichert, W., Paulins, V. and Breddin, H.K.,1983, Laser induced thrombi in rat mesenteric vessels and antithrombotic drugs, Haemostasis, 13:61-71.

Zimmerman, R., Zeltsch, C. and Lange, D.,1979, Estimation of thrombus formation by labelling platelets, red cells and fibrinogen in experimental thrombosis, Thromb.Res., 16:147-158.

597

LUNG

DETERMINATES OF THE LUNG-SURFACE-P0$_2$

H.U. Spiegel, J. Hauss, J. Höpfner, K Schönleben*,
and P.P. Lunkenheimer**

Chirurgische Universitätsklinik,
Jungeblodtplatz 1, D-4400 Münster

*Städtische Krankenanstalten, Chirurgische Klinik
 Bremser Straße 79, D-6700 Ludwigshafen
**Exp. Herz-, Thorax- und Gefaßchirurgie
 Jungeblodt platz 1, D-4400 Münster

During recent years, measurement of the local tissue-p0$_2$ by means of the multiwire surface electrode devised by KESSLER and LÜBBERS and observation of microcirculation changes have been the subject of many surveys (1,2,3).

The present study examines the local p0$_2$ at the lung surface with physiologic and increased oxygen concentration in the respiratory gas. We also followed the influence of the ventilation / perfusion stop on tissue-p0$_2$.

In the present model, the local p0$_2$ of the lung surface is influenced by the following factors (fig. 1):

1) alveolar ventilation
2) oxygen transport via blood and
3) leakage, composed of
   a) the oxygen consumption of the tissue and
   b) the 0$_2$-exchange of the uncoated pleura with the room gas.

Materials and methods

We measured the local lung-surface p0$_2$ of the left upper lobe of the lung of 10 mongrel dogs (mean weight 25

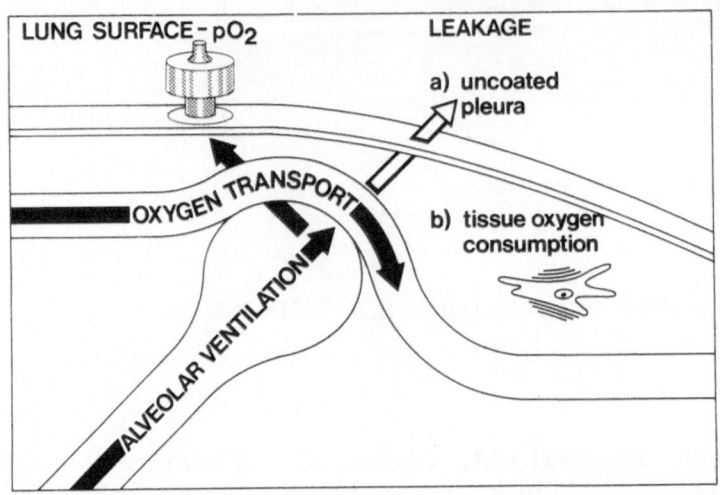

Fig. 1   Model of the measuring localization with those determinants that might influence the local value

kg) who had received sinistro-lateral thoracotomy in the
4th to 5th ICS by means of the multiwire surface electrode
devised by KESSLER and LÜBBERS (4).   Under high doses of
Piritramid basis anesthesia the animals were supplied with
room air and with a PEEP of 3 cm H_2O.   In order to measure hemodynamic and respiratory depending parameters,
pulmonary, left ventricular and vena cava catheters were
placed.   Arterial pressure, heart frequency and arterial
blood temperature were registered <u>continuously</u>.

        Cardiac output, pulmonary-capillary pressure, arte-
rial and mixed-venous pO_2, pCO_2 and pH-values, O_2-content,
hemoglobin, hematocrit, electrolytes, lactate and pyruvate
were determined <u>discontinuously</u>.

        The 5 animals forming the normoxia-group received
20.9 % O_2 for 4 hours under control. pO_2-histograms were
established every hour. In the hyperoxia-group the O_2-
content in the respiratory gas was increased hourly in 3
steps starting at 20.9 %, then reaching 30 % O_2, 60 % O_2
and finally 100 % O_2. pO_2-histograms were established
every 30 minutes following the increase in respiratory
O_2-contnet.   Then the local pO_2 with short term ventilation stop while maintaining perfusion and with perfusion
stop while maintaining ventilation was registered.

Short term <u>perfusion stop</u> was achieved by intravenous injection of acetylcholin, final perfusion stop by injecting 20 mmol/l potassium chloride.

In order to achieve the <u>ventilation stop</u> a special doublebarrelled tubus was introduced into the trachea and the lumen of the left primary bronchus was closed at the end of the inspiration.

Results

1. Lung-surface-pO_2 with normoxia and hyperoxia

Fig. 2a shows a summary of lung-surface pO_2 histograms with 20.9 % O_2-ventilation. The mean value of the local tissue-pO_2 in this normoxia-group is about 100 mm Hg. The pO_2-histograms are subsequently used as contron configuration. They remain nearly unchanged during the 4 hours of testing. Blood and circulation parameters are normal. In the hyperoxia-group (fig. 2b) the mean tissue-pO_2 climbs from 98 mm Hg to 614 mm Hg as respiratory O_2-content and arterial pO_2 increase. The pO_2-histograms are sufficiently normal.

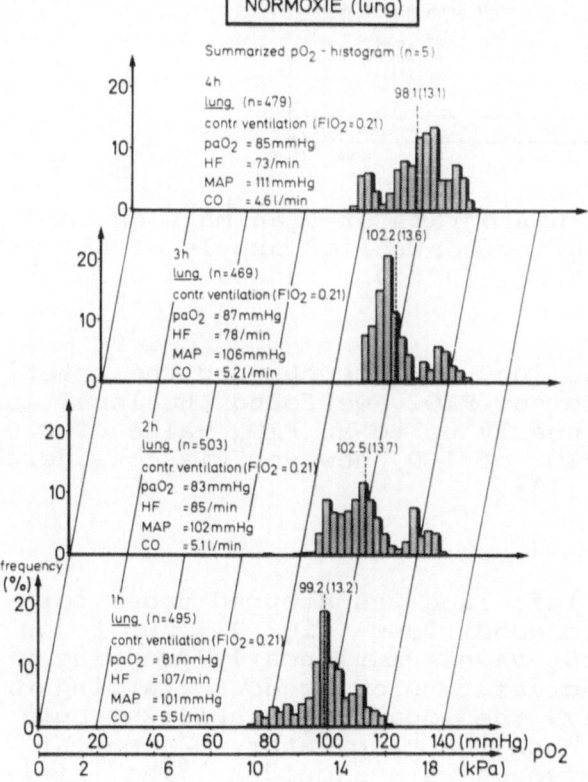

NORMOXIE (lung)

Fig. 2a:
Summarized pO_2-histograms of 5 animals on the lung surface during controlled supply of air with 20.9 % O_2. From bottom to top: Initial histograms, histogram after 2 hrs, 3 hrs, 4 hrs.

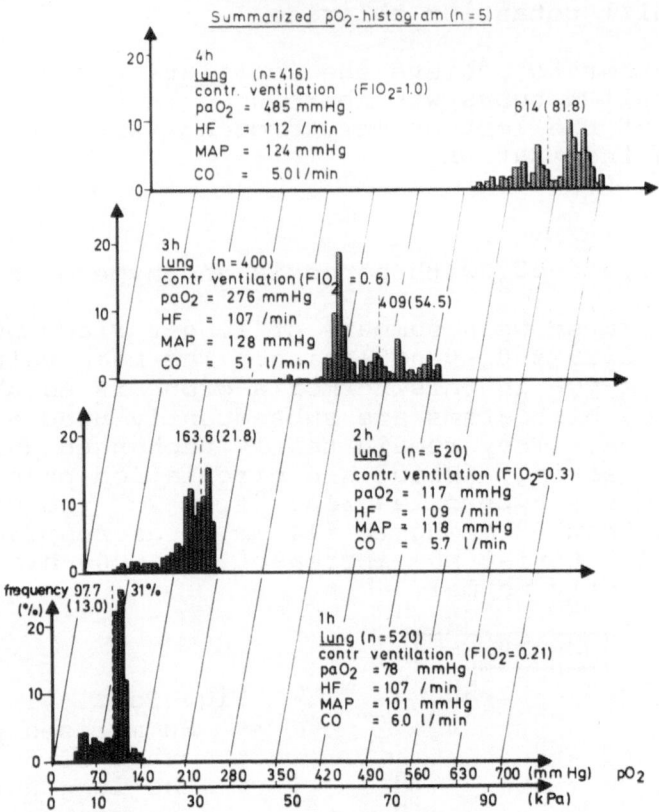

Fig. 2b: Summarized pO_2-histograms of 5 animals on the
lung surface during controlled supply of air with
20.9 % O_2, 30 % O_2, 60 % O_2, and 100 % O_2.

When comparing the lung surface pO_2 and the arterial pO_2 (fig. 3) in different FIO_2, we found the local lung
surface pO_2 to climb linearly up to an FIO_2 value of 0.6.
The pO_2-value with an FIO_2 of 1.0, however, is considerably below this straight line.

2. Ventilation stop

The ventilation of the left lung was stopped under normoxic and under hyperoxic conditions (fig. 4). Up to an
FIO_2 of 0.6 the local pO_2-values are linearly dropping to
about 45 mm Hg. This decrease is slowing down starting at
about 45 mm Hg. Finally, the local pO_2 stabilizes between 25 and 35 mm Hg. When the respiratory O_2-content
exceeds 60 % O_2, the curve shows a shoulder. The initi-

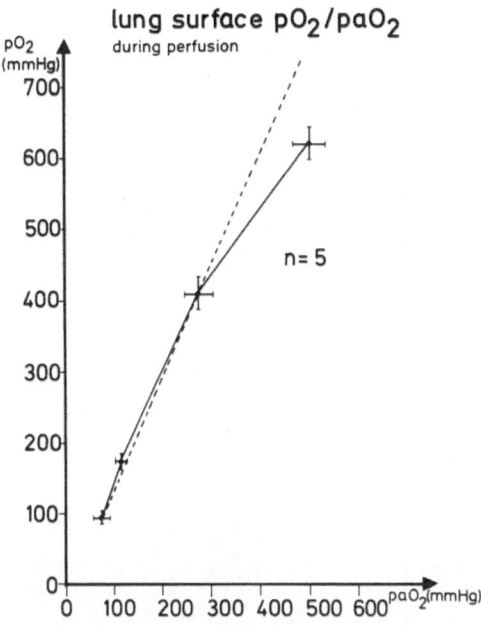

lung surface pO_2/paO_2
during perfusion

n= 5

Fig. 3: Mean value of the lung surface pO_2 and the arterial pO_2 with an FIO_2 of 0.21, 0.3, 0.6, 1.0. The ordinate shows the lung surface pO_2, the abscissa the arterial pO_2.

al pO_2-decrease is delayed. This is followed by a very rapid decrease which is slowing down after reaching values of 50 mm Hg. Finally the local pO_2-values stabilize between 30 - 40 mm Hg. In less than 2 minutes after the onset of ventilation the pO_2 reaches its starting value before ventilation stop.

3. Perfusion stop

Both reversible (fig. 5a) and definitive perfusion stop (fig. 5b) through cardiac arrest show an increase of the lung surface pO_2 of about 10 - 15 mm Hg, the pO_2 thus coming close to the respiratory gas pO_2, which is about 150 mm Hg with 20.9 O_2. After the onset of circulation the pO_2 falls to about 20 mm Hg below the starting point, beginning slightly to increase after 90 seconds. With a latency of 4 minutes the local pO_2 finally reaches its starting value. During the final perfusion stop the surface pO_2 maintains its value, which is by then increased by about 10 mm Hg.

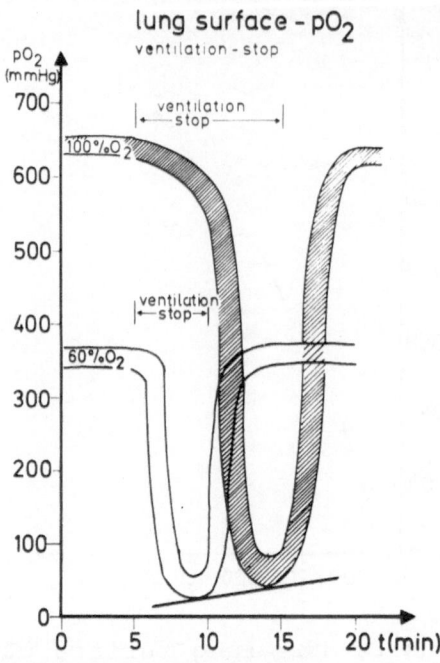

Fig. 4: Measuring the local tissue-pO_2 on the lung surface after closing the left bronchus. The lower
curve has been established with a supply of 60 %
O_2, the upper curve shows the supply of 100 % O_2.

4. Comparison perfusion - perfusion stop

When comparing the perfused to the non-perfused lung (fig.
6), the respiratory O_2-content increased in three steps of
20.9 % O_2 up to 30 %, 60 % and finally up to 100 % in intervals of five minutes each. The local pO_2 of the non-
perfused lung climbs linearly with the increasing respiratory O_2-content and is approx. 15 mm Hg over the local
pO_2 of the perfused lung.

Discussion

The canine pleura visceralis consists of a layer of mesothe-
lial cells and a comparatively thin layer of connective
tissue with small blood vessels and lymphatic cells (6). The
reported alteration of the local pO_2 with perfusion and
ventilation changes suggests the correspondence between
the local pO_2 and the alveolar capillary pO_2. According

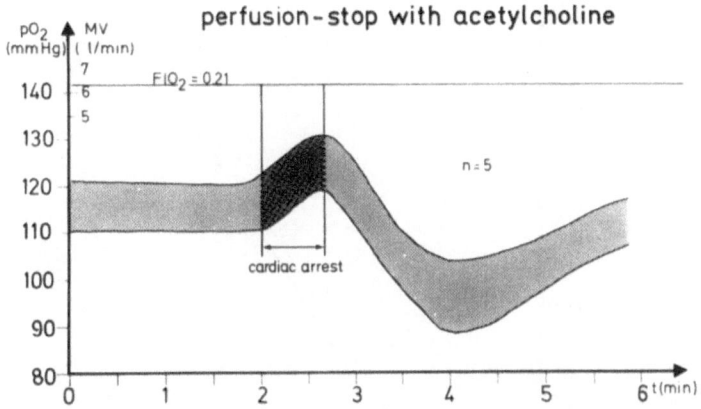

Fig. 5a: Measuring of the local tissue-pO_2 on the lung
surface immediately before cardiac arrest and
after recommencing lung perfusion.

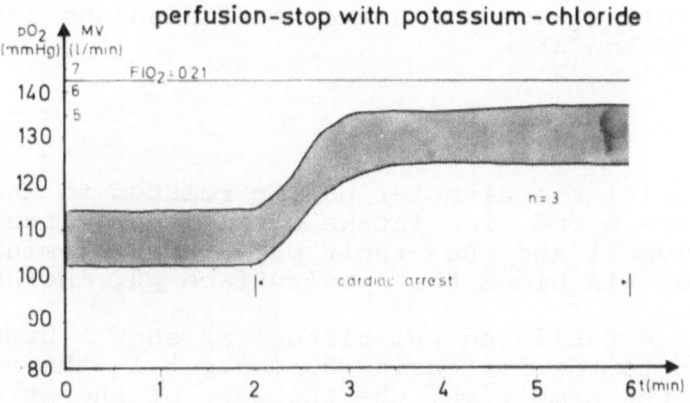

Fig. 5b: Measuring of the local tissue-pO_2 on the lung
surface before and during lung perfusion stop.

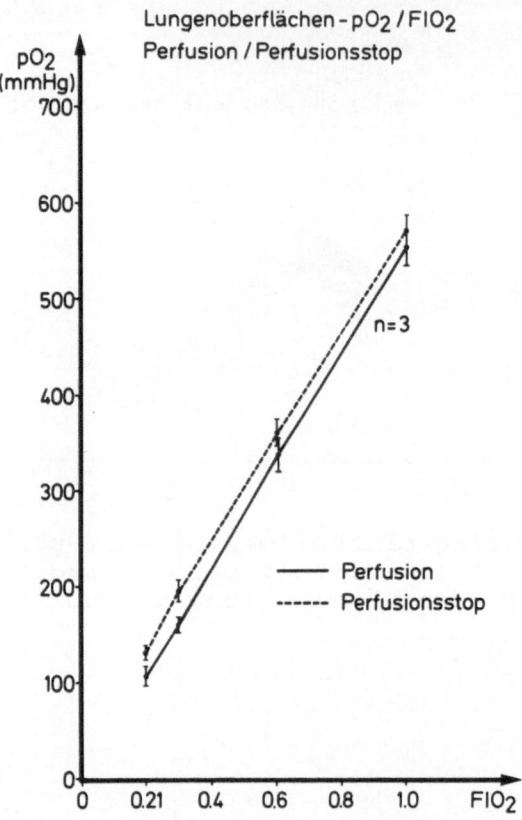

Fig. 6: Mean values of the lung surface pO_2 and respiratory O_2-content during perfusion and after perfusion stop.

to PIIPER (7) the alveolar pO_2 is related to the O_2-intake through the blood. The intake of O_2 reduces the O_2-content of the alveoli and thus their pO_2. When eliminating the O_2-removal via blood the lung-surface pO_2 increases.

The established pO_2-histograms show a broadening connected to the increasing O_2-content in the respiratory gas. At the same time, the increase of the straight surface-pO_2/FIO_2 diminishes starting at an FIO_2 of 0.6. This may be caused by the comparatively slight ventilation of ventral parts of the lung in the supine position described by several authors (7,8,9,10,11). Higher diffusion of O_2 over the uncoated pleura with increased O_2-gradients may have the same effect.

SHEPPARD (12) reports an increase of nearly 100 % of O_2-consumption with equal increases of the O_2-gradient between lung and surrounding gas when he measured the O_2-consumption of the non-perfused lung. An increase of the irregular distribution of ventilation (13) with increased O_2-content in the respiratory gas can also be connected to the broadening and the decrease of the rise. These results tally with a theory (14) suggesting that in areas of a low V/Q-ratio with high O_2-concentrations shunts occur in larger numbers. This corresponds with the established increase of the alveolar-arterial O_2-difference.

The delayed pO_2 decrease found under ventilation stop with continuing circulation points to antecedent storage, followed by the recommencing release of O_2 from the muscular tissue. This underlines the idea that the alveolar pO_2 depends on the O_2-transport in the blood. The O_2-consumption of the lung tissue and the diffusion of O_2 over a freely diffusible lung surface are further, at this stage not yet quantifiable determinates.

Disregarding free diffusion into the surrounding areas as well as the O_2-consumption of the lung tissue we regard the lung surface pO_2 as a new index for the ratio of ventilation/perfusion.

References

1. D.W. Lübbers, Methods of measuring oxygen tensions of blood and organ surfaces, in: "A symposium on oxygen measurement and their significance", J.P.Payne, D. Hill, ed., Churchill, London (1966)
2. J. Hauss, K. Schönleben, H.U. Spiegel, Therapiekontrolle durch Überwachung des Gewebe-pO_2, Hans Huber-Verlag, Bern (1982)
3. K. Schönleben, B. Krumme, H. Bünte, M. Kessler, Kontrolle der Intensivbehandlung durch Messung von Mikrozirkulation und O_2-Versorgung. In: Langenbecks Arch. Chir. (Suppl), Forum 76, 72 (1976)
4. M. Kessler, D.W. Lübbers, Aufbau und Anwendungsmöglichkeiten verschiedener pO_2-Elektroden. Pflügers Arch. Ges. Physiol. R. 82: 291 (1966)
5. H.U. Spiegel, J. Hauss, M. Bergermann, K. Schönleben, Die hochdosierte Piritramid-Basisanästhesie als tierexperimentelles Standardmodell bei der Untersuchung von Hämodynamik und Mikrozirkulation. Der Anästhesist, Suppl. Bd. 32: 143 (1983)
6. D.B. Daly, C. Hebb, Pulmonary and bronchial vascular Systems. Edward Arnold, London, p. 38 (1966)
7. J. Piiper, Blood-gas equilibration in lungs and pul-

monary diffusing capacity. Prog. Resp. Res. 16: 115 (1981)

8. A.C.Bryan, L.G. Bentivoglia, F. Beecel, H. MacLeish, A. Zidulka, D.V. Bates, Factors affecting regional distribution of ventilation and perfusion in the lung. J. Appl. Physiol. 19 (3): 395-402 (1964)

9. H. Rahn, B. Sadoul, L.E.Farhi, J. Shapiro, Distribution of ventilation and perfusion in the lobes of the dog's lung in the supine and erect position. J. Appl. Physiol. 8 (1): 417-426 (1958)

10. J. Milic-Emili, J.A.M. Henderson, M.B. Dolovich, D. Trop, K. Kaneko, Regional distribution of inspired gas in the lung. J. Appl. Physiol. 21 (3): 749-759 (1966)

11. A.C. Bryan, J. Milic-Emili, D. Pengelly, Effect of gravity on the distribution undpulmonary ventilation tion. J. Appl. Physiol. 21 (3): 778-784 (1966)

12. J.W. Shepard jr., V.D. Mink, G.F. Dolan, Gas exchange in non-perfused dog lungs. J. Appl. Physiol.: Resp. Environ. Exercise Physiol. 51 (5): 1261-1267 (1981)

13. P.D. Wagner, R.B. Laravuso, E. Goldzimmer, P.F. Naumann, J.B. West, Distributions of ventilation-perfusion ratios in dogs with normal and abnormal lungs. J. Appl. Physiol. 38 (6): 1099-1109 (1975)

14. D.R. Dantzker, P.D. Wagner, J.B. West, Instability of lung units with low V_A/Q ratios. J. Appl. Physiol. 38 (5): 886-895 (1975)

CONVECTION/DIFFUSION INTERACTIONS IN OXYGEN TRANSPORT:

EFFECT OF FLOW REVERSAL IN LUNG AIRWAYS

Hugh D. Van Liew and Kenneth R. Murray

Department of Physiology
University at Buffalo, SUNY
Buffalo, NY, 14214

Transport of oxygen to alveoli through the airway tree and to tissues through the vascular arborization both involve convection in large vessels followed by diffusion to the final O_2 sink. At the transition between convection and diffusion, there is a steep drop of O_2 concentration in the flowing medium. Gas in airways differs from the blood in that flow is bidirectional. We use a relatively simple computer model to demonstrate behavior of the steep drop when flow changes direction at end-inspiration.

Diffusive phenomena in lung airways, both during flow and when there is no flow, have been studied by mathematical models. During inspiratory flow, the major characteristic of diffusion/convection interaction is that the zone between the two processes, with its steep drop of O_2 concentration, tends to remain in one place in the airway tree, a "stationary front"; convective delivery of unmixed inspired air to the zone equals the diffusive dispersion of O_2 into peripheral airways (Baker et al., 1974; Cumming et al., 1971; Pack et al., 1977; Paiva, 1973; Paiva et al., 1976; Scherer et al., 1972). Other mathematical models showed that when diffusion occurs without convection, there is a mouthward movement of any gradient of gas concentration (LaForce and Lewis, 1970; Cumming et al., 1966). The goal of the present study is to estimate how events in the flow/no flow transition can affect gas exchange effectiveness.

METHODS

Our program assumes symmetric dichotomous branching of the Weibel morphometric model "A" (Weibel, 1963), assumes axial diffusion only, and makes no provision for differences of function of parallel pathways, for volume changes of the lung, nor for passage of O2 across the alveolocapillary membrane. It can account indirectly for convective flow. We use the diffusivity of O2, 0.25 cm^2/sec, but to avoid the complication of resident O2 in the lung, we present our results as amounts of "inspirate", as though inspired air were an indicator gas which has zero concentration in the lung before a breath. Our model appears to be adequate to describe the phenomena under study despite its simplicity; we obtain essentially the same results as calculations by other mathematical methods when we simulate mixing during inspiratory flow with no end-inspiratory pause (Paiva, 1973) or in the absence of flow after imposing a certain pattern of concentration in the lung (LaForce and Lewis, 1970).

The model consists of a number of separate compartments, one for each generation of lung airways. Oxygen can diffuse in the axial direction from a generation to the adjacent one according to a simplified version of Fick's law of diffusion:

$$(V/T)_i = (DA_i/L_i)(C_i - C_{i+1})$$

where D is diffusivity of the inspired gas, Ai is sum of the cross-sectional area of all airways in generation i (symbol Gi), Ci and C(i+1) are concentrations in Gi and G(i+1), and Li is length of airways in Gi. The quantity (V/T)i is amount of inspirate to diffuse per time interval from Gi to G(i+1); the equation gives diffusive movement that would occur under steady-state conditions if concentrations were held at Ci and C(i+1). This approach is equivalent to treating diffusion in a series of disks, where area of each disk represents summed cross-sectional area of all airways of the same generation number. See the inset of Fig. 1 for perspective on the sizes of the various generations.

RESULTS AND DISCUSSION

Figure 1 illustrates the behavior of the steep concentration drop during inspiration. This concentration/cumulative-volume coordinate system has two distinct advantages. First, the area under a curve on the diagram is equivalent to an amount of gas; changes of amount of inspirate in the lung with time are differences of area under the curves. Second, the intrapulmonary profile of the diagram can be correlated with the concentration-vs-volume pattern that would be seen at the mouth during expiration. The very first part of an expiration is made up of pure inspirate with C/C_I of 1.0

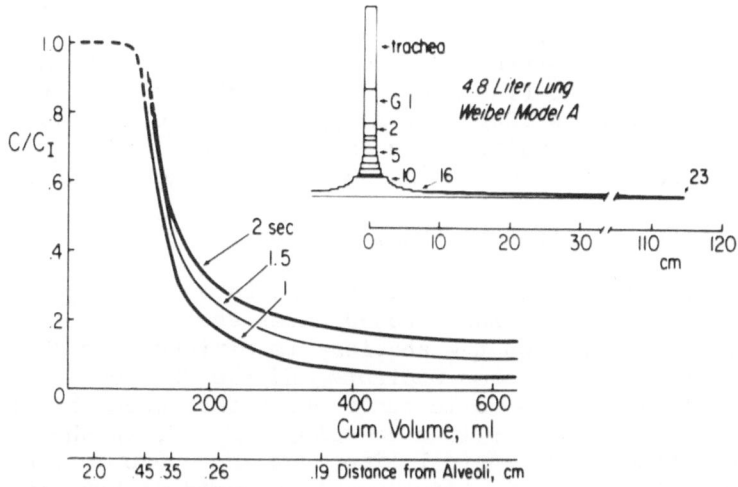

Fig. 1.   Relative concentration of inspired gas during inspiratory
convection is plotted against cumulative volume (zero
volume is at the mouth).   Times are after beginning of
inspiration.   For the simulation, the lung was structured
to a total volume of 2650 ml (2150 ml functional residual
capacity (FRC) plus 500 ml inspirate).   Inset, scale model
of the lung geometry.   Length of airway paths in the model
is 27 cm.

(called Phase I of expiration) followed by a steep fall (Phase II)
and an "alveolar plateau" (Phase III).

     The profiles of Fig. 1 show results for a constant flow of 250
ml/sec of inspired air (a 500 ml inspiration that lasts 2 sec).   To
run the simulation, generations 0-17 were filled with inspirate as
an initial condition; we then simulated convective delivery of air
through the upper airways by adding an appropriate amount of inspirate into G17 in each time interval.   Generation 17 was chosen because its conductance, DA_i/L_i, is 488 ml/sec, so that diffusion out
of the generation can be somewhat larger than the entire 250 ml/sec
that is being put into it.   Results are not appreciably different if
G16, with DA_i/L_i of 225 ml/sec, is the entry port.   The figure shows
that, as expected, the steep drop tends to remain at a fixed
position but the profiles change with time since the added gas
raises the level in the well-mixed lower generations.

     The location of the steep gradient during inspiratory flow is
determined by the relative magnitudes of diffusive conductance and

convective flow. It will be deeper in the lung if flow is high (as in exercise), and if diffusivity is low (as with gases in a hyperbaric environment (Van Liew et al., 1981) or with heavy gases in normal environments (Engel et al., 1979)). It will be more centrally located if diffusive conductance is appreciably enhanced by convective processes such as cardiac mixing (Engel et al., 1973).

Effect of an End-inspiratory Pause

Figure 2 illustrates how the profile becomes changed by diffusion when there is no flow. Coordinates are as in Fig. 1 but the cumulative lung volume on the abscissa is divided into the inspirate volume that will become expirate and the FRC portion, which will not be expired. The solid curve shows that when the inspiratory flow has ended, there is a downslope of C/C_I in the alveolar gas to the left of the vertical line, but the curve is essentially flat in the FRC. If expiration were to proceed without further mixing, an observer would see a Phase I of about 175 ml, a Phase II that extended to 500 or 600 ml, and series dead space would be estimated at about 400 ml. There would be considerable slope in Phase III.

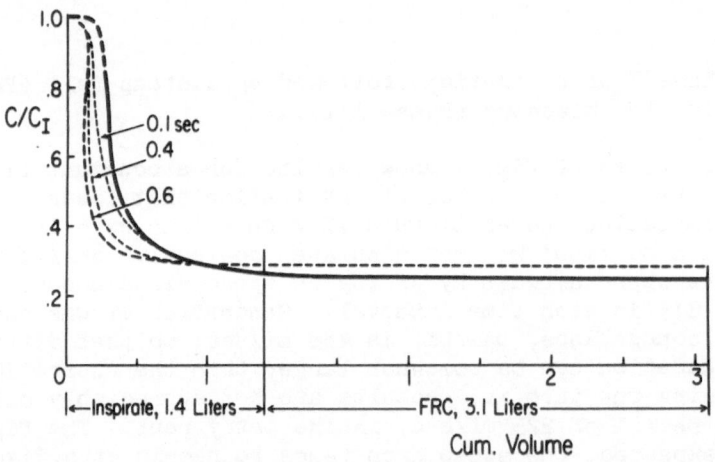

Fig. 2. Effect of an end-inspiratory breathhold on diffusive transport of inspired gas into the FRC of the lung. Solid curve, profile after 3 sec of inspiratory flow. Dashed curves, results of inspiratory breathholds, started from the solid curve. Tidal volume 1.4 liters; inspiratory flow 0.47 l/sec.

After convection stops, diffusion changes both the profile that would be seen at the mouth during expiration and the amount of inspirate in the FRC (dashed curves, Fig. 2). The breathhold rapidly sharpens the angle between Phases II and III and moves Phase II mouthward. For the case shown, the area between the solid inspiratory flow curve and the 0.6 sec breathhold curve is equivalent to 90 ml of inspirate added to the FRC, raising its relative concentration from 0.25 to 0.28. We discuss Fig. 2 as though the transition between inspiration and expiration occurred in a stepwise fashion, with constant inspiratory flow giving way abruptly to an end-inspiratory pause. We believe that a virtual end-inspiratory breathhold, as in the Fig. 2 simulation, is a fair approximation of the more likely sequence of slowing, stopping and reversal of flow of a real breath.

The amount of inspired gas added to the FRC during the end-inspiratory pause is not a matter of equalization of two gas quantities, but rather is due to translocation of the stratification in central airways that exists at the end of flow. The mouthward movement is a propagated phenomenon in that pure inspired gas in the particular airways nearest the steep gradient region approaches concentration equilibrium with the large volume of well-mixed peripheral units; this moves the steep gradient mouthward to the next group of units, which in turn equilibrate with the periphery, and so on. In experiments with dogs, live and postmortem, Engel et al. (1973) were able to observe the mouthward movement during breathholds after inspiration; according to their data, the action of the heart makes the movement about 5 times faster than it would be if mixing were by molecular diffusion alone.

Dead space, estimated in various ways, has been found to be large for poorly-diffusing gases (Okubo and Piiper, 1974; Sikand et al., 1976; Van Liew et al., 1981). Paiva (1973) computed an approximately hyperbolic relation between dead space (by the Bohr formula) and period of a breath with his model, such that dead space is large when period is very small but falls and levels off as period increases. The profiles of Fig. 2 illustrate why: If diffusivity is low or if there is little time in the end-inspiratory pause, a greater amount of indicator is to the left of the steep gradient when expiration occurs. A longer duration resembles a longer pause, so series dead space is smaller, but when time or diffusivity is large enough that the steep gradient is in the uppermost, low-conductance airways, further time makes little difference. Thus, series dead space is a variable that is a function of central airway geometry, time, and effective diffusivity, and its maximal range is between the inspiratory mode profile and the profile corresponding to such low-conductance airways that further time makes no appreciable difference. Because it contains a high concentration of inspirate, series dead space can contribute inspirate to the rest of the airway path if time allows.

Amounts added to the FRC

Figure 3 illustrates the addition of inspirate to the FRC as a function of inspiratory rate and end-inspiratory pause duration. The solid curve is for no pause; if a certain tidal volume is inspired rapidly, less indicator gas enters the FRC during the flow phase than when inspiration is slow. Dashed curves show that additional amounts enter the FRC if there is an end-inspiratory pause. To take the example seen before in Fig. 2 (inspiratory duration of 3 sec), amount of inspirate to reach the FRC is 750 ml, equivalent to perfect mixing with a series dead space of almost 400 ml. The additional mixing due to a pause of only 1 sec decreases the series dead space to about 100 ml.

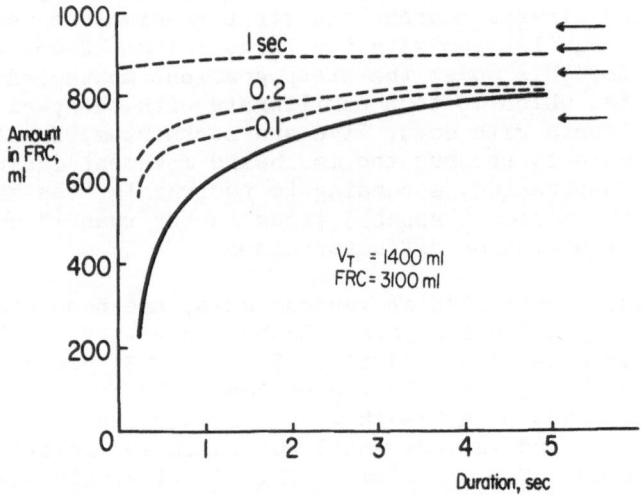

Fig. 3. Effects of inspiratory rate and inspiratory pauses. Amount of inspirate that is in the FRC is plotted against duration of a constant-flow inspiration when tidal volume is kept constant. Solid curve, amount of inspirate in the FRC at the end of the flow phase; vertical distances from the solid curve to the dashed curves are amounts added by inspiratory pauses. Horizontal arrows show results of perfect mixing of the inspired gas with the FRC gas except for series dead spaces of, from the top, 0, 100, 200 and 400 ml.

The effect of a given pause is greater when inspiratory flow has been high (at the left of Fig. 3); when the stationary front is deep in the lungs, it is in a high-conductance region. For example, during 0.1 sec of breathhold after an inspiratory duration of 1.0 sec, 100 ml of inspirate is added to the FRC whereas if duration is 4.0 sec, the amount is only 10 ml. With additional time, the dashed curves flatten because the Phase II front moves into the uppermost airways.

The left-hand region of the solid curve of Fig. 3 approximates the minimal amount of gas exchange that would occur during rapid breathing if the effective diffusivity is the molecular diffusivity. According to the figure, breath effectiveness for rapid inspirations would be considerably less if no inspirate were transported to the FRC by an end-inspiratory pause, or its equivalent due to slowing and stopping of flow. For example, at a rate of 1.4 l/sec (0.7 sec duration) only 600 ml of the 1400 ml of inspirate has entered the FRC at the end of the flow phase; 100 ml more enters in 0.1 sec of pause, and an additional 200 ml enters by the end of 1.0 sec. Thus 1.0 sec of diffusion at end-inspiration increases gas exchange per breath by 300 ml; a third of the total exchange would occur during the pause.

If effective diffusivity is greater than molecular diffusivity because of convective processes during inspiration, the solid curve of Fig. 3 will be higher at every point; if convective mixing is important during the inspiratory pause, the dashed curves will move farther from the solid curve for a given short time interval. It has been observed that time for a breath (in exercise) and gas-phase diffusivity (in hyperbaric environments) can decrease by factors of 5 or 10 without causing severe impairment of gas exchange. Our simulations illustrate why changes of time for diffusion, diffusivity, or effective diffusivity can be expected to have minimal effect on amount of gas that exchanges between inspirate and FRC. The concentration profiles set up during inspiration are largely over-ridden by mixing in the end-inspiratory pause; no matter where the front is positioned, a short interval of slow flow or a pause allows mouthward movement into the low-volume low-conductance upper airways that constitute the series dead space.

REFERENCES

Baker, L. G., Ultman, J. S., and Rhoades, R. A., 1974, Simultaneous gas flow and diffusion in a symmetric airway system: a mathematical model, Respir. Physiol., 21:119.
Cumming, G., Crank, J., Horsfield, K., and Parker, I., 1966, Gaseous diffusion in the airways of the human lung, Respir. Physiol., 1:58.

Cumming, G., Horsfield, K., and Preston, S. B., 1971, Diffusion
    equilibrium in the lungs examined by nodal analysis, Respir.
    Physiol., 12:329.
Engel, L. A., Paiva, M., Siegler, D. I. M., and Fukuchi, Y., 1979,
    Dual tracer single breath studies of gas transport in the
    lung, Respir. Physiol., 36:103.
Engel, L. A., Wood, L. D. H., Utz, G., and Macklem, P. T., 1973,
    Gas mixing during inspiration, J. Appl. Physiol., 35:18.
LaForce, R. C., and Lewis, B. M., 1970, Diffusional transport in the
    human lung, J. Appl. Physiol., 28:291.
Okubo, T., and Piiper, J., 1974, Intrapulmonary gas mixing in
    excised dog lung lobes studied by simultaneous wash-out of
    two inert gases, Respir. Physiol., 21:223.
Pack, A., Hooper, M. B., Nixon, W., and Taylor J. C., 1977, A
    computational model of pulmonary gas transport incorporating
    effective diffusion, Respir. Physiol., 29:101.
Paiva, M., 1973, Gas transport in the human lung, J. Appl. Physiol.,
    35:401.
Paiva, M., Lacquet, L. M., and van der Linden, L. P., 1976, Gas
    transport in a model derived from Hansen-Ampaya anatomical
    data of the human lung, J. Appl. Physiol., 41:115.
Scherer, P. W., Shendalman, L. H., and Greene, N. M., 1972,
    Simultaneous diffusion and convection in single breath lung
    washout, Bull. Math. Biophys., 34:393.
Sikand, R. S., Magnussen, H., Scheid, P., and Piiper, J., 1976,
    Convective and diffusive gas mixing in human lungs:
    experiments and model analysis, J. Appl. Physiol., 40:362.
Van Liew, H. D., Thalmann, E. D., and Sponholtz, D. K., 1981,
    Hindrance to diffusive gas mixing in the lung in hyperbaric
    environments, J. Appl. Physiol., 51:243.
Weibel, E. R., 1963, "Morphometry of the Human Lung," Springer-
    Verlag, Berlin.

CONSEQUENCES OF THE O_2-CO_2 DISSOCIATION CURVES FOR GAS EXCHANGE IN AVIAN AND MAMMALIAN LUNG AT VARIOUS ALTITUDES

Aart Zwart* and Ed Hoorn

Dept. of Plumonary Diseases, Pathophysiological Laboratory
Erasmus University, P.O. Box 1738, 3000 DR Rotterdam
*Present Address: Lab of Inhalation Toxicology, CIVO-TNO
Utrechtseweg 48, 3704 HE Zeist

ABSTRACT

Gas exchange in avian and mammalian lung was studied with computer simulations using mutually dependent O_2-CO_2 dissociation curves. The mammalian lung was simulated with an ideal mixing unit. The model of the avian lung consisted of 25 ideal mixing units placed in series with respect to the ventilation but placed in parallel with respect to the perfusion (cross-current arrangement). The consequence of the right shift in the avian oxygen dissociation curve, if compared with the human dissociation curve, was studied by application of both dissociation curves to the avian lung model. The influence of a decreased tension of oxygen in the inspired air was studied under conditions of constant $P_{\bar{v}}CO_2$ (48 mmHg), $P_{\bar{v}}O_2$ (30 mmHg), RQ (0.70) and approximately constant levels of P_aCO_2.
At sea-level the avian lung needs 80 per cent of the alveolar ventilation and 64 per cent of the cardiac output to transport the same amount of gas if compared with the mammalian lung. The difference in the need for cardiac output resulted from the right shift in the dissociation curve of avian blood.
Changing P_IO_2 from 115 mmHg (2000 m) to 100 mmHg (3000 m) showed a dramatic difference in the performance of the two lung models. The mammalian lung model needed a more than eight fold increase in cardiac output whereas the avian lung model needed less than a three fold increase to maintain a RQ of 0.7. This difference could be ascribed to the Haldane effect in combination with the cross-current arrangement. The Haldane effect was also responsible for an end expired CO_2 tension which exceeded the mixed venous CO_2 tension.

This investigation was partly financed by a grant from ZWO

619

INTRODUCTION

Hazelhoff (1943, 1951) described the unique property of the unidirectional gas flow through the parabronchi of the avian lung during inspiration and expiration. Scheid and Piiper (1970) drew the consequence of this property and showed that the gas exchange in the avian lung could be described as a cross-current arrangement. They described the gas exchange properties of such a system for gases having constant blood-gas partition coefficients. The cross-current gas exchange arrangement is more efficient than the co-current gas exchange arrangement with which the mammalian lung can be described but this does not guarantee a better adaptation to changes in inspired oxygen levels when exercising at different altitudes. We investigated the changes in $\dot{V}/\dot{Q}$ ratio needed to maintain normal levels of CO_2 in arterial and venous blood. The use of two sets of dissociation curves adapted to human and duck blood enabled the investigation of the effect of the right shift in duck blood on gas transfer.
Davies and Dutton (1975) observed a reversal in the difference between the CO_2 tension in the expired gas and in the mixed venous blood. This effect was explained with the charged membrane hypothesis proposed by Gurtner et al. (1969). We investigated whether this observation could be explained with the Haldane effect.

METHODS

Lungmodels: The basic unit of the mammalian and avian lung model is the ideal mixing box or co-current gas exchanger (Fig. 1). For the mammalian lung one unit is used to model the alveolar gas exchange where the tensions of CO_2 and O_2 in the air leaving the unit ($P_{\bar{E}}$) are in equilibrium with the arterial tensions (P_a).
The avian lung is built up with a series of the same ideal mixing units but now placed in series with respect to the ventilation and in parallel with respect to the perfusion. The arterial content results from a weighted summation of the content in blood leaving each unit. From this arterial content we calculated the arterial

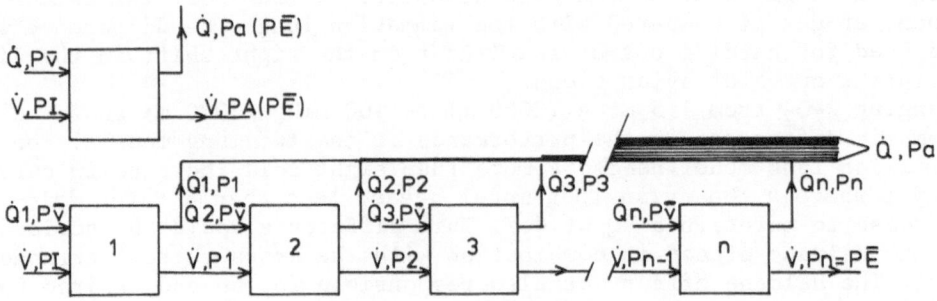

Fig. 1. Set up of lung models for the mammalian lung consisting of one unit and the avian lung consisting of n units.

partial pressure, P_a. The expired tension, $P_{\bar{E}}$, was taken as the tension in the last unit. The model consisted of 25 compartments which yielded output tensions differing less than one promille from the output of a cross-current model with an infinite number of compartments for gases with constant blood-gas partition coefficients.

Dissociation curves: Kinne and Seagrave (1974) described the human dissociation curves of O_2 and CO_2 as follows:

$$c_{O_2} = C_{max} (u/1 + u) + 10^{-5} P_{O_2} \tag{1}$$

$$c_{CO_2} = (0.145 - 0.017 (u/1 + u) P_{CO_2}{}^{0.36} \tag{2}$$

$$u = 0.925 y + 2.8 y^2 + 30 y^3 \tag{3}$$

$$y = (0.004273 + 0.04326 P_{CO_2}{}^{-0.535}) P_{O_2} \tag{4}$$

where: c_{O_2}, c_{CO_2} = content of oxygen and carbon dioxide, resp. (ml/ml)

C_{max} = maximum transport capacity of blood by haemoglobin

P_{O_2}, P_{CO_2} = tension of oxygen and carbon dioxide, resp. (mmHg)

u, y = auxiliary variables

The constants in eqs. 2 and 3 were adapted for duck blood using the data of Scheipers et al. (1975), yielding:

$$c_{CO_2} = (0.195 - 0.019 (u/1 + u)) P_{CO_2}{}^{0.31} \tag{2a}$$

$$u = 0.04802 y + 1.5025 y^2 + 9.3212 y^3 \tag{3a}$$

The O_2 dissociation curves for human and duck blood are shown in Fig. 2 at two levels of P_{CO_2} (40 and 50 mmHg).

Calculations: Mammalian lung (1 unit). Eqs. 1, 2, 3 and 4 were entered in a computer program which calculated the output values of P_{O_2} and P_{CO_2} on the basis of the mass balance for both gases simultaneously in an iterative process. Input values of $P_{\bar{v}}O_2$, $P_{\bar{v}}CO_2$, P_IO_2, P_ICO_2 and $\dot{V}/\dot{Q}$ were entered. After establishment of the mass balance we calculated the RQ. If the RQ differed more than 0.01 from 0.70 then a new $\dot{V}/\dot{Q}$ value was entered and the program restarted.
Avian lung (25 units). The iterative loop of the mammalian lung was also used for the avian lung, calculating the 25 units in succession since the input values of each unit, except for the first, were obtained from the preceeding unit. Now RQ was calculated when all 25 units were ready and the program restarted with a new $\dot{V}/\dot{Q}$ when RQ differed more than 0.01 from 0.70. In the iterative loop we could choose between eqs. 2 and 3 (human dissociation curve) or eqs. 2a and 3a (avian dissociation curve).

P_I, $P_{\overline{E}}$, $P_{\overline{v}}$ and P_a were used to calculate the excretion $(E) = (P_{\overline{E}} - P_I)/$
$(P_{\overline{v}} - P_I)$ and the uptake $(U) = (P_a - P_{\overline{v}})/(P_I - P_{\overline{v}})$. These variables were
plotted in the uptake-excretion diagram. E and U are fully compati-
ble with Δp_{vent} (E) and Δp_{perf} (U) as defined by Piiper and Scheid
(1975). The use of the diagram is discussed in detail by Zwart and
Luijendijk (1982) with as main properties:

1. from the mass balance we obtain $E = (\lambda \dot{Q} / \dot{V}) U$
2. for one ideal mixing unit $E = 1-U$ and
3. for the cross current arrangement $E = 1 - \exp(-\lambda \dot{Q}/\dot{V})$ if the blood-
   gas partition coefficient λ obeys Henry's law.

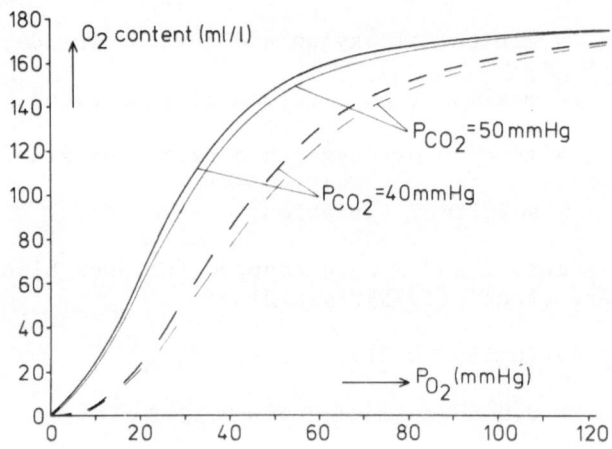

Fig. 2.   Dissociation curves used in our simulations for human blood
(solid curves) and duck blood (dashed curves).

RESULTS

A computer output for the 25 compartment avian lung at $P_IO_2 =$
100 mmHg (± 3000 m altitude) is given in Table I. L_jO_2 and L_jCO_2 are
the effective blood-gas partition coefficients of compartment j using
the formula $L_j = (C_j - C_{\overline{v}})/(P_j - P_{\overline{v}})$.
Note that in unit 8 L_{CO2} becomes negative which corresponds to P_{CO2}
exceeding the $P_{\overline{v}}CO_2$. From unit 13 on L_{CO2} becomes positive again but
now the RQ is negative due to reabsorption of CO_2 ($C_jCO_2 < C_{\overline{v}}CO_2$). At
the output of the model $P_{\overline{E}}CO_2$ still exceeds the $P_{\overline{v}}CO_2$.
The overall behavior of the avian lung model and the mammalian lung

Table I. Output of computer program for the avian lung model at an altitude of ca 3000 m, V_E/Q = overall ventilation-perfusion ratio, V_A/V_T = fraction of ventilation entering the gas exchanger, V_j/V_E = fraction of total ventilation entering compartment j, VQ_{alv} = ventilation-perfusion ratio in gas exchanging units. $P(..)$ = tension in mmHg, $C(..)$ = content in ml/ml, $L(..)$ = compartmental blood-gas partition coefficient, RQ = compartmental respiratory quotient $(P_j - P_{j-1})CO_2/(P_{j-1} - P_j)O_2$.

```
VE/Q   , VA/VT                :      0.45        1.00
VJ/VT  , QJ/QT  , VQalv       :      1.00        0.04      11.250
PIO2   , PICO2                :    100.00        0.00
PVO2   , PVCO2                :     30.00       48.00
HB     , Dissociation curv:          13.00       Bird

VENOUS    CO2,CCO2            :      0.048       0.566
```

J	PO2	PCO2	CO2	CCO2	LO2	LCO2	RQ
1	91.739	15.156	0.171	0.342	1.505	5.166	1.826
2	84.003	25.352	0.163	0.414	1.611	5.075	1.321
3	76.829	32.705	0.155	0.457	1.723	5.399	1.023
4	70.267	38.108	0.146	0.486	1.833	6.115	0.819
5	64.358	42.046	0.136	0.507	1.935	7.469	0.669
6	59.127	44.922	0.126	0.523	2.021	10.500	0.549
7	54.568	46.970	0.116	0.535	2.088	22.323	0.448
8	50.649	48.385	0.106	0.545	2.135	-41.170	0.359
9	47.317	49.309	0.098	0.552	2.165	-7.969	0.278
10	44.506	49.876	0.090	0.557	2.180	-3.413	0.203
11	42.147	50.185	0.083	0.561	2.185	-1.586	0.131
12	40.174	50.308	0.078	0.564	2.182	-0.600	0.062
13	38.527	50.304	0.073	0.566	2.174	0.018	-0.002
14	37.151	50.218	0.069	0.567	2.163	0.440	-0.063
15	36.003	50.080	0.065	0.568	2.151	0.747	-0.120
16	35.044	49.915	0.063	0.568	2.139	0.977	-0.173
17	34.242	49.737	0.060	0.568	2.127	1.156	-0.223
18	33.571	49.558	0.058	0.568	2.116	1.297	-0.267
19	33.008	49.384	0.057	0.568	2.106	1.410	-0.308
20	32.535	49.221	0.055	0.568	2.096	1.503	-0.345
21	32.139	49.071	0.054	0.568	2.087	1.580	-0.379
22	31.805	48.934	0.053	0.568	2.079	1.642	-0.409
23	31.524	48.812	0.053	0.567	2.072	1.696	-0.436
24	31.288	48.703	0.052	0.567	2.066	1.740	-0.460
25	31.088	48.607	0.051	0.567	2.061	1.779	-0.482

```
EXPIRATOIR       PEO2,PECO2  :    31.088     48.607
ARTERIAL         PAO2,PACO2  :    42.840     44.921
                 CAO2,CACO2  :     0.089      0.537
RESP.QUOTIENT                :     0.704
```

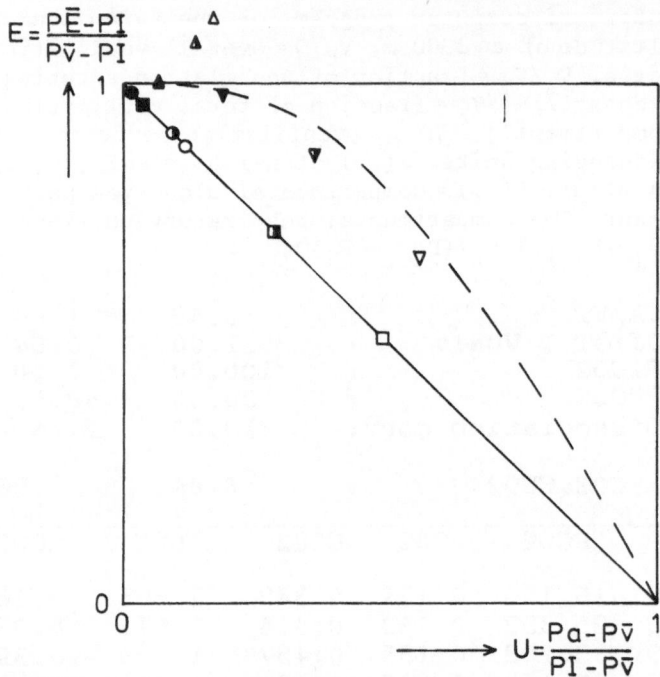

Fig. 3.   Uptake-excretion diagram for gas exchange simulations at
          three altitudes. Sea level open symbols, 2000 m half filled
          symbols, 3000 m filled symbols. Mammalian lung: characte-
          ristic curve = solid line, O_2 squares and CO_2 circles.
          Avian lung (duck dissociation curve) characteristic curve =
          dashed line, O_2 triangles top down and CO_2 triangles top up.

model for O_2 and CO_2 at different altitudes are displayed in the U-E
diagram (Fig. 3). For comparison the characteristic lines of the gas
exchange arrangements are also entered. The $P_{\bar{E}}CO_2$ exceeds the $P_{\bar{v}}CO_2$
in all three simulations of the avian lung which results in an
excretion value larger than one. The U,E points for CO_2 are therefore
located outside the U-E diagram with its boundaries $0 \leqslant U,E \leqslant 1$.
Note that for the mammalian lung with decreasing P_IO_2 the uptake of
O_2 decreases but the excretion of CO_2 increases. In the avian lung
the decrease in O_2 uptake is accompanied by a decrease in CO_2 excretion. This difference in behavior between the mammalian lung and the
avian lung leads to a considerably decreased need for perfusion at

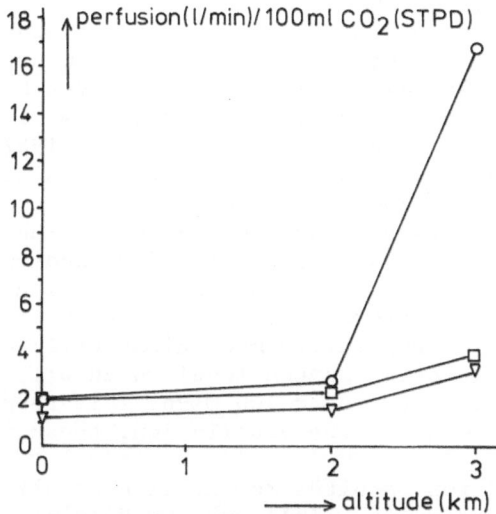

Fig. 4. Perfusion (l/min) needed for the transport of 100 ml CO_2 (STPD) at three different altitudes in the mammalian lung (circles) and in the avian lung for human blood (squares) and duck blood (triangles).

increased altitudes for the avian lung at the same CO_2 production as shown in Fig. 4. The dissociation curves for human blood and duck blood give very similar results on gas exchange in the avian lung simulations. In the mammalian lung simulation at 3000 m altitude we find a more than eight fold increase in the perfusion with approximately the same ventilation as on sea level.

DISCUSSION

During migration birds may perform long lasting exercise at altitudes higher than 2000 m especially when passing medium level mountain ranges. Under such conditions no short lasting altitude adaptation in blood transport properties has been proposed. We investigated the contribution of the construction principle of the lung and the O_2-CO_2 dissociation curve to the better adaptation of bird to exercise at these levels. We supposed venous O_2 and CO_2 levels to be the same at sea level and at altitude and a RQ of 0.70. The dissociation curves given by Kinne and Seagrave (1975) were used and adapted for bird blood, using the data of Scheipers et al. (1975), which were measured in a domestic form of the Muscovy duck, Cairina Moschata. The dissociation curves given by Kinne and Seagrave are well suited for model simulations with iterative processing in contrast to those of Kelman (1966, 1967), which are based on the Henderson-Hasselbalch equation and need pH as input variable. The formulations of Kinne and Seagrave in their present form, however, fail when metabolic changes in the acid-base balance occur during hypoxic conditions. With $P_{\bar{v}}CO_2$ and $P_{\bar{v}}O_2$ unchanged, the transport capacity of CO_2 of both the ventilation and the perfusion remains the same at increased altitudes but the transport capacity of O_2 decreases. The regulatory mechanisms will therefore respond to the decreased arterial oxygen level which will happen at inspired oxygen levels of around 100 mmHg. This response to hypoxia results in an increase in the ventilation, thus disturbing the P_aCO_2 and pH.

The better adaptation of birds to exercise at altitude results from both, the construction principle and the Haldane effect. This is illustrated in Table I, where the P_{CO_2} in the gas entering the successive units first increases and from unit 8 on even exceeds $P_{\bar{v}}CO_2$. From unit 8 on the driving force for transport of CO_2 from the venous blood to the air phase in our model is entirely due to the Haldane effect. Since the Haldane effect gradually decreases in the following units due to a continued decrease in the O_2 tension, a reversal takes place between unit 12 and 13 after which the CO_2 is reabsorbed in the blood shown as a decrease in P_{CO_2}. Total transport of CO_2 between units 9 and 25 is zero and only the first 8 compartments contribute to the CO_2 transport in the avian lung at the given input conditions. The units 9 through 25 contribute 28 per cent of the total O_2 transport.

At sea level the O_2 tensions remained high enough to prevent reabsorption of CO_2 and the Haldane effect resulted in a $P_{\bar{E}}CO_2$ of 54.39 mmHg with a $P_{\bar{v}}CO_2$ of 48 mmHg. Thus, at higher altitudes only part of the avian lung contributes to CO_2 excretion whereas the entire lung contributes to the uptake of O_2. The reversal of the $P_{\bar{E}}CO_2 - P_{\bar{v}}CO_2$ difference is in good agreement with the experimental data from Davies and Dutton (1975). We see no reason to interpret their results as supporting the charged membrane hypothesis of Gurtner et al. (1969). As a result of the Haldane effect we have to accept the strange fact that without an energy demanding active process the CO_2 tension in the alveolar air may become higher than in mixed venous blood due to the oxygen uptake. The Haldane effect may also cause negative values for actual compartmental blood-gas partition coefficients of CO_2. Reabsorption of CO_2 is the cause of negative values of compartmental RQ.

Our simulations show that in adapting to decreased oxygen levels the cardiac output should be increased instead of the ventilation. Such an adaptation should be more pronounced in the mammalian system than in the avian system as can be concluded from the increase of the perfusion shown in Fig. 4 for the mammalian and the

avian lung. Such an adaptation of increasing cardiac output at constant ventilation has never been reported to our knowledge.
The right shift in the O_2 dissociation curve of the duck blood contributed little to the altitude adaptation of birds but allowed a considerably lower cardiac output at sea level. The right shift therefore seems to be mainly an adaptation to the high energy use of birds in general.

REFERENCES

Davies, G.D., and Dutton, R.E., 1975, Gas-blood P_{CO_2} gradients during avian gas exchange, J Appl Physiol 39: 405-410.

Gurtner, G.H., Song, S.H., and Farhi, L.E., 1969, Alveolar to mixed venous P_{CO_2} differences under conditions of no gas exchange, Respir Physiol 7: 173-187.

Hazelhoff, E.H., 1943, Structure and function of the lung of birds, Versl. Gewone Vergad. Afd. Natuurk, Kon Ned Akad Wet 52: 391-400 (Poultry Sci 1951, 30: 3-10, English translation).

Kelman, G.R., 1966, Digital computer subroutine for the conversion of oxygen tension into saturation, J Appl Physiol 21: 1375-1376.

Kelman, G.R., 1967, Digital computer procedure for the conversion of P_{CO_2} into blood CO_2 content, Respir Physiol 3: 111-115.

Kinne, F.L., and Seagrave, R.C., 1974, Effects of mixing patterns in respiratory gas exchange, J Appl Physiol 36: 698-705.

Piiper, J., and Scheid, P., 1975, Gastransport efficacy of gills, lung and skin: Theory and experimental data, Respir Physiol 23: 209-221.

Scheid, P., and Piiper, J., 1970, Analysis of gas exchange in the avian lung: theory and experiments in the domestic fowl, Respir Physiol 9: 246-262.

Scheipers, G., Kawashiro, T., and Scheid, P., 1975, Oxygen and carbon dioxide dissociation of duck blood, Respir Physiol 24: 1-13.

Zwart, A., and Luijendijk, S.C.M., 1982, Excretion-retention diagram to evaluate gas exchange properties of vertebrate respiratory systems, Am J Physiol (Regulatory Integrative Comp Physiol 12): R 329 - R 338.

THE CONTROVERSY ABOUT BLOOD–GAS CO_2 EQUILIBRIUM IN LUNGS: REINVESTIGATION BY PROLONGED CO_2 REBREATHING IN AWAKE DOGS DURING REST AND EXERCISE

P. Scotto, H. Rieke, J.A. Loeppky, M. Meyer,
and J. Piiper

Abteilung Physiologie
Max-Planck-Institut für experimentelle Medizin
Göttingen, FRG

INTRODUCTION

When pulmonary diffusing capacity for O_2 is to be determined in lungs with unequal distribution of alveolar ventilation to pulmonary perfusion it is common practice to correct arterial PO_2 for the shunt effect and the end-tidal PO_2 for alveolar dead space ventilation. The latter correction is based on the assumption that PCO_2 in end-capillary blood is in equilibrium with alveolar gas (Riley and Cournand, 1949). It appears to follow from this assumption that in conditions of no gas exchange, such as rebreathing, PCO_2 in alveolar gas should be equal to that in arterial blood. Thus the finding of negative blood-to-gas PCO_2 differences during rebreathing in dogs (Gurtner et al., 1969) and in man (Jones et al., 1969, 1972; Denison et al., 1971) has challenged the fundamental concepts of pulmonary gas exchange. However, these results could not be reproduced by others (Scheid et al., 1972).

Scheid and Piiper (1980) in their review of these controversial findings concluded that some of the discrepancies found in the literature could be attributed to experimental error in the measurement of PCO_2 in blood and gas phase. However, negative arterial-to-end-expired PCO_2 differences have been observed recently in resting goats during prolonged rebreathing where PCO_2 in lung gas and in arterial blood increases steadily (Steinbrook et al., 1983) although particular efforts were made to eliminate the sources of directional error listed by Scheid and Piiper (1980). Using similar experimental procedures, we have attempted to reproduce these findings in unanesthetized dogs during rest and exercise.

METHODS

Eight dogs, weighing 25-36 kg (average 29.8 kg) were utilized in the experiments. They were prepared with a chronic tracheostomy and an exteriorized carotid artery loop as described by Jennings et al. (1982). Five dogs were studied during rest and six during exercise. Running was performed on a motor-driven treadmill with a 5% incline at three speeds (km/hr): 5.0 (A), 6.3 (B), and 7.9 (C). The dogs were trained to run on the treadmill 3-5 hours per week for a period of two months.

Experimental set-up and protocol

For the experiment a cuffed tracheostomy tube was inserted into the trachea and connected to a three-way stopcock allowing changeover from open-circuit breathing to rebreathing from a flexible container. For measurements at rest the rebreathing container was filled with 12%, 21% or 39% O_2, 6 to 8% CO_2, and 1% He in N_2. A rebreathing gas mixture containing 20% O_2, 9-10% CO_2, and 1% He in N_2 was used during exercise. A 16-gauge teflon cannula was inserted percutaneously into the exteriorized carotid artery. The cannula was connected to a three-way stopcock modified for withdrawal of blood samples into heparinized glass capillaries.

Prior to onset of rebreathing the dogs breathed in open circuit an O_2 mixture similar to that prepared for rebreathing. The open-circuit breathing lasted about 10 min at rest and 5 min at each level of exercise in order to achieve a steady O_2 uptake. Rebreathing was started by changeover to the rebreathing container at end-expiration. During rebreathing 3 to 5 arterial blood samples were obtained. Rebreathing was terminated after 4-5 min at rest and 1-2 min during exercise during which period PCO_2 increased up to about 70 Torr and dogs became agitated. Oxygen uptake was estimated from the amount of pure O_2 supplied continuously to the rebreathing circuit to keep FIO_2 constant. At the end of each rebreathing period, the temperature in the carotid artery was measured by a calibrated thermistor probe.

Analytical techniques

Fractional concentrations of O_2, CO_2, He, and N_2 were continuously measured by a high-performance respiratory mass spectrometer (cf. Scheid, 1983) sampling close to the proximal end of the tracheal cannula. Before and after each rebreathing period, the mass spectrometer was calibrated by gas mixtures provided by precision gas mixing pumps. Recording sensitivity was 10 mm pen deflection for 1% CO_2, 2% O_2, and 0.2% He, repectively. Fractional concentrations of O_2 and CO_2 were converted into partial pressures assuming full water vapor saturation at the measured arterial temperature.

Partial pressures of O_2 and CO_2, and pH of the arterial samples were measured immediately after sampling by an automatic pH-blood gas analyzer (ABL 30, Radiometer, Copenhagen, Denmark) maintained at 37°C.

Calibration of the electrodes was obtained by analyzing blood samples equilibrated at 37°C with the same gas mixtures used for calibration of the mass spectrometer. Corrections for differences between blood temperature in the carotid artery (see above) and the electrodes (37°C) were applied to PO_2 according to Severinghaus (1979) and to PCO_2 according to Siggaard-Andersen (1974).

RESULTS

The differences between simultaneous measurements of PCO_2 in arterial blood and end-tidal gas are compiled in Table 1 for resting conditions, and in Table 2 for the three exercise levels. The following features are evident.

Table 1. PCO_2 differences between arterial blood (Pa) and end-tidal gas (PE´) in resting dogs during prolonged rebreathing at different levels of inspired O_2 (FIO_2). Mean values $\pm$ SD; RB, number of rebreathing periods; n, number of measurements.

FIO_2	0.12	0.21	0.39
(Pa-PE´)CO_2 (Torr)	0.1 ± 0.7	-0.6 ± 1.4	0.2 ± 1.7
RB	9	38	23
n	32	143	91

(1) At rest, there is no correlation between $(Pa-PE')CO_2$ and inspired PO_2 in the range from 70 to 330 Torr.

(2) The overall mean $\pm$ SD of all 246 measurements is -0.3 ± 1.4 Torr.

(3) A very small, but statistically significant ($P<0.05$), PCO_2 difference between arterial blood and end-tidal gas could be detected for all levels of exercise (up to 40% of $\dot{V}O_{2max}$), the overall mean $\pm$ SD of $(Pa-PE')CO_2$ differences was -1.0 ± 1.2 Torr ($n = 153$).

Table 2. PCO_2 differences between arterial blood (Pa) and end-tidal gas (PE') during rebreathing at three levels of exercise in 6 dogs. Mean values $\pm$ SD; RB, number of rebreathing periods; n, number of measurements. A, B, and C refer to running speeds of 5.0, 6.3, and 7.9 km/hr, respectively, at a + 5% incline.

Exercise level	A	B	C
$\dot{V}O_2$ (ml·min^{-1}·kg^{-1})	14.6 $\pm$ 1.2	20.7 $\pm$ 2.6	29.9 $\pm$ 3.8
$(Pa-PE')CO_2$ (Torr)	-1.5 $\pm$ 1.4	-0.8 $\pm$ 1.2	-0.9 $\pm$ 1.1
RB	7	21	18
n	26	70	57

DISCUSSION

Circulation time

Since during prolonged rebreathing, i.e. rebreathing extended beyond recirculation, alveolar and arterial PCO_2 rose steadily, corrections had to be applied for the transit time from the pulmonary capillaries to the site of sampling in the carotid artery. The average rate of rise of PCO_2 was 4.5 Torr/min at rest and 13.2 Torr/min during exercise. According to Lange et al. (1966) the mean transit time from the lungs to the carotid artery is about 6 sec. This value was used in our calculations for resting dogs while a transit time of 4.5 sec was considered reasonable for correction of measurements during exercise. No correction should be considered for the gas phase since, at a breathing frequency of 90-120 breaths/min, the transit time from the alveoli to the measuring site is less than 0.3 sec. Applying these corrections for the estimated transit time delay the mean $(Pa-PE')CO_2$ difference for rest became +0.1 Torr and −0.1 Torr for exercise.

$(Pa-PE')CO_2$ at rest

The finding of no measurable $(Pa-PE')CO_2$ differences during prolonged rebreathing is in agreement with previous studies in dogs from this laboratory both during rebreathing (Scheid et al., 1972) and during steady state open-circuit breathing of hypercapnic mixtures (Scheid et al., 1979; Jennings et al., 1982). They are also consistent with a recent study on anesthetized dogs during rebreathing (Clark et al., 1984) but in disagreement with the results of Steinbrook et al. (1983) in unanesthetized resting goats where $(Pa-PE')CO_2$ differences up to −12 Torr were reported. There are some differences between their procedures and ours: breathing mask vs. endotracheal tube; infrared CO_2 analyzer vs. mass spectrometer; blood sampling with syringes and temporary storage vs. glass capillaries used for blood sampling and immediate analysis; measurement of rectal vs. arterial blood temperature. However, it remains unclear whether any of these differences in techniques may have caused systematic errors leading to spurious blood-gas PCO_2 differences amounting to −12 Torr.

$(Pa-PE')CO_2$ during exercise

Jones et al. (1967, 1969, 1972) have reported blood PCO_2 lower than gas PCO_2 by as much as 15 Torr in healthy exercising man rebreathing at zero CO_2 exchange. In a similar study values up to −26 Torr were observed in adults and children (Godfrey et al., 1971). Denison et al. (1971) found negative $(Pa-PE')CO_2$ differences during prolonged rebreathing, ranging from 0 to −12 Torr. A common feature of all these studies has been the increase of negative $(Pa-PE')CO_2$ differences with work load and gas phase PCO_2. Since the CO_2 output is increased during exercise, the finding of negative blood-gas PCO_2 differences has been interpreted as a physiological adjustment of the body to increased work loads. It is of interest to note that Jones et al. (1979) have not found negative $(Pa-PE')CO_2$ differences at exercise during steady state breathing.

In the present study appreciable negative $(Pa-PE')CO_2$ differences were not observed and the slight differences obtained without correction for circulation time did not correlate with the O_2 uptake or with the level of hypercapnia.

In summary, our results obtained in resting and exercising dogs show that the arterial-to-alveolar difference for PCO_2 during rebreathing is nearly zero, supporting the concept that, in equilibrium, PCO_2 in end-capillary blood is equal to PCO_2 in alveolar gas.

REFERENCES

Clark, J.S., A.G. Cutillo, M.J. Criddle, D.V. Collins, F.L. Farr, A.H. Bigler, and A.D. Renzetti, 1984, Gas-blood PCO_2 and PO_2 equilibrium in a steady-state rebreathing dog preparation, J. Appl. Physiol. 56: 1229-1236.

Denison, D., R.H. Edwards, G. Jones, and H. Pope, 1971, Estimates of the CO_2 pressures in systemic arterial blood during rebreathing on exercise. Respir. Physiol. 11: 186-196.

Godfrey, S., R. Katzenelson, and E.Wolf, 1971, Gas to blood PCO_2 differences during rebreathing in children and adults, Respir. Physiol. 13: 274-282.

Gurtner, G.H., Song, S.H., and L.E. Farhi, 1969, Alveolar to mixed venous PCO_2 difference under conditions of no gas exchange, Respir. Physiol. 7: 173-187.

Jennings, D.B., M. Meyer, T. Stokke, J. Piiper, and P. Scheid, 1982, Blood-gas CO_2 equilibration in lungs of unanesthetized dogs during hypercapnia. J. Appl. Physiol. 52: 1177-1180.

Jones, N.L., E.J. Campbell, R.H. Edwards, and W.G. Wilkoff, 1969, Alveolar-to-blood PCO_2 difference during rebreathing in exercise. J. Appl. Physiol. 27: 356-360.

Jones, N.L., E.J. Campbell, G.J. McHardy, B.E. Higgs, and M. Clode, 1967, The estimation of carbon dioxide pressure of mixed venous blood during exercise. Clin. Sci. 32: 311-327.

Jones, N.L., D.G. Robertson, and J.W. Kane, 1979, Difference between end-tidal and arterial PCO_2 in exercise, J. Appl. Physiol. 47: 954-960.

Jones, N.L., D.G. Robertson, J.W. Kane, and E.J. Campbell, 1972, Effect of PCO_2 level on alveolar-arterial PCO_2 difference during rebreathing. J. Appl. Physiol. 32: 782-787.

Lange, R.L., J.D. Horgan, J.T. Botticelli, T. Tsagaris, R.P. Carlisle, and H. Kuida, 1966, Pulmonary to arterial circulatory transfer function: importance in respiratory control. J. Appl. Physiol. 21: 1281-1291.

Riley, R.L., and A. Cournand, 1949, "Ideal" alveolar air and the analysis of ventilation-perfusion relationships in the lungs, J. Appl. Physiol. 1: 825-847.

Scheid, P., 1983, Respiratory mass spectrometry. In: "Measurement in clinical respiratory physiology", G. Laszlo and M.F. Sudlow, ed., Academic Press, London, pp. 131-166.

Scheid, P., M. Meyer, and J. Piiper, 1979, Arterial-expired PCO_2 differences in the dog during acute hypercapnia. J. Appl. Physiol. 47: 1074-1078.

Scheid, P. and J. Piiper, 1980, Blood/gas equilibrium of carbon dioxide in lungs. A critical review. Respir. Physiol. 39: 1-31.

Scheid, P., J. Teichmann, F. Adaro, and J. Piiper, 1972, Gas-blood CO_2 equilibration in dog lungs during rebreathing. J. Appl. Physiol. 33: 582-588.

Severinghaus, J.W., 1979, Simple, accurate equations for human blood O_2 dissociation computations. J. Appl. Physiol. 46: 599-602.

Siggaard-Andersen, O., 1974, The Acid-base Status of the Blood. Copenhagen, Munksgaard, pp. 51 and 89.

Steinbrook, R.A., V. Fencl, R.A. Gabel, D.E. Leith, and S.E. Weinberger, 1983, Reversal of arterial-to-expired CO_2 partial pressure differences during rebreathing in goats. J. Appl. Physiol. 55: 736-741.

HYPOXIC PULMONARY VASOCONSTRICTION IN THE NEWBORN PIG - AN EXPERIMENTAL MODEL

E.I. de Stoppelaar*, F.G. Leicher**, G.J. Rees*,
W. Erdmann*, N.S. Faithfull* and H. van der Zee***

Departments of Anaesthesia* and Cardiothoracic
Surgery**, Erasmus University, Rotterdam, The
Netherlands and Department of Anaesthesia***
Albany Medical College, New York

During the process of birth, drastic changes occur in the
environment of the foetus as its oxygen supply changes from one
delivered by extracorporeal circulation through the umbilical cord
to oxygen supply (and carbon dioxide removal) via its own lungs.
These changes are accompanied by well-documented alterations in
pulmonary haemodynamics (Nelson,1976). Little is known about the
mediating factors which induce these changes and the aim of this
study was to gain more insight into some of the factors involved
in this physiological process.

During foetal life the pulmonary circulation is a high
pressure/low flow system and the amount of blood reaching the left
atrium via the pulmonary veins is very small. After birth, there
is a sudden decrease in pulmonary vascular resistance and the
system becomes a low pressure/high flow circuit containing, under
normal physiological conditions, enough blood (about 10% of the
total blood volume) to serve as a reservoir for the left ventricle
(Fishman,1961a).

The state of the pulmonary vasculature in the newborn
contrasts with the situation in the adult in that the pulmonary
vessels are as elastic as the aorta and the small arterioles are
richly supplied with sympathetic nerve endings. The vessel walls
contain a large amount of muscle, which rapidly involutes after
birth. Neonatal asphyxia leads to hypoxia and respiratory and
metabolic acidosis. This leads to a rise in the pulmonary artery
pressure (PAP) due to renewed vasoconstriction of the pulmonary

arterial bed. In addition, hypoxic conditions may delay involution of the muscular walls of the pulmonary vasculature (Naeye 1961, Naeye and Letts,1962).

Hypoxia and acidosis cause relaxation of the systemic vascular smooth muscle, whereas the intact pulmonary vascular bed constricts under the same circumstances. However, in vitro, denervated preparations of pulmonary smooth muscle (when completely stripped from its surroundings) also relax under conditions of hypoxia and acidosis (Lloyd,1967). This is in contrast to the situation in denervated preparations left in situ in the animal; in this case vasoconstriction again occurs under the influence of alveolar hypoxia. Thus pulmonary vasoconstriction seems to be a locally mediated response (v Euler and Liljestrand,1946; Fishman,1961b).

Thromboxane A_2 is a strong candidate for the role of chemical transmitter in hypoxic pulmonary vasoconstrictive reactions as it is known to be synthesized particulary in lung tissue (Hamberg and Samuelsson,1974a). Production also occurs in the umbilical cord (Tuvemo et al.,1976), the cerebral cortex (Wolfe et al.,1976), spleen and platelets (Hamberg and Samuelsson,1974b)

Thromboxane A_2 (and its metabolite thromboxane B_2) are products of prostaglandin endoperoxide metabolism and are known to be potent vasoconstrictors (Hamberg and Samuelsson,1974a and b). Thromboxane A_2 has a very short half-life of about 32 seconds, which suggests that it will act locally rather than systemically. Thromboxane B_2, on the other hand, is chemically stable and possesses similar, but less potent, vasoconstrictive properties (Friedman et al.,1979). If thromboxanes actually do, in fact, play an important role, inhibitors blocking the overall synthesis of the Thromboxanes A_2 and B_2 should also block hypoxic pulmonary responses (Cassin, 1980). To study this hypothesis a neonatal pig model was developed in which vascularly isolated lungs were perfused in situ.

MATERIALS AND METHODS

Ten neonatal piglets (of either sex) less than 24 hours old, weighing 1000-2000 grams, were anaesthetised with fluothane vaporised in a gas mixture containing 70% nitrous oxide and 30% oxygen. A tracheostomy was performed and the animals were intubated with a size 3 Ruch endotracheal tube. The animals were relaxed with pancuronium bromide in a dose of 0.2 mg kg^{-1} administered either via a peripheral abdominal vein, or the internal jugular vein. The piglet was then ventilated with a volume cycled Roche Baby Kontrol ventilator at a rate of 40 breaths per minute. The tidal volume was set so that maximum end

638

inspiratory airway pressure amounted to 18 cm of water. A positive end expiratory pressure (PEEP) of 4 cm of water was applied. During surgery, anaesthesia was maintained with 0.5% fluothane, vaporised in 70% nitrous oxide and 30% oxygen.

The animals were placed in a right lateral position and a left lateral thoracotomy was performed through the 4th intercostal space. After the left lung had been anteriorly retracted, the mediastinum over the aorta was opened. The ductus Botalli was dissected free and ligated with two silk ligatures. The pericardium was opened and a ligature was passed around the main pulmonary artery and the aorta. After heparinisation (3 mg/kg bodyweight), the main pulmonary artery and the left atrium were cannulated. The ligature around the pulmonary artery proximal to the cannulation site was tied and the animal was exsanguinated via free drainage of the left atrial cannula. The pulmonary vessels were flushed with 150-200 ml of Haemaccel$^{(R)}$ and both the arterial and venous side were connected to the perfusion system.

The perfusion system contained a reservoir filled with 200 ml of Haemaccel which was maintained at a temperature of 37.5°C $\pm$ 0.5°C. The hydrogen ion concentration was adjusted to a pH of 7.45 $\pm$ 0.05 by the addition of small quantities of sodium bicarbonate. The flow of the calibrated Dreissen roller pump was adjusted to deliver a flow rate of 100 ml kg^{-1} min^{-1}. A needle was introduced through the cannula into the pulmonary artery to facilitate pressure recording. All pressure tracings (airway, pulmonary artery, phasic and mean) were recorded on a 6 channel Grass 7D polygraph and ink writing oscillograph. The lungs, continuously ventilated by the Roche Baby Kontrol ventilator, served as the oxygenator of the circuit.

During the experiment, the preparation was ventilated with gas mixtures containing nitrogen, oxygen and carbon dioxide, the compositions of which were verified using a Gould Godart capnograph Mark III and an Instrument Laboratory type 404 oxymeter. Ten minutes after each change of the ventilating gas mixture, acid/base and gas analyses of the perfusate were performed. The end inspiratory ventilation pressure was maintained at 18 cm H_2O (with a PEEP of 4 cm H_2O) and the respiratory rate was reduced to 20-25 breaths per minute, since higher frequencies tended to cause harmonic interference with the pressure oscillations caused by the roller pump.

The preparation was ventilated with two different gas mixtures and each animal served as its own control. Initial ventilation was with a mixture of 50% oxygen, 45% nitrogen and 5% carbon dioxide ("normoxia"). After the preparation had been left to stabilize for 20 minutes the gas mixture was changed to one containing 5%

oxygen, 90% nitrogen and 5% carbon dioxide ("hypoxia"). The pulmonary arterial pressure reached a stable value after about 10 minutes. The gas mixture was then changed to normoxic and the decrease in mean PAP was observed.

Following the above treatment, which was designed to ensure that the model was functioning satisfactorily, inspired oxygen concentration was again reduced to hypoxic levels. When the PAP had reached a final stable peak value, 5 mg of the thromboxane synthetase inhibitor (TSI) UK 38485 was introduced into the circulation and the response was observed. After the PAP had stabilised, the preparation was again ventilated with the normoxic gas mixture and the PAP returned to base-line. At the end of the experiment the locations of the tips of the cannulas were checked and if they appeared to be in an incorrect position the results of the experiment were discarded.

In those animals having little or no response to TSI, isoprenaline was injected to demonstrate the reversibility of the hypoxic pulmonary vasoconstriction. In those animals which showed a lower PAP following TSI administration than in the control period, adrenaline or noradrenaline was injected to show that the vasoconstrictive properties were still intact. The statistical significance of changes in PAP was assessed using paired Student t tests and the nul hypothesis was rejected at $p < 0.05$.

RESULTS

The mean baseline PAP was 26.2 mm Hg ($\pm$ 2.1 SEM) during ventilation with normoxic gas mixtures. After changing to the hypoxic gas mixture the mean PAP showed a statistically significant increase to 36.7 mm Hg ($\pm$ 4.16 SEM), $p < 0.01$. Significant decreases in PAP to 25.6 mm Hg ($\pm$ 2.0 SEM) were observed when the normoxic gas mixture was again respired, $p < 0.01$. The last value of the mean PAP was not significantly different from the pre-hypoxic mean PAP (fig. 1).

Significant increases in pressure to 42.5 mm Hg ($\pm$ 4.37 SEM) again occurred during ventilation with hypoxic mixtures ($p < 0.01$). TSI was then injected (5 mg) in the proximal tubing. In 6 animals a decrease in PAP was seen, commencing within 1 minute and then slowly and constantly declining over the next 15-20 minutes. In two animals the decrease in PAP was less marked and in another two animals no change was observed following TSI. Nevertheless, the overall response from all 10 experiments showed that a statistically significant decrease in the level of PAP to 36.6 mm Hg ($\pm$ 2.57 SEM) was produced ($p < 0.05$) and that this PAP value is not significantly different from the pre-hypoxic value (fig. 2).

640

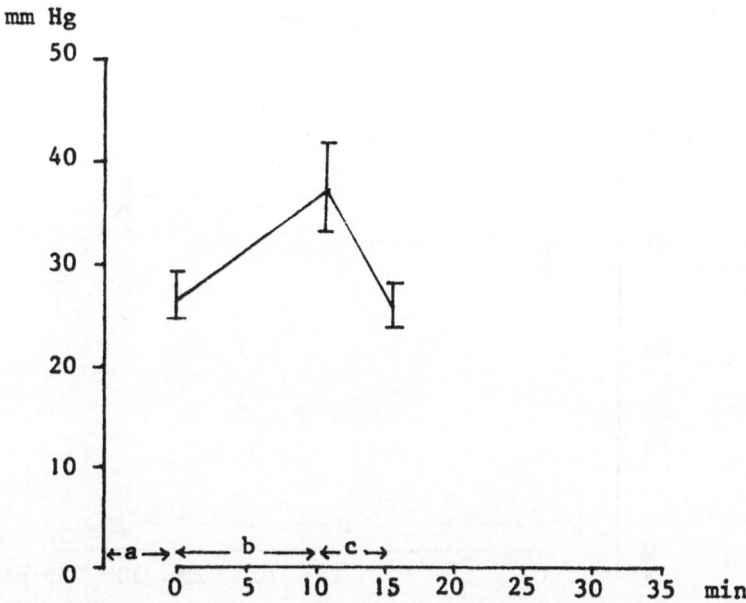

Fig 1. Responses of mean pulmonary artery pressure to changes in inspired gas mixtures. During periods a and c the preparation was ventilated with 50% oxygen, 45% nitrogen and 5% carbon dioxide. During period b the respired gas consisted of 5% oxygen, 90% nitrogen and 5% carbon dioxide.

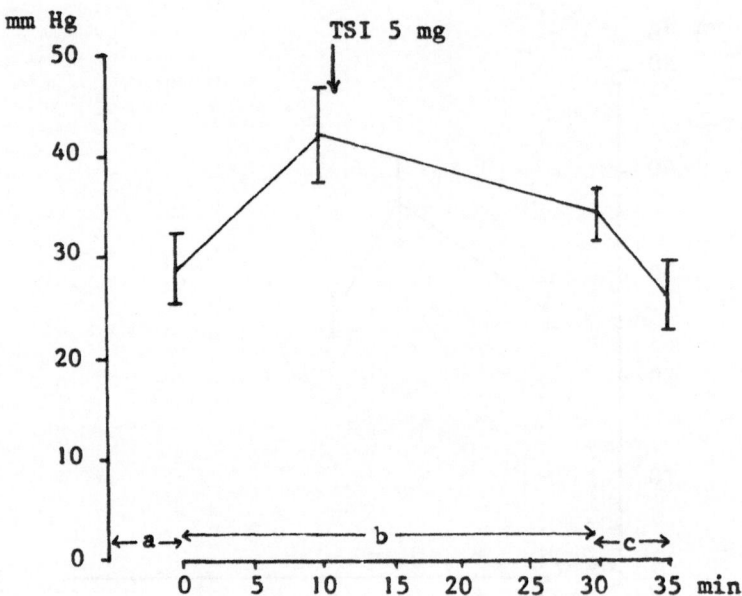

Fig 2. Responses of mean pulmonary artery pressure to changes in
inspired gas mixtures and the effect of the administration of 5 mg
of the thromboxane blocker, UK 38485. During periods a and c the
preparation was ventilated with 50% oxygen, 45% nitrogen and 5%
carbon dioxide. During period b the respired gas consisted of 5%
oxygen, 90% nitrogen and 5% carbon dioxide.

It has to be noted that 6 of the experiments were very positive, while less convincing responses were observed in 4 experiments, which were performed in the last two months of the experimentation period (although these 4 experiments were made within the official expiration date of the drug). In these experiments with little or no response to TSI, isoprenaline was injected at peak hypoxic PAP value. This produced an immediate decrease in PAP, in 3 cases to pre-hypoxic levels. In 1 animal, though this level was not reached, a marked decrease in pressure was observed. In those experiments in which a marked response to TSI was observed, adrenaline (0.1 mg) or noradrenaline (0.01 mg) was given at 50% or at 5% inspiratory oxygen concentration. An immediate increase in PAP was observed in every case.

DISCUSSION

Pulmonary vascular resistance is dependent upon many other factors apart from locally mediated vasoconstrictive and vaso-dilatory properties of the pulmonary vascular bed. For example, nervous stimulation, hormones, cardiac action and blood viscosity are all of considerable importance. In this model, neural and humoral influences originating from the systemic circulation were excluded. Only the lungs were perfused and systemic blood flow, including the bronchial blood flow, was arrested. Thus the preparation can be considered as denervated (Sykes et al.,1973) and, after pH had been corrected with sodium bicarbonate, the viscosity of the perfusate was kept constant.

It is, of course, unphysiological to perfuse the pulmonary artery with a hyperoxic perfusate containing little or no blood. However, the preparation proved to respond to hypoxic gas mixtures in a physiologically predictable mannner. The only exception was that the base-line PAP showed a slow upward drift of approximately 5 mm Hg per hour and hence the TSI experiments, which were performed approximately 1-2 hours after the start of the control experiments, showed slightly increased base-line levels. Since ventilation pressure, perfusate flow and left atrial pressure were kept constant throughout the experiment, the observed increases in PAP under the influence of hypoxia could only be due to vasocon-striction of the pulmonary bed.

The administration of TSI at peak hypoxic response, in 10 animals, led to a significant lowering in PAP - in spite of 4 preparations which showed little or no response. Since these 4 experiments were in the latter stage of the series it might be possible that the drug had reduced potency (although it was used within the official expiration date). Another possibility might be

that, since prostaglandin production undergoes great changes
during labour and in the first hours after birth, the age of the
animals (in hours) might influence the response to hypoxia. It was
impossible to ascertain the actual time of birth of the animals
since farmers generally do not know the exact time.

At the end of all experimental procedures a check was made to
see if the preparation retained its normal pharmacological
response to vasoconstrictive drugs. Adrenaline or noradrenaline
(both acting as alpha stimulating agents on the neonatal pulmonary
vascular bed) was injected in those preparations having a good
response to TSI. The PAP showed an immediate rise, indicating
that the vasoconstrictive properties were still intact.
Isoprenaline (a beta adrenergic agonist which causes vasodilation in most tissues) given at peak hypoxic response to the 4
animals with little response to TSI, caused an immediate decrease
in PAP, thus indicating the possibility of influencing hypoxic
pulmonary vasoconstriction by direct vasodilation of the pulmonary
vascular bed.

In conclusion, this work suggests that thromboxanes play an
important role in hypoxic pulmonary vasoconstriction. It must be
assumed that thromboxanes are being synthesized in the lung tissue
itself, since the systemic circulation was stopped and, whilst the
lung was perfused with Haemaccel, no (thromboxane releasing)
thrombocytes were present.

REFERENCES

Cassin, S., 1980, Role of Prostaglandins and Thromboxanes in the
    control of the pulmonary circulation in the fetus and
    newborn, Semin in Perinatol., 4: 101.
v Euler, U.S. and Liljestrand, G., 1946, Observations on the
    pulmonary arterial blood pressure in the cat, Acta Physiol
    Scand., 12: 301.
Fishman, A.P., 1961 a, The clinical significance of the pulmonary
    collateral circulation, Circulation., 24: 677.
Fishman, A.P., 1961 b, Respiratory gases in the regulation of the
    pulmonary circulation, Physiol Rev., 41: 214.
Friedman, L.S., Fitzpatrick, T.M., Bloom, M., Ramwell, P.W., Rose,
    J.W. and Kot, P.A., 1979, Cardiovascular and pulmonary effects
    of Thromboxane B_2 in the dog, Circul Res., 44: 748.
Hamberg, M. and Samuelsson, B., 1974 a, Prostaglandin endoper-
    oxides. VII. Novel transformations of arachidonic acid in
    guinea pig lung, Biochem Biophys Res Commun., 61: 942.
Hamberg, M., and Samuelsson, B., 1974 b, Prostaglandin endoper-
    oxides. Novel transformations of arachidonic acid in human
    platelets., Proc Natl Acad Sci USA., 71.

Lloyd, T.C. Jr., 1967, Influence of PO2 and pH on resting and
    active tensions of pulmonary arterial strips, J Appl
    Physiol., 22: 1101.
Naeye, R.L., 1961, Arterial changes during the perinatal period,
    Arch Path., 71: 121.
Naeye, R.L. and Letts, H.W., 1962, The effects of prolonged
    neonatal hypoxemia on the pulmonary vascular bed and heart,
    Pediatrics, 30: 902.
Nelson, N.M., 1976, Respiration and circulation before birth, in:
    "Physiology of the newborn infant", Nelson, N.M. and Smith,
    C.A., eds., Thomas, Springfield, 4th edition.
Sykes, M.K., Davies, D.M., Chakrabarti, M.K. and Loh, L., 1973,
    The effects of halothane, trichloroethylene and ether on the
    hypoxic pressor response and pulmonary vascular resistance in
    the isolated perfused cat lung, Brit J Anaesth., 45: 655
Tuvemo, T., Strandberg, K., Hamberg, M. and Samuelsson, B., 1976,
    Formation and action of prostaglandin endoperoxides in the
    isolated umbilical artery, Acta Physiol Scand., 96: 145.
Wolfe, L.S., Rostworowski, K. and Marion, J., 1976, Endogenous
    formation of the prostaglandin endoperoxide metabolite,

Acknowledgement : UK 38485 was kindly supplied by the Pfizer
Pharmaceutical Company.

THE EFFECT OF PHYSICALLY DISSOLVED OXYGEN ON THE P_{CO_2} IN VENOUS BLOOD AND IN BRAIN TISSUE

J.H.G.M. van Beek[*], J. DeGoede, A. Berkenbosch and
C.N. Olievier

Laboratory of Physiology, University Medical Centre
Leiden and [*] Laboratory for Physiology, Free University
Amsterdam, The Netherlands

INTRODUCTION

The transport of CO_2 from tissue is influenced by oxygen through changes in tissue blood flow and in the magnitude of the Haldane effect, even when the arterial CO_2 tension is kept constant. The increase in ventilation following hyperbaric O_2 breathing, seen in human beings, has been ascribed to the increase in CO_2 tension at the central chemosensitive structures which results from these effects of O_2 on CO_2 transport (Lambertsen et al., 1953). In this paper we develop a simple mathematical model for CO_2 transport from tissue which incorporates the influences of O_2 on CO_2 transport. The changes in CO_2 tension due to the reduction of the Haldane effect by physically dissolved O_2 during hyperoxia are calculated and compared with measurements of venous and cerebrospinal fluid CO_2 tensions.

MATHEMATICAL MODEL FOR CO_2 TRANSPORT FROM BRAIN TISSUE

In the steady state the production of CO_2 equals the transport via blood:

$$\dot{V}_{CO_2} = \dot{Q}.(Cv_{CO_2} - Ca_{CO_2}) \qquad (1)$$

(for the meaning of the symbols see Table 1).
Similarly for O_2 we have

$$\dot{V}_{O_2} = -\dot{Q}.(Cv_{O_2} - Ca_{O_2}) \qquad (2)$$

647

Table 1. List of symbols

c_{Hb}	concentration of haemoglobin	$g.ml^{-1}$
C_{CO_2}	total content of CO_2	$ml.ml^{-1}$
C_{O_2}	total content of O_2	$ml.ml^{-1}$
m	slope of CO_2 dissociation curve	$ml.ml^{-1}.kPa^{-1}$
n	extrapolated value for C_{CO_2} at $PCO_2 = 0$, $S_{O_2} = 0$	$ml.ml^{-1}$
$\dot{Q}$	specific blood flow	$ml.g^{-1}.min^{-1}$
R	respiratory quotient i.e. $\dot{V}_{CO_2} / \dot{V}_{O_2}$	dimensionless
S_{O_2}	fractional saturation of haemoglobin	dimensionless
$\dot{V}_{CO_2}$	metabolic CO_2 production	$ml.g^{-1}.min^{-1}$
$\dot{V}_{O_2}$	metabolic O_2 consumption	$ml.g^{-1}.min^{-1}$
α	solubility coefficient for oxygen	$ml.ml^{-1}.kPa^{-1}$
β	O_2 binding capacity of haemoglobin	$ml.g^{-1}$
γ	Haldane factor	$ml.ml^{-1}$
ξ	fraction of O_2-uptake provided by the physically dissolved oxygen	dimensionless

subscripts

a	arterial	t	mean brain tissue
v	venous	c	mean capillary
csf	cerebrospinal fluid		

For the relation between CO_2 content and CO_2 tension in blood we use

$$c_{CO_2} = m \cdot P_{CO_2} + n - \gamma \cdot c_{Hb} \cdot \beta \cdot S_{O_2} \tag{3}$$

which is an empirical linear approximation for the CO_2 dissociation curve in the physiological range (Visser, 1960). For the O_2 content:

$$c_{O_2} = \alpha \cdot P_{O_2} + c_{Hb} \cdot \beta \cdot S_{O_2} \tag{4}$$

The two terms on the right hand side of Eq. (4) represent the physically dissolved and haemoglobin-bound O_2 respectively. Introducing the respiratory quotient R, this set of equations yields

$$Pv_{CO_2} = Pa_{CO_2} + \frac{1}{m} \left\{ \frac{\dot{V}_{CO_2}}{\dot{Q}} \left(1 - \frac{\gamma}{R}\right) + \gamma \cdot \alpha \cdot (Pa_{O_2} - Pv_{O_2}) \right\} \tag{5}$$

We remark that $\dot{Q}$ depends on Pa_{O_2}, Pa_{CO_2} and the local rate of metabolism (Siesjö, 1978). We assume that $\dot{V}_{O_2}$ and $\dot{V}_{CO_2}$ are not altered following moderate changes in blood gas tensions. Indeed, oxygen consumption in brain tissue does not change following hypercapnia, hypocapnia, hypoxia and hyperoxia (Siesjö, 1978; Lambertsen et al., 1953).

We will now derive a formula for the mean tissue P_{CO_2} (Pt_{CO_2}). Using the Krogh model, Pontén and Siesjö (1966) derived that Pt_{CO_2} is equal to the mean capillary P_{CO_2} (Pc_{CO_2}) plus a term d which represents the small P_{CO_2} gradient between tissue and capillaries:

$$Pt_{CO_2} = Pc_{CO_2} + d \tag{6}$$

For the term d they calculated an order of magnitude of 0.1 kPa. We will calculate Pc_{CO_2} using the following simplifying assumptions: the physically dissolved O_2 that is delivered during hyperoxia is extracted from the blood in the first part of the capillary (Lambertsen, 1965), and in the rest of the capillary haemoglobin is deoxygenated. During hyperoxia there is no contribution of the Haldane effect to the buffering of CO_2 in the first part of the capillary since there is no deoxygenation of haemoglobin. The P_{CO_2} rises therefore faster in this first part than in the second part of the capillary where haemoglobin is deoxygenated (see fig. 1). At a point x along the capillary the deoxygenation of haemoglobin starts. The P_{CO_2} at x is

$$P_{CO_2}(x) = Pa_{CO_2} + \frac{\xi \cdot \dot{V}_{CO_2}}{m \cdot \dot{Q}} \tag{7}$$

in which ξ is the fraction of $\dot{V}_{CO_2}$ that is taken up by the blood in the first part of the capillary. Eq. (7) is derived by applying Eqs. (1) and (3) and setting $S_{O_2}(x)$ equal to Sa_{O_2}. The venous P_{CO_2} is

$$Pv_{CO_2} = P_{CO_2}(x) + (1 - \xi) \cdot \frac{\dot{V}_{CO_2}}{m.\dot{Q}} \cdot (1 - \frac{\gamma}{R}) \qquad (8)$$

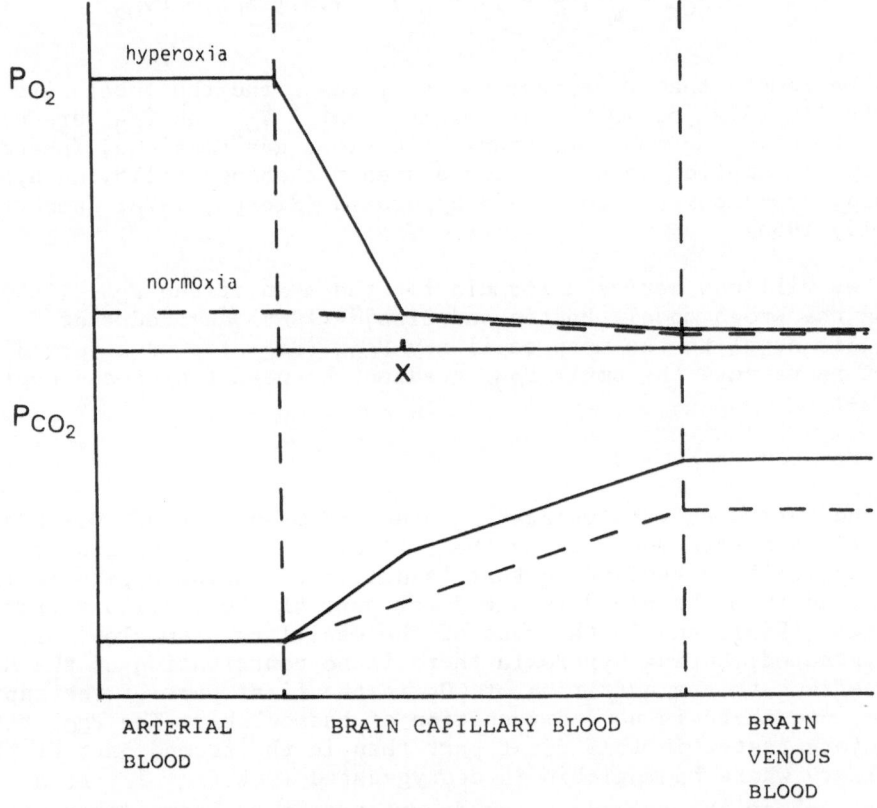

Fig. 1. Schematic representation of the change in P_{O_2} and P_{CO_2} in blood traversing brain tissue. It is assumed that the O_2 uptake and CO_2 delivery per unit of length is the same at all places along the capillary. The broken line is for normoxic arterial blood, the drawn line for hyperoxic arterial blood. At the point x the deoxygenation of haemoglobin starts.

which follows from Eq. (5) if we set $P_{O_2}(x)$ equal to Pv_{O_2} and insert $P_{CO_2}(x)$ for Pa_{CO_2}. Equating Eq. (8) to Eq. (5) we find

$$\xi = \frac{\alpha \cdot (Pa_{O_2} - Pv_{O_2})}{\dot{V}_{O_2}} \cdot \dot{Q} \qquad (9)$$

Therefore ξ is the amount of delivered physically dissolved O_2 divided by the total O_2 uptake, as it should.

From geometric considerations (see fig. 1) it follows that the mean capillary P_{CO_2} is given by

$$Pc_{CO_2} = \xi(0.5\ Pa_{CO_2} + 0.5\ P_{CO_2}(x)) + (1-\xi)(0.5\ P_{CO_2}(x) + 0.5\ Pv_{CO_2}) \qquad (10)$$

Substituting Eqs. (7), (8) and (9) into Eq. (10) and also using Eq. (6) we get

$$Pt_{CO_2} = Pa_{CO_2} + \frac{0.5\dot{V}_{CO_2}}{\dot{Q} \cdot m} \cdot (1-\frac{\gamma}{R}) + (1-0.5\xi) \cdot \frac{\gamma\alpha}{m} \cdot (Pa_{O_2} - Pv_{O_2}) + d \qquad (11)$$

Using Eq. (3), the CO_2 dissociation curve at equilibrium, we have assumed that the chemical processes involved in the buffering of CO_2 are fast compared with the transit time of blood in the capillaries. Pontén and Siesjö (1966) found that the measured mean tissue P_{CO_2} was close to the value expected from calculations for diffusion in the Krogh cylinder with instantaneous chemical reactions. This suggests that the speed of these chemical reactions is not a limiting factor in CO_2 transport.

Eqs. (5) and (11) are the main results derived from our model. From Eq. (5) it follows that the arterial-to-venous P_{CO_2} difference is diminished by

$$\frac{\gamma}{m}(\frac{\dot{V}_{O_2}}{\dot{Q}} - \alpha(Pa_{O_2} - Pv_{O_2})) = \frac{\gamma}{m} \cdot \frac{\dot{V}_{O_2}}{\dot{Q}} \cdot (1 - \xi)$$

due to the Haldane effect. When there is no contribution of physically dissolved molecules to O_2 delivery (ξ equal to zero) the Haldane effect is greatest. On the other hand, a high Pa_{O_2} in the range where haemoglobin is fully saturated and where there is much physically dissolved O_2 will lead to a reduction of the Haldane effect resulting in an increased Pv_{CO_2} at a fixed Pa_{CO_2}, as was already described by Gesell (1923). It can be seen from Eq. (5) that Pv_{CO_2} is increased by $\alpha \cdot \gamma \cdot m^{-1} \cdot (Pa_{O_2} - Pv_{O_2})$, due to the utilization of physically dissolved O_2. Eqs. (11) and (5) predict that the increase in Pt_{CO_2} with Pa_{O_2} at a fixed Pa_{CO_2} is less than the increase in Pv_{CO_2} by a factor $(1 - 0.5\xi)$.

THE VENOUS P_{CO_2} DURING HYPEROXAEMIA

Lambertsen et al. (1953) measured the arterial and the internal jugular P_{CO_2} of men during air breathing and during hyperbaric oxygen breathing at 3.5 atm. They found for the difference between Pv_{CO_2} and Pa_{CO_2} ($Pv_{CO_2} - Pa_{CO_2}$) an average value of 1.5 kPa (11 mmHg) during air breathing. Following hyperbaric oxygen breathing this value increased to 2.5 kPa (19 mmHg), while Pa_{O_2} was 280 kPa (2100 mmHg). Pv_{O_2} was still only 10 kPa (75 mmHg). Part of the increase in $Pv_{CO_2} - Pa_{CO_2}$ following hyperbaric oxygen breathing was due to a decrease in blood flow by 25%, ascribed by Lambertsen et al. (1953) to hypocapnia. This change in blood flow accounts for a 0.5 kPa (3.7 mmHg) increase of $Pv_{CO_2} - Pa_{CO_2}$, according to Eq. (5). The reduction of the Haldane effect is calculated from $\alpha . \gamma . m^{-1} . (Pa_{O_2} - Pv_{O_2})$, using for the parameters: $\gamma = 0.28$ ml.ml^{-1} and $m = 0.030$ ml.ml^{-1}.kPa^{-1} (Loeppky et al., 1983). The reduction of the Haldane effect amounts to 0.58 kPa (4.4 mmHg). The total increase in Pv_{CO_2} of 8.1 mmHg (1.1 kPa) derived from Eq. (5) is close to the 8 mmHg increase actually measured.

CHANGES IN $Pcsf_{CO_2}$ DUE TO THE HALDANE EFFECT

There is a clear increase in cerebrospinal fluid P_{CO_2} ($Pcsf_{CO_2}$) when Pa_{O_2} is changed from normoxia to hyperoxia (Olievier et al., 1982). In this section the contribution of the Haldane effect to this increase in $Pcsf_{CO_2}$ will be calculated from data on cat blood. We make use of the finding of Pontén and Siesjö (1966) that the average brain tissue P_{CO_2} (Pt_{CO_2}) and the $Pcsf_{CO_2}$ are equal.

We fitted the CO_2 content data of Bartels and Harms (1959) for cat blood with Eq. (3), using multiple regression analysis. We chose those data points where the CO_2 dissociation curve is almost linear (Pa_{CO_2} in the range 4-11 kPa). For 7 cats the average values for m and γ were 2.5×10^{-2} (SD=0.17×10^{-2}) ml.ml^{-1}.kPa^{-1} and 0.36 (SD=0.04) ml. ml^{-1} respectively. Inserting these values into Eq. (11) it follows that the increase in the $Pcsf_{CO_2}$ -to- Pa_{CO_2} difference, due to the Haldane effect, is about 0.12 kPa (1 mmHg) when going from Pa_{O_2} = 13 kPa (100 mmHg) to Pa_{O_2} = 50 kPa (375 mmHg), on the assumption that the blood flow is constant. For Pv_{O_2} a fixed value of 5.3 kPa (40 mmHg) was chosen since changes in Pv_{O_2} are relatively small as long as there is desaturation of haemoglobin. An increase in $Pcsf_{CO_2}$ of 0.2 kPa (1.5 mmHg) was measured when Pa_{O_2} was changed from about 13 to 50 kPa in our experiments on cats (Olievier et al., 1982). The $Pcsf_{CO_2}$ -to- Pa_{CO_2} difference, however, increased by about 0.14 kPa (1.0 mmHg) since there was on the average a slight increase in Pa_{CO_2} (see fig. 5, Olievier et al., 1982). This measured value is about equal to the calculated one, suggesting that the the reduction of the Haldane effect plays an important role in the $Pcsf_{CO_2}$ change following O_2 breathing. Although such a small change in $Pcsf_{CO_2}$ may seem unimportant it should be realized that it gives rise to an increase in ventilation of the order of one fifth of its resting value (Olievier et al., 1982).

CONCLUSIONS

The transport of CO_2 from tissue has been modeled in a simple way, including the effects of O_2 on CO_2 transport. The model quantitatively explains the marked increase in brain venous P_{CO_2} following hyperbaric O_2 breathing. The increase in brain tissue P_{CO_2} caused by hyperoxia can for a major part be attributed to a reduction of the Haldane effect. Although the changes in brain tissue P_{CO_2} following normobaric O_2 breathing are small, they have an appreciable influence on ventilation via the central chemosensors.

ACKNOWLEDGEMENTS

Part of this research was supported by the Foundation for Medical Research FUNGO (grant no. 13-36-37). We thank Dr. P. Rispens for valuable suggestions concerning the model.

REFERENCES

Bartels, H., and Harms, H., 1959, Sauerstoffsdissoziationskurven des Bluttes von Säugetieren, Pflügers Archiv., 268: 334-365.

Gesell, R., 1923, On the chemical regulation of respiration. I. The regulation of respiration with special reference to the metabolism of the respiratory center and the coordination of the dual function of hemoglobin, Am. J. Physiol., 66: 5-49.

Lambertsen, C.J., 1965, Effects of oxygen at high partial pressure, in: "Handbook of Physiology. Section 3: Respiration, Vol. II," W.O. Fenn and H. Rahn, eds., American Physiological Society, Washington.

Lambertsen, C.J., Kough, R.H., Cooper, D.Y., Emmel, G.L., Loeschcke, H.H., and Schmidt, C.F., 1953, Oxygen toxicity. Effects in man of oxygen inhalation at 1 and 3.5. atmospheres upon blood gas transport, cerebral circulation and cerebral metabolism, J. Appl. Physiol., 5: 471-486.

Loeppky, J.A., Luft, U.C. and Fletcher, E.R., 1983, Quantitative description of whole blood CO_2 dissociation curve and Haldane effect, Respir. Physiol., 51: 167-181.

Olievier, C.N., Berkenbosch, A., van Beek, J.H.G.M., de Goede, J., and Quanjer, Ph.H., 1982, Hypoxia, cerebrospinal fluid P_{CO_2} and central depression of ventilation, Bull. Eur. Physiopath. Respir., 18 (Suppl. 4): 165-172.

Pontén, U. and Siesjö, B.K., 1966, Gradients of CO_2 tension in the brain, Acta Physiol. Scand., 67: 129-140.

Siesjö, B.K., 1978, "Brain Energy Metabolism," John Wiley, Chichester.

Visser, B.F., 1960, Pulmonary diffusion of carbon dioxide, Physics in Medicine and Biology, 5: 155-166.

ENDOTOXIN PROTECTION AGAINST OXYGEN TOXICITY AND ITS REVERSAL

BY SALICYLATE

J. Klein and A. Trouwborst

Department of Anaesthesia, Erasmus University
Rotterdam, The Netherlands

INTRODUCTION

It has long been recognised that prolonged exposure to high inspired oxygen concentrations can produce pulmonary damage. Exposure to 100% O_2 at 1 atm. of pressure is lethal to most mammalian species after a period of days to weeks (1). While the potential dangers of hyperoxia on the lung are generally recognised, administration of above ambient O_2 tensions remains a necessity in the treatment of severe hypoxemia caused by respiratory failure or acute lung injury.

It has been reported that the administration of small doses of bacterial endotoxin markedly increased the survival rate of adult rats exposed for periods that are normally lethal (60-72 hrs) to 98% O_2 (2,3,4,5).

Details concerning the mechanism and even the cellular site or sites of the action of endotoxin are not yet known, but several viable possibilities exist.

Evidence has been accumulating to show that the pulmonary responses which occur following bacterial endotoxin administration are due to substances derived from arachidonic acid (6) and that the endotoxin induced responses are prevented by concurrent treatment with various cyclo-oxygenase inhibitors (7). Therefore we attempted to investigate the involvement of these deratives in the mechanism of endotoxin's protective action against pulmonary toxicity, by combined treatment with the soluble lysine salt of acetylsalicylic acid (L-ASA).

METHODS

Male Sprague-Dawley rats (TNO, Rijswijk, NL) weighing 250-300 g and maintained on a standard laboratory diet (Hope Farms rat food, Woerden, NL) were assigned at random to four different groups: one endotoxin treated group, one control group, one endotoxin treated group concommitantly treated with L-ASA and one L-ASA treated group.

Endotoxin treated rats were given a single intraperitoneal (i.p.) injection of 1 mg kg^{-1} body wt. of endotoxin (Salmonella typhimurium lipopoly- saccharide, phenol water extraction: Sigma Chemical Co., London, UK) dissolved in normal saline.
Control rats received an equal volume i.p. normal saline.
L-ASA treated rats received 100 mg kg^{-1} L-ASA subcutaneously (s.c.), 30 min before the i.p. endotoxin or saline administration, and every 24 hrs thereafter.

Directly after the i.p. endotoxin or saline administration, half of the rats of each group (chosen at random) were exposed to compressed air at 1 ATA, the other half of each group were exposed to 100% O_2 at 1 ATA for 7 days. This was performed in special airtight cages with an overflow hole. The O_2 concentration was continuously measured by means of an Instrumental Laboratory oxygen monitor and was constantly higher than 95% in the oxygen perfused cages. The CO_2 concentration was held constant at a level similar to that of room air (0.033%) by means of a high oxygen flow (7-8 complete gas changes per hour) and by placing containers of soda lime chips in the chamber. The chamber temperature was held constant between 23-26°C. Water and food were provided ad libitum. The chambers were opened once a day for a 10-15 min period to faciltiate injection, replenishment of food and water, and waste removal. Survival was monitored on a daily basis. Changes in duration of survival were reflected in a shift of the survival curve to the right or left. To determine whether such shifts were statistically significant, we used the Wilcoxon test (8). The level of statistical significance for a change in duration was established as $p < 0.05$.

RESULTS

The survival of the rats exposed to 100% O_2 for 7 days is shown in the figure. Although the saline treated rats and the L-ASA treated rats (100 mg kg^{-1} 24 hrs^{-1}) all died within 3 days, 83% of the endotoxin treated rats (1 mg kg^{-1}) survived for 7 days. Of the rats treated with endotoxin (1 mg kg^{-1}) plus L-ASA (100 mg kg^{-1} 24 hrs^{-1}), 25% survived for 7 days. No deaths were observed in identically treated control groups, of 6 rats each, exposed to compressed air (data not shown in figure).

The survival curve for rats pre-treated with 1 mg kg^{-1} endotoxin is significantly shifted to the right of the survival curve for saline treated rats, which indicates prolonged survival ($p < 0.01$). This prolonged survival is partly reversed by concurrent treatment with 100 mg kg^{-1} L-ASA per 24 hrs ($p < 0.05$).

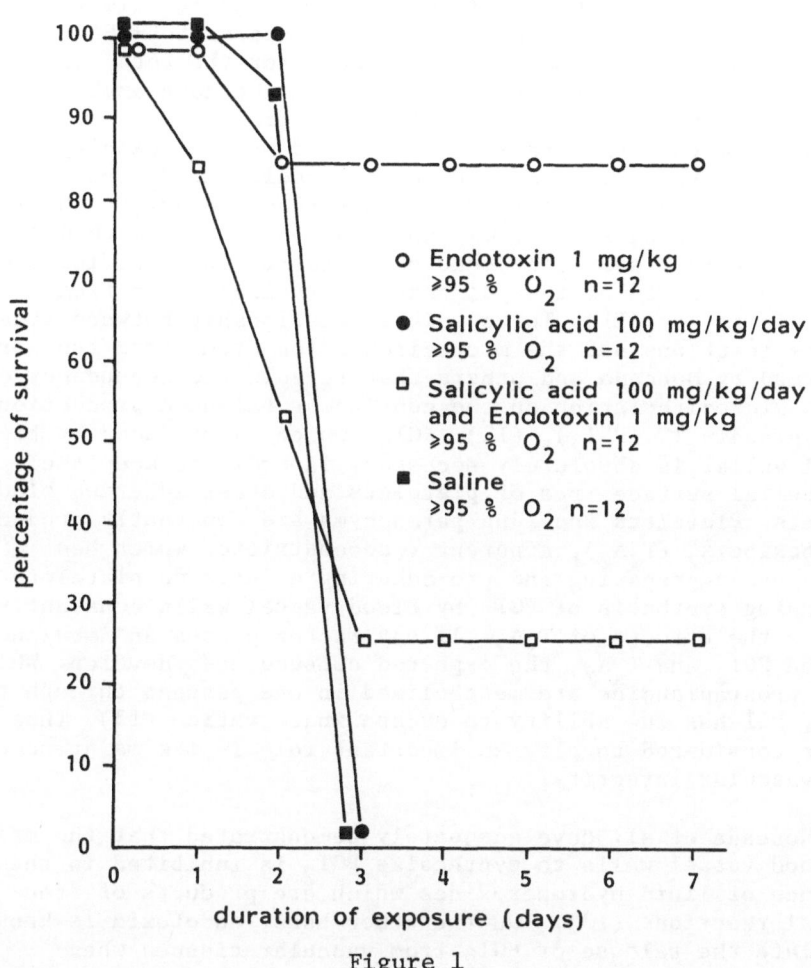

Figure 1

DISCUSSION

The present study confirms earlier observations that endotoxin protects against hyperoxic injury. We found that repeated administration of L-ASA (100 mg kg^{-1}) could partly reverse endotoxin induced protection. Frank and Roberts (2) also administered a cyclo-oxygenase inhibitor to their endotoxin

treated rats exposed to >95% O_2 (a single i.p. dose of
Indomethacin 3 mg kg^{-1}), but they did not find any detrimental
effect on the endotoxin induced protection expressed as survival.
Although this discrepancy is difficult to interpret, one of the
explanations might possibly be that a single dose of Indomethacin
of 3 mg kg^{-1} is not sufficient to block the enzyme
cyclo-oxygenase for the total period endotoxin is able to
'activate' this enzyme, whereas repeated doses of L-ASA (100 mg
kg^{-1}) inhibit the enzyme cyclo-oxygenase for the total period
the rats are exposed to >95% O_2. L-ASA in the dose employed
inhibits cyclo-oxygenase for at least 24 hrs (9).
According to the 'free radical theory' of oxygen toxicity,
exposure to hyperoxia elevates the intracellular O_2 concentration
and increases the production of highly reactive oxygen species
such as superoxide anion ($^-O_2$) and hydrogen peroxide (H_2O_2),
(10). It seems likely that endotoxin excerts its beneficial effect
via the protection of the pulmonary microcirculation from
hyperoxic injury (11). The possible relationship between free
radical reactions and the microcirculation stems from the work
performed by Moncada and others that reveals the dependency of a
patent microcirculation on the continuing balanced production of
prostaglandin I_2 (PGI_2), (12). PGI_2, which is produced by blood
vessel walls, is absolutely necessary in order to keep the
endothelial surface free of platelets and other adhering blood
elements. Platelets and lung paranchyma are constantly producing
Thromboxane A_2 (T_xA_2), a potent vasoconstrictor which has
marked pro-aggregating and pro-adhering effects on platelets. The
continuing synthesis of PGI_2 by blood vessel walls constantly
opposes the effects of T_xA_2. If any factor causes an imbalance
between PGI_2 and T_xA_2, the expected consequences develop. While
other prostaglandins are metabolised in one passage through the
lungs, PGI has the ability to escape inactivation (13). Thus PGI_2
may be considered to play an important role in the maintenance of
microvascular integrity.

Moncada et al. have adequately demonstrated that the ability
of blood vessel walls to synthesize PGI_2 is inhibited in the
presence of lipid hydroperoxides which are products of free
radical reactions (12). On the other hand, endotoxin is known to
stimulate the release of PGI_2 from vascular tissues when
administered in a single dose (14).

Therefore, the present study was designed to determine
whether endotoxin protects against pulmonary microcirculatory
injury by an interaction with the prostaglandin metabolism. The
results indicate that prostaglandin metabolism may indeed play an
important role in the protective action of endotoxin during
hyperoxia.

REFERENCES

1. Clark JM and Lambersten CG. Pulmonary oxygen toxicity, a review. Pharmacol Rev 23; 37-113 (1971).
2. Frank L and Roberts RJ. Oxygen toxicity: protection of the lung by the bacterial lipopolysaccharide (endotoxin). Toxicol Appl Pharmacol 50; 371 (1979).
3. Frank L and Roberts RJ. Endotoxin protection against oxygen-induced acute and chronic lung injury. J Appl Physiol 47; 577 (1979).
4. Frank L, Summerville J, Massaro D. Protection from oxygen toxicity with endotoxin: role of the endogenous antioxidant enzymes of the lung. J Clin Invest 65; 1104 (1980).
5. Frank L, Yam J, Roberts RJ. The role of endotoxin in protection of adult rats from oxygen-induced lung toxicity. J Clin Invest 61; 269 (1978).
6. Coker SJ, Hughes B, Parratt JR, Rodger IW, Zeitlin IJ. The release of prostanoids during the acute pulmonary response to E.coli endotoxin in anaesthetized cats. Br J Pharmac 78; 561-570 (1983).
7. Parratt JR and Sturgess RM. E.coli endotoxin shock in the cat; treatment with indomethacin. Br J Pharmac 53; 485-488 (1975).
8. Wilcoxon F. Some rapid approximate statistical procedures. Stamford, Conn: American Cyanamid Co (1949).
9. Villa S and de Gaetano G. Prostacyclin-like activity in rat vascular tissues. Fast, long-lasting inhibition by treatment with lysine acetylsalicylate. Prostaglandins 14;6,1117 (1977).
10. Freeman BA and Crapo JD: Hyperoxia increases oxygen radical production in rat lungs and lung mitochondria. J Biol Chem 256; 21, 10986-10992 (1981).
11. Crapo JD, Freeman BA, Barry BE, Turrens JF, Young SL. Mechanisms of hyperoxic injury to the pulmonary microcirculation. The Physiologist 26; 3, 170-175 (1983).
12. Moncada S, Gryglewski RJ, Buntin J, Vane JR. A lipid peroxide inhibits the enzyme in blood vessel microsomes that generates from prostaglandin endoperoxides the substance (prostaglandin X) which prevents platelet aggregation. Prostaglandins 12; 5, 715-737 (1976).
13. Slotman GJ, Machiedo GW, Casey KF, Lyons MJ. Histologic and hemodynamic effects of prostacyclin and prostaglandin El f following oleic acid infusion. Surgery 92; 1, 93-100 (1982).
14. Villa S, de Gaetano G, Semeraro N. Increased vascular prostacyclin activity in rats after endotoxin administration. Experientia 37; 494-495 (1981).

MISCELLANEOUS ORGANS AND TISSUES

OXYGEN TENSION IN THE FETAL SCALP DURING LABOUR

J.G. Aarnoudse, M. Cornel, T.M. Smits

Dept. of Obstetrics & Gynaecology
University Hospital
Groningen, The Netherlands

During labour uterine contractions cause a decrease in utero-placental blood flow that results in a reduction of the transfer of oxygen from maternal to fetal blood. Under normal circumstances this intermittent reduction in oxygen supply is well tolerated by the fetus and does not lead to hypoxia and fetal acidosis. If, however, the uteroplacental circulation is already compromised, as in preeclampsia or fetal growth retardation, normal uterine contractions may result in fetal hypoxia and acidosis with temporary or even permanent damage to the central nervous system.

Until recently, fetal oxygenation in the human could only be monitored continuously by indirect methods, e.g. fetal heart rate monitoring or intermittently by fetal scalp blood sampling. The introduction of the transcutaneous (tc) oxygen electrode made it possible to measure fetal oxygen tension (PO_2) continuously during labour[1]. This new technique certainly has enlarged our knowledge of the physiology and the pathophysiology of fetal oxygen supply during labour. The transcutaneous method, however, has some dis-advantages, which become particularly evident when the tc electrode is used during labour. First, the relatively large size of the tc electrode requires a cervical dilatation of at least 4 cm, the scalp has to be shaven locally, and the tc electrode has to be carefully glued onto the skin. Second, the transcutaneous electrode can only function properly if local skin blood flow is augmented considerably. However, experimental and clinical work has provided sufficient evidence now, that fetal scalp blood flow decreases in the course of labour[2,3,4]. This is most probably the result of engagement of the fetal head in the birth canal, the pressure exerted by the cervical ring on scalp tissue impeding blood flow within the ring[2,5].

We have developed a small needle electrode that can be easily applied in early labour and does not require a heat-induced increase in local blood flow[6]. This polarographic needle electrode measures PO_2 in the subcutaneous (sc) tissue of the scalp. This chapter deals with a brief description of the construction and the characteristics of the electrode and summarizes the most relevant clinical findings under normal and pathological conditions.

THE OXYGEN ELECTRODE

The oxygen electrode consists of a 50 μm glass-insulated platinum cathode, covered with polystyrene and mounted in a stainless steel needle with an outer diameter of 0.4 mm (fig. 1). The needle is fitted in an epoxy holder which also contains two spirals for fetal ECG-recording and anchoring of the electrode. With the aid of a specially designed applicator, the electrode assembly is anchored in scalp tissue by rotating it over 270 degrees. This method has proved to be safe, simple and effective in clinical obstetrics, where similar spiral electrodes are used for routine fetal heart rate monitoring. If necessary, application is possible at the beginning of labour through a small amnioscope with a smallest inner diameter of 1 cm. A disposable self-adhesive Ag/AgCl electrode, attached to the lower abdomen of the mother, is used as a reference.

The electrodes are sterilized by immersion in a 2% glutaraldehyde solution for 20 min, after which they are carefully rinsed with sterile saline solution. This method of sterilisation did not influence the calibration values. In practice, zero current of the electrodes appeared to be low (less than 0.005 nA) and very stable. At PO_2 = 150 mmHg most electrodes produce a current between 2.5 and 5 nA.

Fetal heart rate (FHR), intra-uterine pressure (IUP) and fetal scalp $scPO_2$ were recorded on a 4 channel recorder (HP 7754A). Data were acquired on line in a microcomputer system (Apple Europlus) using a sample frequency of 0.2 Hz for $scPO_2$ and IUP. The data stored on discette were analyzed by using a special program for the microcomputer and then displayed in frequency distribution histograms, compressed data plots of $scPO_2$ and IUP and scatter diagrams of $scPO_2$ versus IUP.

In all patients, umbilical arterial and venous blood samples were taken anaerobically within 2 min after delivery from a double clamped cord segment and immediately analyzed on an AVL-940 automatic blood gas analyzer. Quality control of this analyzer was maintained daily with special attention to the calibration of the oxygen electrode at PO_2 values between 0 en 50 mmHg.

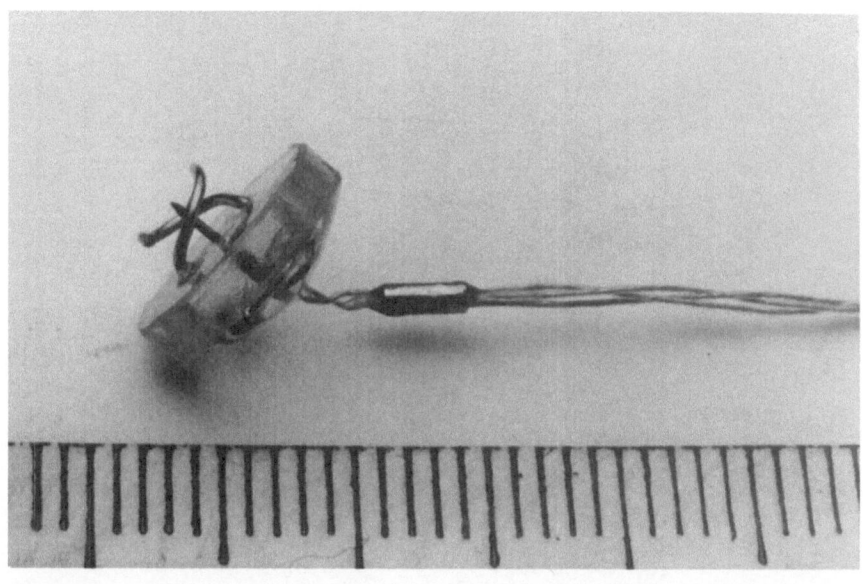

Figure 1. The oxygen needle electrode mounted in the centre of the spirals. The latter are for fetal ECG recording and to anchor the electrode assembly in fetal tissue.

FETAL scPO$_2$ DURING LABOUR

Until now we have obtained 40 successful recordings, about half of which were derived from high risk patients. The average recording time in this group studied was 4.5 h (range 1-11 h) and the mean cervical dilatation at the time of application was 2.5 cm. Figure 2 shows a representative example of a recording obtained during the first stage of an uncomplicated normal labour. It demonstrates the most commonly observed changes in fetal scPO$_2$ caused by a single uterine contraction. During the first half of a contraction, scPO$_2$ slightly increases, whereas scPO$_2$ falls during and after the second half of a contraction, the PO$_2$ level more or less slowly recovering to the baseline towards the following contraction. Under normal circumstances this transient decrease in scPO$_2$ usually did not exceed 5 mmHg. However, uterine hyperactivity, e.g. coupling of uterine contractions, was usually followed by a much greater fall in scPO$_2$. In general, fetal scPO$_2$ fell when uterine activity (total area of IUP) increased (fig. 3). Figure 4 is an example of the frequency distribtuion of fetal scPO$_2$ of a patient during a normal labour.

Abnormal FHR patterns during labour were often associated with lower scPO$_2$ values, either by a more pronounced transient decrease

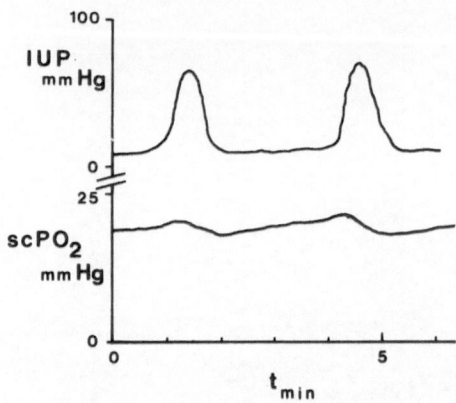

Figure 2. The most commonly observed pattern of
changes in scPO$_2$ in relation to a normal uterine
contraction.

of scPO$_2$ following a contraction (fig. 5), or by persistently low
scPO$_2$ levels of < 10 mmHg. Table I shows the distribution of fetal
scPO$_2$ values in 10 min periods during normal and abnormal FHR of
34 women in labour. There was a significant increase (χ^2 test, p <
0.001) in the incidence of abnormal FHR patterns at lower scPO$_2$
levels.

The trend of fetal scPO$_2$ when labour progresses is best
illustrated in fig. 6. This figure shows the course of scPO$_2$ in 7
women with uncomplicated labour, where scPO$_2$ could be recorded
for at least 4 hours. After an initial stabilization period of
15-30 min, which was not included, the scPO$_2$ remains fairly
stable during the first stage of labour. In most patients, however,
scPO$_2$ fell more or less shortly before the onset of bearing down
contractions and continued to fall in the second stage towards
delivery. As shown in table I, this long term decrease in the
scPO$_2$ "baseline" level was highly associated with the occurrence of
abnormal FHR when labour progresses.

After birth, the umbilical arterial and venous blood PO$_2$
values were compared with the scPO$_2$ values during the last 5 min
prior to delivery. For both the arterial and venous PO$_2$ values a
good correlation was found with scPO$_2$ (r values of 0.76 and 0.75
respectively) over a wide range of umbilical PO$_2$ values (5-35 mmHg).

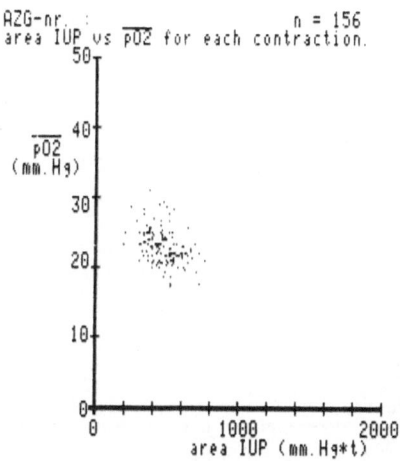

Figure 3. Relationship between uterine contractility, indicated as total area of IUP, and fetal
scPO$_2$ in one patient. scPO$_2$ is calculated as the
average value from the beginning of a contraction
to the start of the next contraction.

Table I. Incidence of abnormal fetal heart rate (FHR) patterns at
various fetal scalp scPO$_2$ levels of 34 patients during labour.
(n = number of 10 min periods of recording.

scPO$_2$ (mmHg)	% abnormal FHR
0-10 (n= 93)	52
10-20 (n=166)	31
> 20 (n=303)	7

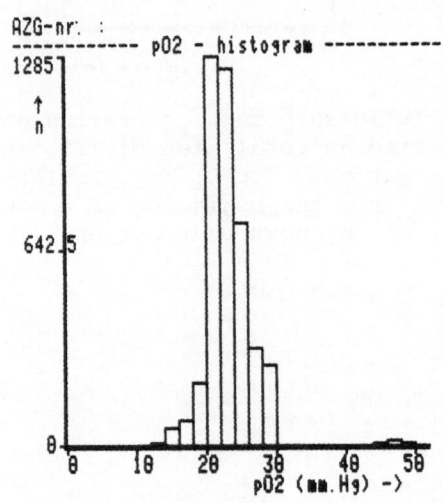

Figure 4. Frequency distribution of fetal scPO$_2$ values during normal labour.

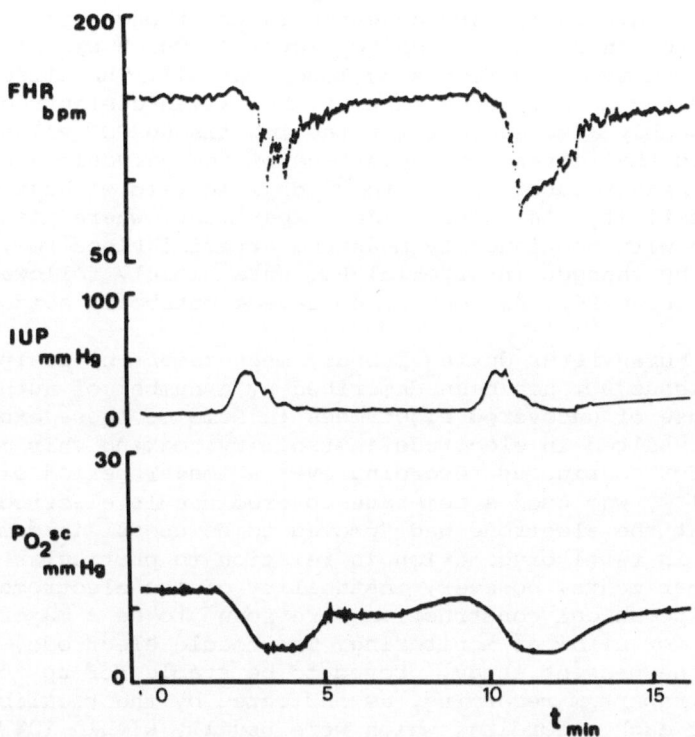

Figure 5. Fetal scPO₂ during abnormal FHR in early
labour. Note the considerable reduction in scPO₂ .

There are relatively few studies of tissue PO_2 in the fetus. In the chronically catheterized fetal lamb Towell et al[7,8], using galvanic oxygen electrodes, have investigated tissue PO_2 in muscle, brain cortex and subcutaneous tissue. Fetal subcutaneous scalp tissue PO_2 has been measured during acute experiments in the sheep by polarographic oxygen electrodes[9,10]. With the latter, higher PO_2 values were reported in the sheep than with galvanic electrodes, which is partly explained because polarographic electrodes have been used exclusively during acute experiments. Under these circumstances, hyperaemia and anaesthesia are thought to be responsible for increased tissue PO_2 levels[8], which was also demonstrated in the experiments by Towell et al[8]. The different construction and mode of operation of the galvanic electrodes, however, probably also account for the low tissue PO_2 values recorded with the latter. The advantage of the galvanic electrodes is that they can be used for up to 73 days in vivo without undue loss of sensitivity. In those animal experiments where tissue PO_2 was compared with continuously measured arterial blood PO_2, it was found that the changes in arterial PO_2 were closely followed by changes in tissue PO_2, as long as no severe metabolic acidosis occurred[9].

In the human fetus during labour, measurement of scalp sub-cutaneous tissue PO_2 has been described by a number of authors[11,12,13]. The use of uncovered electrodes in some of these experiments inevitably resulted in electrode instability, making this method unsuitable for continuous recording over a longer period of time. Walker et al[11], who used a membrane-covered needle electrode, reported that the electrode had "proved to be useful in demonstrating changes in fetal oxygenation in relation to particular events". In their experiments, however, instability of the electrode and its complicated technical construction were found to be a major restriction for clinical monitoring. The needle electrode, which we used in the present study, proved to be stable for up to 11 hours of intrapartum recording, as indicated by the recalibration values after each recording, which were usually within 10% of the initial calibration value.

The in vivo performance of the electrodes for several hours is best illustrated in fig. 6. The question whether the decrease in fetal scalp $scPO_2$ towards the end of the first stage of labour, which continues during the second stage, is really caused by a decrease in fetal arterial PO_2 or is the result of other factors, e.g. local tissue damage, cannot be answered directly, becasue direct comparison with the arterial PO_2 values is impossible in the human fetus.

The relatively large cathode used in the needle electrode

obtains 95% of its oxygen from an area within 200 μ of the cathode. Since the mean intercapillary distance in the subcutaneous tissue of the fetal scalp is 76 μm[11], the electrode is supplied from a number of capillaries and measures an average tissue PO_2.

There are 2 arguments indicating that even after several hours of recording, the $scPO_2$ values are still representative for the arterial PO_2 values of the fetus and that local tissue damage or electrode drift does not become an important limiting factor. First, there was a good correlation between umbilical blood PO_2 values measured at delivery and the $scPO_2$ values during the last 5 minutes prior to delivery. Second, no evidence could be found in the present study that a longer recording time was associated with lower $scPO_2$ levels at the end of a recording.

Continuous measurment of fetal tissue PO_2 makes it possible now to get a better understanding of fetal oxygenation during several types of abnormal FHR. Until recently, information on fetal oxygenation during abnormal FHR had to be based mainly on secondary changes in fetal pH, measured in micro blood samples from the scalp. The results of the present study confirm previous observations in animal studies that some abnormal FHR patterns are the result of reduced oxygen supply to the fetus, irrespective whether acidosis is present or not. So far, continuous measurement of fetal tissue PO_2 has certainly enlarged our knowledge of the physiology and the pathophysiology of fetal oxygenation during labour.

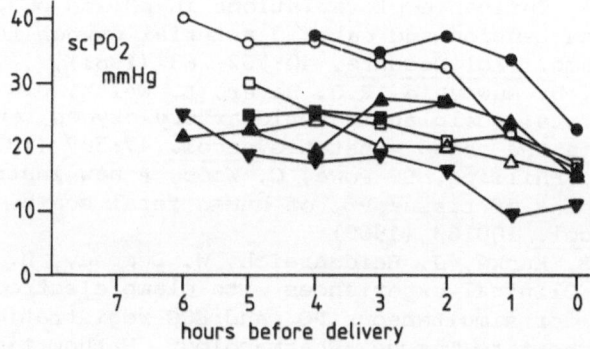

Figure 6. The trend of fetal $scPO_2$ during the course of labour in 7 patients where recording was done for at least 4 hrs.

REFERENCES

1. A. Huch, R. Huch, H. Schneider, G. Rooth, Continuous transcutaneous monitoring of fetal oxygen during labour, Br.J.
Obstet.Gynaecol. 84:suppl.1,1-37 (1977).
2. J.G. Aarnoudse, J.C.W. Crawley, P.A. Flecknell, F.E. Hytten,
Scalp blood flow measured by the Xenon clearance technique
and transcutaneous PO_2 in the fetal lamb. Pediat.Res. 17:982-
985 (1983).
3. C.A.M. Jansen, P.W. Nathanielsz, Pressure related changes in
fetal transcutaneous PO_2 measurements. J.Physiol. 308:29
(1980).
4. T.M. Smits, J.G. Aarnoudse, Variability of fetal scalp blood
flow during labour: continuous transcutaneous measurement by
the laser Doppler technique. Br.J.Obstet.Gynaecol. 91:524-531
(1984).
5. M.C. O'Connor, F.E. Hytten, G.D. Zanelli, Is the fetus 'scalped'
in labour? Lancet ii, 947-949 (1979).
6. J.G. Aarnoudse, H.J. Huisjes, B. Oeseburg, W.G. Zijlstra, Subcutaneous oxygen tension in the fetal scalp during labour.
Continuous monitoring with a needle electrode. Br.J.Obstet.
Gynaecol. 88:517-524 (1981).
7. M.E. Towell, I. Regier, I. Lysak, D. Saÿler, S.P. Bessman,
Maternal and fetal tissue PO_2 in the pregnant ewe, measured
with galvanic PO_2 electrodes, in: Oxygen transport to tissue
- IV. H.I. Bicher and D.F. Bruley, eds., Adv. Exper. Med. Biol.,
Vol. 159, Plenum Press, New York and London, p. 37-48 (1983).
8. M.E. Towell, J. Johnsen, K. Smedstad, M. Andrew, T.L. Vu, Fetal
blood and tissue PO_2 during maternal oxygen breathing.
J.Developm.Phys., in press.
9. J.G. Aarnoudse, B. Oeseburg, G. Kwant, A. Zwart, W.G. Zijlstra,
H.J. Huisjes, Influence of variations in pH and pCO_2 on scalp
tissue oxygen tension and carotid arterial oxygen tension in
the fetal lamb. Biol.Neonate, 40:252-263 (1981),
10. K.J. Staisch, B. Nuwayhid, R.O. Bayer, L. Welsh, C.R. Brinkman,
Continuous fetal scalp and carotid artery oxygen tension
monitoring in the sheep. Obstet.Gynecol. 47:587 (1976).
11. A. Walker, L. Phillips, L. Powe, C. Wood, A new instrument for
the measurement of tissue PO_2 of human fetal scalp. Am.J.
Obstet.Gynecol. 100:63 (1968).
12. W. Erdmann, S. Kunke, J. Heidenreich, W. Dempsey, H. Günther,
H. Schäfer, Clinical experiences with clamp electrodes in
fetal scalp for simultaneous PO_2 and ECG-registration, in:
Oxygen Transport to Tissue. Pharmacology, Mathematical Studies,
and Neonatology", D.F. Bruley and H.I. Bicher, eds., Adv.Exper.
Med. Biol., Vol. 37b, Plenum Press, New York - London, p.1129-
1133 (1973).
13. H. Belleé, V. Schönjahn, Verhalten des Sauerstoffpartialdruckes
in der Kopfschwarte des Feten während der physiologischen
Uteruskontraktion. Zentbl.Gynäk. 97:413 (1975).

14. L.S. James, H.O. Marishima, S.S. Daniel, E.T. Bowe, H. Cohen, W.H. Niemann, Mechanism of late deceleration of the fetal heart rate. Am.J.Obstet.Gynecol. 113:578 (1972).

PERFUSATE OXYGENATION AND RENAL FUNCTION IN THE ISOLATED RAT KIDNEY*

Gernot Gronow   and Herbert Kossmann

Physiologisches Institut der Universität Kiel
Olshausenstr. 40, D-2300 Kiel 1, FRG

INTRODUCTION

Measurements of glomerular and tubular function in the hypoxic kidney were complicated in vivo by the effects of increased levels of circulating vasoconstrictory hormones and a raised sympathetic nervous activity. In consequence, a severe renal vasoconstriction and the resulting reduction in renal blood flow restrained glomerular and tubular functions at very low oxygen tensions (Bursaux et al., 1976; Zillig et al., 1978). Even in vitro, without nervous interference, the perfusion of an isolated kidney preparation with whole blood (Nizet et al., 1967) or Ringer solutions (Ross, 1978) was often hampered by a long lasting vasoconstriction which reduced perfusion flow rate and kept glomerular filtration and tubular Na^+ reabsorption far below their physiological levels (Maack, 1980).

However, recent experiments with an isolated rat kidney preparation indicate that, at a physiological perfusion pressure of about 100mmHg, normal rates of glomerular filtration and Na^+ reabsorption may be obtained by the use of hyperbaric oxygenated Ringer solutions (pO_2 in the range of 600-700mmHg) which contain physiological colloids (albumin/globulin) and exogenous substrates such as glucose and amino acids (Maack, 1980; Swanson et al., 1981). Moreover, the observation that even in extreme hypoxia ($pO_2 < 1$mmHg) the perfusion flow rate in an isolated kidney preparation did not decrease (Gronow and Cohen, 1984) made it now possible to vary systematically oxygen transport to renal tissue without concomitant cessation of the perfusate flow in the renal vascular tree.

------

*Supported by the Deutsche Forschungsgemeinschaft

MATERIAL AND METHODS

The right kidney of fed, male Sprague-Dawley rats (mean BW±SD=385 ±31g) was by recirculation perfused with a 250ml Ringer-bicarbonate medium at pH 7.3-7.4, 38°C, and a mean ±SD "arterial" pressure of 100±4mmHg. The perfusate contained 6g/dl albumin and, if not otherwise stated, 10mM glucose in combination with a mixture of amino acids (Maack, 1980), 2mM each. The preparation and cannulation of the kidney have been described elsewhere (Gronow and Cohen, 1984). Modifications from the previous technique were as follows: 1. the albumin (Serva, Heidelberg, FRG) which contained about 8% αglobulin and 3-5mg/g fatty acids was dialyzed at 4°C overnight against the final Ringer solution; 2. the cannulated kidney was placed on the bottom of a stainless-steel chamber which was inserted into the front edge of a water-thermostated perspex box; 3. the perspex box contained submers two twin circuits with a venous reservoir , a Millipore-filter (0.8μm, Bedford, Mass., USA), an artificial lung (two 5m coils of silicon tubing in parallel, ID: 1.5mm, OD: 1.9mm), and an arterial reservoir; 4. the perfusate flow was directed alternatively either through the oxygenated (95% O_2 : 5% CO_2) or deoxygenated (95% N_2 : 5% CO_2) branch of the twin circuit to an "arterial" or "venous" roller pump (Verder, Düsseldorf, FRG) outside of the perspex box; 5. measuring devices in close proximity of the renal cannulas were: a hydrostatic pressure transducer (Statham, USA), an electromagnetic flow probe (Narcomatic RT 510, Hugo Sachs, March-Hugstetten, FRG), "arterial" and "venous" oxygen electrodes (Eschweiler, Kiel, FRG), a pH electrode (Schott, Hofheim, FRG), and a temperature probe (Esters Elektronik, Rodgau, FRG).

Glomerular filtration rate was assumed to be equal to the clearance of alkali-stable inulin. Samples of the perfusate and the urine were analyzed for Na^+ by flame photometry (Eppendorf, Hamburg, FRG), for inulin by the "direct" diphenyl-amine method (Gronow and Cohen, 1984), for protein content and enzymatic activities of lactate dehydrogenase (EC 1.1.1.27) and of γglutamyl-transferase (EC 2.3.2.2) according to standard assays (Bergmeyer, 1974). A P-value of 0.05 or less (Student's t-test) was considered to indicate a significant difference.

RESULTS AND DISCUSSION

CONSTANT OXYGEN TENSIONS: In a first series of experiments, the oxygen pressure in the perfusate was held constant throughout the entire perfusion (90min). When isolated rat kidneys were perfused at a pO_2 of about 680mmHg, variations in glomerular filtration rates (GFR) occurred in parallel with different degrees of perfusion flow rates (PFR) up to 45min after cannulation (Fig. 1A). Apparently, an about 6-fold higher PFR (31ml $\cdot g^{-1} \cdot min^{-1}$) than in vivo (about 5ml $\cdot g^{-1} \cdot min^{-1}$) was necessary to achieve a physio-

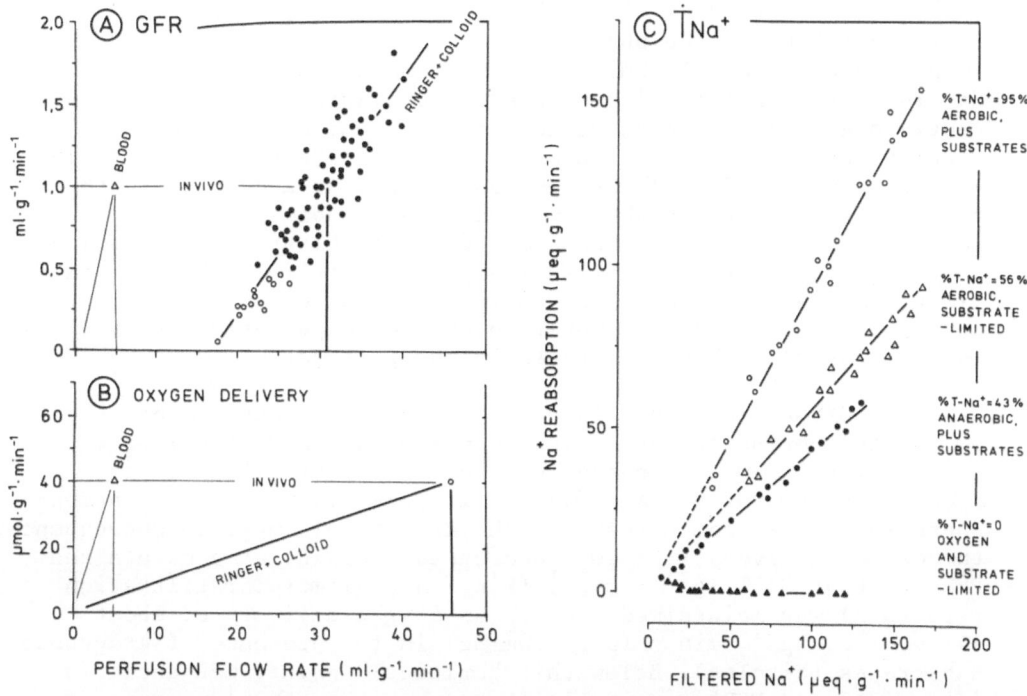

Fig. 1 Dependency of (A) glomerular filtration rate (GFR) and of oxygen delivery (B) on spontaneous variations in perfusion flow rate ($pO_2 \sim 680$mmHg), and of (C) the absolute rate of Na^+ reabsorption ($T-Na^+$) on GFR-dependent variations in filtered Na^+ (open symbols: $pO_2 \sim 680$mmHg; closed symbols: $pO_2 < 1$mmHg) in the isolated perfused rat kidney at a mean ±SD perfusion pressure of 100 ±4mmHg (38°C). Substrates: 10mM glucose in combination with 9 amino acids, 2mM each (circles). No substrates added: triangles. Each point represents a single observation. (A:n=80; C:n=20).

logical GFR of about $1 \text{ml} \cdot g^{-1} \cdot \text{min}^{-1}$. At this level, the oxygen delivery ($\alpha \cdot$PFR) in the oxygen carrier-free perfusate (Fig. 1B) did not approach the physiological value of about $40 \mu \text{mol } O_2 \cdot g^{-1} \cdot \text{min}^{-1}$. However, in view of the "excess" renal blood flow in vivo (about $5 \text{ml} \cdot g^{-1} \cdot \text{min}^{-1}$) it appears not surprising that an about 30% lower oxygen delivery in the cell-free perfusate did not limit GFR and Na^+ reabsorption in the isolated rat kidney (Fig. 1C).

According to spontaneous variations in GFR, the absolute rate of Na^+ reabsorption ($T-Na^+$) paralleled all resulting changes in filtered Na^+ up to the physiological level of about $150\mu eq$ $Na^+ \cdot g^{-1} \cdot min^{-1}$ (open circles). This glomerulotubular balance kept fractional Na^+ reabsorption ($\%T-Na^+$) independent of variations in GFR significantly higher ($\sim 95\%$) than without glucose and amino acids ($\sim 56\%$, open triangles) in the perfusate. Even at an "arterial" $pO_2 < 1mmHg$ (closed circles) $\%T-Na^+$ was constantly held at about 43% in the presence of substrates which may yield anaerobically formed ATP (Gronow and Cohen, 1984). However, when no substrates were added to the perfusate (closed triangles), $\%T-Na^+$ fell in the substrate limited kidney to zero. Thus, an insufficient oxygen delivery to an isolated rat kidney preparation may be compensated for, at least in part, by anaerobic substrates in the perfusate.

VARIABLE OXYGEN TENSIONS: In a second series of experiments the pO_2 in the perfusate was varied stepwise in 12min time intervals (change within 2min, constant pO_2 for 10min) by mixing in increasing volume of 95% N_2 : 5% CO_2 with the 95% O_2 : 5% CO_2 atmosphere in the gas compartment of the artificial lung. In consequence, the oxygen delivery (and pO_2) decreased stepwise at a maintained PFR of about $31ml \cdot g^{-1} \cdot min^{-1}$ (Fig. 2A): glomerular filtration rate (GFR) was maintained down to an oxygen delivery of about 14 μmol $O_2 \cdot g^{-1} \cdot min^{-1}$ ($pO_2 \sim 370mmHg$) in the presence of exogenous substrates (circles). Below this "critical" point, GFR declined (at maintained PFR) exponentially by more than 50%. Omission of the exogenous substrates in the perfusate (triangles) significantly shifted GFR to a lower and less stable level. In contrast, fractional Na^+ reabsorption ($\%T-Na^+$, Fig. 2B) was maintained in the presence of exogenous substrates (circles) until a lower delivery of oxygen was reached ($\sim 10\mu mol$ $O_2 \cdot g^{-1} \cdot min^{-1}$). Interestingly enough, this "critical" value was very similar to the observed rates of oxygen consumption ($9.7\mu mol$ $O_2 \cdot g^{-1} \cdot min^{-1}$) at "normal" ($pO_2 > 370mmHg$) oxygenation of the perfusate. Omission of glucose and the mixture of amino acids (triangles) significantly reduced $\%T-Na^+$ to a lower and less constant level.

The absolute rate of Na^+ reabsorption ($T-Na^+$) as well as the oxygen consumption in the isolated rat kidney (Fig. 2C) were maintained fairly constant in the presence of exogenous substrates (circles) at a $T-Na^+/Q-O_2$ ratio of about 14.7. Below an oxygen delivery of $\sim 14\mu mol$ $O_2 \cdot g^{-1} \cdot min^{-1}$ ($pO_2 < 370mmHg$), however, $T-Na^+$ and oxygen consumption declined nearly parallel to the observed reduction in GFR (Fig. 2A). When virtually no oxygen was present in the perfusate ($pO_2 < 1mmHg$), $T-Na^+$ approached the level of support by anaerobic metabolic energy (Gronow and Cohen, 1984), and $Q-O_2$ declined to zero. Without addition of substrates to the perfusate (triangles), $T-Na^+$ started at about half of the values obtained in the presence of substrates, and declined steadily to zero in extreme hypoxia.

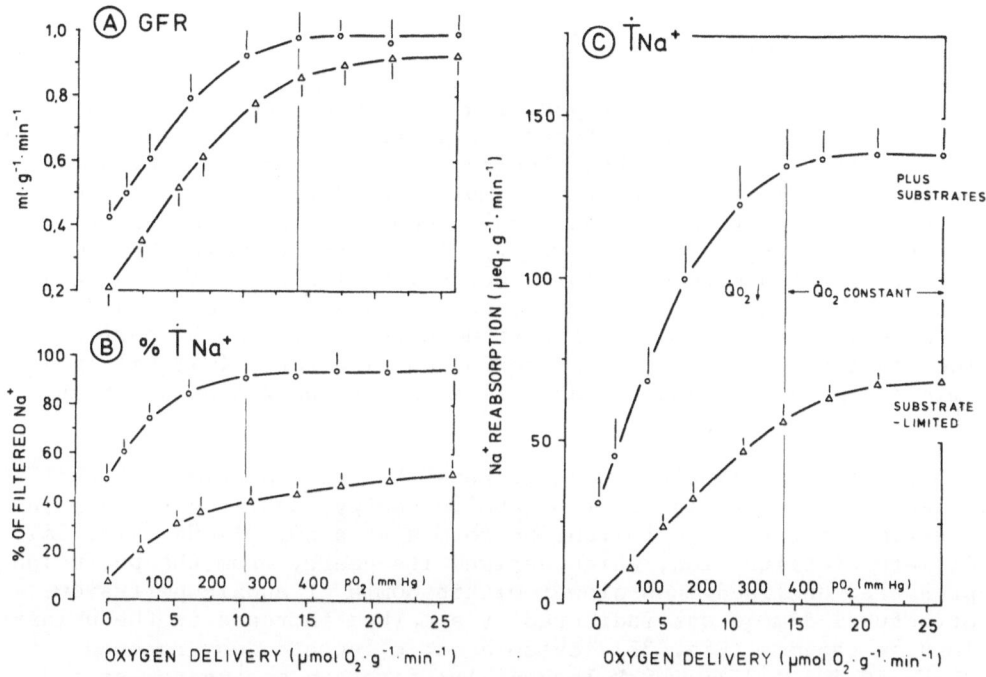

Fig. 2 Limitation of glomerular filtration (GFR =A), fractional
(%T-Na$^+$ =B), and absolute rate of Na$^+$ reabsorption
(T-Na$^+$ =C) by decreasing rates of oxygen delivery in the
perfusate of the isolated rat kidney (38°C). Oxygen
delivery was calculated for an observed mean perfusion
flow rate of 31ml ·g^{-1} ·min^{-1}. Substrates: 10mM glucose
in combination with 9 amino acids, 2mM each (circles).
No substrates added: triangles ($\bar{x}$±SD, n=7).

If one takes a mean perfusion flow rate of 31ml ·g^{-1} ·min^{-1} into
account, then an O_2 delivery of >14µmol O_2 ·g^{-1} ·min^{-1} (or a perfusate pO_2 >400mmHg) appeared to be sufficient to maintain a
physiological rate of glomerular filtration and Na$^+$ reabsorption
in the isolated perfused rat kidney. Interestingly, this "reduced"
pO_2 exerted a beneficial effect on tissue damage which may have
been induced at higher oxygen tensions (pO_2 ∿680mmHg) by the
deleterious action of free oxygen radicals (Gauduel and Duvelleroy,
1984), as indicated by a significantly smaller loss of urinary
γglutamyltransferase (γGT, EC 2.3.2.2) in kidneys perfused constantly at a pO_2 of 450mmHg (1.5±0.6 mUγGT ·g^{-1} ·min^{-1}, n=4) in

comparison to kidneys which were perfused at ~680mmHg
(5.3 ±2.0 mU γGT $\cdot$g^{-1} $\cdot$min^{-1}, n=7).

In isolated kidney preparations with much lower perfusion flow
rates, however, even a perfusate oxygenation of ~680mmHg may be not
sufficient to maintain physiological rates of renal function. At
an about 50% reduced PFR, for example, the "critical" point in
oxygen delivery (Fig. 2) would have been shifted to the right
(at PFR =15ml $\cdot$g^{-1} $\cdot$min^{-1} to a pO_2 >680 mmHg). Accordingly, Franke
et al. (1976) observed at lower perfusion flow rates local areas
of hypoxia in the cortex of isolated rat kidneys, and the addition
of an oxygenated emulsion of perfluoro-chemicals to the perfusate
increased at nearly identical perfusion flow rates (~13.8ml $\cdot$g^{-1}
$\cdot$min^{-1}) oxygen consumption as well as Na$^+$ reabsorption by about
80% (Franke et al., 1978).

ANOXIA AND POST-ANOXIC RECOVERY: Renal Na$^+$ reabsorption, which
depends on the provision of metabolic energy, declined rapidly in
the time course of perfusions performed at a pO_2 <1mmHg (Fig. 3A).
Glomerular filtration, which derived its energy from the perfusion
pressure, declined much slower within 60min of anoxic perfusion.
Structural damage was indicated by a marked increase in the urinary
loss of enzymes (Fig. 3B): cytoplasmatic lactate dehydrogenase
(LDH, EC 1.1.1.27), which leaked also into the perfusate, at a
lower rate than γGT from intraluminal brush border microvilli.
Similar time courses of enzyme leakage have been observed in
anoxic tubular segments from the rat kidney cortex (Gronow et al.,
1985), indicating that disruptive swelling at the cellular level
also limited organ functions in the anoxic rat kidney.

The urinary loss of protein was even more striking (Fig. 3B),
indicating that, at decreasing glomerular filtration rates, a
marked increase in the glomerular sieving coefficient (GSC)
occurred during anoxia (aerobic controls: 20.1µg protein $\cdot$g^{-1}
$\cdot$min^{-1}; GSC $\cdot$100 =0.05%; 60min anoxia: 80mg$\cdot$protein $\cdot$g^{-1}$\cdot$60min^{-1};
GSC $\cdot$100 =1.2%). This reduced efficiency of the glomerular filter
in restricting the passage of high molecular proteins has also
been observed in the rat kidney in vivo during surgical treatment
(Baumann, 1981), indicating again a high susceptibility of the
rat kidney to experimental conditions which may induce renal
hypoxia (Balaban and Sylvia, 1981).

To test whether the post-anoxic reversibility of renal functions correlated with the observed urinary loss of cell consti-
tuents, glomerular filtration rate (GFR) and Na$^+$ reabsorption
(T-Na$^+$, %T-Na$^+$) were measured after up to 60min of normothermic
anoxia and subsequent reoxygenation (Fig. 3C). Apparently, all 3
functional parameters correlated in an exponential manner with
the urinary loss of γGT (and thus also with the preceding anoxic
time interval). Thus, the observed significant depression of renal
functions during acute anoxia (Fig. 3A) was reversible only up

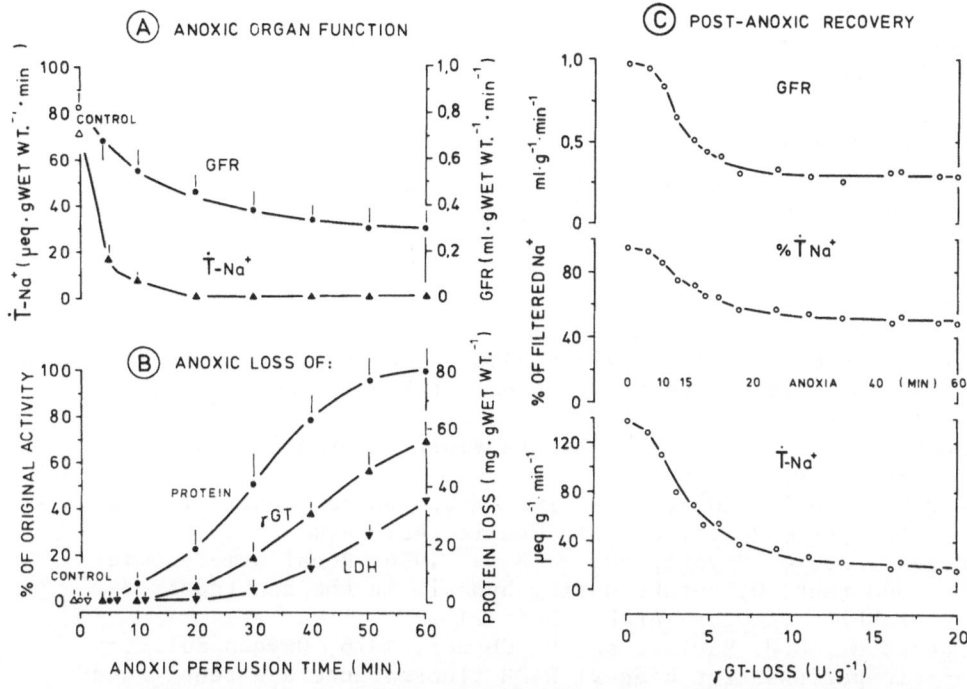

Fig. 3 Anoxic organ functions (a) and urinary loss of protein
and enzymes (B) in the time course of 60min of anoxic
perfusion (pO$_2$ <1mmHg), and (C) post-anoxic recovery of
renal functions (pO$_2$∿680mmHg) in relation to the cumulative
loss of γGT (=γglutamyltransferase, EC 2.3.2.2) in the
isolated perfused rat kidney (38°C). Mean ±SD perfusion
pressure 100 ±4mmHg; A+B: no substrates added, C: in the
presence of 10mM glucose and 9 amino acids, 2mM each.
LDH =lactate dehydrogenase (EC 1.1.1.27), GFR =glomerular
filtration rate, T-Na$^+$ =absolute, and %T-Na$^+$ =fractional
rate of Na reabsorption ($\bar{x}$±SD, n=7).

to 5min after the onset of anoxia, or when the cumulative γGT-loss
did not exceed 1 U γGT·g^{-1}. The presence of oxygen radical scaven-
gers (10mM mannitol, 5mM arginine, 5mM methionine) and of oxygen
radical converting enzymes (100mU superoxide dismutase ·ml^{-1};
100mU catalase ·ml^{-1}) in the perfusate of a post-anoxic (20min)
rat kidney did not only reduce significantly the urinary loss of
γGT by -22.8 ±4.6% (n=4), but increased also GFR (+14.3 ±3.7%) and
the absolute rate of Na$^+$ reabsorption (+11.9 ±4.5%) in comparison
to 5 kidneys which were reoxygenated with a perfusate containing
no additives. Thus, similar to the effect of hyperbaric reoxygenation on myocardial cells (Gauduel and Duvelleroy, 1984), the observed irreversible reduction of renal functions after 20min of

anoxia appeared to me bediated, at least in part, by the toxic act-
tion of hyperbaric oxygen in the perfusate of the isolated perfused
rat kidney.

ACKNOWLEDGMENT

The excellent technical assistance of Mrs. M. Quinten is gratefully
acknowledged.

REFERENCES

Balaban, R.S., and A.L. Sylvia, 1981, Spectrophotometric monitoring
    of O_2 delivery to the exposed rat kidney. Am. J. Physiol.,
    241: F257.
Baumann, K., 1981, in: "Renal transport of organic substances",
    Springer, Berlin.
Bergmeyer, H.U. (Ed.), 1974, in: "Methoden der enzymatischen
    Analyse", Vol. I and II, Chemie, Weinheim.
Bursaux, E., C. Poyart, and B. Bohn, 1976, Renal hemodynamics
    and renal O_2 uptake during hypoxia in the anesthetized
    rabbit. Pflügers Arch., 365: 213.
Franke, H., C.H. Barlow, and B. Chance, 1976, Oxygen delivery
    in perfused rat kidney: NADH fluorescence and renal func-
    tional state. Am. J. Physiol., 231: 1082.
Franke, H., M. Mályusz, and D. Runge, 1978, Improved sodium and
    PAH transport in the isolated fluorocarbon-perfused rat
    kidney, Nephron, 22: 423.
Gauduel, Y., and M.A. Duvelleroy, 1984, Deleterious effects of
    oxygen radicals on reoxygenated myocardial cells.
    Adv. Exp. Med. Biol. 169: 421.
Gronow, G., P. Benk, and H. Franke, 1985, Effects of anaerobic
    substrates on post-anoxic cellular function in isolated
    tubular segments of rat kidney cortex. in: "Oxygen transport
    to tissue", Vol. VI, Adv. Exp. Med. Biol., Plenum, New York
    (in print).
Gronow, G.H.J., and J.J. Cohen, 1984. Substrate support for renal
    function during hypoxia in the perfused rat kidney.
    Am. J. Physiol. (in print).
Maack, T., 1980, Physiological evaluation of the isolated perfused
    rat kidney. Am. J. Physiol., 238: F71.
Nizet, A., Y. Cuypers, P. Deetjen, and K. Kramer, 1967, Functional
    capacity of the isolated perfused dog kidney. Pflügers Arch.
    296: 179.
Ross, B. D., 1978, The isolated perfused rat kidney. Clin. Sc.
    Molec. Med. 55: 513.
Swanson, I.W., A. Besarab, P.P. Pomerantz, and A. DeGuzman, 1981,
    Effect of erythrocytes and globulin on renal functions of the
    isolated rat kidney. Am. J. Physiol., 241: F139.
Zillig, B., G. Schuler, and B. Truninger, 1978, Renal function
    and intrarenal hemodynamics in acutely hypoxic and hypercapnic
    rats. Kidney Int., 14: 58.

REGULATION OF REACTIVE HYPERAEMIA IN THE KIDNEY

M. Kessler[*], J. Höper[*], B. Chance[**],
D.W.Lübbers[***], K.Messmer[****],
and E. Sinagowitz[*]

[*] Institut für Physiologie und Kardiologie
der Universität Erlangen-Nürnberg
Waldstrasse 6, D-8520 Erlangen, FRG
[**] Johnson-Research Foundation
Philadelphia, USA
[***] Max-Planck-Institut für Systemphysio-
logie, Dortmund, FRG
[****] Institut für chirurgische Forschung
Heidelberg, FRG

INTRODUCTION

As shown by Sinagowitz et al. (1977) the behaviour of
postischaemic hyperaemia in the kidney is complex, and
depends on the duration of the ischaemic period. In
order to investigate the relation between the total
renal blood flow (RBF), local oxygen supply and oxygen
uptake rate under these conditions, experiments were
performed in the kidneys of anaesthetized dogs.

METHODS

Twenty experiments were performed in the kidneys of 20
mongrel dogs of both sexes. Mean weight of the animals
was 24.6±5 kg. The animals were anaesthetized with an
intraperitoneal injection of Na-pentobarbital (30mg/kg).

Then, they were intubated and mechanically ventilated with a gas mixture of N_2O and oxygen (3:1). Flow in the renal artery was measured continuously with an electromagnetic flowmeter (Statham SP 1200).
Oxygen uptake was calculated from renal arterial and renal venous oxygen contents determined with a Lex-O_2-Con, and from RBF.
Local pO_2 in the cortex of the kidney was measured by a pO_2-multiwire surface electrode (Kessler and Lübbers, 1966). Intracapillary haemoglobin oxygenation and the redox-state of cytochrome aa_3 were measured with the Rapidspectrometer according to Lübbers and Niesel (1959).
During the postischaemic reactions, 50 spectra/sec were recorded on-line with a Honeywell 560 computer and evaluated after the end of each reaction.
NAD(P)H fluorescence was registered with a fluorometer according to Chance and coworkers (1974). To perform the measurements of NAD(P)H and cyt aa_3 it was necessary to lower the haematocrit of the animals to 10%. Therefore, isovolaemic haemodilution with Dextran-solution was performed at the beginning of the experiment and was kept constant throughout.
In one series of experiments the renal artery was clamped for 1, 10, 20 or 30 min and the postischaemic reactions of RBF, local pO_2 and O_2-uptake were measured. In a second series of experiments, the renal artery was clamped for 60 sec. After application of the clamp, 100 ml Dextran-solution, saturated either with N_2 or with CO were infused into the kidney. 1 min after occlusion, the clamp was released and the above listed parameters were investigated.

RESULTS

In the first series of experiments, in which the renal artery was clamped for different times, RBF, local pO_2 and O_2-uptake were measured during the postischaemic period. Fig. 1 shows the relation between RBF and local pO_2 during the postischaemic period after clamping the artery for 1 min and 30 min; when tissue pO_2 reached control values, RBF also returned to a normal range after an initial hyperaemic period. Fig.2 presents the corresponding values of O_2-uptake, measured 30 and 120 sec after release of the clamp; during the early postischaemic period, O_2-uptake was diminished after renal ischaemia of 20 or 30 min.

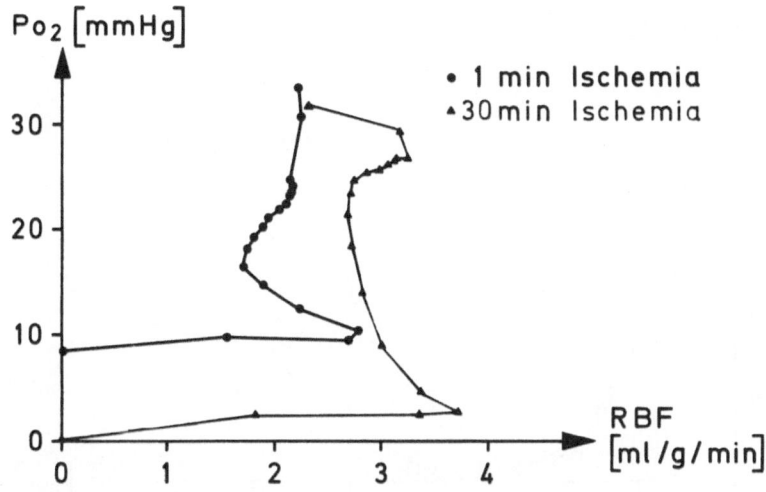

Fig. 1: Relation between RBF and local pO_2

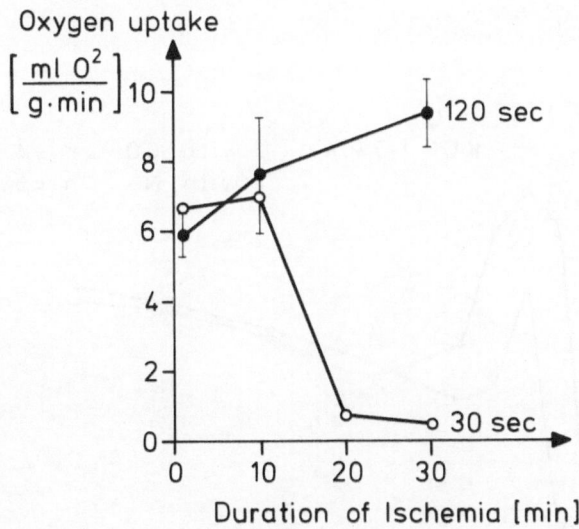

Fig. 2: Postischaemic oxygen uptake of the kidney, measured 30 and 120 sec after release of the clamp.

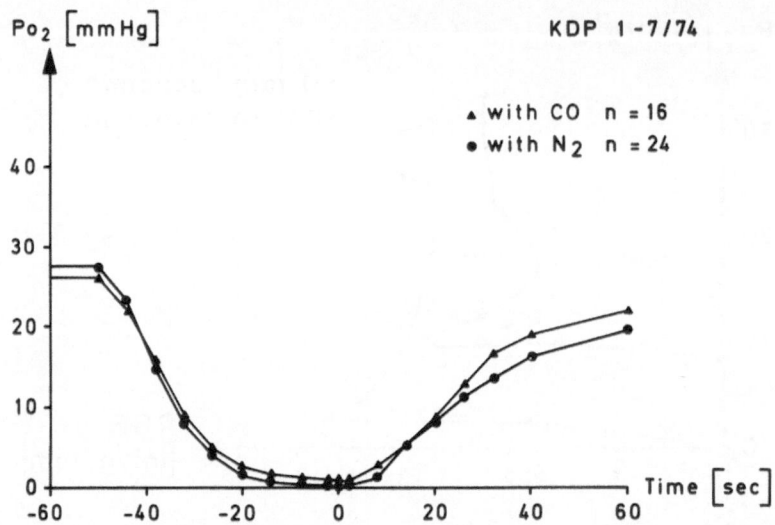

Fig. 3: Change in local pO_2 during (-60 to 0 sec) and after the infusion of N_2- or CO- saturated Dextran-solution into the renal artery proximal to the occlusion. The infusion lasted one minute; after this time ("0" time) the clamp of the renal artery was released.

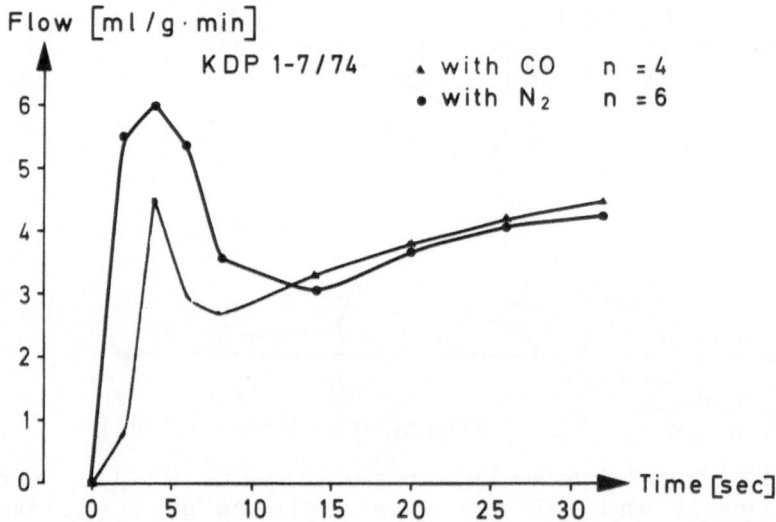

Fig. 4: Increase in RBF after release of the clamp. These reactions were measured simultaneously with the pO_2 values shown in fig. 3 (from "0" time on).

In the second series of experiments, a one minute occlusion of the renal artery was performed. After application of the clamp, 100 ml haemoglobin free solution were infused into the renal artery proximal to the occlusion. The perfusate (Dextran-solution) was saturated with either N_2 or CO.

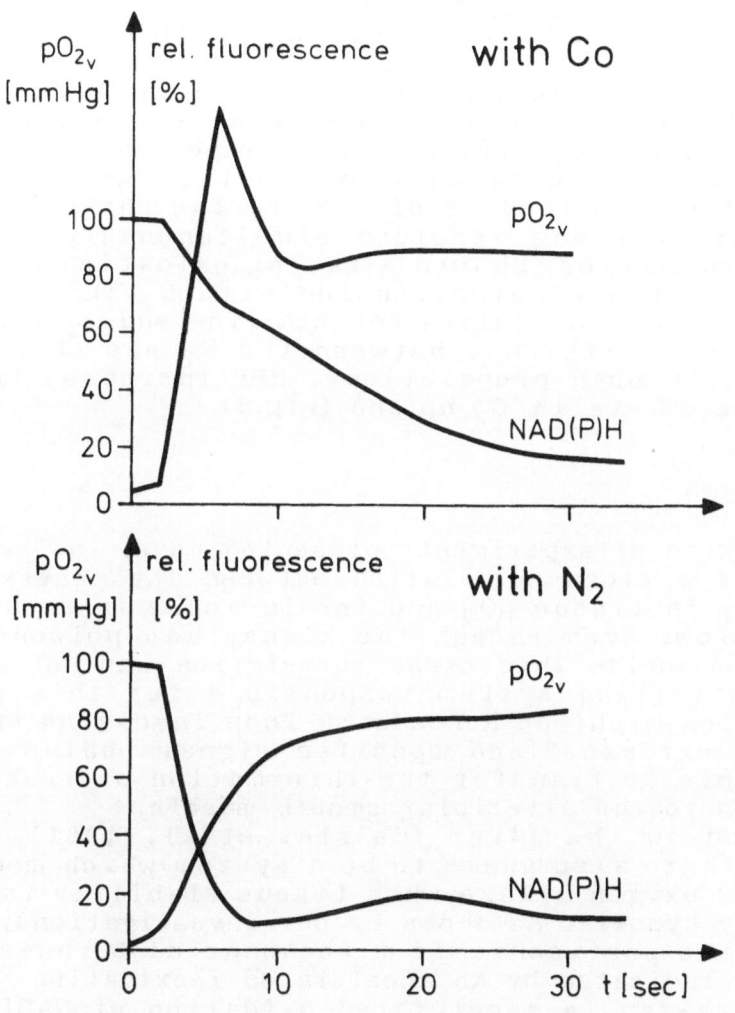

Fig. 5: Simultaneous measurements of NAD(P)H and venous pO_2 after release of the arterial clamp.

In fig.3 the mean values of pO_2 measured in 7 experiments are shown; there were no differences between the two experimental groups. Fig. 4 presents the corresponding postischaemic increase in RBF; the reactive hyperaemia was reduced after infusion of CO-saturated dextran-solution.

Fig.5 depicts the postocclusion changes of venous pO_2 and relative NAD(P)H fluorescence . After infusion of CO-saturated Dextran-solution, the reoxidation of NAD(P)H was much slower than after infusing the N_2-saturated solution. While there was a continuous increase in venous pO_2 after N_2-perfusion, venous pO_2 had an overshoot after perfusion with CO-saturated perfusate.

Fig. 6 shows the results obtained with the Rapidspectrometer. After equilibration with CO a rapid reoxygenation of haemoglobin was observed upon reperfusion, while in the N_2 model a delayed reoxygenation was found. In contrast to the results of fig. 6, the change in redox state of cyt aa_3 recorded simultaneously with the Rapidspectrometer, showed a faster oxidation after CO-perfusion than after perfusion with N_2 (Fig. 7). The postocclusive correlation between flow and O_2-uptake did not show a difference between the N_2 and CO perfused kidneys; in both preparations, RBF increased linearly with increments in O_2-uptake (Fig.8).

DISCUSSION

The results of experiments presented here, indicate that there is a close correlation between the postischaemic recovery in tissue pO_2 and the increase in total renal blood flow. Even though the kidney was poisoned with carbon monoxide this close correlation was not altered. The controlling system responsible for this precise regulation might be a feedback loop involving specific "signal oxidases" and specific signal chains (Höper, 1984) able to transfer the information of tissue oxygenation to the arteriolar smooth muscle.

As found in the liver (Kessler et al. 1981), in the kidney there also seems to be a system which modulates cellular oxygen uptake when tissue viability is threatened by hypoxia. As shown by our investigations, CO can affect the postischaemic mitochondrial turnover rate; this is indicated by an accelerated reoxidation of cytochrome aa_3 and a decelerated oxidation of NAD(P)H. Our

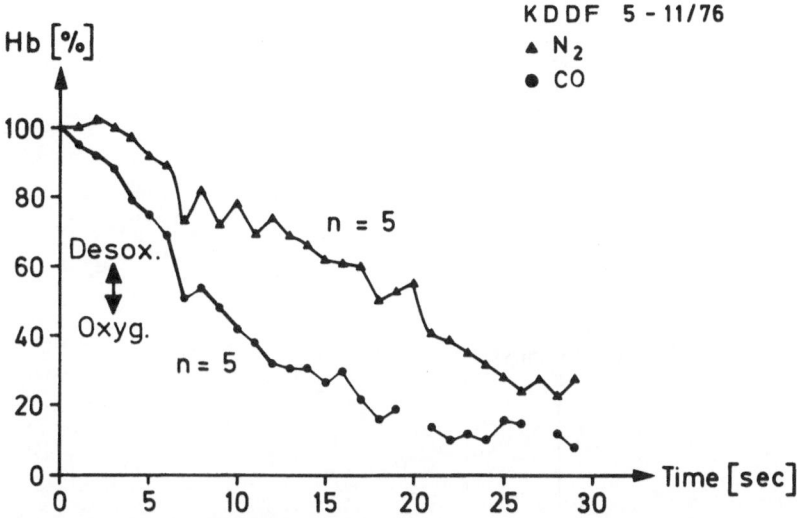

Fig. 6: Reoxygenation of haemoglobin during the postischaemic period.

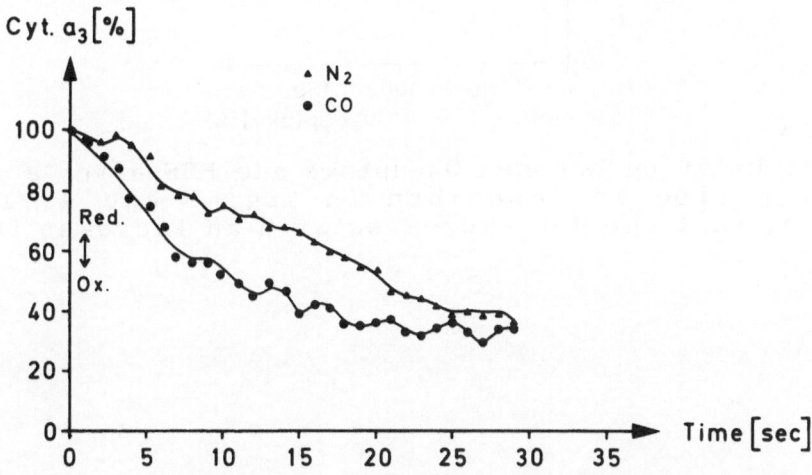

Fig. 7: Postischaemic reoxidation of cyt aa_3. In contrast to the slow oxidation of $NAD(P)H$; the oxidation of cyt.aa_3 occured faster after CO-anoxia.

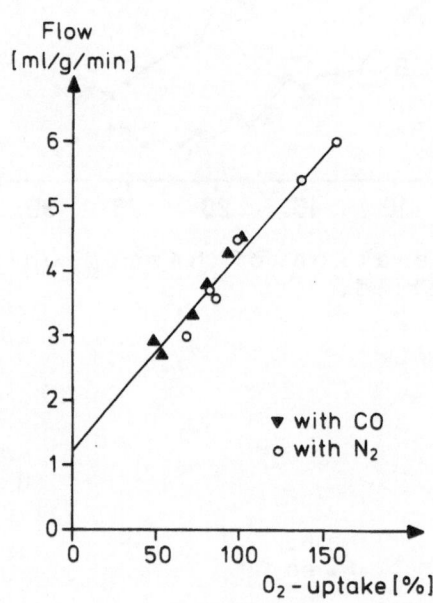

Fig. 8: Relation between O_2-uptake and RBF after a short anoxic period as described in fig. 3 and 4. It is evident, that the RBF increases with an increase in O_2-uptake.

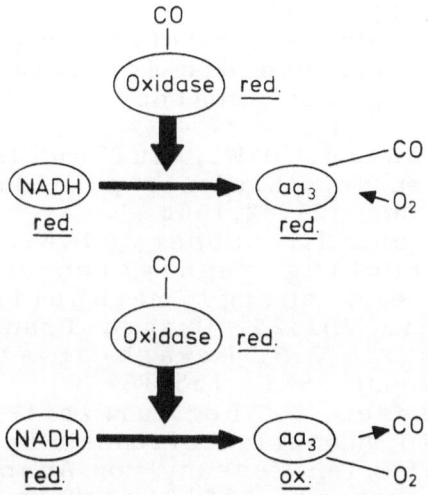

Fig. 9: CO seems to be able to influence the turnover rate of the respiratory chain by a mechanism independent of the redox state of cytochrome oxidase.

observation seems to support the concept that a mitochondrial "signal oxidase" may exist, which can decrease the rate of cellular oxygen uptake.

Our findings are summarized in a hypothetical scheme (Fig. 9): A modulating "signal oxidase" which could be located at the outer mitochondrial membrane, may influence the electron flow through the respiratory chain.

REFERENCES

Chance, B., Mayewsky, A., Goodwin, C., Mela, L.,
    Factors in oxygen delivery to tissue. Microvasc.
    Res., 8,276-282,1974
Höper, J., Einfluß der Sauerstoffversorgung auf das
    Membranpotential und die intercelluläre elektri-
    sche Koppelung von Hepatocyten, Thesis, Erlangen
    1984
Kessler, M., Lübbers, D.W., Aufbau und Anwendungs-
    möglichkeiten verschiedener pO_2-Elektroden.
    Pflügers Arch. 291,82,1966
Kessler, M., Höper, J., Lübbers, D.W., Ji, S. Local
    factors affecting regulation of microflow,
    O_2 uptake and energy metabolism. In: Adv.
    Physiol. Sci. Vol.25. Oxygen Transport to
    Tissue. Eds.: A.G.B. Kovach et al., Akademiai
    Kiado, Budapest 1981, 155-162
Lübbers, D.W., Niesel, W., Der Kurzzeit-Spektralana-
    lysator. Ein schnellarbeitendes Spektralphotome-
    ter zur laufenden Messung von Absorptions- bzw.
    Extinktionsspektren. Pflügers Arch. 268,
    286-295, 1959
Sinagowitz, E., Höper, J., Krumme, B., Kessler, M.,
    Postischemic regulation of oxygen supply in
    the renal cortex. Urol. Res. 5,39,1977.

692

CONTROL OF O_2 SUPPLY TO THE STIMULATED EXOCRINE PANCREAS

H.J.M. Beijer, A.J.G. Holtgrefe, and M. Woerlee

Exp. Lab. Peripheral Circulation and
Dept. of Theoretical Biology, University of Utrecht
Catharijnesingel 101, Utrecht, The Netherlands

The involvement of blood flow in metabolic activity was investigated in the exocrine pancreas in the anesthetized dog using secretin as the specific stimulus. After a bolus injection of secretin (1 U/kg) the exocrine secretion as well as the O_2 consumption were increased in the same way. The increased O_2 supply was accomplished by changes of blood flow and/or O_2 extraction: during the build-up of the response (first 2 min) blood flow was increased before or simultaneous with the increase of secretion. At the same time O_2 extraction decreased, which is quite unexpected during stimulation of the metabolic O_2 demand. During the 2nd phase (2-16 min) blood flow returned to its initial level very rapidly, while O_2 extraction continued to rise. During the 3rd phase (16-30 min) secretion returned to its initial level, as did O_2 consumption and O_2 extraction. The explanation of these phenomena was sought in the theory of the metabolic control of tissue oxygenation, which describes flow and diffusion capacity being controlled by the tissue PO_2: a lowering of tissue PO_2 to a level below which the O_2 availability limits the effective aerobic ATP production will create a feedback signal that lowers arteriolar resistance and/or increases the diffusion capacity of the tissue, thus increasing the O_2 supply and maintaining the tissue oxygenation. This explanation was evaluated by computer-simulation of data: RESULTS. The build up of the responses could be mimicked completely by setting the time constants so that the blood flow was increased 8 to 16 times faster than the diffusion capacity was. Thus the contradictory lowering of the O_2 extraction during the build-up of the O_2 demand could be explained by assuming: 1. a slowly increasing diffusion capacity (that is the main source of O_2 supply during the 2nd and 3rd phase) and 2. a fast increase of blood flow, that is the main source of O_2 supply during the first phase. During steady state secretion (2-16 min) the simulation yielded data different from the experimental data: because of the lowered tissue O_2 level in this interval, the model maintains a feedback signal to both arteriolar resistance and diffusion capacity. Thus blood flow is calculated to be enhanced. In the experiments blood flow returns to its initial level at about 10 min. Therefore either another control system may maintain blood flow at its initial level, or arteriolar resistance and diffusion capacity exhibit different sensitivities to the mediators of the feedback signal, or different mediators may be involved in the control of resistance and diffusion.

CONCLUSIONS. 1. The theory of the metabolic control of tissue oxygenation provides a good explanation for the observed increase in blood flow and change in O_2 extraction in the stimulated pancreas. 2. Long term control is exerted mainly by a change of the diffusion capacity of the tissue. 3. Short term control - if needed - is exerted by change of arteriolar resistance.

In previous studies [2,3] we have observed that secretin - the hormone specifically stimulating the exocrine pancreas- induces an increase in the exocrine secretory activity as well as an increase in blood flow to the pancreas. This increased blood flow was confined to the pancreas.[1] The increase in metabolic activity was seen at lower stimulus levels than an increase in blood flow. If - at high stimulus level- an increase in blood flow occurred, this increased blood flow took place a few tens of seconds before the increase in metabolic activity.[2] These observations suggested that the metabolic rate is involved in the control of blood flow of the pancreas. Therefore a study was performed to outline the relation between metabolic rate, O_2 supply and O_2 demand in the exocrine pancreas.[3]

METHODS. Eleven dogs were used, anesthesia was performed with sodium pentobarbital. Arterial pressure was measured and found constant throughout the entire experiment. The three arteries supplying the pancreas were dissected free. Measurement of blood flow was performed with electromagnetic flowmeters (Skalar). Blood samples from the venous outflow of the pancreas and arterial blood samples were analyzed on an Acid Base Laboratory 2 (Radiometer), yielding the $a-vO_2$ concentration difference (= O_2 extraction). Instantaneous flow times instantaneous O_2 extraction yielded O_2 consumption. The main pancreatic duct was cannulated, to measure secretory flow by drop counting. The HCO_3^- concentration in the secretory juice was measured. Secretin (1 U/kg.i.v.) was used to stimulate the secretory process.

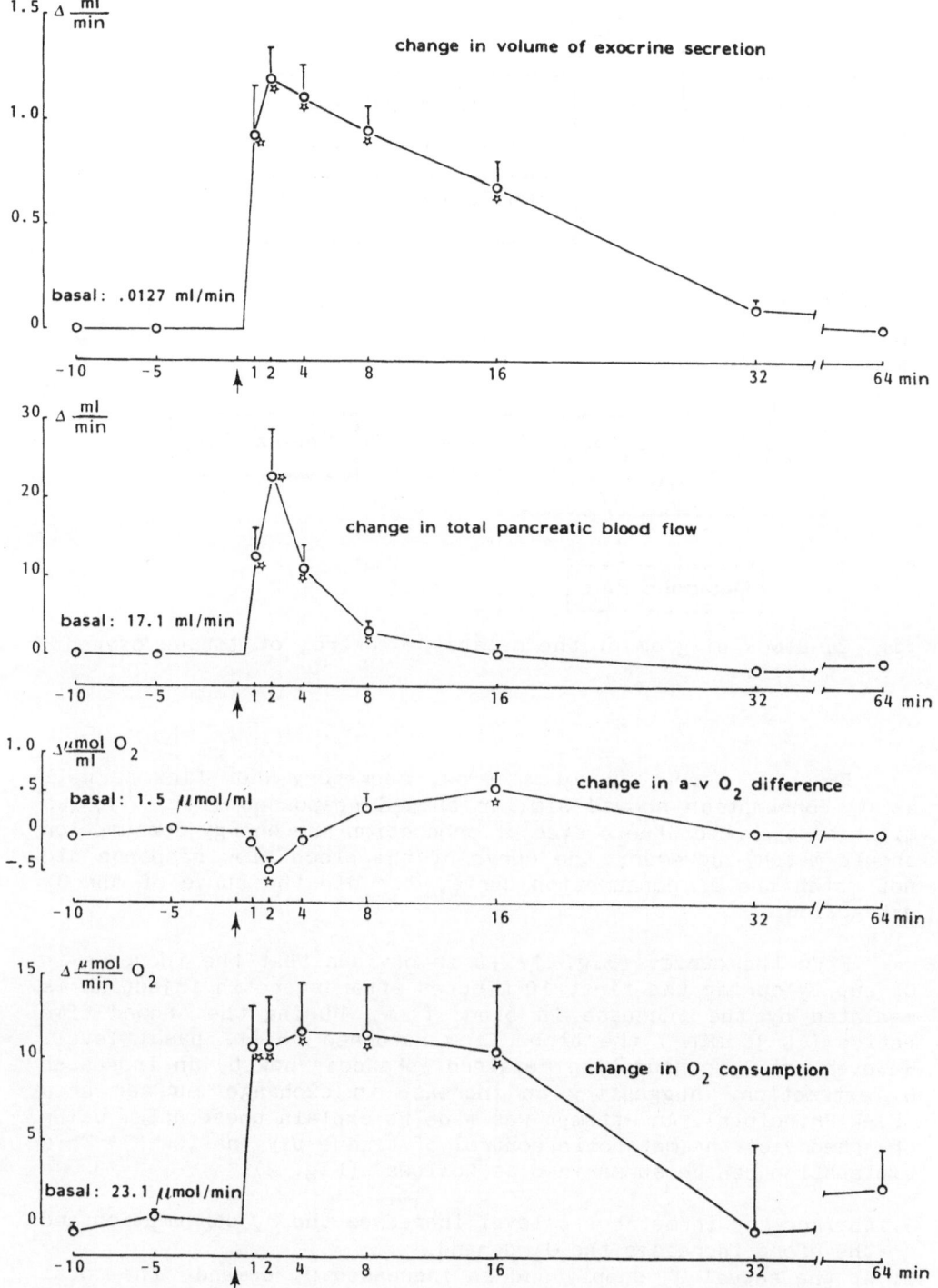

Fig. 1. Changes in the metabolic variables of the pancreas, as stimulated by secretin (1 U/kg, i.v., at arrow).

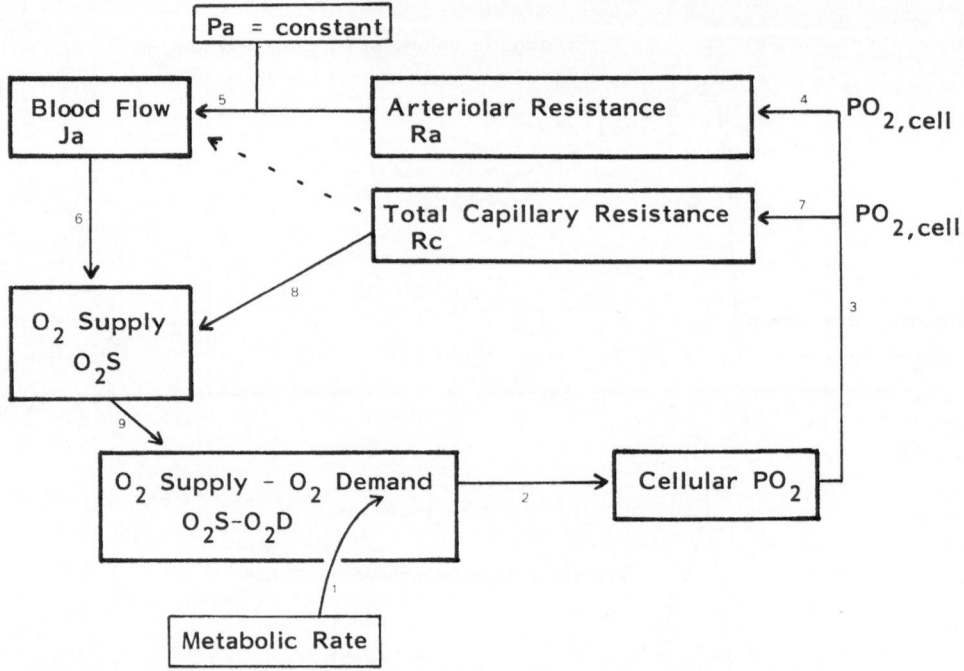

Fig. 2. Block diagram of the metabolic control of tissue oxygenation.

RESULTS. Secretory volume flow, secretory HCO_3^- flow as well as O_2 consumption showed similar shaped responses (Fig. 1), as might be expected: the curves of production and energy consumption should match. However, the curve of the blood flow response did not match the O_2 consumption curve, nor did the curve of the O_2 extraction.

From the curves (Fig. 1) it is obvious that the increase in O_2 supply during the first 10 minutes after secretin injection is mediated by the increase in blood flow. During the second time period (10-30 min.) the blood flow returned to its basal level. However the O_2 consumption remained enhanced, now by an increased O_2 extraction, suggesting an increase in exchange surface area (Fick Principle). An attempt was made to explain these data, using the theory of the metabolic control of tissue oxygenation.[4-9] This explanation can be summarized as follows[3] (Fig. 2).

1. An increase in metabolic level increases the O_2 consumption and therefore increases the O_2 demand.
2. At the actual O_2 supply and an increased O_2 demand, the local cellular PO_2 will decrease.

3. The pivotal idea of the theory of the metabolic control of the tissue oxygenation is that upon a decrease of the cellular PO_2, the organ responds with a feedback, that will:
4. Decrease in the arterial resistance (thus 5: increasing blood flow i.e. 6: increasing O_2 supply) and 7: will increase capillary density (i.e. increase in the exchange surface area), and thus 8: will increase the O_2 supply to the tissue. An increase in O_2 supply together with the increased O_2 demand will restore cellular PO_2 towards normal values. Thus the tissue is capable to prevent a deleterious cellular hypoxia.

The cellular PO_2 is of crucial importance: the metabolic control mechanisms maintain the cellular PO_2 above its critical level, i.e. above that PO_2 level below which O_2 availability limits the efficient aerobic production of ATP.

In our experiments this explanation may be applied, although the increase of arterial blood flow and the increase of exchange surface area presumably show no concomitant rises because increase of blood flow occurred before the increase of O_2 extraction (an increased O_2 extraction at constant blood flow indicates an increase in exchange surface area, with an increase in metabolic level).

However there is a snake in the grass: against this - only qualitative - explanation there may be expressed a serious objection. In our experiments, the O_2 extraction was significantly decreased during the maximum increase of blood flow at 2 minutes after the injection of secretin. This may be explained as an uncontrolled response. Arteriolar resistance then would decrease to an absolute minimum, allowing the blood to flow very fast through the capillary bed. Thus the blood would leave the exchange area rather unused. Even a shunting phenomenon, i.e. opening of non-nutritive channels, may explain the decrease of O_2 extraction.

Thus the question raised was: can the controversial decrease of O_2 extraction be explained by the theory of the metabolic control of tissue oxygenation, or: is the decrease in O_2 extraction seriously contradicting a metabolic control?

We have tested this controversy, using the mathematical model of the metabolic control of tissue oxygenation (Fig. 3), kindly provided by Dr. AP Shepherd and Dr. HJ Granger. This program was implemented on a PDP 11/55 in the Computer Department of the University Hospital Utrecht. The program describes the model of metabolic control in the skeletal muscle. Of course the organ parameters of a skeletal muscle and a pancreas are different, so first we calibrated basal values of the blood flow, O_2 extraction and O_2 consumption in the mathematical model to the basal values observed

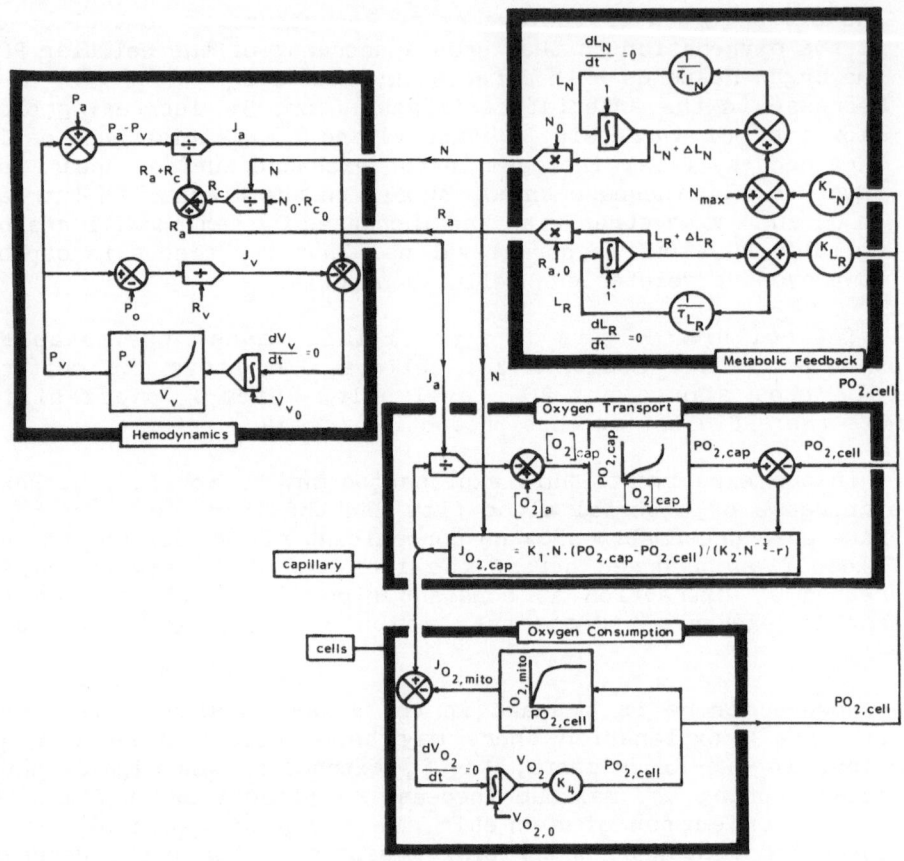

Fig. 3. System diagram, showing the interrelationship between hemodynamics, O_2 transport, O_2 consumption and metabolic control of arterioles and precapillary sphincters, modified after Shepherd and Granger.

in the experiments:

variable	basal values exp.	model
blood flow	28.5	28.6 ml/min/100 g
O_2 extraction	0.0382*	0.0341
O_2 consumption	0.980	0.976 ml/O_2/min/100 g

*In the experiments the mean value of the O_2 extraction (0.0382) was slightly different from mean O_2 consumption/mean blood flow (0.98/28.5 = 0.0344). This is caused by the variations between the individual experiments, i.e. by the more or less skewness of the distributions of the blood flow data and the O_2 extraction data. So the simulation of the basal values yielded a fit that was quite good.

Simulation of the responses required adjustments in a different section: the feed back section. In this section the parameters are:
KLR and KLN: the coefficients for the participation of arteriolar
resistance (KLR) and capillary density (KLN) in the local control
of the O_2 supply. The response is rather insensitive to changes
in KLR or KLN.

τLR = time constant for the rate of the arteriolar resistance
        response.
τLN = time constant for the rate of the capillary density respon-
        se.
These parameters determine the shape of the response, i.e. the
rate at which a new equilibrium is achieved. They do not affect
the values of the new equilibrium.

The application of the secretin stimulus was simulated in the
model by increasing the O_2 consumption stepwise from 0.98 to 1.48
ml O_2/min/100 g. The simulation was continued for 16 minutes i.e.
as long as the O_2 consumption in the experiments remained fairly
constant (Fig. 4).

The model calculates the mitochondrial O_2 consumption (=J02M)
and the O_2 flux from the capillaries to the tissue (=J02C). In the
second box (Fig. 3) the J02M and the J02C curves are plotted together.

At the moment of the stimulation, the mitochondrial O_2 consumption is increased stepwise, as instructed. The next half
minute the mitochondria consume nearly all the O_2 that is dissolved in cell plasma, while the increase in O_2 flux from the capillaries into the tissue still only is in its starting phase. Therefore the local -small- storage of O_2 is depleted, i.e. the mitochondrial O_2 consumption (box 2) is lowered, as well as cellular
PO_2 (box 4), that is lowered from 4.5 to 1.1 mmHg. In the model
this lowering of PO2CEL is the pivotal stimulus for the feed back,
to lower arteriolar resistance and to increase capillary density,
leading to an increase in O_2 flux from capillary to tissue (box
3). After 1 minute the O_2 flux from the capillaries to the tissue
rises above the mitochondrial O_2 consumption. From this moment on
there is a small overshoot of O_2, repleting the small store of O_2
dissolved in the cell plasma and thus increasing the PO2CEL (box
4).

The increase in O_2 supply is achieved by an increase of blood
flow and an increase in capillary density. If the time constants
(τLR and τLN) for these responses were set equal, then the increase in blood flow and the increase in O_2 extraction, respectively the increase in capillary density occurred simultaneously: no
decrease of O_2 extraction was calculated by the model. However, if

699

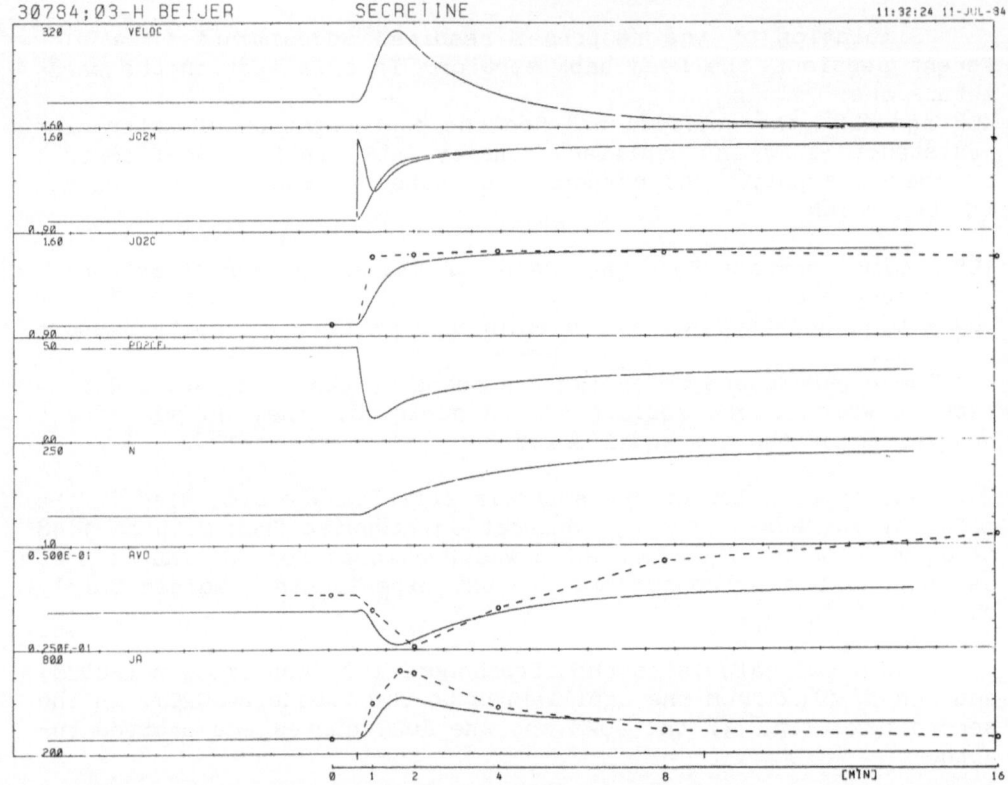

Fig. 4. Simulation of the experimental data by the mathematical
        model of the metabolic control of tissue oxygenation.
        Dotted lines = experimental data
        Solid lines = simulated curves

the response rate of the arteriolar resistance was set faster
than the response rate of the capillary density, then an initial
lowering of O_2 extraction was calculated by the model. Thus if the
response rate of the arteriolar resistance was set 16 times faster
than the response rate of the capillary density, a rather good fit
of the blood flow and O_2 extraction curves was obtained, at least
for the first 5 minutes after the stimulation. Between 5 and 16
minutes, the simulation yielded a blood flow higher than basal
level. This contrasts with the experiments, in which the blood
flow did return to its basal level at about 10 minutes and remained constant. A corresponding contrast is seen in the O_2 extraction curves: the higher blood flow and the identical oxygen
consumption in the simulated curves, compared to the experimental
ones, yielded a lower O_2 extraction in the simulated curves.

700

	Steady state at 16 minutes	
variable	exp.	model
blood flow	28.7	37.4 ml/min/100 g
O_2 extraction	0.0524	0.0397
O_2 consumption	1.417	1.482 ml/O_2/min/100 g

Trying to understand this phenomenon, we may postulate a few explanations:

a. The pancreas may possess another feed back system - probably a neural one - that is trying to maintain the blood flow at its basal level.

b. May be the - unknown - mediators of the feed back signal are different in nature, or may be the sensitivity of the two effector systems (arteriolar resistance and capillary density) to these mediators are different, so that in the long run the arteriolar resistance is rather insensitive to the feed back mediator, compared to the capillary density.

These experiments suggest that when the metabolic level is increased at steady state, the increase in O_2 supply is completely provided by the increase in the exchange surface area. But the process of increasing this exchange surface area seems to be a slow one, compared to the increase of blood flow. These experiments also suggest that this increase in blood flow is called upon when the metabolic level is increasing so fast that the increase of the exchange surface area is not able to cope with the required increase in O_2 demand.

It is concluded that:

1. The theory of the metabolic control of tissue oxygenation can explain the observed increase in blood flow, the controversial decrease of O_2 extraction and the increase of O_2 extraction in the secretin stimulated pancreas.

2. Long term control of tissue oxygenation is achieved mainly by changing the diffusion capacity of the tissue, but this process is a rather slow one.

3. Short term control of tissue oxygenation may be achieved by a change in arteriolar resistance, leading to an increase in blood flow. This process is a rather fast one and may be called upon at a fast stimulation of the metabolic O_2 demand.

Literature

1. H.J.M. Beijer, P.F. Hulstaert, F.A.S. Brouwer and G.A. Charbon. The effect of secretin on peripheral arterial blood flow. Arch. Int. Pharmacodyn. Ther. 240: 269-277, 1979.

2. H.J.M. Beijer, F.A.S. Brouwer and G.A. Charbon. Time course and sensitivity of secretin-stimulated pancreatic secretion and blood flow in the anesthetized dog. Scand.J. Gastroent. 14: 295-300, 1979.

3. H.J.M. Beijer, A.H.J. Maas and G.A. Charbon. Pancreatic O_2 consumption and CO_2 output during secretin-induced, exocrine secretion from the pancreas in the anesthetized dog. Pflügers Arch. 400: 318-323, 1984.

4. H.J. Granger and A.P. Shepherd. Intrinsic microvascular control of tissue oxygen delivery. Microvasc. Res. 5: 49-72, 1973.

5. H.J. Granger and A.P. Shepherd. Dynamics and control of the microcirculation. Adv. Biomed. Engin. 7: 1-63, 1979.

6. H.J. Granger and R.A. Nyhof. Dynamics of intestinal oxygenation: interactions between oxygen sypply and uptake. Am. J. Physiol. 243: G91-G96, 1982.

7. A.P. Shepherd and H.J. Granger. Autoregulatory escape in the gut: a systems analysis. Gastroenterology 65: 77-91, 1973.

8. A.P. Shepherd. Local control of intestinal oxygenation and blood flow. Ann. Rev. Physiol. 44: 13-27, 1982.

9. A.P. Shepherd. Role of capillary recruitment in the regulation of intestinal oxygenation. Am. J. Physiol. 242: G435-G441, 1982.

INFLUENCE OF PORTOCAVAL ANASTOMOSIS (PCA) ON TISSUE PO$_2$ OF RENAL CORTEX AND SKELETAL MUSCLE IN RATS WITH LIVER CIRRHOSIS

T. Brendler, R. Heinrich, S. Dette, M. Günderoth-Palmowski, M. Grein, E. Huber, W. Grauer, W. Fleckenstein, and H. Schomerus

Medizinische Universitätsklinik Tübingen
Otfried-Müller-Strasse 10, 74 Tübingen (FRG)

Portocaval anastomosis in the rat leads to a time-limited hyperperfusion of the skeletal muscle due to an increase of cardiac output. Although it is known that PCA in rats changes intrarenal perfusion to dimished relative cortical perfusion (Grün et al., 1976) resembling cirrhosis-induced perfusion changes in man (Kew et al., 1971), there is no influence on PO$_2$ distribution and mean tissue PO$_2$ on the renal cortex (Grein et al., 1984). Pharmacologically induced liver cirrhosis with spontaneous portal hypertension and consecutive portosystemic shunting in rats also leads to an increase of mean muscular PO$_2$ but mean PO$_2$ on the renal cortex declines (Dette et al., 1984).

The purpose of this study was to find out what influence PCA has on PO$_2$ distribution in skeletal muscle and renal cortex of rats with liver cirrhosis.

MATERIAL AND METHODS

To induce liver cirrhosis, 500 mg Thioacetamid (TAA) per liter drinking water were administered to 25 Sprague-Dawley rats for a total of 146 days. A prestage of cirrhosis (direct hepatotoxic damage with fatty degeneration of liver cells) is present after 40 - 50 days; hepatic fibrosis/cirrhosis after 90 days of administration (Bachmann et al., 1980; Brodehl, 1961). In fourteen rats a PCA was performed 90 days after starting TAA according to the procedure described by Bismuth et al. (1963). Eleven rats were sham operated (clamping of the portal vein for 10 to 15 min). All rats were kept under constant environmental conditions, normal daylight rhythm, feeding ad libitum, room temperature of 26° C, constant air humidity. Two animals were kept in one cage. PO$_2$ measurements were done with a platinum multiwire surface electrode according to Kessler and Lübbers (1966). PO_2 histograms were taken between the 7th and 56th postoperative day. Separate recordings were done for right and left abdominal wall muscle and renal cortex. All measurements were done during the steady state of continuous ether anesthesia.

RESULTS

Fig. 1 shows the pooled PO_2 histograms recorded on the surface of the abdominal wall muscle of rats with liver cirrhosis and PCA (right) as well as from sham-operated animals with liver cirrhosis (left) at different postoperative time intervals.

Seven days after PCA mean PO_2 was approximately 41 Torr. With increasing postoperative interval, mean PO_2 rose to 45 Torr (day 22) and decreased to 37 Torr (day 56). Mean muscular PO_2 was approximately 30 Torr at all investigated time intervals after sham operation.

Fig. 2 shows the pooled PO_2 histograms recorded on the renal cortex of rats with liver cirrhosis and PCA (right) and sham operation (left) at different postoperative intervals. After operation mean PO_2 decreased from 38 Torr (day 7) to 32 Torr (day 22). Fifty-six days after PCA mean PO_2 was about 28 Torr.

The mean PO_2 of the sham operated animals is 43 Torr, significantly higher than in the PCA group ($p<0.05$, one tailed t-test) on day 7. In the postoperative course mean PO_2 changed to 39 Torr (day 22) and 35 Torr (day 56). The values are significantly higher than in the PCA group ($p<0.01$ on day 22; $p<0.05$ day 56).

DISCUSSION

PCA in rats leads to a time-limited hyperperfusion of skeletal muscle. In rats with preexisting cirrhosis, an additional PCA leads to a time-limited slight increase of mean muscular PO_2. The postoperative change in muscular PO_2 in these animals resembles that in rats with PCA without liver cirrhosis but is not that marked (Heinrich et al., 1984). This might be due to the hyperdynamic circulation associated with liver cirrhosis. PCA in rats does not influence mean PO_2 and PO_2 distribution on the renal cortex (Grein et al., 1984). Furthermore, pharmacologically induced liver cirrhosis with consecutive spontaneous portosystemic shunting is associated with a decrease of mean PO_2 on the renal cortex with signs of maldistribution. An additional PCA in rats with preexisting liver cirrhosis does not change the continuous decrease of mean PO_2 on renal cortex. This might indicate that only the deterioration of liver function (as a consequence of cirrhosis) leads to changes in mean PO_2 and oxygen distribution of the renal cortex.

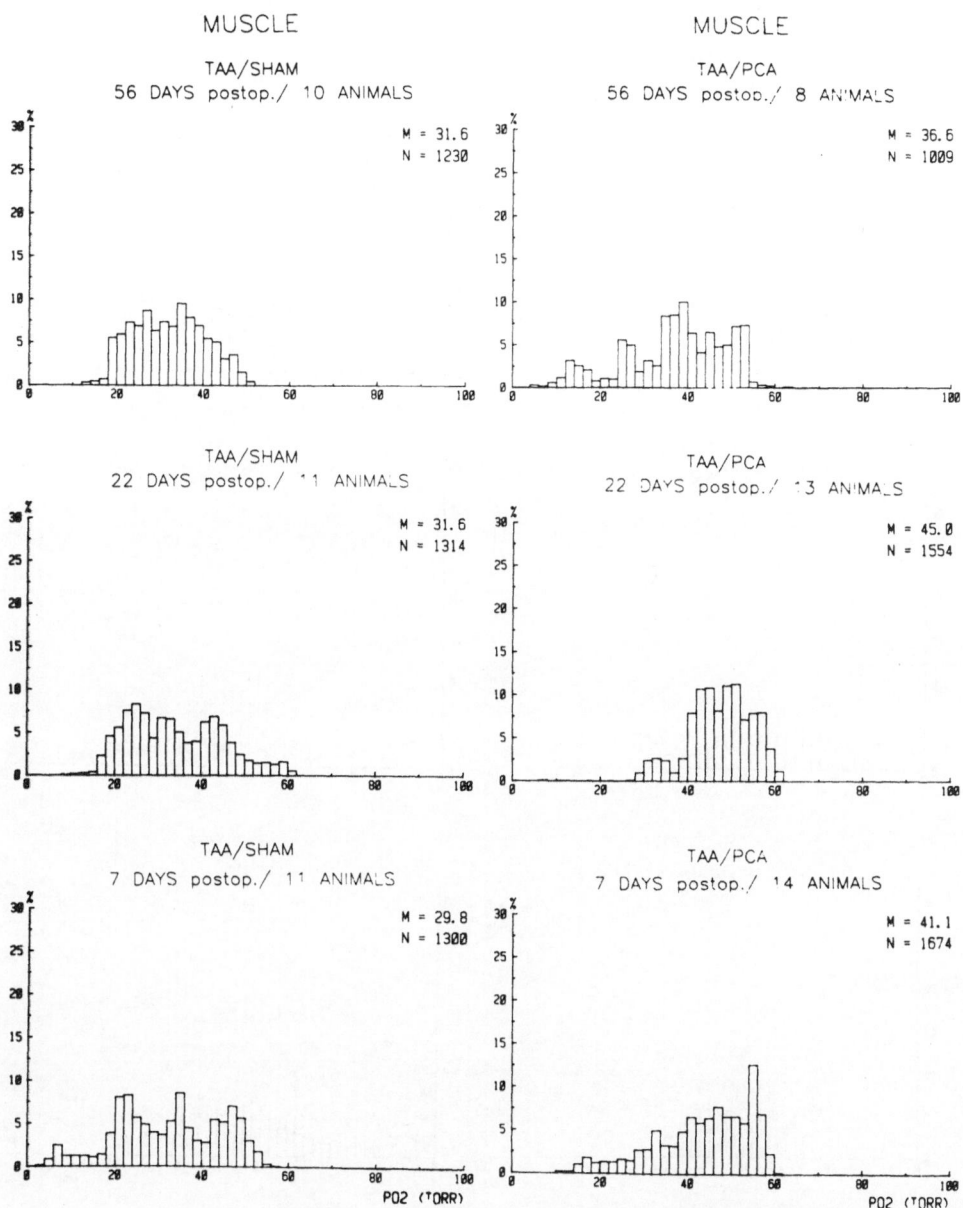

Fig. 1. Pooled histograms of muscle PO_2 at different postoperative intervals. Right side: rats with liver cirrhosis and PCA. Left side: rats with liver cirrhosis and sham operation. N: number of single measurements, M: mean tissue PO_2.

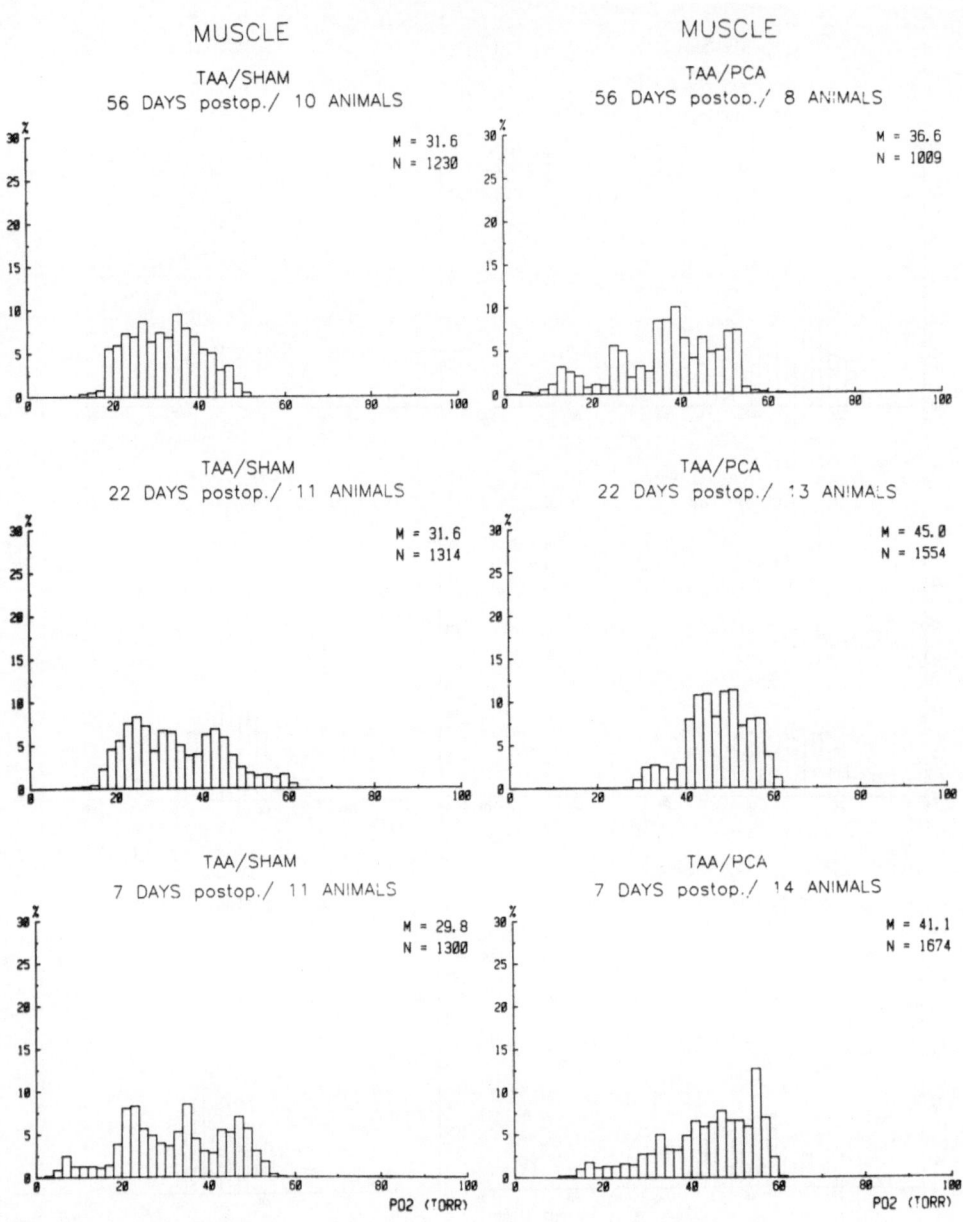

Fig. 2. Pooled PO_2 histograms of renal cortex at different post-operative intervals. Right side: rats with liver cirrhosis and PCA. Left side: rats with liver cirrhosis and sham operation. N: Number of points measured, M: mean tissue-PO_2.

REFERENCES

Bachmann, E., Lindner, J., Grasedyck, K., Eurich, R., 1980, Ratten-
    kollagen bei protrahierter Thioacetamidintoxikation, Arzneim.
    Forsch., 28:226.
Bismuth, H., Benhamou, J.P., Lataste, J., 1963, L'anastomose porto-
    cave expérimental chez le rat normal. Technique et résultats
    préliminaires, Presse Med., 71:1859.
Brodehl, J., 1961, Thioacetamid in der Leberforschung, Klin. Wschr.,
    39:956.
Dette, S., Heinrich, R., Grein, N., Günderoth-Palmowski, M., Grauer,
    W., Schomerus, H., 1984, Messung des Sauerstoffdrucks im
    ruhenden Skelettmuskel und der Niere bei Thioacetamid (TAA)
    behandelten Ratten, Verh. Dtsch. Ges. Inn. Med., 90:1755.
Grein, N., Heinrich, R., Grauer, W., Dette, S., Günderoth, M.,
    Schomerus, H., 1984, Lokaler pO_2 auf der Nierenrinde bei
    Ratten mit portocavaler Anastomose (PCA), Verh. Dtsch. Ges.
    Inn. Med.,90:1523.
Grün, M., Liehr, H., Thiel, H., Rasenack, U., 1976, Effekt einer
    Endotoxinämie auf die renale und intrarenale Hämodynamik
    bei Ratten mit und ohne portokavale Anastomose, Z. Gastro-
    enterol., 76:285.
Heinrich, R., Grauer, W., Schomerus, H., Günderoth, M., Höper, J.,
    Kessler, M., 1984, Measurements of local pO2 in resting
    skeletal muscle of rats with portocaval anastomosis (PCA)
    under normoxic conditions, in: "Oxygen Transport to Tissue-
    VI", D. Bruley, H.I. Bicher and D. Reneau, eds., Plenum
    Publishing Corporation, New York, pp. 623-628.
Kessler, M., and Lübbers, D.W., 1966. Aufbau und Anwendungsmöglich-
    keiten verschiedener pO2 Elektroden. Pflüg. Arch., 291:82.
Kew, M., Brunt, P.W., Varma, R.R., Hourigan, K.J., Williams, H.S.,
    Sherlock, S., 1971, Renal and intrarenal blood flow in
    cirrhosis of the liver, Lancet II:504.

ACKNOWLEDGMENT

This study was supported by grant HE 1293-1 from the Deutsche
Forschungsgemeinschaft.

EXTRACELLULAR pH RESPONSES TO DIFFERENT STIMULI IN THE SUPERFUSED

CAT CAROTID BODY

Marco A. Delpiano and Helmut Acker

Max-Planck-Institut für Systemphysiologie,
Rheinlanddamm 201, D-4600 Dortmund (F.R.G.)

INTRODUCTION AND METHODS

The superfused carotid body responds to a Po_2 decrease or a Pco_2 increase in the superfusion medium with an increase of the chemosensory activity of the sinus nerve. Although many hypotheses have tried to give an adequate explanation, the intrinsic mechanism of the chemoreception has not been elucidated. Among these hypotheses (for review see Belmonte and Gonzalez, 1983), the metabolic hypothesis originating from the Russian school (Anichkov and Belen'kii, 1963) has yielded strong evidence for a linkage between chemoreception and the metabolic energy production in the last years (Joels and Neil, 1963, 1968; Krylov and Anichkov, 1968; Mulligan and Lahiri, 1981; Mulligan et al., 1981). Perturbation of mitochondrial respiration and energy metabolism produced by a Po_2 decrease could be responsible for the neurohumoral secretion from cells, that at last creates chemoreception (Mills and Jöbsis, 1972; Purves, 1970). The implication of the glycolytic pathway in this hypothesis was never seriously considered, since most of the experimental evidence is based on blockers of the mitochondrial respiratory chain and uncouplers of the oxidative phosphorylation (Anichkov and Belen'kii, 1963).

Using double barrelled pH glass microelectrodes (Acker et al., 1982) with a mean tip diameter of 3 /um and inserted in the carotid body tissue via a step motor driven manipulator (Science Trading) we could find that hypoxia caused changes in the pH signal indicating an acidification of the tissue. We would like to present experimental data that hypoxic and hypercapnic chemoreception need glucose for the generating process. Furthermore, we like to discuss a possible synergic interconnection of glycolysis and mitochondrial respiration during the chemosensory process.

The superfused carotid bodies and the recording of the chemosensory nerve activity were prepared as reported elsewhere (Delpiano and Acker, 1980; Eyzaguirre and Lewin, 1961).

Tissue pH was measured in the carotid body under constant pH (7.45 ± 0.02), temperature ($35^{\circ}C$), flow (3.6 ml/min), and osmolality (300 mOsml) of the medium. Change of the Po_2 in the medium from about 188 Torr to 35 or 12 Torr was called hypoxia. Increase of Pco_2 in the medium from about 20 Torr to 70 Torr was called hypercapnia. The pH in the medium was monitored with a pH-macro-electrode (Ingold). The Po_2 in the medium was controlled by a Po_2-needle electrode (Lübbers et al., 1969)

A modified Locke's solution (NaCl, 128; KCl, 5.6; $CaCl_2$, 2.1; D-glucose, 5.5; $NaHCO_3$, 10 and HEPES; 7.0 mmol/l) was freshly prepared before each experiment under constant pH, osmotic, and temperature conditions. In some experiments D-glucose (a. grade, Serva) was replaced by 2-deoxy-D-glucose (grade II, Sigma) or pyruvate (sodium salt, Boehringer) or iodoacetic acid (free acid, Sigma), or succinate (disodium salt, Sigma).

RESULTS AND DISCUSSION

Fig. 1a shows the decrease of the extracellular pH (pHe) and the chemosensory nerve response (nerv. resp.) during hypoxia by lowering the Po_2 in the medium (PmO_2) and during hypercapnia by increasing the Pco_2 in the medium measured as a pH decrease of the medium (pHm) under normal glucose concentration. Immediately after onset of hypoxia, it can be seen in Fig. 1a that the pHe starts to decrease. The pHe decrease amounts to 0.07 units during hypoxia (Fig. 1a). However, changes of about 0.1 pH units were observable dependent on the stimulus intensity. It can also be observed that during hypercapnia the pHm declines by about 0.2 pH units. This pHm change could explain the strong acidification of the tissue observed in Fig. 1a. When the glucose was removed from the Locke's solution and replaced by sucrose to maintain the osmolality constant (300 mOsml), the chemosensory nerve response to hypoxia was inhibited in a time-dependent manner, as shown in Fig. 1b. Not shown here is that the chemosensory nerve response to hypercapnia was also inhibited with zero glucose. Together with the gradual reduction of the hypoxic nerve response, the pHe is also reduced under zero glucose (Fig. 1b). After 3 hours of glucose deprivation, the carotid body was again superfused with normal glucose concentration and both chemosensory nerve response and pHe change were restored, as shown in Fig. 1b. This experiment demonstrates that the Po_2 decrease in the medium induces activation of glycolysis. In this case the pHe decrease may represent lactate production. The glycolysis seems to exist in the carotid body at

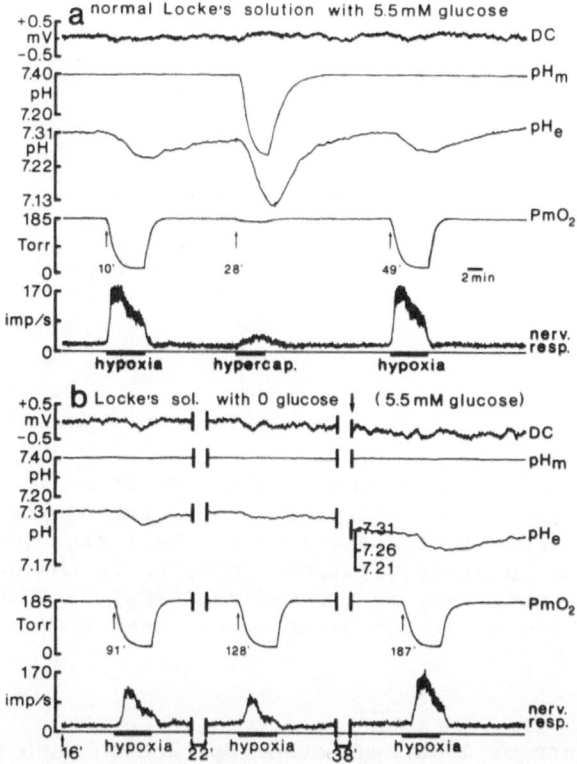

Fig. 1. Chemoreceptor response to hypoxia and hypercapnia during superfusion with normal glucose concentration (5.5 mmol/l) or zero glucose in the medium. Traces from top to below: biopotential signal from DC channel of the pH glass electrode (DC), pH in the medium (pHm), extracellular pH in the carotid body (pHe), Po_2 in the medium (PmO_2), and counted impulses per second of the sinus nerve activity (nerv. resp.). Fig. 1a shows hypoxic and hypercapnic response with normal glucose concentration. Fig. 1b shows time-dependent depression of the hypoxic chemosensory and pHe response during zero glucose.

high Po_2, because, as shown in Fig. 1a, the pHe starts to decrease during hypoxia almost immediately when PmO_2 is still sufficient to maintain tissue oxygenation, as known from earlier studies (Delpiano and Acker, 1980). To prove this hypothesis we blocked glycolysis with 2-deoxyglucose and mono-iodoacetate.

Fig. 2 shows the effect of 2-deoxyglucose when it replaces glucose. After 1 hour, the chemosensory nerve activity is reduced about 50% and after 2 hours about 90%. The pHe change is almost abolished after 2 hours. It is interesting to observe

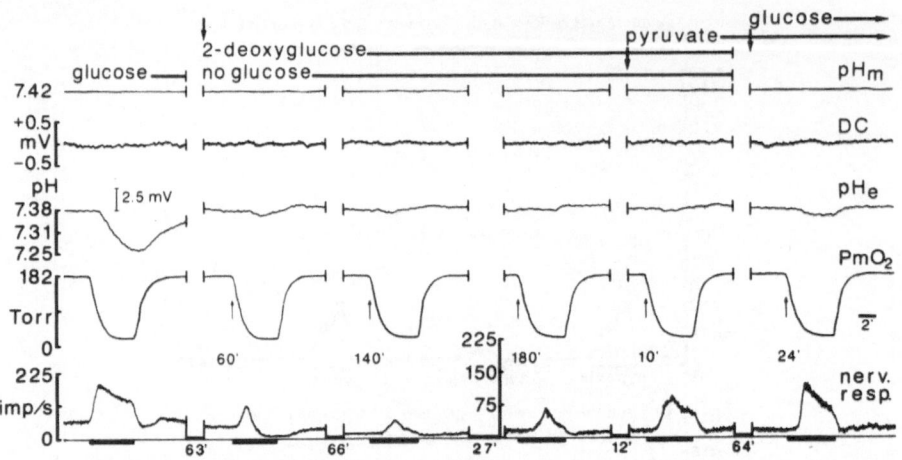

Fig. 2.   Effects of 2-deoxyglucose (5.5 mmol/l) on the extracellular pH and chemosensory nerve activity during hypoxia.
Traces from top to below: pH in the medium (pHm), DC signal from pH glass electrode (DC), pH in the carotid body
tissue (pHe), Po_2 in the medium (PmO_2), and counted impulses per second of the sinus nerve activity (nerv. resp.).

that after 3 hours of 2-deoxyglucose application when the glycolysis is presumably inhibited the chemosensory nerve response is
also substantially inhibited. 2-deoxyglucose also inhibits the
hypercapnic nerve response but not the pHe changes (not shown). Addition of pyruvate to the medium restores partially the hypoxic
chemosensory response but no significant change in the pHe response
could be observed compared with the addition of glucose after 3
hours of 2-deoxyglucose application (Fig. 2). According to this
experiment glucose has two effects on chemoreception: firstly, it
restores lactate production, and secondly, it enhances nerve response at higher Po_2 values than during 2-deoxyglucose application
where the chemosensory response starts slowly at very low PmO_2
values, as shown in Fig. 2.

Fig. 3 shows the effect of iodoacetate on hypoxic and hypercapnic nerve response and pHe changes, respectively. Iodoacetate
blocks irreversibly the nerve chemoreceptor activity and pHe
changes during hypoxia. Anichkov and Belen'kii (1963) could observe
the same effect. They also observed that the acetylcholine response,
which is produced by direct effect on nerve endings, was also depressed. Iodoacetate abolished the spontaneous nerve activity
(Fig. 3), which could be indicative for an additional non-specific
effect on nerve excitability. This could probably then explain an
absence of effect of pyruvate with an iodoacetate concentration of
5.0 mmol/l. The pHe change during hypercapnia is not abolished, because it is only reflecting the pHm change. Finally, the short ini-

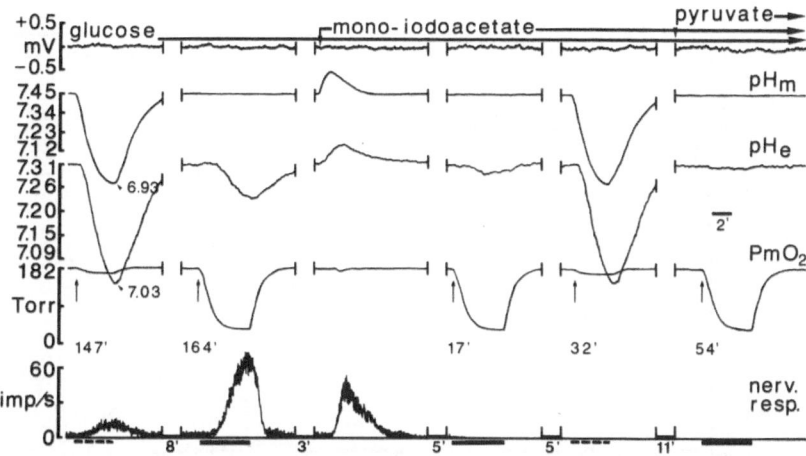

Fig. 3. Effects of mono-iodoacetate (5.0 mmol/l) on extracellular pH and chemosensory nerve activity during hypoxia
and hypercapnia. The parameters from top to bottom are the
same as in Fig. 1.

tial activation of the spontaneous nerve activity produced by iodoacetate could be explained as a Crabtree-like effect, as postulated
in other tissues (Hackenbrock et al., 1971; Packer and Golder,
1960).

The experiments with inhibitors of glycolysis demonstrated
that tissue acidification during hypoxia probably results from
glucose breakdown to lactate formation. This interpretation confirms the findings of other authors who worked with the same glycolytic inhibitors and postulated that a normal course of carbohy-
drate metabolism is indispensable for chemoreceptor excitability
(Winder, 1937; Landgren et al., 1954; Anichkov and Belen'kii, 1963).

The question arises now how pyruvate can overcome glucose deprivation or glycolytic inhibition with 2-deoxyglucose to restore
partially chemosensory nerve response. Fig. 4 shows that pyruvate
restores principally the initial increase of the hypoxic chemosensory nerve response, but this declines very fast during hypoxia
when the low PmO_2 values indicate anaerobic conditions of the
tissue. From this it seems that maintenance of a high response rate
from the nerves during low Po_2 is dependent on an intact anaerobic glucose utilization. From the experiments with 2-deoxyglucose
(Fig. 2) it seems unlikely that pyruvate restores chemoreceptor response through conversion to glucose and further utilization to
lactate pathway or to the pentose cycle, since both are depressed
by this inhibitor (Stanbrook and McMurtry, 1983; Webb, 1966).
Direct conversion of pyruvate to lactate seems to be negligible, as

713

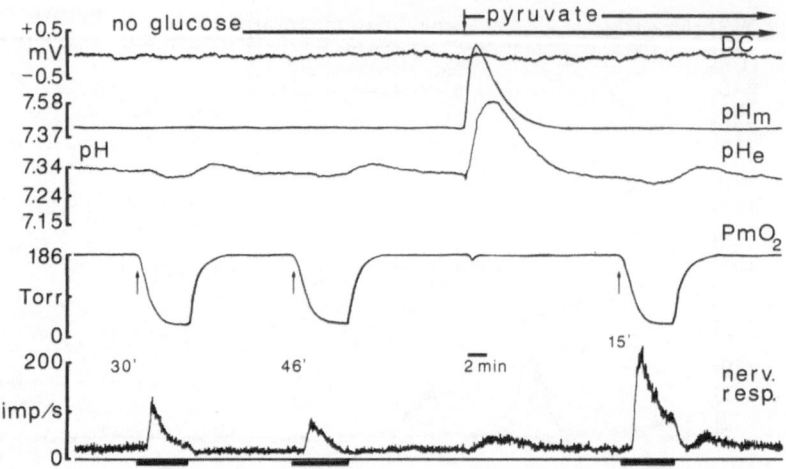

Fig. 4.   Effect of pyruvate (5.5 mmol/l) addition after superfusion
with zero glucose on the extracellular pH and chemosensory response to hypoxia. Traces same as Fig. 1.

the absent pHe response under pyruvate application illustrates
(Fig. 4). More probably, it could be an oxidation of pyruvate in
the citric acid cycle producing CO_2 and providing reducing substrates for mitochondrial respiration.

Bartels (1979) found in the bullock carotid body, which has a
high glycolytic capacity, that succinate increases the O_2 consumption 4-fold compared with the O_2 consumption under glucose conditions. Furthermore, he could show that pyruvate did not change the
oxygen consumption rate. In our case we could observe that succinate instead of glucose inhibits completely the chemosensory nerve
response to hypoxia and hypercapnia, but not the pHe response
during hypoxia as Fig. 5a illustrates. Pyruvate restores again the
hypoxic nerve response and partially the hypercapnic nerve response
after two and a half hours superfusion with succinate (Figs. 5a and
5b). Again it can be observed in Fig. 5a that pyruvate does not influence the pHe during hypoxia and that the gradual hypoxic pHe decrease is due to glucose deficiency. Removal of pyruvate during
succinate superfusion as shown in Fig. 5b leads to a very fast di-
minishing of the chemosensory nerve response. New addition of glucose after about six hours of succinate superfusion restores the
pHe decrease during hypoxia but only 30% of the chemosensory nerve
activity. This probably results from the long duration of the experiments (Fig. 5b). Figs. 5a and 5b illustrate that the pHe decrease during hypoxia continues for a long time during the succinate effect. This could mean that succinate does not perturb glycolysis per se and the inhibitory effect of succinate on the chemo-

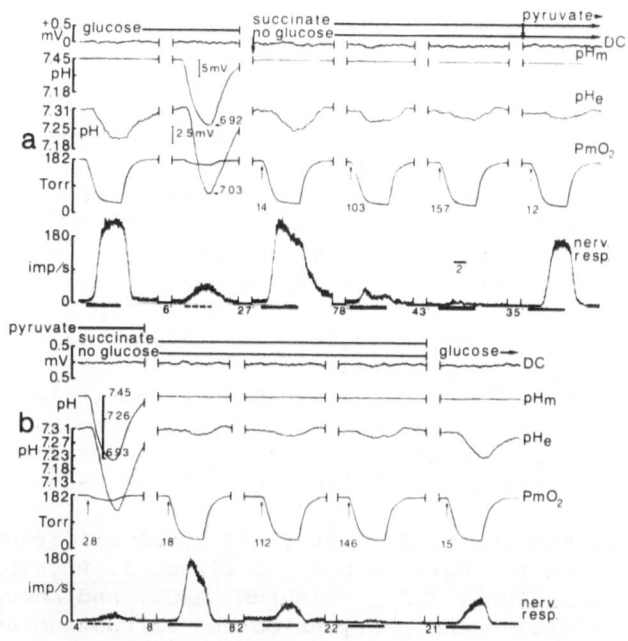

Fig. 5. Influence of succinate (5.5 mmol/l) on the extracellular
pH changes and on the chemosensory nerve response during
hypoxia and hypercapnia. Traces are the same as in Fig. 1.
Fig. 5a illustrates the effect of succinate on the extracellular pH and chemoreceptor response to hypoxia during
zero glucose and during addition of pyruvate. Fig. 5b
shows the effect of pyruvate on chemosensory response
during hypercapnia and the effect of removal of pyruvate
during succinate superfusion and new glucose addition.

receptor nerve activity needs to be clarified with respect to the
mitochondrial respiration. At present, we can neither explain the
pyruvate restoration nor the succinate inhibition of the chemoreceptive response. However, taking into account the findings of
Bartels (1979) in the bullock carotid body, it is possible to
speculate on the conception that both glycolysis and mitochondrial
respiration contribute in a synergistic form to the expression of
chemoreception. Possibly, both metabolic pathways converge to a
common mechanism related to the regulation of the intracellular
calcium, which is necessary for transmitter release (Delpiano and
Acker, 1983).

REFERENCES

Acker, H., Holtermann, G., and Carlsson, J., 1982, Microelectrode
    measurements of pH in cellular spheroids, Pflügers Arch.
    Suppl., R31:394.

Anichkov, S.V., and Belen'kii, M.L., 1963, "Pharmacology of the Carotid Body Chemoreceptors", Pergamon Press, Oxford, 164 pp.

Bartels, J., 1979, Enzymaktivitätsmuster des energieliefernden Stoffwechsels und Sauerstoffverbrauch im Glomus caroticum des Rindes, Dissertation, Hamburg.

Belmonte, C., and Gonzalez, C., 1983, Mechanism of chemoreception in the carotid body: possible models, in: "Physiology of the Peripheral Arterial Chemoreceptors", H. Acker, and R.G. O'Regan, eds., Elsevier, Amsterdam, 197 pp.

Delpiano, M.A., and Acker, H., 1980, Relationship between tissue Po_2 and chemoreceptor activity of the cat carotid body in vitro, Brain Res., 195:85.

Delpiano, M.A., and Acker, H., 1983, The extracellular Ca^{++} and K^+ activities in the cat carotid body in vitro and their relationship to chemoreception, in: "The Peripheral Arterial Chemoreceptors", D.J. Pallot, ed., Croom Helm, London, 101 pp.

Eyzaguirre, C., and Lewin, J., 1961, Effect of different oxygen tensions on the carotid body in vitro, J. Physiol., 159:238.

Hackenbrock, C.R., Rhen, T.G., Weinbach, E.C., and Lemasters, J.J., 1971, Oxidative phosphorylation and ultrastructural transformation in mitochondria in the intact ascites tumor cells, J. Cell Biol., 51:123.

Joels, N., and Neil, E., 1963, The excitation mechanism of the carotid body, Br. Med. Bull., 19:21.

Joels, N., and Neil, E., 1968, The idea of a sensory transmitter, in: "Arterial Chemoreceptors", R.W. Torrance, ed., Blackwell Scientific Publication, Oxford, 153 pp.

Krylov, S.S., and Anichkov, S.V., 1968, The effect of metabolic inhibitors on carotid chemoreceptors, in: "Arterial Chemoreceptors", R.W. Torrance, ed., Blackwell Scientific Publication, Oxford, 103 pp.

Landgren, S., Liljestrand, G., and Zottermann, Y., 1954, Impulse activity in the carotid sinus nerve following intracarotid injections of sodium-iodo-acetate, histamine hydrochloride, lergitin and some purine and barbituric acid derivates, Acta Physiol. Scand., 30:149.

Lübbers, D.W., Baumgärtl, H., Fabel, H., Huch, A., Kessler, M., Kunze, K., Riemann, H., Seiler, D., and Schuchardt, S., 1969, Principles of construction and application of various platinum electrodes, Prog. Resp. Res., 3:136.

Mills, E., and Jöbsis, F.F., 1972, Mitochondrial respiration chain of carotid body and chemoreceptor response to changes in oxygen tension, J. Neurophysiol., 35:405.

Mulligan, E., and Lahiri, S., 1981, Dependence of carotid chemoreceptor stimulation by metabolic agents on PaO_2 and $PaCO_2$, J. Appl. Physiol., 50:884.

Mulligan, E., Lahiri, S., and Storey, B.T., 1981, Carotid body O_2 chemoreception and mitochondrial oxidative phosphorylation, J. Appl. Physiol., 51:438.

Packer, L., and Golder, R.H., 1960, Correlation of structural and metabolic changes accompanying the addition of carbohydrates to Ehrlich ascite tumor cells, J. Biol. Chem., 235:1234.

Purves, M.J., 1970, The effect of hypoxia, hypercapnia and hypotension upon carotid body blood flow and oxygen consumption in the cat, J. Physiol., 209:395.

Standbrook, H.S., and McMurtry, I.F., 1983, Inhibition of glycolysis potentiates hypoxic vasoconstriction in rat lungs, J. Appl. Physiol., 55:1467.

Webb, J.L., 1966, "Enzyme and Metabolic Inhibitors", Academic Press, New York.

Winder, C.V., 1937, On the mechanism of stimulation of carotid gland chemoreceptors, Am. J. Physiol., 118:389.

Acknowledgement

The authors are indebted to Frau Menne, Frau Schebaum, and Frl. Rathke for preparing this manuscript and to Dr. K. Amsler for kindly reviewing the English.

717

MATHEMATICAL ANALYSIS OF PO_2 AND LOCAL FLOW DISTRIBUTION IN THE

CAROTID BODY

F. Degner and H. Acker

Max-Planck-Institut für Systemphysiologie
Rheinlanddamm 201, 4600 Dortmund 1, FRG

INTRODUCTION

The local environment of chemoreceptor elements in the carotid body with regard to oxygen supply is of importance for the receptor mechanism. In the literature the absolute figures of tissue Po_2, local flow, and oxygen consumption are not described clearly.

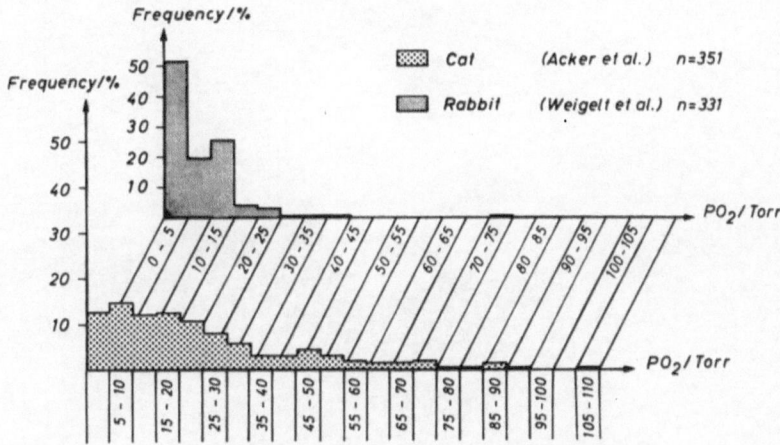

Fig. 1. Frequency distribution of tissue Po_2 found in carotid bodies of cats and rabbits. On the X-axis the Po_2 is given in different classes; on the Y-axis the frequency is given in per cent; n=number of measurements. (Weigelt and Acker, 1977).

Whalen et al. (1981) showed tissue Po_2 values near the arterial Po_2, whereas Weigelt and Acker (1977) found values below the mixed venous Po_2 (Fig. 1).

Since Daly et al. (1954), the local flow is assumed to be about 2000 ml/100g/min, but Acker and O'Regan (1981) described already a local flow only 5% of the total flow.

The oxygen consumption is measured between 0.6 and 6 ml O_2/100g/min (Daly et al., 1954; Fay, 1970; Leitner and Liaubet, 1971; Starlinger and Lübbers, 1976; Acker and Lübbers, 1977).

Some authors found an oxygen consumption dependent on the actual local Po_2 leading to an increased oxygen consumption with elevating the Po_2. In order to get an impression of the relations among these local conditions we tried to describe them in a model.

METHOD

By serial reconstruction of one capillary loop Seidl (1975) defined the functional unit of the carotid body as a glomoid, which is shown in Fig. 2. The specific tissue surrounds the capillary which runs in a tortuous way in the tissue.

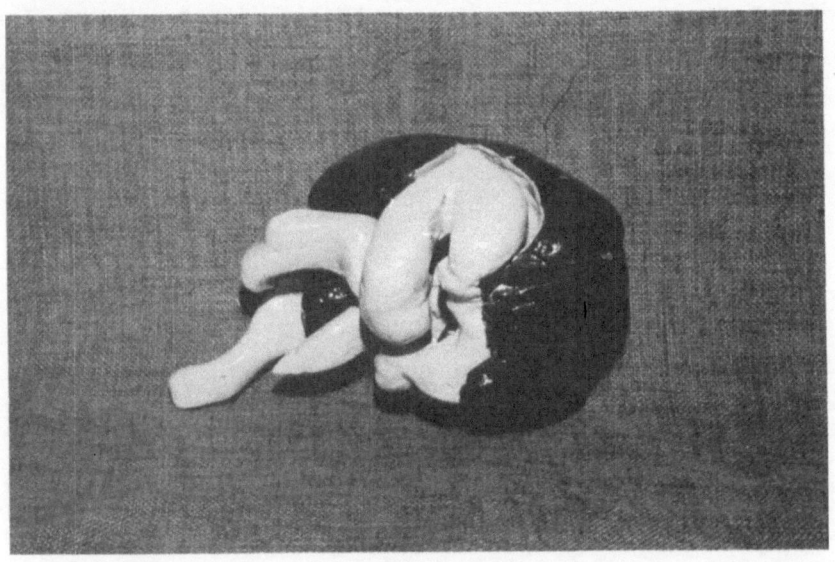

Fig. 2. Reconstruction of a glomoid with the specific tissue surrounding the capillary (Seidl, 1975).

With a mathematical model of Metzger (1969) one can calculate a three-dimensional Po_2 distribution in this glomoid for the capillary region and for the tissue region, according to the formulas shown in Fig. 3. The velocity of the streaming blood, the hematocrit, and the radius of the vessel influence the Po_2 decrease in the course of the vessel, whereas diffusion of oxygen in tissue and the oxygen consumption are responsible for the Po_2 distribution in the tissue.

A second serial reconstruction was done to get information about the capillary arrangement in the carotid body. Without this information one could only make simplified assumptions of the vascular arrangement. Glomoids can be connected in series or in parallel.

One example of a connection of the arterial and venous end found by the reconstruction is transformed in an electrical current circle. The various elements of vessels with their length

$$\text{VESSEL:} \quad K \cdot v \cdot \alpha \cdot \frac{\partial Po_2}{\partial l} = D \cdot \alpha \cdot d \cdot \frac{\partial Po_2}{\partial n}$$

with $K = 1,34 \cdot HK \cdot N/(\alpha \cdot 10000)$ with HK = hematocrit

N = slope of the oxygen dissoziation curve

α = oxygen solubility coefficient

v = velocity of the streaming blood

α = oxygen solubility coefficient

$\frac{\partial Po_2}{\partial l}$ = partial derivation of Po_2 in the direction of the vessel

D = diffusion coefficient of oxygen

d = length of one side of the quadratic assumed vessel

$\frac{\partial Po_2}{\partial n}$ = partial derivation of Po_2 in the four directions, perpendicular on the vessel

$$\text{TISSUE:} \quad D \cdot \alpha \cdot \Delta Po_2 - R(Po_2) = 0$$

with
D = diffusion coefficient of oxygen
α = oxygen solubility coefficient
ΔPo_2 = second partial derivation in three directions
$R(Po_2)$ = oxygen consumption per time and per volume

Fig. 3. Differential equations (Metzger, 1969) to describe the Po_2 distribution in a three dimensional tissue and capillary area.

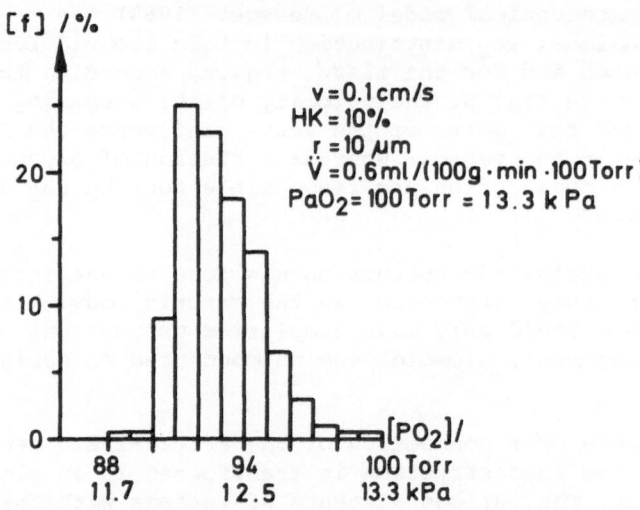

Fig. 4. Calculated P_{O_2} histogram of a single glomoid. The parameters are v = flow velocity, r = radius of the capillary, $\dot{V}$ = oxygen consumption, P_aO_2 = arterial P_{O_2}

Table 1. Frequency of different streaming velocities depending on the arterio-venous blood pressure difference, the viscosity, and the radius of the input arteriole.

Blood Pressure in Torr	Viscosity in Ns/m$_2$	V<0.02 cm/s	V0.02 cm/s< – 0.05 cm/s	V 1>cm/s
100	0.001	53%	7%	40%
100	0.002	58%	19%	23%
100	0.003	60%	24%	16%
100	0.004	70%	14%	16%
50	0.001	58%	19%	23%
50	0.002	70%	14%	16%
50	0.003	77%	9%	14%
50	0.004	84%	9%	7%
10	0.001	84%	9%	7%
10	0.002	93%	7%	0%
10	0.003	95%	5%	0%
10	0.004	98%	2%	0%

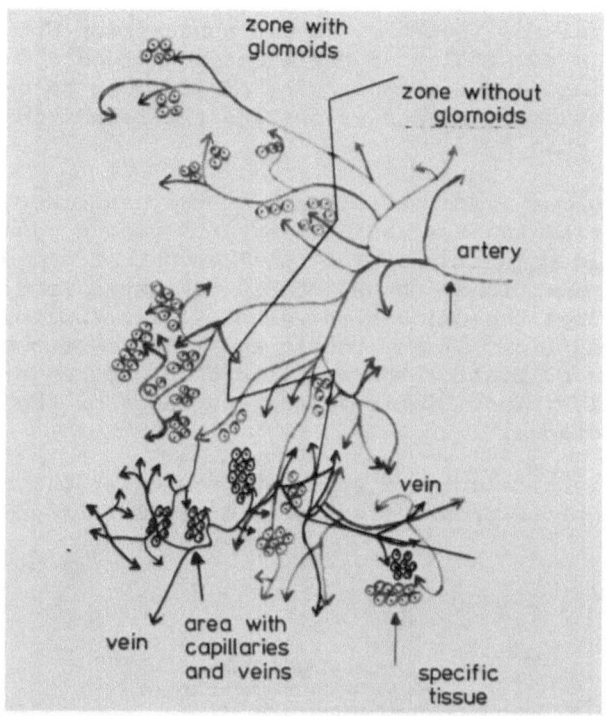

Fig. 5. Schematic drawing of the capillary arrangement due to a serial reconstruction, including the capillary area, and the arterial input area with short arterio-venous connections.

and radius and the viscosity of the streaming blood are substituted by a resistance R according to $R = 8 \eta \, l / \pi r^4 = p/I$) (i.e. the law of Hagen-Poiseuille) with eta = viscosity, l = length of the vessel, r = radius of the vessel, I = flow, p = blood pressure difference between beginning and end of the part of the vessel, and $I = p/R$ (law of Ohm). With the aid of this formula it is possible to calculate the velocity of the streaming blood in different parts of the vessels.

The velocities of the streaming blood allow to obtain a Po_2 distribution of the whole carotid body, assuming a homogeneous distribution of the glomoids along the course of the reconstructed vessel with the knowlegde of the total number of glomoids in the reconstructed tissue volume.

RESULTS AND DISCUSSION

Fig. 4 shows a Po_2 histogram for one glomoid for the conditions: arterial P_{O_2} 100 Torr, oxygen consumption 0.6 ml O_2/100g/min/100 Torr and velocity of the streaming blood 0.1 cm/s. One can see a reduction of the arterial P_{O_2} of 100 Torr to a venous P_{O_2} of 88 Torr. By assuming higher velocities the reduction decreases to values lower than 5 %.

Fig. 5 shows a schematic graph of the capillary arrangement and the arterial input with short arterio-venous connections in the carotid body tissue. The total amount of glomoids and their interconnections can be roughly estimated from this graph. Table 1 displays the calculated velocity distributions under different conditions of hematocrit and arterio-venous blood pressure difference. Most of the values are in the range of common capillary velocities. Higher values are those of the short arterio-venous connections.

Fig. 6 is a calculated P_{O_2} histogram under the condition arterio-venous blood pressure difference of 70 Torr and a hematocrit

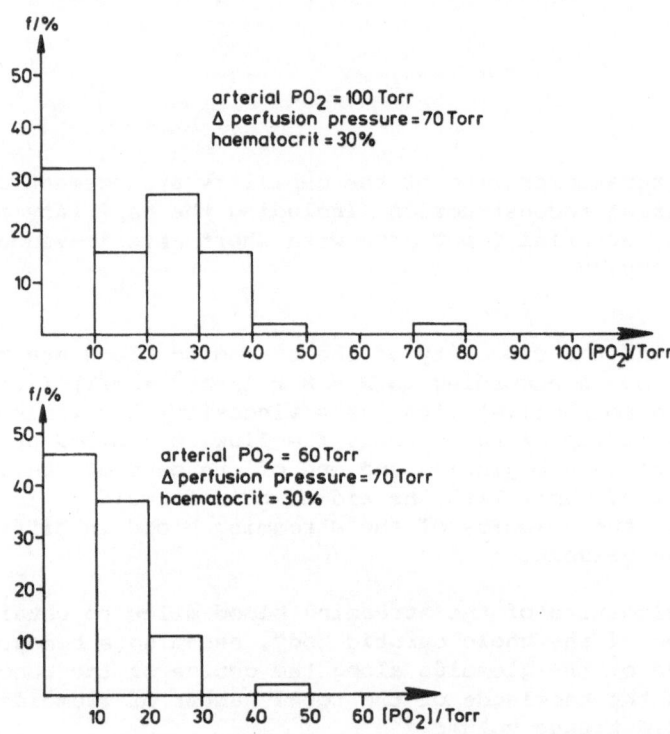

Fig. 6.   Calculated P_{O_2} histograms on the basis of the calculated flow velocity distribution (Fig. 6) with the parameters arterial P_{O_2} 60 Torr and 100 Torr, arterio-venous blood pressure difference of 70 Torr, and hematocrit of 30 %.

of 30 %. The number of glomoids is assumed to be 420, as it is figured out from the reconstruction. One can see a left-shifted Po_2 histogram with a median Po_2 between 20 and 30 Torr. A hypothetical slight variation of the vascular arrangement leads to a Po_2 distribution known from Whalen (Acker et al., 1983). Although the number of short capillaries increases, the velocity remains in the range of common capillary velocities.

SUMMARY

A common capillary velocity of streaming blood, i.e. a common local flow combined with the geometry of the vascular elements already explains the measured left-shifted Po_2 histogram. A slight variation of the vascular arrangement can also explain higher Po_2 values without the assumption of a very high flow in the capillaries.

REFERENCES

Acker, H., Delpiano, M., and Degner, F., 1983, The meaning of the pO_2 field in the carotid body for the chemoreceptive process, in: "Physiology of the Peripheral Arterial Chemoreceptors," H. Acker, R.G. O'Regan, eds., Elsevier Comp., Amsterdam, pp. 89-119.

Acker, H., and Lübbers, D.W., 1977, The kinetics of local tissue pO_2-decrease after perfusion stop within the carotid body of the cat in vivo and in vitro, Pflügers Arch., 369:135-140.

Acker, H., and O'Regan, R.G., 1981, The effects of stimulation of autonomic nerves on carotid body flow in the cat, J. Physiol., 315:99-110.

Daly, M., Lambertsen, C.J., and Schweitzer, A., 1954, Observations on the volume of blood flow and oxygen utilization of the carotid body in the cat, J. Physiol., 125:67-89.

Fay, F.S., 1970, Oxygen consumption of the carotid body, Am. J. Physiol., 218:518-523.

Leitner, L.M., and Liaubet, M.J., 1971, Carotid body oxygen consumption of the cat in vitro, Pflügers Arch., 323:315-322.

Metzger, H., 1969, Distribution of oxygen partial pressure in a two-dimensional tissue supplied by capillary meshes and concurrent and countercurrent systems, Math. biosc., 5:143-154.

Seidl, E., 1975, On the morphology of the vascular system of the carotid body of cat and rabbit and its relation to the glomus type-I cells, in: "The Peripheral Arterial Chemoreceptors," M.J. Purves, ed., Cambridge University Press, London, pp. 293-299.

Starlinger, H., and Lübbers, D.W., 1976, Oxygen consumption of the isolated carotid body tissue (cat), Pflügers Arch., 366: 61-66.

Weigelt, H., and Acker, H., 1977, Comparative measurements of tissue pO_2 in the carotid body, in: "Chemoreception in the Carotid Body," H. Acker et al., eds., Springer, Berlin, pp. 244-249.

Whalen, W.J. et al., 1981, Cat carotid body: Oxygen consumption and other parameters, J. Appl. Physiol., 50:129-133.

MEMBRANE POTENTIAL AND Ca INFLUX IN HYPOXIC AND NORMOXIC CAROTID BODY TYPE-I CELLS

F. Pietruschka and A. Acker

Max-Planck-Institut für Systemphysiologie
Rheinlanddamm 201, 4600 Dortmund, FRG

INTRODUCTION

The carotid body is described as being a chemoreceptor since 1928 (de Castro). Under hypoxia, the natural stimulus, transmitter like dopamine, and Ach are released (Fidone et al., 1982; Eyzaguirre et al., 1965) and chemoreceptor discharge is increased (Delpiano and Acker, 1980). Till now it is not clear, whether this chemoreceptive process is located in the glomus cell membrane or in the adjacent nerve endings. Working with cells in primary tissue culture we can investigate the stimulation process on isolated carotid body cells. As previous studies showed (Pietruschka and Schäfer, 1976) fine structure of these cells, especially the dense cored vesicles, is preserved in culture.

Cultivation of the cells under different O_2 concentrations should show, whether there is any influence of this stimulus on electrical membrane properties by ion movements across the cell membrane. Therefore, carotid body cells were impaled with micro-electrodes after a 2 day culturing under normoxic or hypoxic conditions.

Another set of experiments dealt with calcium influx measurements as a proof for the primary stimulus of a secretory process in carotid body cells under various oxygen conditions. In carotid bodies of the rat Grönblad et al. (1979) could show that a rise in intracellular calcium induces exocytotic membrane profiles in type-I cells. The direct proof, however, was still missing, that glomus cells take up calcium under hypoxia.

727

MATERIAL AND METHODS

Carotid body cells were prepared from rabbit embryos. The cells were dissociated by trypsin/collagenase and plated either directly in multiwell plastic culture dishes (^{45}Ca-influx experiments) or on polystyrene cover slips coated with reconstituted rat-tail collagen (for impalement).

Glioma cells were derived from the rat glioma cell line C_6.

IMPALEMENT

The cells originating from one pool of embryos were cultivated for 2 days under normoxic (21% O_2, 10% CO_2, rest N_2) or hypoxic (5% O_2, 10% CO_2, rest N_2) conditions. For impalement the cover slip with the cells was transferred to a perfusion chamber through which the culture medium without serum was circulating (10 ml/min). The cells could be identified by an inverted microscope, which was connected to a TV system. Intracellular recordings from type-I cells were obtained with microfilament glass microelectrodes (Albrecht, Munich) filled with 3 mol l^{-1} KCl. The electrode resistance varied between 20-50 MΩ and the tip potential between 1-5 mV.

^{45}Ca UPTAKE

^{45}Ca uptake experiments were performed by a method analogous to the method described by Barnes et al. (1981). The culture medium was removed from the cells and the cells were washed twice with HEPES-buffered saline (incubation medium containing 136 mmol l^{-1} NaCl, 5.4 mmol l^{-1} KCl, 1.4 mmol l^{-1} MgCl$_2$, 1.2 mmol l^{-1} Ca Cl$_2$, 1.0 mmol l^{-1} NaH$_2$PO$_4$, 10 mmol l^{-1} glucose, 20 mmol l^{-1} HEPES, and having pH 7.4) and pre-incubated in this medium on a rocker platform at 37°C. After one hour, the culture dishes were transferred to an exsiccator in an atmos bag, an inflatable polyethylene chamber. After having filled this bag with either air or N_2, the dishes were attached to a shaker and medium changed to an incubation medium (as above) containing ^{45}CaCl$_2$. Uptake experiments lasted for half an hour. They were terminated by cooling the culture dish on an ice-cold metal plate and washing 4 times with ice-cold stop-solution (similar to the incubation medium, but NaCl concentration raised to 150 mmol l^{-1}). Cells were detached by trypsin/collagenase, counted under a microscope and then digested in 0,5n NaOH.

Blank values were obtained with cooled cultures and culture dishes without cells incubated for half an hour at 37°C. Both blanks representing calcium bound to cell membranes and to culture dishes were substracted from the experimental values.

RESULTS

   Carotid body type-I cells could be impaled under our experimental conditions after they had been clearly identified by
microscopy. The cells were always punctured near the nucleus,
since the cells have there the biggest elevation.

   Firstly, we proved the dependence of the type-I cell membrane
potential on the cultivation time in tissue culture. Fig. 1 summarizes the results. Comparable mesasurements were done between
type-I cells of the cat and the rat carotid body. The tendency to
higher membrane potential values after 2-3 days cultivation is
clearly seen. The values are comparable with data for type-I cells
in the in vitro preparation given by Eyzaguirre et al. (1977). For
further experiments rabbit carotid body cells were used, since it
is easier to get embryonic tissue probes from that animal over the

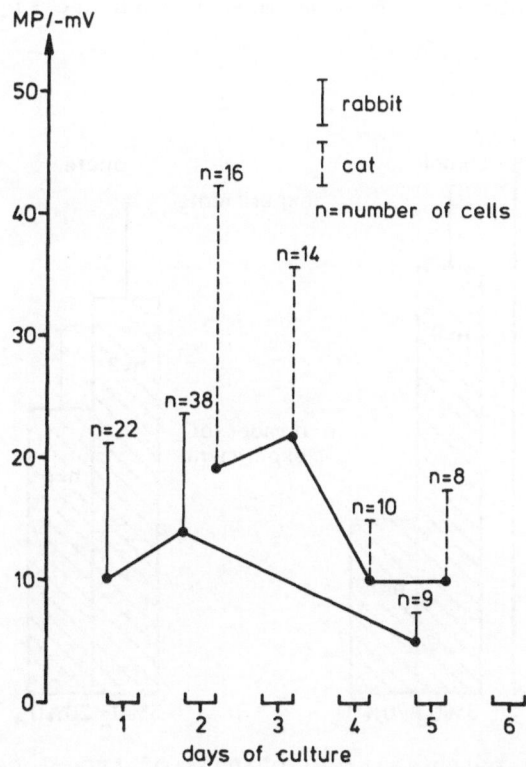

Fig. 1.   Membrane potentials (MP) of type-I cells of the cat and
          rabbit carotid body maintained in tissue culture for
          different times.

whole year. However, the comparable data between cat and rabbit, as shown in Fig. 1, permit perhaps a generalization of the experimental results.

Two days of cultivation were chosen as standard time, to prove the influence of hypoxia on the membrane characteristics of type-I cells. This was done in a second step. Type-I cells were cultivated under normoxic (21% O_2, 10% CO_2, 68% N_2) and hypoxic (5% O_2, 10% CO_2, 85% N_2) conditions for two days simultaneously. The cells were kept then in the perfusion chamber under the same conditions for the impalement on the same date. Fig. 2 shows the results. 70 type-I cells were punctured under normoxic conditions in 14 experiments (chronic experiments).

The mean value of the membrane potential was about -11 mV with a standard error of estimate of about $\pm$ 1.8. 65 type-I cells were punctured under hypoxic conditions in 9 experiments. The mean values increased to about -27 mV with a standard error of estimate of about $\pm$ 5. The two mean values are significantly

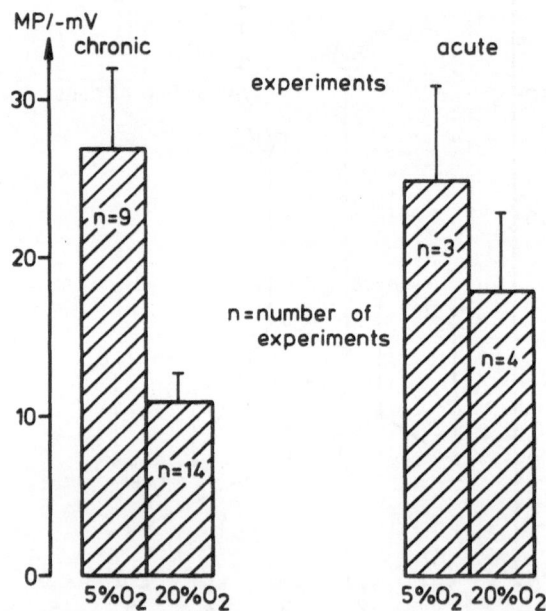

Fig. 2. Membrane potential (MP) changes of type-I cells cultured for 2 days under normoxic and hypoxic conditions (chronic experiments) as well cultured for 2 days under hypoxic conditions and exposed for 1 h to normoxia (acute experiments).

different at the 99% level using the U-test according to Wilcoxon et al. (1978).

These findings were confirmed with cells cultivated under hypoxic conditions and impaled after one hour of normoxia (acute experiments). The cells show also the tendency to lower membrane potentials when returned to normoxic conditions with values decreasing from -25 mV $\pm$ 6 to - 18 mV $\pm$ 5. This may indicate that the increase of membrane potential is a reversible process.

To measure directly the ion movements across the cell membrane, possibly responsible for these electrical events, experiments with exchangeable $^{45}Ca^{++}$ were performed on carotid body cells. Especially, the control of the calcium influx seemed to us important, since an increase of the cytosolic calcium could act as a coupling factor between hypoxia and transmitter secretion.

To study this first we had to show the pool of exchangeable cell calcium under steady state conditions. Therefore, we incubated glomus cells (Fig. 3) and rat glioma cells (Fig. 4) in ^{45}Ca for 1 minute to 3 hours, when isotopic equilibrium seemd to be reached. Fig. 5 shows that calcium exchange is more rapid in glomus than in glioma cells and that the amount of exchangeable calcium is higher, too. In carotid body cells we find values of 3 nm $\pm$ 0.86/10^6 cells compared to 2.3 nm $\pm$ 0.23/10^6 cells in glioma cells. Based on the

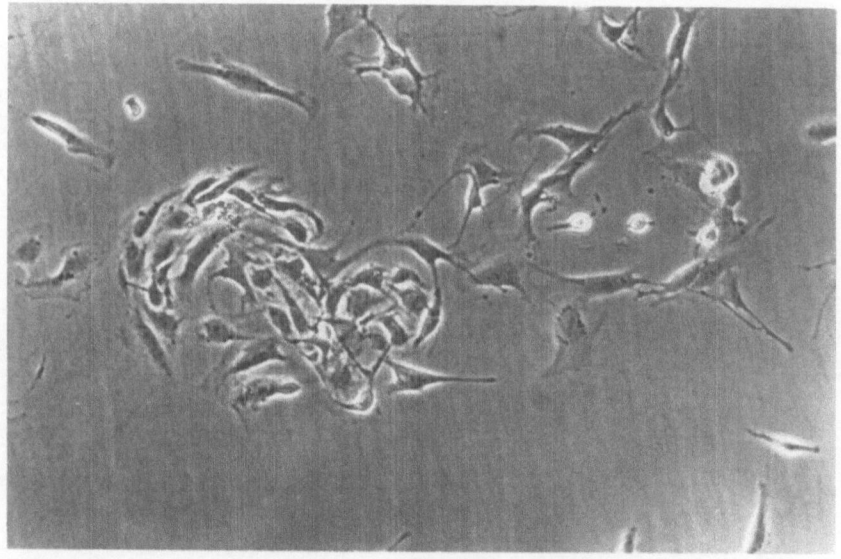

Fig. 3. Carotid body cells in culture after completion of the uptake experiment and washes (x186).

731

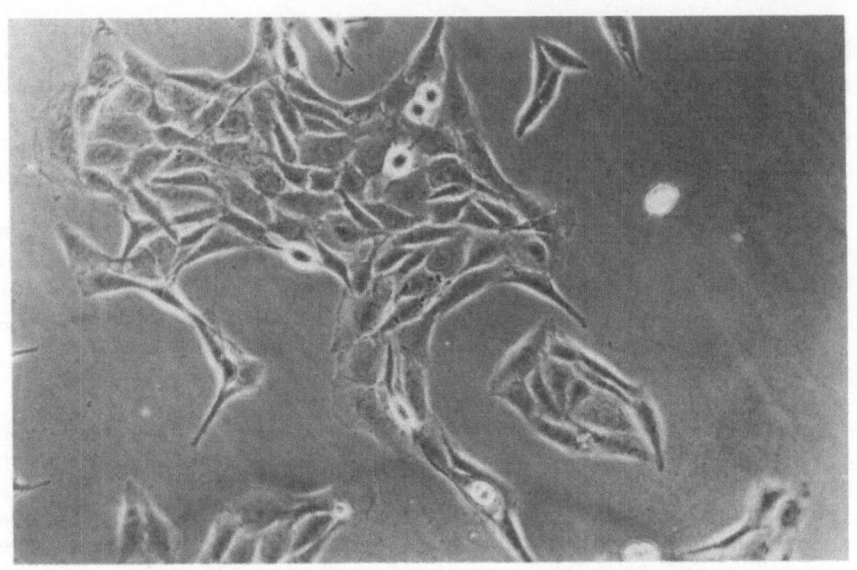

Fig. 4. Gioma cells in culture after completion of uptake
experiment and washes (x 186).

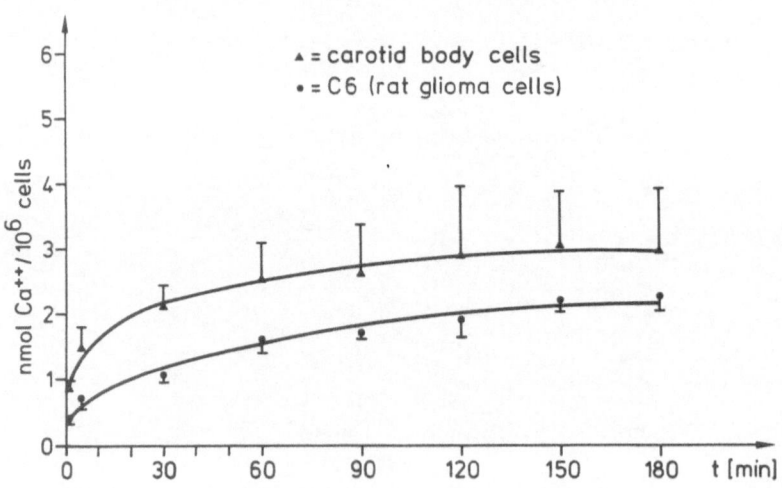

Fig. 5. $^{45}Ca^{++}$ uptake under steady-state conditions by glomus
cells and glioma cells.

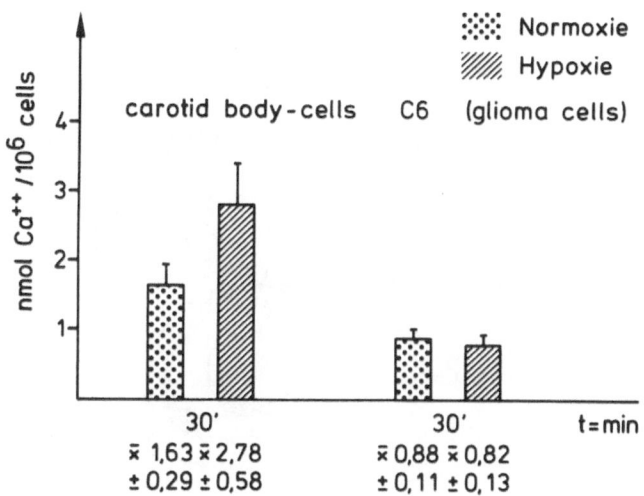

Fig. 6. Effect of hypoxia on $^{45}Ca^{++}$ uptake by glomus and glioma cells.

cell volume this difference is even greater, because glioma cells are 1.8 times bigger than glomus cells. The cells showed different behaviour (Fig. 6), also with reduction of pO_2 nearly to zero for half an hour.

In glomus cells there is a marked increase (170%) of the calcium influx during hypoxia compared to normoxic cells. This increase is significant (λ98%) and similar to that obtained with acetylcholine stimulation. Rat glioma cells treated in the same way as carotid body cells do not show a comparable difference in Ca^{++} influx under hypoxic and normoxic conditions.

DISCUSSION

The described results indicate two different points. Firstly, glomus cells are able to respond in some way to changes in pO_2 independent of any nervous supply. Secondly, calcium plays a role in the process of chemoreception. With our methods we cannot distinguish whether there is a short and transient increase in intracellular cytosolic calcium content under hypoxia or an augmented exchange of calcium through the cell membrane. As glioma cells do not show any increase in calcium influx under the same conditions this seems to be a specific process related to chemore-ception in carotid body cells. From cells of adrenal medulla it is known (Schneider et al., 1981) that increased calcium influx is coupled with catecholamine release. Since Fidone et al. (1982) could demonstrate that during hypoxia dopamine and Ach are released in the carotid body these data fit well the scheme of McDonald and Mitchell (1975) for chemoreception (Fig. 7). With a decreased pO_2

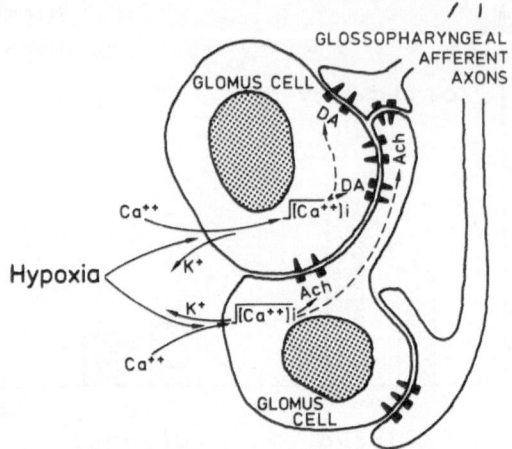

Fig. 7. Action of hypoxia on ion movement across type-I cell membrane. It is supposed that hypoxia opens calcium channels
by an unknown mechanism. The consequently increased
cytosolic calcium firstly induces transmitter release to
nerve endings and adjacent glomus cells and secondly acti-
vates potassium channels (adapted from McDonald and
Mitchell).

calcium uptake is increased and transmitters are secreted from
glomus cells. The transmitters act on sensory nerve endings as well
as on neighbouring type-I glomus cells, where acetylcholine receptors could be localized (Chen and Yates, 1984; Dinger et al.,
1981). Since it was found that the potassium activity increases
under hypoxia in the carotid body extracellularly (Acker, 1978) the
described hyperpolarization of type-I cells could be explained by
calcium activated potassium channels under chronic as well as under
acute hypoxia conditions. Further experiments have to be performed
to clarify the location and the action of the primary process,
which enhances the calcium influx in carotid body cells, mainly responsible for a transmitter release, stimulating nerve endings, and
transducing pO_2 changes into a nervous signal.

REFERENCES

Acker, H., 1978, Measurements of potassium activity in the cat
carotid body under hypoxia and hypercapnia, Pflügers Arch.,
375:229-232.
Barnes, E.M., Mandel, Jr., and Mandel, P., 1981, Calcium transport
by primary cultured neuronal and glial cells from chick
embryo brain, J. Neurochem. 36:82-85.

Chen, I., and Yates, R.D., 1984, Two types of glomus cells in the rat carotid body as revealed by α-bungarotoxin binding, J. Neuropathol., 13:281-302.

De Castro, F., 1928, Sur la structure et l'innervation du sinus carotidien de l'homme et des mammifères. Nouveaux faits sur l'innervation et la fonction du glomus caroticum, Trav. Lab. Rech. Biol. Univ. Madrid, 25:330-380.

Delpiano, M.A., and Acker, H., 1980, Relationship between tissue pO_2 and chemoreceptor activity of the carotid body in vitro, Brain Res., 195:85.

Dinger, B., Gonzalez, C., Yoshizaki, K., and Fidone, S., 1981, Alpha-bungarotoxin binding in cat carotid body, Brain Res., 205:187-193.

Eyzaguirre, C., Baron, M., and Gallego, R., 1977, Intracellular studies of carotid body cells: effects of temperature, "natural" stimuli and chemical substances, in: "Tissue Hypoxia and Ischemia", Adv. Exp. Med. Biol., Vol. 78, M. Reivich, R. Coburn, S. Lahiri, and B. Chance (eds.), Plenum Press, New York-London, pp.209-223.

Eyzaguirre, C., Koyano, H., and Taylor, J.R., 1965, Presence of acetylcholine and transmitter release from carotid body chemoreceptors, J. Physiol. (Lond.), 178:463-476.

Fidone, S., Gonzalez, C., and Yoshizaki, K., 1982, Effects of low oxyen on the release of dopamine from the rabbit carotid body in vitro, J. Physiol., 333:93-110.

Grönblad, M., Akerman, K.E., and Eränkö, O., 1979, Induction of exocytosis from glomus cells by incubation of the carotid body of the rat with calcium and ionophore A 23187, Anat. Rec., 195:387-395.

McDonald, D.M., and Mitchell, R.A., 1975, The innervation of glomus cells, ganglion cells, and blood vessels in the rat carotid body: a quantitative ultrastructural analysis, J. Neurocytol., 4:177-230.

Pietruschka, F., and Schäfer, D., 1976, Fine structure of chemosensitive cells (glomus caroticum) in tissue culture, Cell Tiss. Res., 168:55-63.

Schneider, A.S., Cline, H.T., Rosenheck, K., and Ionenberg, M., 1981, Stimulus secretion coupling in isolated adrenal chromaffin cells: Calcium channel activation and possible role of cyto-skeletal elements, J. Neurochem., 37:567-575.

HUMAN MAMMARY CARCINOMAS IN NUDE RATS - A NEW APPROACH FOR INVESTIGATING OXYGEN TRANSPORT AND SUBSTRATE UTILIZATION IN TUMOR TISSUES[*]

P. Vaupel[1], F. Kallinowski[1], S. Dave[1], H. Gabbert[2], and G. Bastert[3]

[1]Dept. Applied Physiology, and [2]Dept. Pathology University of Mainz, D- 6500 Mainz, FRG
[3]Dept. Gynaecology and Obstetrics, University of Frankfurt, D- 6000 Frankfurt/Main, FRG

INTRODUCTION

An understanding of tumor pathophysiology with respect to blood flow, oxygenation status, pH distribution and utilization of the relevant substrates which, all together, critically influence growth kinetics and the efficiency of nonsurgical therapeutic modalities in vivo requires information derived directly from human malignant tissues. At present, only inadequate knowledge of the relevant physiological factors in tumor tissues of patients are accessible. The little data available to date were obtained from clinical observations rather than from systematic studies, i.e., data were collected from various tumor types with differing staging and grading. For this reason generally valid statements concerning the above mentioned parameters cannot be made.

The only results derived from systematic investigations on human tumor tissue oxygenation were published by Wendling et al. (1984). In this paper tissue oxygenation was measured in 10 patients with a differentiated adenocarcinoma in a very localized region of the rectum, at a distance of 5 - 8 cm from the anus (grade I - II according to Mason, and Dukes stage B). From the data obtained it was concluded that the oxygenation of differentiated rectal adenocarcinomas is distinctly lower than

---

[*]Supported by Deutsche Forschungsgemeinschaft (Va 57/2-4)

that of the normal rectal mucosa. Tissue hypoxia or even anoxia were common features in these tumors. Considerable inter- individual differences among tumors of the same clinical staging and histological grading were evident. Furthermore, substantial intra- individual heterogeneities in the oxygenation existed within the same tumor and even within neighbouring microareas of the tissue, therefore implying that the commonly used classifications do not allow any conclusions concerning the oxygenation status, and thus probably the radiosensitivity of a tumor.

Earlier investigations on tissue oxygenation in human tumors must either be considered as more or less informative case reports or were performed to test the efficacy of therapeutic measures. Invasive measurements of O_2 tensions were performed in miscellaneous malignant tumors by Urbach (1956), Urbach and Noell (1958), Cater and Silver (1960), Evans and Naylor (1963), Jamieson and van den Brenk (1965), Bergsjø et al.(1967), Bergsjø and Evans (1968, 1971), Kolstad (1968), Badib and Webster (1969), Mundinger and Hahn (1972), Bicher et al.(1980), and Pappova et al.(1982). Surface oxygen tension measurements on normal gastric mucosa and on a gastric carcinoma were presented by Endrich (1984). Oxygenation data from studies on tumors of the oral cavity in humans were published by Mueller- Klieser et al.(1981). In this study, as a measure of the oxygenation status, the oxyhemoglobin saturation of single red blood cells within tumor microvessels was determined.

Only a few reports on pH values in human tumors are available. Whereas the data of Millet (1928) and Meyer et al.(1948) do not reflect physiological conditions because the pH readings were taken from surgical specimens after removal from the body, all other measurements were performed with macroelectrodes so that only integrating pH values could be observed and thus information concerning the heterogeneous pH distribution within microareas of a single tumor could not be obtained (Naeslund and Swenson, 1953; Inch, 1954; Pampus, 1963; Ashby, 1966; van den Berg et al., 1982; Wike- Hooley et al., 1984).

The literature dealing with the quantification and dynamics of tumor blood flow has also until recently been rather sparse (for reviews see Peterson, 1979, and Vaupel, 1982). Using the 133-Xenon-clearance technique, blood flow in human tumors was assessed by Nyström et al.(1969), Bru et al.(1970), Tanaka (1974), Mäntylä et al.(1976, 1982), Boneu et al.(1977), and Mäntylä (1979). Johnson (1976) reported on tumor blood flow values in 5 patients using a thermodynamic method. Regional blood flow was studied in 8 patients with brain tumors (Ito et al., 1982) and in 9 patients with breast carcinoma (Beaney et al., 1984) by means of the 15-Oxygen steady state inhalation technique and positron emission tomography.

From this compilation of previous data on human tumors there is clear evidence that a certain standardization is lacking. This is due to a broad variability of parameters such as histological type, growth characteristic and anatomical site. An attractive approach to overcome some of the difficulties mentioned may be the study of human tumor xenografts in immune- deficient laboratory animals such as athymic mice and rats. The main advantage of the new model is that it is possible to standardize the above outlined parameters so that systematic studies concerning tumor pathophysiology can be performed. One of the problems still remaining with this model is that, although the tumor cells are of human origin, the tumor stroma is (at least partially) provided by the host animal. This has to be taken into consideration, although tumor cells are able to establish their own extracellular matrix (Angello and Hosick, 1982).

ANIMALS AND TUMORS

The athymic rat used in our laboratory is known as the Rowett nude (rnu/rnu) mutation. This immune- deficient hairless rat mutation was first observed in 1953 in a colony of outbred rats maintained at the Rowett Research Institute in Aberdeen (UK) but died out in the early 1960s. Homozygous individuals were recovered in 1975 and a breeding colony was established thereafter (Festing et al., 1978; Festing, 1981). A breeding nucleus of Rowett nude rats was obtained from the MRC Laboratory Animal Centre (M.F.W. Festing). Nude rodents have a depressed or absent T- cell function as there is only a small and highly abnormal thymus rudiment with a depletion of lymphocytes in T-cell- dependent regions of the lymphatic tissues (Rygaard, 1981). Compared to nude mice, the nude rats are more convenient for all investigations involving microsurgery and monitoring of the relevant systemic parameters. Furthermore, they have a better survival than nude mice and appear to be more robust.

All animals are housed within laminar air flow racks (Makrolon[R] cages provided with dust- free wood granulate bedding), are fed on Altromin[R] 1410 tpf. diet ad libitum and are supplied with drinking water containing oxytetracycline (0.3 g/l; pH = 2.5). For further details concer-

ning breeding and maintainance of rnu/rnu- rats see Fortmeyer and Bastert (1981).

Data on the heterotransplantation of human tumors in
nude rats have started to appear in the literature since
1978 indicating that these animals support the growth of
tumor tissue derived from human cancers (Festing et al.,
1978; Salomon et al., 1980; Colston et al., 1981; Bastert
et al., 1981 b; Stark and Schlipköter, 1981; Stragand et
al., 1982; Williams et al., 1984; Giovanella et al., 1984;
for a review see Bastert et al., 1981 a). The data available so far showed unequivocally that tumors retain their
individual characteristics in the host animals. Therefore,
it may be expected that the results collected from human
tumors in immune- deficient laboratory animals are applicable in human oncology.

Since in recent years mammary carcinomas have aroused
special interest in oncology because of their frequency
and problematic prognosis, in a first series of experiments the O_2 transport and related supply parameters were
investigated in human breast cancer. Of 20 primary human
mammary carcinomas xenografted, 6 tumors were able to sur-
vive and to thrive in rnu/rnu- rats. Hereby, for xenotransplantation all carcinomas were cut into 5 x 5 x 1 mm
pieces, put in TCM 199- medium and implanted under sterile
conditions into female or castrated male animals, which
were approx. 8 - 10 weeks old and weighing between 80 and
160 g. In general, the growth rate of the xenografts was
slower in rnu/rnu- rats than in nude mice. This holds also true for 8 human mammary carcinomas which grew in nude
rats only after serial passages in nude mice. The average
tumor volume doubling time (t_D) was 5 - 6 days. This value
fits quite well with the data obtained for human colonic
adenocarcinoma (t_D = 5.5 days for cell line SW 620; Stragand et al., 1982) but is somewhat lower than that for
DUB human breast carcinoma (t_D = ca. 9 days) observed by
Giovanella et al.(1984). The tumor volume doubling time
for the xenografts mentioned above, however, is distinctly shorter than that obtained from primary breast carcinomas in patients (breast adenocarcinomas: mean t_D = ca.
74 days; soft- tissue metastases of breast carcinomas:
mean t_D = approx. 19 days; for a review see Steel, 1977).
The tumors xenotransplanted were either medullary or anaplastic carcinomas of the breast whose steroid hormone
receptor capacity, cytostatic sensitivity and radiosensitivity were known in each individual case.

TUMOR MODELS

Tumor oxygen supply studies as well as blood flow measurements by means of venous outflow sampling were performed in vivo using an epigastric pouching technique. Subcutaneous heterotransplants of the same tumors were also used for indirect measurements of tumor blood flow by means of a thermo- clearance technique as well as for evaluation of tumor tissue oxygenation and pH distribution using microtechniques.

Subcutaneous Tumor Xenografts (see Fig. 1)

Tumors were cut into 5 x 5 x 1 mm pieces and were implanted subcutaneously in the anterior milk line (sterile conditions, ether anaesthesia). At the time of implantation the animals were approx. 60 days old. After a mean tumor growth period of 29 days the tumors reached an average wet weight of ca. 2.9 g (t_D = approx. 5 days) and were subjected to the experimental procedures mentioned above. At the end of the experiments the tumors were always excised and subsequently examined by standard histological techniques.

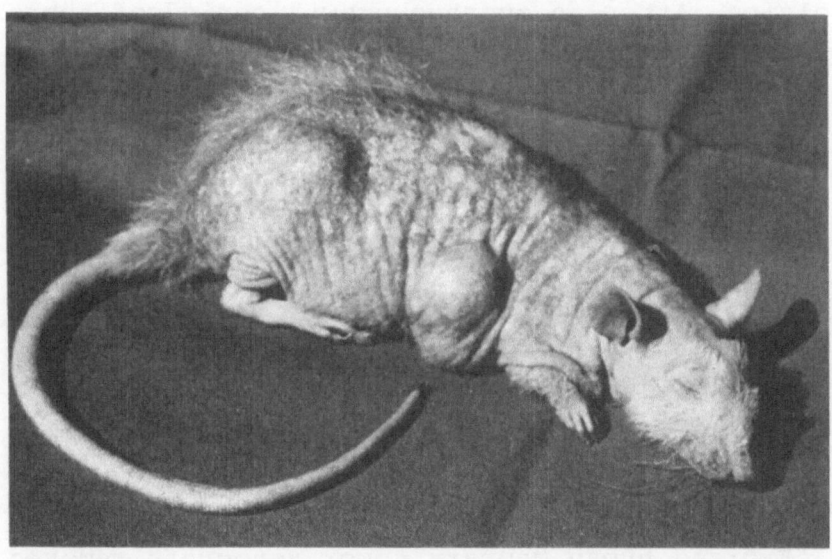

Fig.1. Thymusaplastic rnu/rnu- rat 4 weeks after s.c. xenotransplantation of a human mammary carcinoma.

Epigastric Pouching Technique

Using the epigastric pouching technique it is possible to obtain a tissue- isolated tumor preparation, in which one artery and one vein are the only vascular connection between host and tumor (Grantham et al., 1973; Steinau et al., 1981; Sauer et al., 1982).

The vascular supply of the lower abdominal wall of rats is mainly provided by the superficial epigastric artery and vein paired in a relatively long pedicle which can be severed without any disturbances of the blood supply due to numerous anastomoses. For tumor implantation the animals were anaesthetized (Pentobarbital- Na, 30 mg per kg body weight, i.p.), and the groin was opened by an incision over the inguinal crease. Afterwards the vascular pedicle containing the superficial epigastric vessels was carefully dissected up to its origin at the femoral vessels. A 3 mm- cube of tumor material was removed from the donor nude mouse and immediately sutured to the distal end of the pedicle. The tumor xenograft and adjacent pedicle were placed in a thin polyethylene pouch where the human tumor material grew as a tissue- isolated preparation, i.e., the final preparation was a solid tumor growing in a subcutaneous pouch but separated from the surrounding tissues by a polyethylene envelope (see Fig. 2). The rat skin was then closed beyond the pouch with clamps. After an average growth period of approx. 32 days, the carcinomas reached a mean wet weight of ca. 2.4 g (t_D = ca. 6 days).

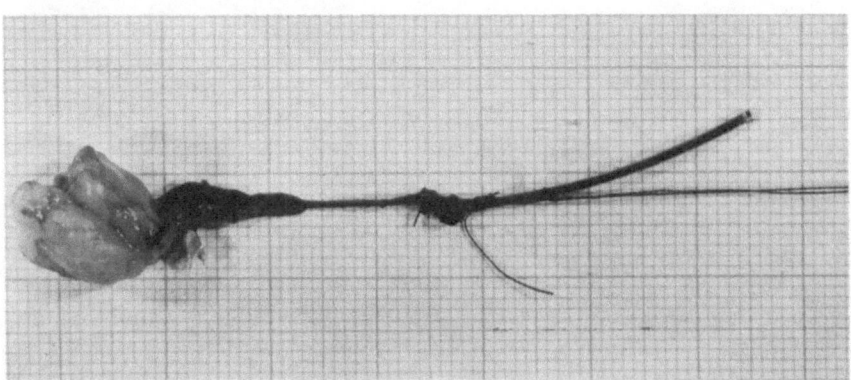

Fig.2. Excised human mammary tumor xenograft removed from the polyethylene sack, showing the vascular pedicle with a cannula for tumor- venous blood sampling.

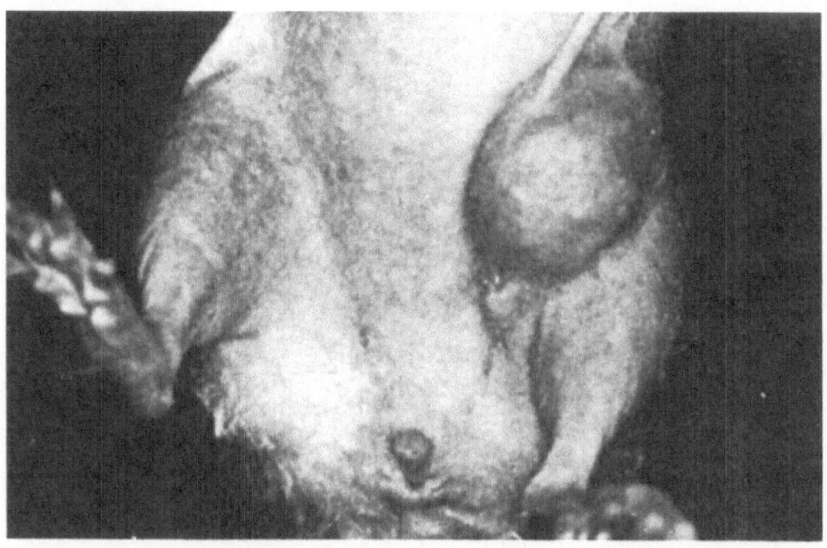

Fig.3. Thymusaplastic nude rat with an epigastric pouch
tumor 4 weeks after xenotransplantation of a human
medullary breast carcinoma.

Animals with a certain tumor size (see Fig.3) were anaesthetized with Pentobarbital- Na (30 mg/kg i.p.) and
placed supine on a heated operating pad that allowed the
rectal temperature to be maintained at or near 37°C. The
left common carotid artery was cannulated in order to
monitor the mean arterial blood pressure in the thoracic
aorta continuously by means of a Statham pressure transducer (see Fig.4). Throughout all experiments the host
animals were breathing room air spontaneously and were
anticoagulated with heparin (300 USP units/kg/hr). In
order to measure tumor blood flow and the relevant parameters of interest in the tumor- venous blood, the tumor
vein (i.e. the former superficial epigastric vein) was
cannulated via the femoral vein using polyethylene tubing
(ID 0.4 mm, OD 0.8 mm). Microsurgical techniques were
used for all vessel preparations (operating microscope,
Olympus MTX). The femoral vein and its major branches
were exposed and cleared of adipose and connective tissue.
In order to insure an exclusive collection of tumorvenous blood, the femoral vein and two deep venous branches (the muscular branch and the profund femoral vein)
were exposed and the latter ligated. The proximal femoral vein was also tied off during sampling (see Fig.5).

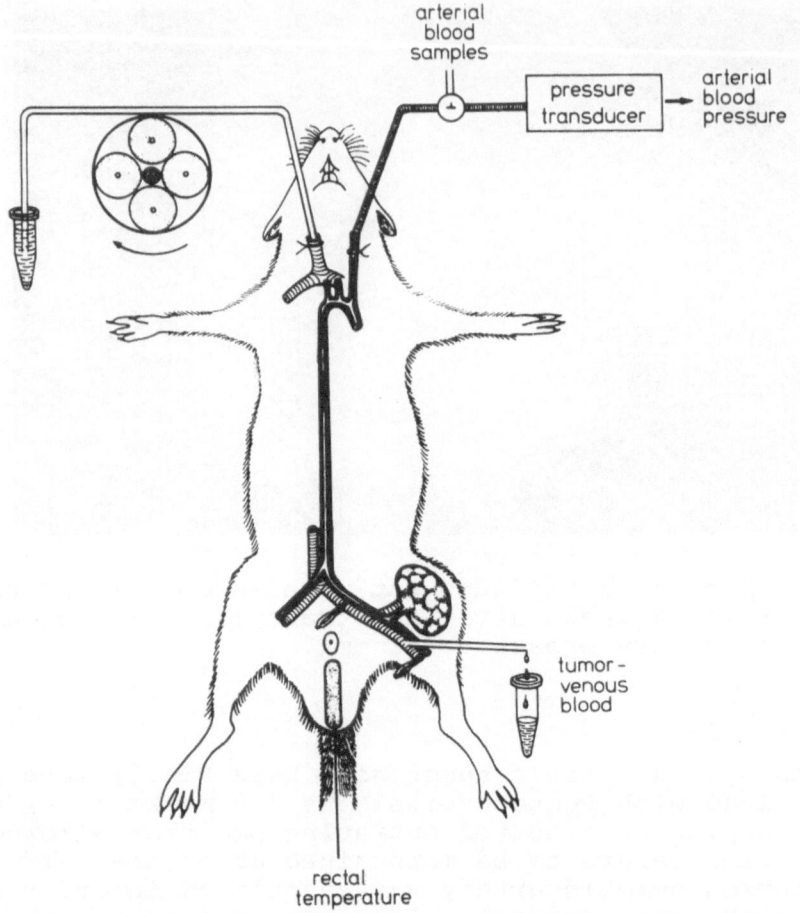

arterial
blood
samples

pressure
transducer

arterial
blood
pressure

tumor-
venous
blood

rectal
temperature

Fig.4. Schematic illustration of the experimental set-up
for measuring the relevant parameters of the respiratory gas exchange and substrate supply of
tumors in situ.

Total tumor blood flow (TBF) was assessed by measuring the
amount of venous blood leaving the tumor within a certain
period of time. To obtain the weight- related (= specific)
tumor blood flow, at the end of each experiment the respective tumor was removed from the host for the determination of its wet weight. Balancing of the blood loss via
the tumor vein throughout the experiments was achieved
by the continuous and adequate transfusion of blood from
donor rats into the right external jugular vein.

In order to get an insight into the substrate utilization for energy production in human tumors in vivo,
arterial and tumor- venous blood samples were taken under

744

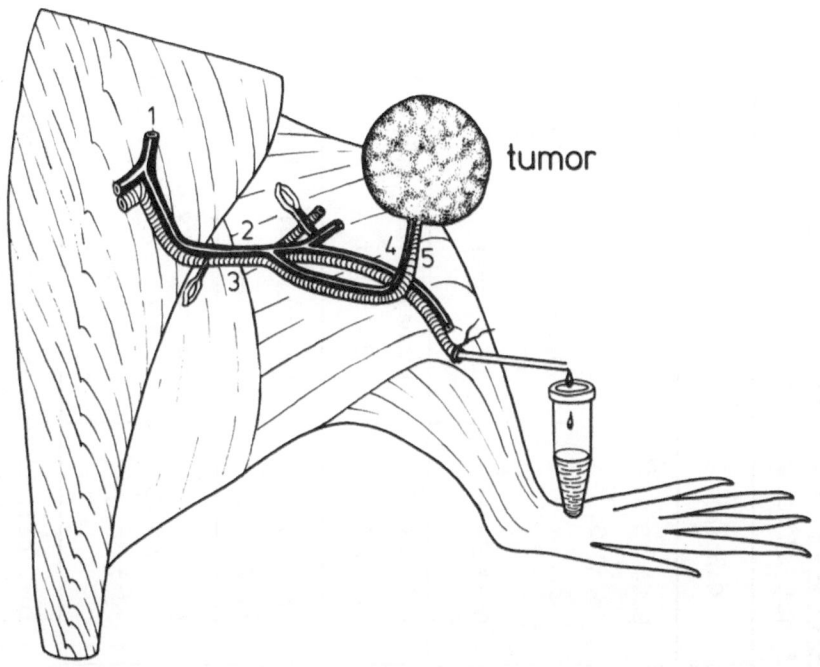

Fig.5. Scheme of the vascular pedicle supplying the human
tumor xenograft.. Collection of tumor- venous blood
by a catheter introduced through the femoral vein.
1: abdominal aorta, 2: femoral artery, 3: femoral
vein, 4: superficial epigastric artery = tumor
artery, 5: superficial epigastric vein = tumor vein.

steady state conditions to assess the relevant parameters
of the respiratory gas exchange, the acid- base status,
the concentrations of whole- blood glucose and lactate,
of amino acids, urea and ammonia, of non- esterified fatty
acids and of the ketone bodies. The respective consumption
or release rates were calculated according to Fick's principle taking into account TBF and the respective concentration differences in the arterial and tumor- venous
blood. In all cases pouches with connective/granulomatous
tissue served as controls.

EXPERIMENTAL RESULTS AND CONCLUSIONS

The experimental results obtained so far are compiled in Table I. For comparison, relevant data collected
from human mammary carcinomas in patients are also given.
From this data collection it can be concluded that tumor

Table 1. Blood flow, O_2 consumption rate, O_2 utilization and pH distribution in human mammary carcinomas (data from patients and from tumor xenografts in nude rats). Values are man ± SD if not otherwise stated.

	Human mammary carcinoma		Control	Author(s)
	in patients	rat xenograft		
Blood flow (ml/g/min)	0.188 ± 0.097 ca. 0.20 0.102 ± 0.082^{b} 0.200 ± 0.146^{c}	0.118 ± 0.102^{d} 0.126 ± 0.080^{e}	0.04 ± 0.01^{a} ca. 0.01^{a} 0.34 ± 0.22^{f}	Beaney et al. (1984) Johnson (1976) Mäntylä et al. (1982) Mäntylä et al. (1982) this paper
Oxygen consumption rate (µl/g/min)	6.6 ± 2.8	8.10 ± 7.73^{d}	4.5 ± 1.0^{a} 11.3 ± 7.2^{f}	Beaney et al. (1984) this paper
Oxygen utilization (%)	23 ± 8	47.0 ± 15.6^{d}	65 ± 10^{a} 21.7 ± 12.9^{f}	Beaney et al. (1984) this paper
Tissue-pH	7.29 ± 0.05 ($\overline{x} \pm$ SEM)	6.79 ± 0.27^{h} 7.06 ± 0.23^{i}	7.63 ± 0.03^{g} ($\overline{x} \pm$ SEM) 7.37 ± 0.03^{g}	van den Berg et al. (1982) this paper this paper

a) normal breast; b) anaplastic carcinomas, breast tumors included; c) differentiated carcinomas, breast tumors included; d) epigastric pouching technique; e) s.c. tumor; f) fat and granulomatous tissue; g) subcutis; h) medullary mammary carcinoma; i) anaplastic mammary carcinoma.

xenografts in nude rats do constitute a valid model to assess tumor blood flow, respiratory gas exchange and substrate supply of human breast carcinomas, and probably of other human tumor types, too.

SUMMARY

A new model is presented for the study of oxygen supply and substrate utilization in human tumor tissue. In this approach human tumor material thrives in immune-deficient nude rats. The host chosen allows the continuous evaluation of all relevant parameters. From the data obtained so far it is concluded that this model is a valid tool in investigation of the metabolic status of human tumors.

REFERENCES

Angello, J.C., and Hosick, H.L., 1982, Glycosaminoglycan synthesis by mammary tumor spheroids, Biochem. Biophys. Res. Comm., 107: 1130 - 1137.

Ashby, B.S., 1966, pH studies in human malignant tumours, Lancet, 2: 312 - 315.

Badib, A.O., and Webster, J.H., 1969, Changes in tumor oxygen tension during radiation therapy, Acta radiol., 8: 247 - 257.

Bastert, G,B., Fortmeyer, H.P., and Schmidt- Matthiesen, H.(eds.),1981a, Thymusaplastic nude mice and rats in clinical oncology, G. Fischer Verlag, Stuttgart, New York.

Bastert, G., Eichholz, H., Fortmeyer, H.P., Michel, R.T., Huck, R., and Schmidt- Matthiesen, H.,1981b, Comparison of human breast cancer xenotransplantation in nu/nu mice and rnu/rnu rats, in: Thymusaplastic nude mice and rats in clinical oncology, G.B. Bastert et al., eds., G. Fischer Verlag, Stuttgart, New York.

Beaney, R.P., Lammertsma, A.A., Jones, T., McKenzie, C.G., and Halnan, K.E., 1984, Positron emission tomography for in- vivo measurements of regional blood flow, oxygen utilisation, and blood volume in patients with breast carcinoma, Lancet, 1: 131 - 134.

Bergsjø, P., and Evans, J.C., 1968, Tissue oxygen tension of cervix cancer, Acta radiol., 7: 1 - 11.

Bergsjø, P., and Evans, J.C., 1971, Oxygen tension of cervical carcinoma during the early phase of external irradiation, Scand. J. clin. Lab. Invest., 27: 71-82.

Bergsjø, P., Christensen, O.J., and Kolstad, P., 1967, Oxygen tension in cancer of the cervix following administration of vasodilator drugs during oxygen inhalation, Cancer, 20: 1625 - 1634.

Bicher, H.I., Hetzel, F.W., Sandhu, T.S., Frinak, S.,
    Vaupel, P., O'Hara, M.D., and O'Brien, T., 1980,
    Effects of hyperthermia on normal and tumor micro-
    environment, Radiology, 137: 523 - 530.
Boneu, A., Bugat, R., Daly, N., Douchez, J., and Combes,
    P.F., 1977, Influence de l'heparinate de calcium sur
    la regression sous irridation d'adenopathies cervi-
    cales metastatiques, in: Radiobiological Research and
    Radiotherapy (vol.2), IAEA, Vienna.
Bru, A., Combes, P.F., Douchez, J., Lucot, H., and Ribot,
    J.F., 1970, Estimation de l'activité circulatoire a
    l'interieur des tumeurs ganglionnaires malignes par
    la mesure du taux d'eputation du xenon-133, in: Dyn-
    amic studies with radioisotopes in medicine, IAEA,
    Vienna.
Cater, D.B., Silver,I.A., 1960, Quantitative measurements
    of oxygen tension in normal tissues and in the tumours
    of patients before and after radiotherapy, Acta rad-
    iol., 53: 233 - 256.
Colston, J., Fjeldsteel, A.H., and Dawson, P.J., 1981,
    Growth and regression of human tumor cell lines in
    congenitally athymic (rnu/rnu) rats, J. Natl. Cancer
    Inst., 66: 843 - 848.
Endrich, B., 1984, Mikrozirkulation maligner Tumoren,
    Habilitationsschrift der Medizinischen Fakultät,
    Heidelberg.
Evans, N.T.S., and Naylor, P.F.D., 1963, The effect of O_2
    breathing and radiotherapy upon the tissue oxygen ten-
    sion of some human tumours, Brit. J. Radiol., 36:
    418 - 425.
Festing, M.F.W., 1981, The Rowett athymic nude rat, in:
    Thymusaplastic nude mice and rats in clinical onco-
    logy, G.B. Bastert et al., eds., G. Fischer Verlag,
    Stuttgart, New York.
Festing, M.F.W., May, D., Connors, T.A., Lovell, D., and
    Sparrow, S., 1978, An athymic nude mutation in the
    rat, Nature, 274: 365 - 366.
Fortmeyer, H.P., and Bastert, G., 1981, Breeding and main-
    tainance of nu/nu mice and rnu/rnu rats, in: Thymus-
    aplastic nude mice and rats in clinical oncology,
    G.B. Bastert et al., eds., G. Fischer Verlag, Stutt-
    gart, New York.
Giovanella, B.C., Stehlin, J.S., and Coil, D., 1984,
    Human tumors heterotransplanted in nude mice and rats,
    Exptl. Cell Biol. 52: 76 - 79.
Grantham, F.H., Hill, D.M., and Gullino, P.M., 1973,
    Primary mammary tumors connected to the host by a
    single artery and vein, J. Natl. Cancer Inst., 50:
    1381 - 1383.

Inch, W.R., 1954, Direct current potential and pH of
    several varieties of skin neoplasms, Can. J. Biochem.
    Physiol., 32: 519 - 525.
Ito, M., Lammertsma, A.A., Wise, R.J.S., Bernardi, S.,
    Frackowiak, R.S.J., Heather, J.D., McKenzie, C.G.,
    Thomas, D.G.T., and Jones,T., 1982, Measurement of
    regional cerebral blood flow and oxygen utilisation
    in patients with cerebral tumours using 15-0 and
    positron emission tomography: analytical techniques
    and preliminary results, Neuroradiol., 23: 63 - 74.
Jamieson, D., and van den Brenk, H.A.S., 1965, Oxygen
    tension in human malignant disease under hyperbaric
    conditions, Brit. J. Cancer, 19: 139 - 150.
Johnson, R., 1976, A thermodynamic method for investiga-
    tion of radiation induced changes in the microcircu-
    lation of human tumors, Int.J. Radiat. Oncol. Biol.
    Phys., 1: 659 - 670.
Kolstad, P., 1968, Intercapillary distance, oxygen tension
    and local recurrence in cervix cancer, Scand. J. clin.
    Lab.Invest., 22 (Suppl. 106): 145 - 157.
Mäntylä, M., 1979, Regional blood flow in human tumors,
    Cancer Res., 39: 2304 - 2306.
Mäntylä, M., Kuikka, J., and Rekonen, A., 1976, Regional
    blood flow in human tumours with special reference
    to the effect of radiotherapy, Brit. J. Radiol.,
    49: 335 - 338.
Mäntylä, M., Toivanen, J.T., Pitkänen, M.A., and Rekonen,
    A.H., 1982, Radiation- induced changes in regional
    blood flow in human tumors, Int. J. Radiat. Oncol.
    Biol. Phys., 8: 1711 - 1717.
Meyer, K.A., Kammerling, E.M., Amtman, L., Koller, M.,and
    Hoffman, S.J., 1948, pH studies of malignant tissues
    in human beings, Cancer Res., 8: 513 - 518.
Millet, H., 1928, Measurements of the pH of normal, fetal,
    and neoplastic tissues by means of the glass electrode,
    J. biol. Chem., 78: 281 - 288.
Mueller- Klieser, W., Vaupel, P., Manz, R., and Schmid-
    seder, R., 1981, Intracapillary oxyhemoglobin sat-
    uration of malignant tumors in humans, Int. J. Radiat.
    Oncol. Biol. Phys., 7: 1397 - 1404.
Mundinger, F., and Hahn, K., 1972, Direct measurement of
    the partial oxygen tension in different cortical and
    subcortical structures of the brain and in gliomas
    during stereotactic operation, Confin. neurol., 34:
    106 - 111.
Naeslund, J., and Swenson, K.E., 1953, Investigations on
    the pH of malignant tumours in mice and humans after
    the administration of glucose, Acta. Obstet. Gynecol.
    Scand., 32: 359 - 367.

Nyström, C., Forssman, L., and Roos, B., 1969, Myometrial
    blood flow studies in carcinoma of the corpus uteri,
    Acta Radiol. Ther. Phys. Biol., 8: 193 - 198
Pampus, F., 1963, Die Wasserstoffionenkonzentration des
    Hirngewebes bei raumfordernden intracraniellen Pro-
    zessen, Acta neurochir., 11: 305 - 318.
Pappova, N., Siracka, E., Vacek, A., and Durkovsky, J.,
    1982, Oxygen tension and prediction of the radiation
    response. Polarographic study in human breast cancer,
    Neoplasma, 29: 669 - 674.
Peterson, H.I. (ed.), 1979, Tumor blood circulation -
    Angiogenesis, vascular morphology and blood flow of
    experimental and human tumors, CRC press, Boca Raton.
Salomon, J.C., Lynch, N., and Prin, J., 1980, Graft sus-
    ceptibility of nude rats and mice to animal and human
    tumors and to hybrid cell lines, in: Immunodeficient
    animals in cancer research, H. Sparrow, ed., Macmil-
    lan, New York.
Sauer, L.A., Stayman, J.W., and Dauchy, R.T., 1982, Amino
    acid, glucose, and lactic acid utilization in vivo
    by rat tumors, Cancer Res., 42: 4090 - 4097.
Stark, M., and Schlipköter, H.W., 1981, The heterogeneity
    of human bronchogenic carcinomas in in-vitro and in-
    vivo models of the nu/nu mouse and rnu/rnu rat, in:
    Thymusaplastic nude mice and rats in clinical onco-
    logy, G.B. Bastert et al., eds., G. Fischer Verlag,
    Stuttgart, New York.
Steel, G.G., 1977, Growth kinetics of tumours, Clarendon
    Press, Oxford.
Steinau, H.U., Bastert, G., Eichholz, H., Fortmeyer, H.P.,
    and Schmidt- Matthiesen, H., 1981, Epigastric pouch-
    ing technique - human xenografts in rnu/rnu rats,
    in: Thymusaplastic nude mice and rats in clinical on-
    cology, G.B. Basert et al., eds., G. Fischer Verlag,
    Stuttgart, New York.
Stragand, J.J., Drewinko, B., Henderson, S.D., Grossie,
    B., Stephens, L.C., Barlogie, B., and Trujillo, J.M.,
    1982, Growth characteristics of human colonic adeno-
    carcinomas propagated in the Rowett athymic rat,
    Cancer Res., 42: 3111 - 3115.
Tanaka, Y., 1974, Regional tumor blood flow and radio-
    sensitivity, in: Fraction size in radiobiology and
    radiotherapy, T. Sugahara et al., eds., Urban &
    Schwarzenberg, München.
Urbach, F., 1956, Pathophysiology of Malignancy.I. Tissue
    oxygen tension of benign and malignant tumors of the
    skin, Proc. Soc. Exptl. Biol. Med., 92: 644 - 649.
Urbach, F., and Noell, W.K., 1958, Effects of oxygen
    breathing on tumor oxygen measured polarographically,
    J. Appl. Physiol., 13: 61 - 65.

Van den Berg, A.P., Wike- Hooley, J.L., van den Berg-Blok, A.E., van der Zee, J., and Reinhold, H.S., 1982, Tumour pH in human mammary carcinoma, <u>Eur. J. Cancer Clin. Oncol.</u>, 18: 457 - 462.

Vaupel, P., 1982, Pathophysiologie der Durchblutung maligner Tumoren, <u>Funktionsanalyse biolog. Systeme</u>, 8: 155 - 170.

Wendling, P., Manz, R., Thews, G., and Vaupel, P., 1984, Heterogeneous oxygenation of rectal carcinomas in humans - a critical parameter for preoperative irradiation, <u>Advanc. Exptl. Med. Biol.</u>, in press.

Wike- Hooley, J.L., van der Zee, J., van Rhoon, G., van den Berg, A.P., and Reinhold, H.S., 1984, Human tumour pH changes following hyperthermia and radiation therapy, <u>Eur. J. Cancer Clin. Oncol.</u>, 20: 619 - 623.

Williams, R.D., Matsumoto, T., and Dombrovskis, S., 1984, Progressive growth of human genitourinary cancer cell lines in young nude rats, <u>Expl. Cell Biol.</u>, 52:80-84.

BLOOD FLOW AND OXYGEN SUPPLY TO HUMAN MAMMARY CARCINOMAS
TRANSPLANTED INTO NUDE RATS[*]

S. Dave, F. Kallinowski, and P. Vaupel

Dept. Applied Physiology, University of Mainz
D-6500 Mainz, W.- Germany

INTRODUCTION

Tumor blood flow (TBF), by itself, greatly influences
the efficiency of nonsurgical therapeutic modalities, especially chemotherapy and hyperthermia. Furthermore, TBF
is one of the most important determinants of tumor tissue
oxygenation in vivo, thus playing a relevant role in tumor
growth kinetics and in the development of regressive changes. In addition, the oxygenation of tumor tissue strongly
determines the efficiency of radiation therapy and to a
certain extent, pharmacodynamics of some antiproliferative
drugs. Despite the considerable information available for
rodent tumor systems, there are only sporadic reports on
blood flow (Beaney et al., 1984, Johnson, 1976, Mäntylä,
1979, Mäntylä et al., 1982) and oxygen supply (Beaney et
al., 1984, Müller- Klieser et al., 1981) in human tumors
mostly derived from clinical observations rather than from
systematic studies. Therefore, using an epigastric pouching technique in immune- deficient (rnu/rnu) rats, TBF
and oxygen utilization were evaluated systematically in
tissue- isolated human mammary tumor heterotransplants.

MATERIALS AND METHODS

A total of 31 immune- deficient (rnu/rnu) rats of
both sexes with a mean body weight of 250 ± 50 g were
used in these experiments. Cancer tissue from 5 patients

[*] Supported by Deutsche Forschungsgemeinschaft (Va 57/2-4)

(anaplastic and medullary carcinomas serially transplanted as 28th to 60th generation heterotransplants in nude animals) was implanted in the epigastric region of these nude rats using a pouching technique. (For details concerning breeding and maintainance of these animals, the pouching technique, the microsurgical preparation and the experimental set- up see Vaupel et al., 1985). TBF was assessed by a direct venous outflow technique. Tumor- venous and arterial blood samples were taken simultaneously under anaerobic conditions. Blood loss due to sampling was compensated by adequate transfusion of blood from donor rats via an external jugular vein.

Measurements were taken repeatedly under steady state conditions only. The oxygen saturation of hemoglobin S_{O_2} in arterial and tumor- venous blood was obtained using actual O_2 and CO_2 partial pressures as well as pH values (blood gas analyzer, type A 3, Eschweiler, Kiel, FRG) and considering respiratory gas/pH- nomograms for rats published by Bork et al.(1975). Hemoglobin concentration [Hb] was determined using a spectrophotometric method (cyanhemiglobin method, Betke and Savelsberg, 1950), and hematocrit values Hct. were obtained utilizing the Hawskley- micromethod. The O_2 concentration $[O_2]$ in the blood was calculated by means of [Hb] and the actual O_2 saturation of the blood as well as the physically dissolved amount of O_2 using the following equation:

$$[O_2] = \frac{1.36 \cdot [Hb] \cdot S_{O_2}}{100} + \frac{pO_2 \cdot \alpha_{O_2} \cdot 100}{760}$$

Hereby, an O_2 solubility coefficient α_{O_2} as given by Zander (1981) is taken into account.

The O_2 consumption rate $\dot{V}_{O_2}$ was then calculated considering the actual TBF and the respective arterio- tumor-venous O_2 concentration differences avD_{O_2}. At the end of the experiments, the pouches were excised, weighed and examined by standard histological techniques. Pouches with fat and/or granulomatous tissue served as controls.

RESULTS

From the 24 tumors studied so far, the results obtained clearly show that TBF decreases from 0.34 to 0.02 ml/g/min with increasing tumor wet weight from 0.15 to 5.47 g (see fig.1). The average TBF is 0.12 $\pm$ 0.10 ml/g per min at a mean wet weight of 2.42 $\pm$ 1.33 g, the average mean arterial blood pressure (MABP) being 125 ± 10 mmHg. For a comprehensive view concerning the relevant parameters investigated see Table I.

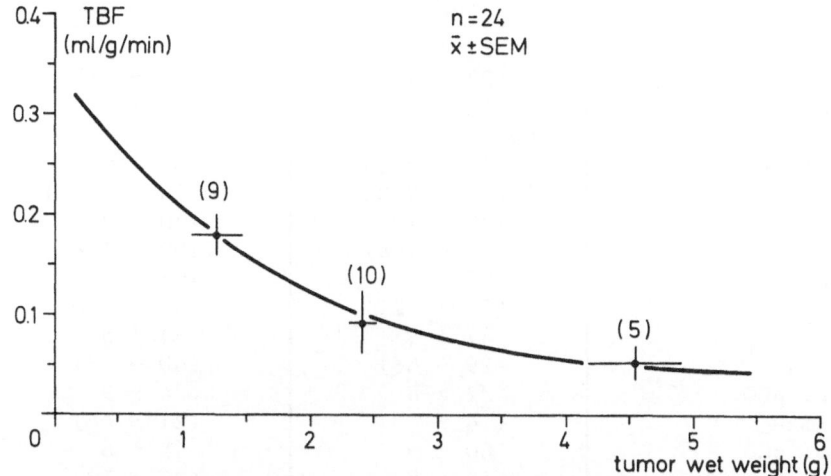

Fig.1. Tumor blood flow (TBF) as a function of tumor wet weight in human mammary carcinoma heterotransplants. Numbers in brackets indicate the respective number of tumors investigated.

The mean O_2 consumption rate $\dot{V}_{O_2}$ of human mammary carcinoma heterotransplants is $8.10 \pm 7.73 \, \mu l/g/min$. With increasing tumor wet weight the consumption rate of O_2 dropped drastically from 25.60 to 0.14 $\mu l/g/min$, as shown in fig.2.

Considering the O_2 consumption rate as a function of the O_2 availability (TBF · art. $[O_2]$), a linear relationship is obtained (see fig. 3). The O_2 availability ranges from 2.2 to 55.9 $\mu l/g/min$, the average value being 17.9 ± 16.9 $\mu l/g/min$.

The O_2 utilization (arterio- tumorvenous O_2 concentration difference/ arterial O_2 concentration) is already high for the tumors of low wet weight, and increases only slightly with increasing tumor wet weight, as shown in fig. 4. The average value for the O_2 utilization of these xenotransplanted tumors is 47 ± 16% (range: 6 to 70%).

TABLE I. Compilation of relevant parameters investigated for the evaluation of TBF and O_2 consumption of human mammary carcinomas heterotransplanted into nude rats. The values are means ± SD. Ranges are given in brackets.

	TUMORS	CONTROLS
Age	32 ± 4	35 ± 4
(days)	(22 – 41)	(30 – 41)
wet weight	2.42 ± 1.33	0.38 ± 0.20
(g)	(0.15 – 5.47)	(0.15 – 0.70)
blood flow	0.12 ± 0.10	0.34 ± 0.22
(ml/g/min)	(0.02 – 0.34)	(0.18 – 0.81)
MABP	125 ± 10	120 ± 8
(mm Hg)	(111 – 148)	(108 – 128)
art. pO_2	97 ± 12	105 ± 17
(mm Hg)	(76 – 121)	(83 – 130)
ven. pO_2	47 ± 9	54 ± 8
(mm Hg)	(29 – 68)	(40 – 63)
art. pCO_2	32 ± 8	34 ± 9
(mm Hg)	(14 – 43)	(21 – 44)
ven. pCO_2	60 ± 9	45 ± 6
(mm Hg)	(42 – 82)	(36 – 53)
art. pH	7.35 ± 0.07	7.39 ± 0.09
	(7.15 – 7.48)	(7.23 – 7.50)
ven. pH	7.14 ± 0.12	7.32 ± 0.04
	(6.84 – 7.34)	(7.27 – 7.38)
art. [Hb]	108.0 ± 19.9	127.9 ± 16.3
(g/l)	(73.0 – 140.3)	(98.0 – 143.5)
ven. [Hb]	114.6 ± 20.9	135.5 ± 17.7
(g/l)	(64.0 – 144.0)	(101.0 – 153.0)
art. Hct	32 ± 6	40 ± 5
(%)	(20 – 42)	(34 – 45)
ven. Hct	34 ± 6	40 ± 7
(%)	(22 – 44)	(28 – 48)
art. S_{O_2}	98 ± 2	99 ± 2
(%)	(93 – 100)	(94 – 100)
ven. S_{O_2}	48 ± 14	74 ± 13
(%)	(15 – 69)	(48 – 86)
art. $[O_2]$	14.3 ± 2.7	17.5 ± 2.5
(ml O_2/dl)	(10.7 – 19.1)	(13.1 – 19.8)
ven. $[O_2]$	7.6 ± 2.7	13.6 ± 2.8
(ml O_2/dl)	(2.2 – 12.5)	(10.1 – 17.5)
avD_{O_2} (ml O_2/dl)	6.8 ± 2.7	3.9 ± 2.6
	(0.73 – 12.63)	(1.63 – 9.56)
$\dot{V}_{O_2}$ (µl/g/min)	8.10 ± 7.73	11.30 ± 7.16
	(0.14 – 25.60)	(6.00 – 24.30)
O_2 utilization	47 ± 16	22 ± 13
(%)	(6 – 70)	(10 – 49)

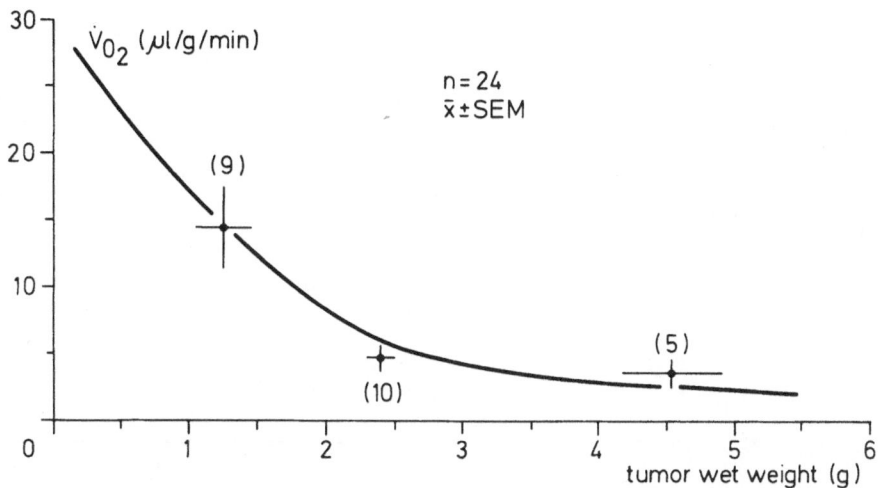

Fig.2. O_2 consumption rate $\dot{V}_{O_2}$ of human mammary tumors as a function of tumor wet weight. Numbers in brackets indicate the respective number of tumors investigated.

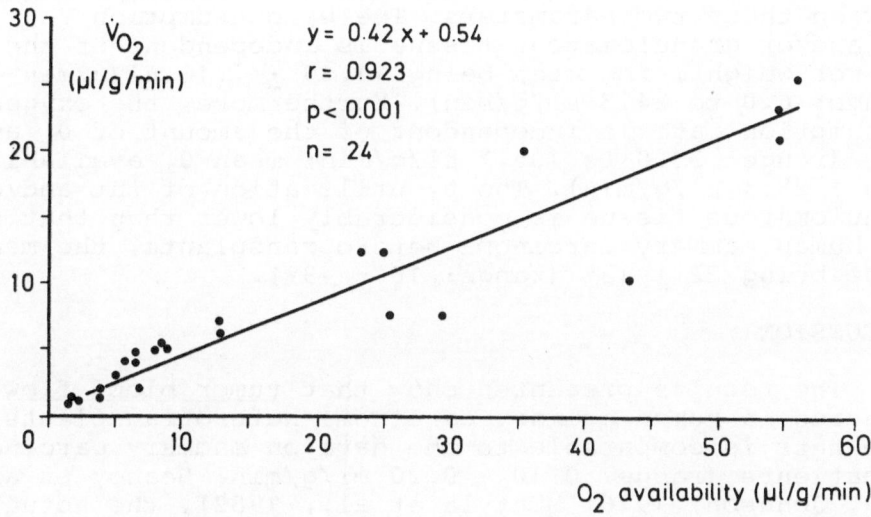

Fig.3. O_2 consumption rate $\dot{V}_{O_2}$ of human breast carcinoma heterotransplants as a function of the oxygen availability.

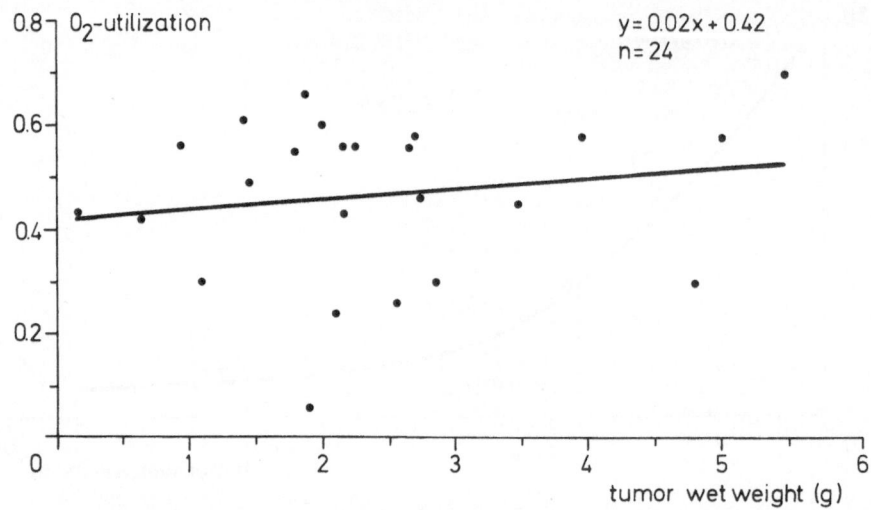

Fig.4. O_2 utilization in human mammary carcinoma heterotransplants as a function of tumor wet weight.

Blood flow in 7 control experiments (fat and/or granulomatous tissue) is 0.34 ± 0.22 ml/g/min (range: 0.18 to
0.81 ml/g/min) at an average tissue wet weight of 0.38 ±
0.20 g (range: 0.15 to 0.70 g). No relationship is found
between these two parameters. The O_2 consumption rate for
fat and/or granulomatous tissue is independent of the tissue wet weight, the mean being 11.30 ± 7.16 µl/g/min
(range: 6.0 to 24.3 µl/g/min). Furthermore, the oxygen
consumption rate is independent of the amount of O_2 available (range: 33.0 to 105.7 µl/g/min; mean O_2 availability:
55.0 ± 25.1 µl/g/min). The O_2 utilization of fat and/or
granulomatous tissue is considerably lower than that of
the human mammary carcinoma heterotransplants, the mean
value being 22 ± 13% (range: 10 - 49%).

DISCUSSION

The results presented show that tumor blood flow
measured in human mammary carcinoma heterotransplants in
nude rats is comparable to the data on mammary carcinomas
in patients (range: 0.10 - 0.20 ml/g/min; Beaney et al.,
1984, Johnson, 1976, Mäntylä et al., 1982), the actual
mean flow value lying in the lower half of the range
given. The TBF obtained for the human mammary carcinoma
heterotransplants is about one third of that reported
earlier in various rat tumor isotransplants using tissue-
isolated preparations (0.34 ml/g/min, Gullino et al., 1967;

0.29 ml/g/min, Vaupel, 1977), and twice as high as the flow estimated from the study by Sauer et al.(1982; 0.06 ml/g/min), again using tissue- isolated rodent isotransplants.

The weight- related TBF decreases with increasing tumor wet weight in human mammary carcinoma heterotransplants, as has been found in tumor isotransplants in rodents as well. In contrast to this, weight- related TBF appears to increase with increasing size of mammary carcinomas of different staging and grading measured in patients by Beaney et al. (1984).The dependancy of tumor blood flow on tumor wet weight found in heterotransplants is in accordance with findings previously reported by Vaupel et al. (1981), stating that during tumor growth typical changes in the microvascular pattern occur, leading finally to a chaotic vascular supply of the tumor mass as well as to a general rarefaction of the terminal vascular bed and concomitant severe disturbances of tumor microcirculation. In the end these disturbances cause growth retardation, appearance of regressive changes and may finally result in the development of ischemic tissue regions and of necrosis. Thus, measuring global tumor blood flow and considering the total tumor mass, both a decrease in weight- related TBF and an increasing underestimation of the perfusion in vital tissue regions has to be expected with increasing tumor weight. Furthermore, on measuring total blood flow, local inhomogeneities which may range from complete ischemia to hyperperfusion (Vaupel, 1982) cannot be evaluated.

The O_2 consumption rate of human mammary carcinoma heterotransplants in nude rats is comparable to that obtained for mammary carcinomas in patients (6.6 µl/g/min; Beaney et al., 1984), but it is 30 to 60% of those for some rodent isotransplants, e.g. hepatomas, Walker carcinoma (Gullino et al., 1967) and DS- Carcinosarcoma (Vaupel, 1977). On the other hand it is approximately twice as high as the oxygen consumption rate of fibrosarcomas (Gullino et al., 1967). Comparable to the results in rodent isotransplants, the oxygen consumption of human mammary carcinoma heterotransplants decreases with increasing tumor wet weight (Vaupel, 1977). Here again, similar to TBF, the measurement of global O_2 consumption does not take into account regional heterogeneities, which were experimentally shown by Constable et al. (1978) for untreated or irradiated Lewis lung carcinoma and for human carcinoma of the cervix.

The O_2 consumption rate is linearly related to the O_2 availability. Since the latter takes into account the arterial O_2 concentration and TBF, and considering that the arterial oxygen concentration remains relatively constant, tumor blood flow is the main determinant and the limiting factor of tumor oxygen supply in vivo. Furthermore, a deterioration of the diffusive O_2 transport due to increased intercapillary distances with increasing tumor mass also restricts the O_2 supply to the tumor cells and superimposes on the already existing disturbances of the convective transport due to the discussed inadequacy of nutritive blood perfusion.

The average O_2 concentrations in the arterial and tumor- venous blood are lower than those in tumor- free animals. This is mostly caused by the lower hemoglobin concentrations in tumor- bearing animals compared to the control animals, chronic anemia being a well documented manifestation of progressive tumor growth. This low O_2 concentration in the arterial blood further restricts the O_2 supply to the tumor cells. Considering all these parameters it can be stated that the actual O_2 consumption rate of the tumor is mostly determined by the O_2 supply and not by the demand of the cancer cells.

The O_2 utilization in human mammary carcinoma heterotransplants is found to be in the same range as that in rodent isotransplants but somewhat higher than that of the mammary carcinomas in patients. Since the oxygen consumption rate lies in the same range and as the mean blood flow is somewhat higher in tumors in patients than in the heterotransplants, a lower utilization has to be expected.

Arterio- venous shunt perfusion, the extent of which is unknown in the individual case, has to be considered when evaluating the O_2 supply to tumor cells. Due to this shunt perfusion, where the arterial blood with a high O_2 content is directly lead into the tumor- venous blood, the O_2 utilization may be considerably higher than the value calculated. The O_2 consumption rate and the oxygen utilization could only be accurately evaluated if either the percentage of shunt flow or the amount of nutritive perfusion are known.

SUMMARY

Blood flow of human mammary carcinomas heterotransplanted into immune- deficient rnu/rnu-rats is low. It decreases further with increasing tumor wet weight, the mean value being comparable to that of mammary carcinomas in patients.

The O_2 consumption rate of the heterotransplanted tumors decreases with increasing tumor wet weight and again is comparable to that of mammary carcinomas in patients. Furthermore, it is directly proportional to the O_2 availability which in turn is mainly determined by TBF.

The O_2 utilization of the human mammary carcinomas heterotransplanted into nude rats is already high in small tumors and increases only slightly with increasing tumor weight.

From these results and taking into account an impairment of convective and diffusive O_2 transport it can be concluded that the O_2 consumption rate of the tumor cells is mostly determined by the the O_2 supply and not by the actual demand of the cancer cells. This finding holds true for different tumor cell lines in different species.

REFERENCES

Betke, K., and Savelsberg, W., 1950, Stufenphotometrische Hämoglobinbestimmung mittels Cyanhämiglobin, Biochem. Zschr., 320: 431.

Beaney, R.P., Lammertsma, A.A., Jones, T., McKenzie, C., and Halnan, K.E., 1984, Positron emission tomography for in vivo measurement of regional blood flow, oxygen utilization and blood volume in patients with breast carcinoma, Lancet, 1: 131.

Bork, R., Vaupel, P., Günther, H., and Thews, G., 1975, Atemgas- pH- Nomogramme für das Rattenblut bei 37°C, Anaesthesist, 24: 84.

Constable, T.B., Rogers, M.A., and Evans, N.T.S., 1978, Comparison between the oxygen removal rate and the histological structure of normal and tumor tissues, Pflügers Arch., 373: 145.

Gullino, P.M., Grantham, F.H., and Courtney, A.H., 1967, Utilization of oxygen by transplanted tumors in vivo, Cancer Res., 27: 1020.

Johnson, R., 1976, A thermodynamic method for investigation of radiation induced changes in the microcirculation of human tumors, Int. J. Radiat. Oncol. Biol. Phys., 1: 659.

Mäntylä, M.J., 1979, Regional blood flow in human tumors, Cancer Res., 39: 2304.

Mäntylä, M.J., Toivanen, J.T., Pitkänen, M.A., and Rekonen, A.H., 1982, Radiation- induced changes in regional blood flow in human tumors, Int. J. Radiat. Oncol. Biol. Phys., 8: 1711.

Müller- Klieser, W., Vaupel, P., Manz, R., and Schmidseder, R., 1981, Intracapillary oxyhemoglobin saturation of malignant tumors in human, Int. J. Radiat. Oncol. Biol. Phys., 7: 1397.

Sauer, L.A., Stayman, J.W., and Dauchy, R.T., 1982, Amino acid, glucose, and lactic acid utilization in vivo by rat tumors, Cancer Res., 42: 4090.

Vaupel,P., 1977, Hypoxia in neoplastic tissue, Microvasc. Res., 13: 399.

Vaupel, P., 1982, Pathophysiologie der Durchblutung maligner Tumoren, Funktionsanalyse biolog. Syst., 8: 155.

Vaupel, P., Frinak, S., and Bicher, H.I., 1981, Heterogeneous oxygen partial pressure and pH distribution in C3H mouse mammary adenocarcinoma, Cancer Res., 41: 2008.

Vaupel, P., Kallinowski, F., Dave, S., Gabbert, H., and Bastert, G., 1985, Human mammary carcinomas in nude rats - a new approach for investigating oxygen transport and substrate utilization in tumor tissues, Advanc. Exptl. Med. Biol., in press.

Zander, R., 1981, Oxygen solubility in normal human blood, Advanc. Physiol. Sci., 25: 331.

GLUCOSE, LACTATE, AND KETONE BODY UTILIZATION BY HUMAN MAMMARY CARCINOMAS IN VIVO[*]

F. Kallinowski[1], S. Dave[1], P. Vaupel[1],
K.H. Baessler[2], and K. Wagner[2]

[1]Dept. Applied Physiology, and [2]Dept. Physiol.
Chemistry, University of Mainz, D-6500 Mainz

INTRODUCTION

Uncontrolled growth, one of the fundamental properties of malignant tumors, requires a great supply of energy. This energy can be derived from the use of a variety
of substrates. Besides glucose oxidation and glucose
breakdown to lactic acid, the turnover of endogeneous
substrates such as amino acids, free fatty acids and ketone bodies is well documented in vitro. However, under
in vivo conditions, only glucose utilization has been investigated in detail, using tumor isotransplants in rodents. For human tumors, only scarce data is available,
derived mainly from clinical observations rather than
from systematic studies.

Therefore, glucose, lactate and ketone body utilization have been studied in human mammary carcinomas
heterotransplanted in immune- deficient (rnu/rnu) rats
using an epigastric pouching technique.

MATERIAL AND METHODS

A total of 31 immune- deficient rats of both sexes
with a mean body weight of 250 ± 50 g were used in these
experiments. Cancer tissue from 5 different patients
(anaplastic and medullary carcinomas, serially transplanted as 28th to 60th generation heterotransplants in

---

[*]Supported by Deutsche Forschungsgemeinschaft (Va 57/2-4)

nude animals) was implanted in the epigastric region of these nude rats using a pouching technique. The experiments were performed approx. 32 $\pm$ 4 days after implantation (for further details concerning breeding and maintainance of these animals, the pouching technique, the microsurgical preparations and the experimental set- up see Vaupel et al., this volume).

Tumor blood flow (TBF) was assessed by a direct venous outflow technique. For the determination of glucose, lactate and ketone bodies blood samples from the tumor vein and the carotid artery were taken at the same time and transferred into ice- chilled $HClO_4$ immediately. Blood loss due to sampling was compensated by adequate transfusion of blood from donor rats via the external jugular vein.

The concentrations of the substrates were determined enzymatically. For determination of the glucose concentration in whole blood the hexokinase/G6P-DH method was used (Glucoquant test combination, Boehringer Mannheim, FRG). For determination of the lactate concentration in whole blood the lactate dehydrogenase method was used (lactate test combination, Boehringer Mannheim, FRG). The concentrations of the ketone bodies (acetoacetate, ß- hydroxybutyrate) were measured by means of 3- hydroxybutyrate- dehydrogenase according to the method described by Stein and Baessler (1968).

The availability of the above substrates to the tumor tissue was calculated taking into account the actual TBF and the respective arterial concentrations. The glucose uptake rate was derived from the arterio- tumorvenous concentration differences and the actual TBF according to Fick's principle. In the same way, according to the arterio- tumorvenous concentration differences of lactate and ketone bodies, release or uptake rates of these substrates was obtained. As a measure of the intramitochondrial redox potential, the ß- hydroxybutyrate/acetoacetate ratio in the tumorvenous blood was calculated.

All relevant parameters were determined repeatedly; in the case of TBF at least 5 times per hour. All measurements were taken under steady- state conditions. At the end of the experiments, the pouches were excised, weighed and examined by standard histological techniques.

Pouches with fat and/or granulomatous tissue served as controls. Measurements on 7 control pouches were performed.

764

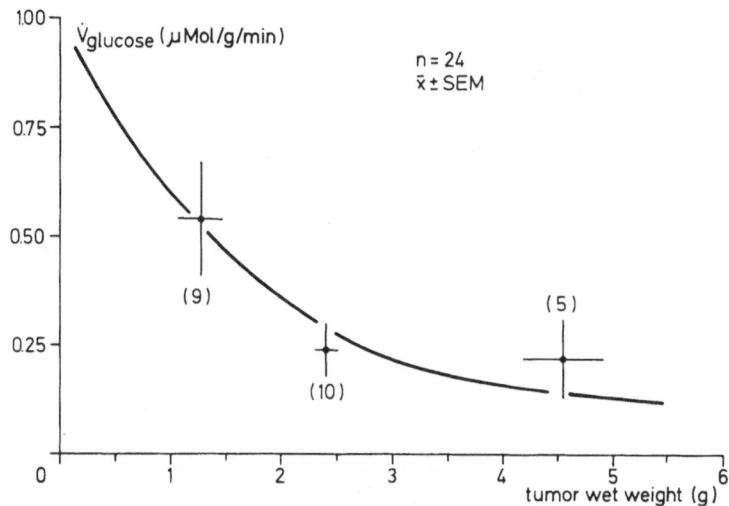

Fig.1. Glucose uptake rate ($\dot{V}_{glucose}$) of human mammary
carcinomas heterotransplanted into nude rats as a
function of tumor wet weight. Numbers in brackets
indicate the respective number of tumors investigated.

RESULTS

From the 24 tumors studied so far the results obtained clearly show that the glucose uptake rate decreases from 1.090 to 0.018 µMol/g/min with increasing tumor
wet weight from 0.15 to 5.47 g (see Fig.1). The average
glucose uptake rate was 0.351 ± 0.311 µMol/g/min at a
mean tumor wet weight of 2.42 ± 1.33 g. The amount of
glucose taken up was linearly related to the amount of
glucose available within the availability range studied
(0.12 to 2.95 µMol/g/min; see Fig.2).

All tumors with the exception of three released lactate. With increasing glucose uptake rate there is a linear rise of the lactic acid output from 23.5 to 779.9
nMol/g/min (mean lactate release: 228.9 ± 253.6 nMol/g/min).
The three exceptions mentioned utilize lactate and inci-
dentally show the highest glucose uptake rate (see Fig.3).

ß- hydroxybutyrate is taken up by most of the tumors
(mean uptake rate: 2.59 ± 3.34 nMol/g/min), the rate of
uptake being linearly related to the amount of ß- hydroxybutyrate available in the availability range studied (Fig.4).

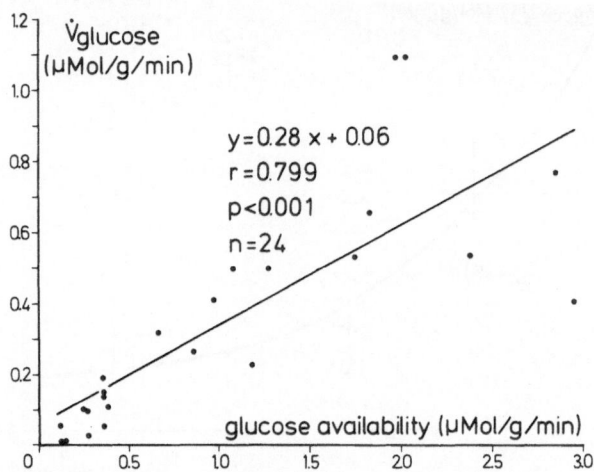

Fig.2. Glucose uptake rate ($\dot{V}_{glucose}$) of human mammary
carcinoma xenotransplants as a function of glucose
availability in the arterial blood.

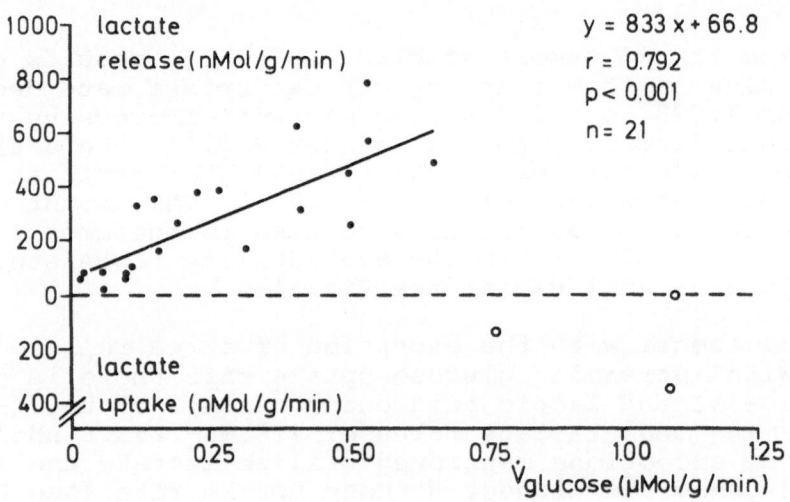

Fig.3. Lactate release (dots) and lactate uptake (circles)
as a function of glucose uptake rate. (The linear
regression line was calculated from the release
data only.)

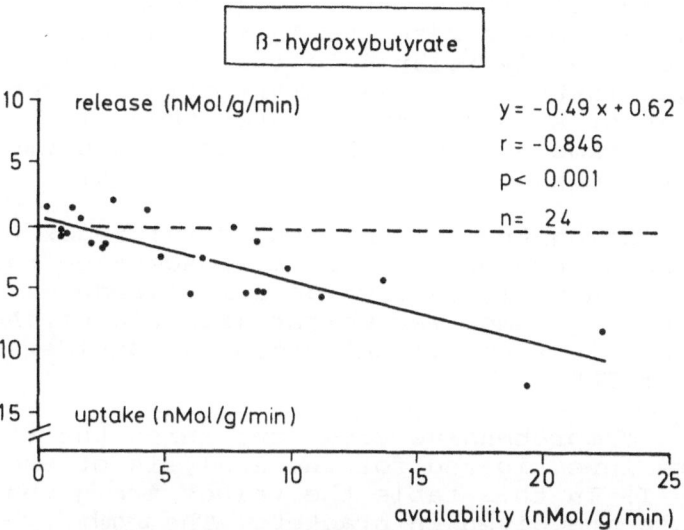

Fig.4. ß-hydroxybutyrate release or uptake by human breast cancers as a function of the ß-hydroxybutyrate availability.

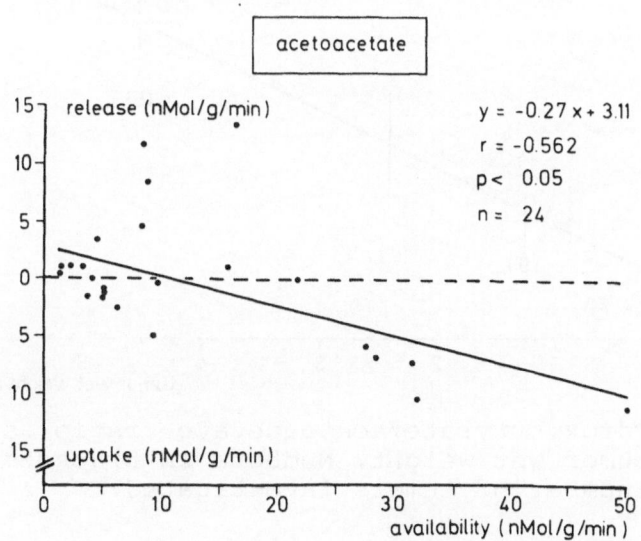

Fig.5. Acetoacetate release or uptake of human mammary carcinomas in nude rats as a function of aceto-acetate availability.

For acetoacetate the pattern is somewhat more complex.
Although the majority of the tumors tend to take up acetoacetate (mean uptake rate: 0.318 ± 6.036 nMol/g/min), the
rate being linearly related to its availability in the
range investigated, several tumors release acetoacetate
in high rates. As a common feature, these latter tumors
at the same time exhibit a high glucose consumption rate
and a sustained lactic acidosis (see Fig.5).

Considering the intramitochondrial redox potential
status, the ß- hydroxybutyrate/acetoacetate- ratio shifts
to higher values, i.e., towards a more reduced state,
with increasing tumor wet weight (see Fig.6). An inverse
relationship is found if the ratio is considered as a
function of TBF.

For a comprehensive view concerning the relevant
parameters investigated for the analysis of energy supply
see Table I. In this table the values are given as means
±SD; ranges are given in brackets. The symbol "-" indicates
a release of the respective substrate.

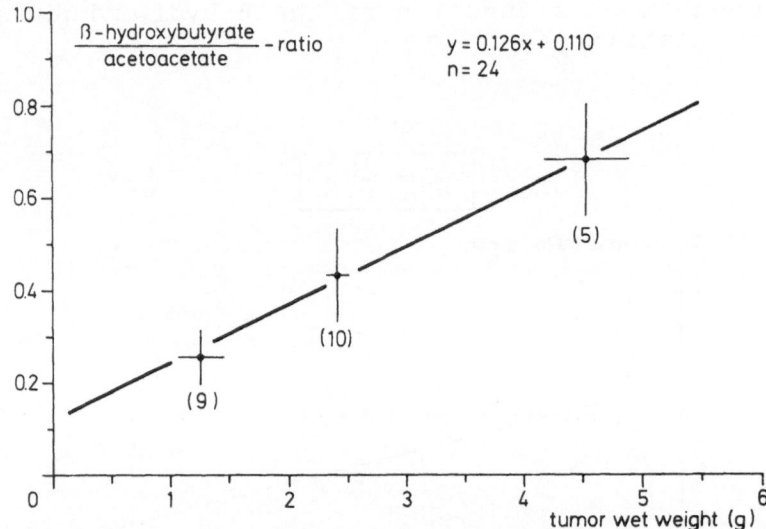

Fig.6. ß-hydroxybutyrate/acetoacetate- ratio as a function
of tumor wet weight. Numbers in brackets indicate
the number of tumors investigated.

Table I. Compilation of the relevant parameters investigated for the analysis of energy supply to human mammary carcinomas heterotransplanted into nude rats.

	tumors	controls
blood flow (ml/g/min)	0.12 ± 0.10 ($0.02 - 0.34$)	0.34 ± 0.22 ($0.18 - 0.81$)
art. C_{gl} ($\mu Mol/ml$)	8.78 ± 2.36 ($4.77 - 14.89$)	7.36 ± 1.24 ($5.86 - 9.53$)
ven. C_{gl} ($\mu Mol/ml$)	5.52 ± 1.22 ($2.83 - 7.66$)	6.03 ± 0.89 ($5.08 - 7.69$)
avD_{gl} ($\mu Mol/ml$)	3.26 ± 1.82 ($0.92 - 7.26$)	1.33 ± 0.77 ($0.28 - 2.60$)
$\dot{V}_{gl}$ ($\mu Mol/g/min$)	0.35 ± 0.31 ($0.02 - 1.09$)	0.39 ± 0.31 ($0.18 - 1.06$)
art. C_{lac} ($\mu Mol/ml$)	5.99 ± 2.79 ($3.00 - 13.45$)	4.40 ± 1.34 ($2.16 - 6.46$)
ven. C_{lac} ($\mu Mol/ml$)	8.84 ± 3.37 ($4.20 - 17.29$)	4.67 ± 1.25 ($3.22 - 6.71$)
vaD_{lac} ($\mu Mol/ml$)	2.84 ± 2.28 ($2.15 - -8.63$)	0.27 ± 1.25 ($1.00 - -2.22$)
$\dot{V}_{lac}$ ($nMol/g/min$)	-228.94 ± 253.59 ($358.00 - -779.90$)	-27.56 ± 297.78 ($211.80 - -497.60$)
art. C_{acac} ($\mu Mol/ml$)	0.114 ± 0.045 ($0.04 - 0.25$)	0.14 ± 0.07 ($0.05 - 0.26$)
ven. C_{acac} ($\mu Mol/ml$)	0.115 ± 0.045 ($0.07 - 0.21$)	0.12 ± 0.06 ($0.07 - 0.11$)
$av D_{acac}$ ($\mu Mol/ml$)	-0.001 ± 0.060 ($0.13 - -0.10$)	0.02 ± 0.04 ($0.08 - -0.03$)
$\dot{V}_{acac}$ ($nMol/g/min$)	-0.32 ± 6.04 ($11.10 - -13.50$)	3.27 ± 12.10 ($21.80 - -11.70$)
art. $C_{\beta- HB}$ ($\mu Mol/ml$)	0.06 ± 0.03 ($0.01 - 0.12$)	0.04 ± 0.02 ($0.03 - 0.09$)
ven. $C_{\beta- HB}$ ($\mu Mol/ml$)	0.04 ± 0.03 ($0.00 - 0.14$)	0.04 ± 0.06 ($0.00 - 0.20$)
$av D_{\beta- HB}$ ($\mu Mol/ml$)	0.02 ± 0.04 ($0.08 - -0.06$)	-0.003 ± 0.073 ($0.07 - -0.15$)
$\dot{V}_{\beta- HB}$ ($nMol/g/min$)	2.59 ± 3.34 ($12.60 - -8.06$)	-0.44 ± 19.74 ($12.90 - -44.40$)

The mean glucose uptake rate of fat and granulomatous tissue (controls, n = 7) was 0.39 ± 0.31 µMol/g/min (range: 0.18 to 1.06 µMol/g/min) at an average tissue wet weight of 0.38 ± 0.20 g (range: 0.15 to 0.70 g) and a mean glucose availability of 2.47 ± 1.45 µMol/g/min (range: 1.22 to 5.50 µMol/g/min). The controls utilized or released lactate with a mean lactate release rate of 27.56 ± 297.78 nMol/g/min. On the whole, the controls appear to release ß- hydroxybutyrate (0.44 ± 19.74 nMol/g/min) but they tend to take up acetoacetate (3.27 ± 12.10 nMol/g/min).

DISCUSSION

The glucose uptake of human mammary carcinomas transplanted into nude rats is in the same range as that obtained on isotransplanted rodent tumors (see Table II). From the results available, it is clear that the glucose consumption in tumors depends on the glucose availability, a finding that has been reported consistently on rodent isotransplants (Gullino et al., 1967; Vaupel, 1974; Sauer et al., 1982, 1983) and holds true for human mammary carcinomas xenografted into nude rats as well. With increasing tumor wet weight, the weight- related glucose consumption of human mammary carcinomas decreases as has been reported previously for rodent isotransplants (Vaupel, 1974) as well as for osteosarcomas in patients (Norton et al., 1980).

Human mammary carcinomas release lactate, the amount of which depends on the rate of glucose consumed, as has been reported previously for rodent isotransplants (Vaupel, 1974). Regarding human mammary carcinomas with lactate uptake, the only common finding is that lactate uptake occurred at the highest glucose consumption rates observed. It has been reported previously for various rodent tumors, that tumors are able to take lactate up at higher arterial lactate concentrations (Sauer et al, 1982). In contrast to this, human mammary carcinomas release lactate at corresponding arterial lactate concentrations.

Rodent tumor isotransplants take up acetoacetate and ß- hydroxybutyrate, the uptake rate being linearly related to the amount supplied. This also holds true for fasted rats in which the supply is approx. ten-fold increased (Sauer et al., 1982). A similar relationship is found for human mammary carcinomas although human mammary carcinomas seem to be able to release acetoacetate and ß- hydroxybutyrate as well as utilize it. This behavior may be a special metabolic feature of mammary tumors as ketogenesis

Table II. Glucose uptake rate ($\dot{V}_{gl}$), glucose availability (gl_{avail}) and tumor wet weight (tww) in various tumors

Tumor type	$\dot{V}_{gl}$ (μMol/g/min)	tww (g)	$gl_{avail.}$ (μMol/g/min)	Author(s)
Walker tumor	0.89 ± 0.18	2.0 - 11.5	3.15 ± 0.46	Gullino et al. (1967)
hepatoma 5123	0.51 ± 0.25	3.4 - 7.0	2.22 ± 0.74	
fibrosarcoma 4956	0.45 ± 0.25	5.0 - 12.7	1.30 ± 0.65	
DS- Carcinosarcoma	0.22 ± 0.10	5.8 ± 1.2	1.28 ± 0.12	Vaupel (1974)
hepatoma 5123c	0.12 ± 0.03	2.5	0.33	Sauer et al. (1982)
hepatoma 7777	0.15 ± 0.06	1.8	0.45	
hepatoma 7288 CTCF	0.18 ± 0.04	1.8	0.45	
Walker tumor	0.23 ± 0.07	1.1	0.74	
Human breast cancers	0.35 ± 0.31	2.42 ± 1.33	1.04 ± 0.90	this paper

has been reported to be a property of normal mammary glands (Terner, 1958). On the other hand, in case of significant acetoacetate release one may speculate that those tumors are in a poor energetic state and thus are forced to convert ß- hydroxybutyrate to acetoacetate. Subsequently they are unable to further oxidize the latter substrate and have to release it.

The ß- hydroxybutyrate/acetoacetate- ratio gives an insight into the intramitochondrial redox state. Since with increasing tumor wet weight TBF and the oxygen consumption rate are progressively reduced (see Dave et al., this volume), it is not surprising that the intramitochondrial redox potential shifts towards a more reduced state with increasing tumor wet weight or decreasing tumor blood flow. Therefore, tumor hypoxia is not only evidenced by a rising lactate/pyruvate- ratio (Vaupel, 1974), but also by a rising ß- hydroxybutyrate/acetoacetate- ratio with increasing tumor wet weight, both alterations directly or indirectly reflecting an impaired intramitochondrial energy production, which in turn can hinder the cytosolic substrate utilization due to proton accumulation.

SUMMARY

1. The glucose uptake rate of human mammary carcinomas transplanted into nude rats is comparable to values obtained in isotransplanted rodent tumors. The glucose uptake decreases with increasing tumor wet weight and is linearly related to the glucose availability.
2. Most tumors release lactate, the rate being linearly related to the glucose uptake rate.
3. Tumors use acetoacetate and ß- hydroxybutyrate as substrates. Additionally, human mammary carcinomas may have the ability for ketogenesis probably depending on the metabolic state.
4. Using the epigastric pouching technique, human mammary carcinoma xenografts in nude rats seem to be a valid model for systematic investigations of the energy supply of human tumors.

REFERENCES

Dave, S., Kallinowski, F., Vaupel, P., 1985, Blood flow and oxygen supply to human mammary carcinomas transplanted into nude rats, Advanc. Exptl. Med. Biol., (in press).
Gullino, P.M., Grantham, F.H., Courtney, A.H., 1967, Glucose consumption by transplanted tumors in vivo, Cancer Res., 27: 1031.

Norton, J.A., Burt, M.E., Brennan, M.F., 1980, In vivo utilization of substrate by human sarcoma-bearing limbs, Cancer, 45: 2934.

Sauer, L.A., Stayman, J.W., Dauchy, R.T., 1982, Amino acid, glucose, lactic acid utilization in vivo by rat tumors, Cancer Res., 42: 4090.

Sauer, L.A., Dauchy, R.T., 1983, Ketone body, glucose, lactic acid, and amino acid utilization by tumors in vivo in fasted rats, Cancer Res., 43: 4397.

Stein, G., and Baessler, K.H., 1968, Mikromethode zur enzymatischen Bestimmung von Acetessigsaeure und D-(-)-ß- Hydroxybuttersaeure in Blut und Geweben, Zschr. Klin. Chem. Klin. Biochem. 6: 27.

Terner, C., 1958, The formation of acetoacetate in homogenates of the mammary gland, Biochem. J., 70, 402.

Vaupel, P., 1974, Atemgaswechsel und Glucosestoffwechsel von Implantationstumoren (DS- Carcinosarkom) in vivo, Funktionsanalyse biolog. Systeme, 1: 1.

Vaupel, P., Kallinowski, F., Dave, S., Gabbert, H., Bastert, G., 1985, Human mammary carcinomas in nude rats - a new approach in cancer research, Advanc. Exptl. Med. Biol., (in press).

CHANGES IN O_2 CONSUMPTION OF MULTICELLULAR SPHEROIDS DURING DEVELOPMENT OF NECROSIS *

W. Mueller-Klieser[1], B. Bourrat[1], H. Gabbert[2], and R.M. Sutherland[1]

[1]Dept. of Applied Physiology, and [2]Dept. of Pathology
University of Mainz, D-6500 Mainz, FRG

INTRODUCTION

Multicellular spheroids are spherical aggregates of cells that are supplied by diffusion of oxygen and substrates from the surrounding growth medium (Sutherland and Durand, 1976). Metabolic waste products are removed from the cells in these aggregates by diffusion into the growth medium. Cells within multicellular spheroids may be exposed to environmental conditions similar to those in tissue located between nutritive microvessels. Thus, tumor spheroids make it possible to study the impact of the tumor-specific micromilieu on cellular metabolism, cell cycle state, cellular viability or response to treatment. Factors in the microenvironment of tumor cells which may be relevant in this regard, are the oxygen tension (P_{O_2}), as well as the concentration of hydrogen ions (pH), of glucose and other nutrients, and of metabolic waste products such as lactate. The distribution of P_{O_2}-values in spheroids has been assessed by several investigators using O_2-sensitive microelectrodes (Carlsson et al., 1979; Kaufman et al., 1981; Mueller-Klieser and Sutherland, 1982a,b, 1983; Mueller-Klieser et al., 1983; Hetzel and Kaufman, 1983; Mueller-Klieser, 1984a,b). The data obtained indicate that the steady state P_{O_2}-distribution in spheroids is determined by the balance between O_2 diffusion from the surrounding

*This work has been supported by grants Mu 576/1 and Mu 576/2-1 from the Deutsche Forschungsgemeinschaft, by grants CA 20329, CA 11198 and CA 11051 from the National Cancer Institute, NIH, and by the "Award for Senior U.S. Scientists" from the Alexander von Humboldt-Stiftung to Robert M. Sutherland as a Visiting Professor at the Department of Applied Physiology, University of Mainz.

medium into the spheroids and the O_2 consumption within the spheroids. It has been demonstrated that a theoretical analysis of steady state P_{O_2}-profiles in multicellular spheroids may result in a quantitative characterization of O_2 metabolism and O_2 diffusion properties in spheroids (Franko and Sutherland, 1979; Freyer, 1981; Bush et al., 1983; Mueller-Klieser, 1984a,b; Franko and Freedman, 1984; Mueller-Klieser and Sutherland, in press). The evaluation of P_{O_2}-profiles in EMT6/Ro-spheroids revealed a decrease in volume-related O_2-consumption rate Q with increasing spheroid size (Mueller-Klieser and Sutherland, in press). The respective data also indicate that this correlation between Q and spheroid diameter may be particularly pronounced in a size range in which the development of central necroses occurs. However, more data from small spheroids without necrosis were needed to support this interpretation of the respective measurements. Therefore, the goal of the present study was to measure P_{O_2}-profiles in small EMT6-spheroids without central necrosis under conditions comparable to those from previous investigations. In the present investigation, the volume-related O_2-consumption rate Q was derived from the measured profiles using a method published previously (Mueller-Klieser, 1984b). In addition, P_{O_2}-values were obtained from spheroids with small central necrotic areas in an early stage of development.

MATERIALS AND METHODS

1. Spheroid Culturing

Culturing of monolayers and multicellular spheroids from EMT6/Ro-cells was performed as described in detail elsewhere (Freyer and Sutherland, 1980). The spheroids were grown in spinner flasks using Eagle's basal medium supported with 15 % (v/v) fetal calf serum. The medium contained 5.5 mM glucose and was equilibrated with air and 3 % (v/v) CO_2 creating a P_{O_2} in the bulk medium in the range of 140-145 mm Hg.

2. Histological investigations

To determine the thickness of the viable rim serial paraffin sections stained with hematoxylin and eosin were prepared from 22 spheroids with diameters in the range of 400-1000 μm. Spheroids were sized before and after histological processing to account for shrinkage artefacts. The thickness of the viable rim in each spheroid was determined through measuring the rim thicknesses in central sections on two orthogonal diameters and taking the mean of these measurements.

3. Measurements of P_{O_2}-profiles in spheroids

P_{O_2}-profiles were recorded in spheroids using O_2-sensitive micro-electrodes with a recessed cathode according to Whalen et al. (1967). Steady state P_{O_2}-distributions were measured on radial tracks through the center of spheroids under conditions that closely match the growth conditions in the spinner flasks. This was achieved by employing a set-up for microelectrode measurements that has been described previously (Mueller-Klieser and Sutherland, 1982a). Unlike in previous studies, the present experimental set-up allowed the continuous monitoring of P_{O_2}, P_{CO_2} and pH in the medium flowing through the measuring chamber. This was made possible by pumping the medium through the measuring system of a blood gas analyzer positioned next to the chamber. The electrode was advanced stepwise from the medium into the spheroid with changing step widths. A steady state reading over a time period of 30-60 s was recorded at each step. Usually, a step width of 10 μm was chosen when the electrode tip approached the surface and penetrated the spheroid, as determined by microscopic observation. Further inside and outside the spheroids the step width was increased to 20-30 μm and 50-60 μm, respectively (see Fig. 1). The P_{O_2}-distributions obtained were characterized by a diffusion-depleted zone around the spheroids with O_2 tensions below the P_{O_2} in the bulk medium and by a parabolic P_{O_2}-profile inside spheroids without necrotic centers. Investi-

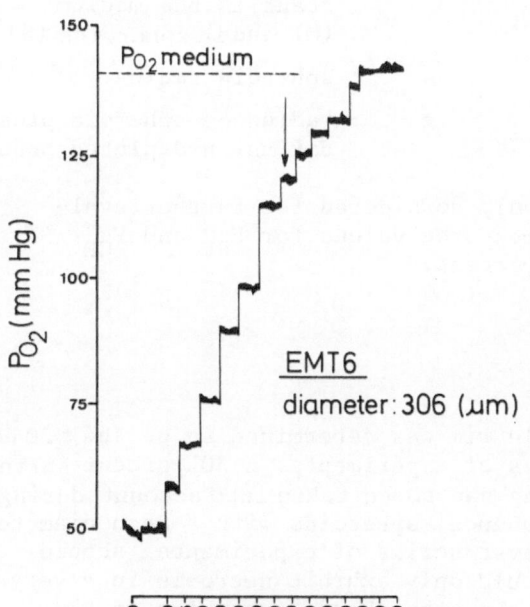

Fig. 1.

Original tracing of P_{O_2}-measurements in multi-cellular spheroids (abscissa to be read from the right to the left); the arrow indicates the spheroid surface.

gations were carried out on two series of spheroids: (i) 16 spheroids with a diameter (mean ± SD) of 291 ± 30 μm (range: 232–347 μm)
showing no central necrosis or only necrosis in a very early stage
of development (ii) 10 spheroids with a diameter (mean ± SD) of
460 ± 29 μm exhibiting central necrosis throughout.

4. Determination of O_2 consumption

The volume–related O_2 consumption rate Q in each individual
spheroid was determined from the P_{O_2}-gradient in the diffusion-
depleted zone around the spheroid using theoretical considerations.
It has been demonstrated that this P_{O_2}-gradient is proportional to
the overall O_2-consumption in the spheroid considered (Mueller-
Klieser, 1984b). Similar considerations lead to the determination
of Krogh's diffusion constant K_S in the spheroid from the P_{O_2}-
gradient in the viable part of the spheroid. To improve the
accuracy of this method the values obtained for Q and K_S were used
to calculate the P_{O_2} at the spheroid surface (P_{SF}) and in the spheroid center (P_{CE}). For spheroids without necrosis the following
equations were applied:

$$(I) \quad P_{SF} = P_M - \frac{Qs^2}{3\,K_M}\left(1 - \frac{s}{g}\right) ; \qquad P_M \quad : P_{O_2} \text{ in the bulk medium}$$

$$K_M, K_S : \text{Krogh's diffusion con-}$$
stant in the medium
(M) and in spheroids (S)

$$(II) \quad P_{CE} = P_{SF} - \frac{Qs^2}{6\,K_S} ;$$

$$s \quad : \text{spheroid radius}$$

$$g \quad : \text{radius of spheroid plus}$$
diffusion-depleted zone

Values for Q and K_S were only considered for further evaluation, if the calculated and measured values for P_{SF} and P_{CE}
did not differ by more than 5 percent.

RESULTS

1. Histological investigations

The thickness of the viable rim was determined to be 164 ± 20 μm
(mean ± SD) in the present series of experiments. A 30 percent shrinkage due to histological processing had to be taken into account during
these measurements. As a consequence, spheroids with a mean diameter
of 291 μm, as studied in the first series of experiments, should
not contain any necrosis or should only exhibit necrosis in a very
early stage of development. On the other hand, spheroids of the
second series of experiments with a mean diameter of 460 μm can be
expected to contain central necrotic areas.

778

2. P_{O_2}-distribution in the spheroids

P_{O_2}-profiles measured were in a good agreement with those recorded in previous studies. Fig. 2 shows the P_{O_2}-values in the center of EMT6-spheroids as a function of spheroid size from the present investigation (dots) and from earlier experiments (circles). It is obvious that the oxygenation of the spheroid centers is similar in both series of experiments indicating a deterioration of O_2-supply with increasing spheroid size. The change in the slope of the P_{O_2}-profile at the spheroid surface of small spheroids was less pronounced than in larger EMT6-spheroids investigated previously.

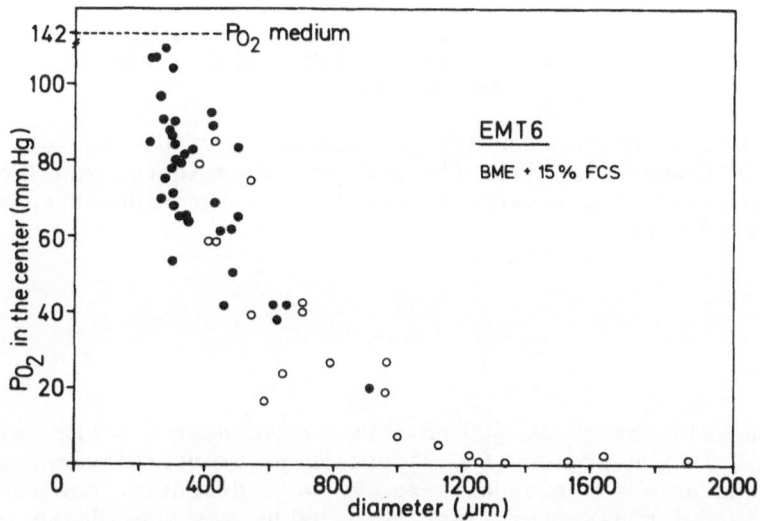

Fig. 2.   Central P_{O_2} in EMT6-spheroids from the present study (dots) and from previous experiments (circles) as a function of spheroid size.

3. O_2 consumption rate

The volume-related O_2-consumption rate Q (mean ± SD) in EMT6-spheroids with a diameter of 291 ± 30 μm was $(7.49 \pm 1.1) \cdot 10^{-4}$ ml $O_2 \cdot$ cm$^{-3} \cdot$s^{-1}. Q dropped to $(4.56 \pm 0.52) \cdot 10^{-4}$ ml $O_2 \cdot$cm$^{-3} \cdot$s^{-1} in spheroids with diameters ranging from 418 μm to 499 μm. In spheroids larger than 1000 μm in diameter an average value for Q of $2.42 \cdot 10^{-4}$ ml $O_2 \cdot$cm$^{-3} \cdot$s^{-1} was found. The data provided evidence for a distinct decrease in Q by a factor of approximately 3 in the diameter range of 200–600 μm with increasing spheroid size (see Fig. 3). Only a slight decrease in Q occurred, when the spheroid diameter

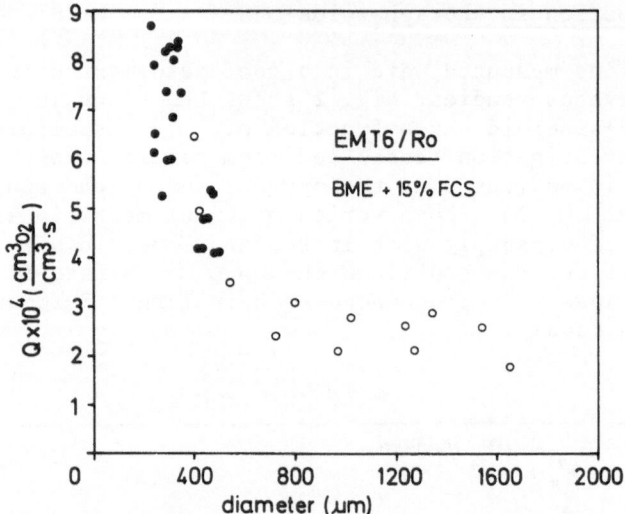

Fig. 3. Oxygen consumption (Q) per volume of viable regions in
EMT6-spheroids from the present study (dots) and from
previous experiments (circles) as a function of spheroid size.

exceeded a value of about 600 µm. Fig. 3 demonstrates the values
found for Q in the present (dots) and in previous (circles) investigations as a function of size. Krogh's diffusion constant K_S
in spheroids with diameters less than 300 µm was considerably higher
than that in larger spheroids (>600 µm), i.e. $3.29 \cdot 10^{-5}$ ml $O_2 \cdot cm^{-1} \cdot$
$min^{-1} \cdot atm^{-1}$ versus $1.87 \cdot 10^{-5}$ ml $O_2 \cdot cm^{-1} \cdot min^{-1} \cdot atm^{-1}$. However, K_S
decreased towards the latter value even in smaller spheroids in the
size range of 400-500 µm. These changes in K_S cannot be explained
on the basis of the present data. The values obtained for Q and K_S
allowed the calculation of P_{O_2}-profiles that closely match the
experimental data from micro-electrode measurements. A representative example is demonstrated in Fig. 4.

DISCUSSION

The present findings suggest that there is a substantial
decrease in the O_2-consumption per volume in viable regions of
multicellular EMT6-spheroids. This change in Q mainly occurs in a

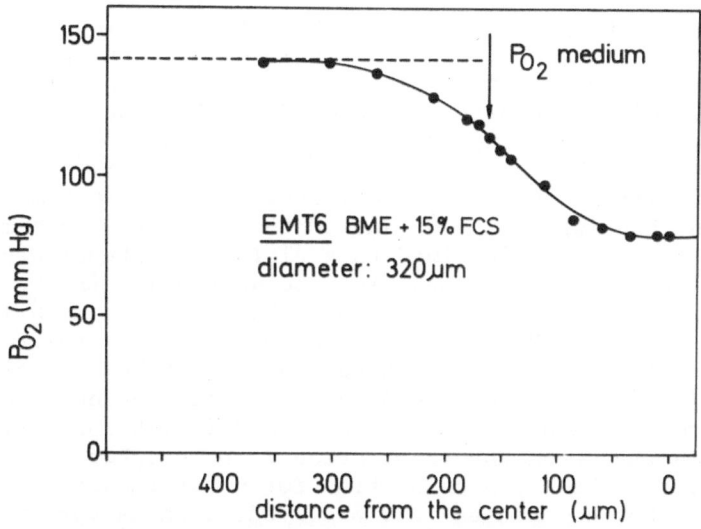

Fig. 4. Calculated (solid line) and measured (dots) P_{O_2} - distribution in an EMT6-spheroid with a diameter of 320 μm. (The arrow indicates the spheroid surface.)

size range in which central necrosis develops. A comparison of the values for Q with the O_2-consumption rate of single cells is difficult on the basis of the data available at present, since the volume fraction of extracellular space is not exactly known, and since the O_2 consumption rate of single cells can vary depending on nutrient supply conditions, such as glucose or glutamine supply. A comparison among the respective O_2 consumption rates on a per cell basis, however, leads to the conclusion that Q in the smallest spheroids investigated is approximately equal to that found for single EMT6-cells (Freyer, 1981; Mueller-Klieser, unpublished data).

Changes in O_2-consumption similar to that found in this investigation have been reported recently for EMT-spheroids (Freyer, 1981) and for V79-spheroids (Freyer et al., 1984) using a polarographic method for O_2 consumption measurements. In the latter study a sharp drop in Q by a factor of four was observed in spheroids with diameters of 200-400 μm. This result could be partially explained by the impact of the microenvironment in spheroids on cellular respiration and by changes in Q due to alterations in the proliferative status of the cells. The decrease in Q with increasing spheroid size registered in the present study seems to be extended over a wider diameter range than in the findings quoted. Also, the change in Q of V79-spheroids occurs before necrosis develops, yet the corresponding decrease of Q in EMT6-spheroids starts before but continues after necrosis has developed. These differences may be indicative of different mechanisms involved in changing Q in V79- and EMT6-spheroids. The same mechanisms may also be involved to a different extent; e.g., it has been found that the differences in Q between cells in the exponential growth phase and in the plateau phase are much less in EMT6-cells than in V79-cells. Thus, changes in the proliferative status of cells may be less critical for Q in EMT6-spheroids than for Q in V79-spheroids. On the other hand, substances from the necrotic area which have no influence on Q in V79-spheroids may well have an impact on the respiration in EMT6-spheroids. Equivalent considerations may also be true for other factors possibly contributing to the changes in Q observed, such as variations in cell packing density or in cell-cell interaction, or such as accumulation of metabolic waste products.

The present results should be taken into consideration when critical diffusion distances are calculated for tumor tissue. If these calculations are performed using the O_2-consumption rate of the respective single cells, the length of diffusion distances will be extremely underestimated. The data presented in this paper also imply that the respiration in tumor tissue may not be a fixed 'intrinsic' characteristic of the particular tumor cell considered, but may be influenced by many physiological parameters and may be changed through mechanisms yet unknown.

Local variations in Q within the spheroids have not been detected in the present study and in previous investigations on EMT6-spheroids (Mueller-Klieser, 1984a,b) whereas other investigators have found such variations in spheroids from several cell lines (Bush et al., 1983; Grossmann et al., 1983). These discrepancies may be elicited in part by the use of different cell lines. Recently, we have recorded P_{O_2}-distributions in spheroids from human coloncarcinoma cells that indicate a decrease of Q in the inner parts of the spheroids. To some extent, the discrepancies mentioned may be attributed to using different culturing and measuring techniques.

Further investigations on factors with possible influence on O_2 consumption in spheroids are required for a better understanding of the mechanisms involved in the changes in Q observed. Observations should be concentrated on cell number per spheroid, mean cell colume, volume fraction of extracellular space, or on diffusion of glucose and other nutrients into the spheroids investigated. These studies should contribute to quantifying the interrelationship among nutrient supply, proliferative status and metabolic rates in solid tumors, thus, characterizing factors which may critically determine tumor growth and tumor response to therapy (Vaupel, 1980).

SUMMARY

Using O_2-sensitive microelectrodes oxygen tension profiles were recorded in EMT6-spheroids either showing no necrosis or having developed a small necrotic area in the center. The profiles obtained were in accordance with those measured in previous investigations under similar conditions. The volume-related O_2-consumption rate Q in the viable parts of the spheroids could be determined through theoretical considerations. The results show that there is a steep decrease in Q by a factor of three when the spheroids grow from diameters of 200 µm to diameters larger than 1000 µm. The drop in Q mainly occurs in a size range in which central necrosis develops in EMT6-spheroids cultured under these particular conditions. Among other factors, changes in the proliferative status, in extracellular volume fraction or in physiological parameters of the micromilieu in spheroids, such as accumulation of metabolic waste products or of toxic substances from the necrotic area may contribute to the variation in Q observed.

REFERENCES

Bush, N.A., Bruley, D.F., and Bicher, H.I., 1983, Identification of viable regions in "in vitro" spheroidal tumors: a mathematical investigation, Adv. Exp. Med. Biol., 157:1.

Carlsson, J., Stalnacke, C.G., Acker, H., Haji-Karim, M., Milsson, S., and Larsson, B., 1979, The influence of oxygen on viability and proliferation in cellular spheroids, Int. J. Radiat. Oncol. Biol. Phys., 5:2011.

Franko, A.J., and Sutherland, R.M., 1979, Oxygen diffusion distance and development of necrosis in multicell spheroids, Radiat. Res., 79:439.

Franko, A.J., and Freedman, H.I., 1984, Model of diffusion of oxygen to spheroids grown in stationary medium - I. Complete symmetry, Bull. Math. Biol., 46:205.

Freyer, J.P., 1981, Heterogeneity in multicell spheroids induced by alterations in the external oxygen and glucose concentration, Thesis, University of Rochester, N.Y.

Freyer, J.P., and Sutherland, R.M., 1980, Selective dissociation and characterization of cells from different regions of multicell tumor spheroids, Cancer Res., 40:3956.

Freyer, J.P., Tustanoff, E., Franko, A.J., and Sutherland, R.M., 1984, In situ oxygen consumption rates of cells in V79-multicellular spheroids during growth, J. Cell. Physiol., 118:53.

Grossmann, U., Carlsson, J., and Acker, H., 1983, Oxygen consumption profiles inside cellular spheroids calculated from P_{O_2}-profiles Adv. Exp. Med. Biol., 159:477.

Hetzel, F.W., and Kaufman, N., 1983, Chemotherapeutic drugs as indirect oxygen radiosensitizers, Int. J. Radiat. Oncol. Biol. Phys., 9:751.

Kaufman, N., Bicher, H.I., Hetzel, F.W., and Brown, M., 1981, A system for determining the pharmacology of indirect radiation sensitizer drugs on multicellular spheroids, Cancer Clin. Trials, 4:199.

Mueller-Klieser, W., 1984a, Microelectrode measurements of oxygen tension distributions in multicellular spheroids cultured in spinner flasks, Rec. Res. Cancer Res., 95:134.

Mueller-Klieser, W., 1984b, A method for the determination of oxygen consumption rates and oxygen diffusion coefficients in multicellular spheroids, Biophys. J., 46:in press.

Mueller-Klieser, W., and Sutherland, R.M., 1982a, Influence of convection in the growth medium on oxygen tensions in multicellular tumor spheroids, Cancer Res., 42:237.

Mueller-Klieser, W., and Sutherland, R.M., 1982b, Oxygen tensions in multicell spheroids of two cell lines, Brit. J. Cancer, 45:256.

Mueller-Klieser, W., and Sutherland, R.M., 1983, Frequency distribution histograms of oxygen tensions in multicell spheroids, Adv. Exp. Med. Biol., 159:497.

Mueller-Klieser, W., and Sutherland, R.M., in press, Oxygen consumption and oxygen diffusion properties of multicellular spheroids from two different cell lines, Adv. Exp. Med. Biol.,

Mueller-Klieser, W., Freyer, J.P., and Sutherland, R.M., 1983, Evidence for a major role of glucose in controlling development of necrosis in EMT6/Ro multicell tumor spheroids, Adv. Exp. Med. Biol., 159:487.

Sutherland, R.M., and Durand, R.E., 1976, Radiation response of multicellular spheroids - an in vitro tumour model, Curr. Top. Radiat. Res., 11:87.

Vaupel, P., 1980, Oxygen supply to malignant tumors, in: "Tumor Blood Circulation: Angiogenesis, Morphology and Blood Flow of Experimental and Human Tumors", H.I. Peterson, ed., CRC Press, Boca Raton.

Whalen, W.J., Riley, J., and Nair, P., 1967, A microelectrode for measuring intracellular P_{O_2}, J. Appl. Physiol., 23:798.

THE BEHAVIOUR OF THE TISSUE pO_2 IN TRANSPARENT CHAMBERS OF RATS WITH AND WITHOUT TUMOUR IMPLANTATIONS

P. Streichhan[1], M. Fischer[2], and H. Acker[1]

[1]Max-Planck-Institut für Systemphysiologie
Rheinlanddamm 201, 4600 Dortmund, FRG
[2]Physiologisches Institut II der Universität (Neuro-
physiologie); Wilhelm Straße 31, 5300 Bonn, FRG

INTRODUCTION

Tissue oxygen partial pressure (p_tO_2) reflects O_2 supply and O_2 consumption of an organ and, hence, has characteristic values in active biological systems (Lübbers, 1981a, 1981b; Kessler et al., 1984). Restorations of an organ-specific O_2 supply after injuries have often been examined, since recovery of O_2 supply is important for the survival of tissue either in natural wounds or clinical surgery (Hunt, 1970, 1973; Hunt et al., 1966, 1972a, 1972b; Goodwin and Heppenstall, 1978; Silver, 1978, Winter, 1978). In order to follow structural and functional changes in wounds simultaneously, recent experimental work in wound healing of subcutaneous tissue was often done by intra-vitalmicroscopy in transparent chambers (van den Brenk, 1956; Endrich et al., 1982). This report deals with the healing of chronic subcutis wounds in dorsal rat skinfolds covered by transparent chambers (TK) (Streichhan and Lübbers, 1982). It is confined to p_tO_2 changes as a function of post-operative age in acute normoxic, hypoxic, and post-hypoxic breathing conditions. Modulations of p_tO_2 under the different conditions by heteroplastic tumour implantations were investigated as a further parameter.

METHODS

Experiments were done on about 6 months old female Wistar rats of roughly 200 g body weight (BW), with or without tissue pockets inside the wound area. The construction of the experimental plexiglass TK is shown in Fig. 1. It was implanted in rats by means of plastic screws and silicon distancers. The animals were shaved

785

and chemically depilated 24 hours before operation. TK implantation resembled the description of Papenfuss et al. (1979) to a large degree. The planed subcutis tissue, which was embedded without contusions, had a thickness of 600-650 μm. In order to avoid foldings because of muscle atrophies inside the skinfolds, the TKs were fixed in their position by adhesive tapes and individually adapted ventral plastic corsets. The TKs and their envelopes had a weight of about 26 g. In intervals of 1 - 3 days TK fitting and regeneration processes were inspected under anesthesia (40-50 mg pentobar-

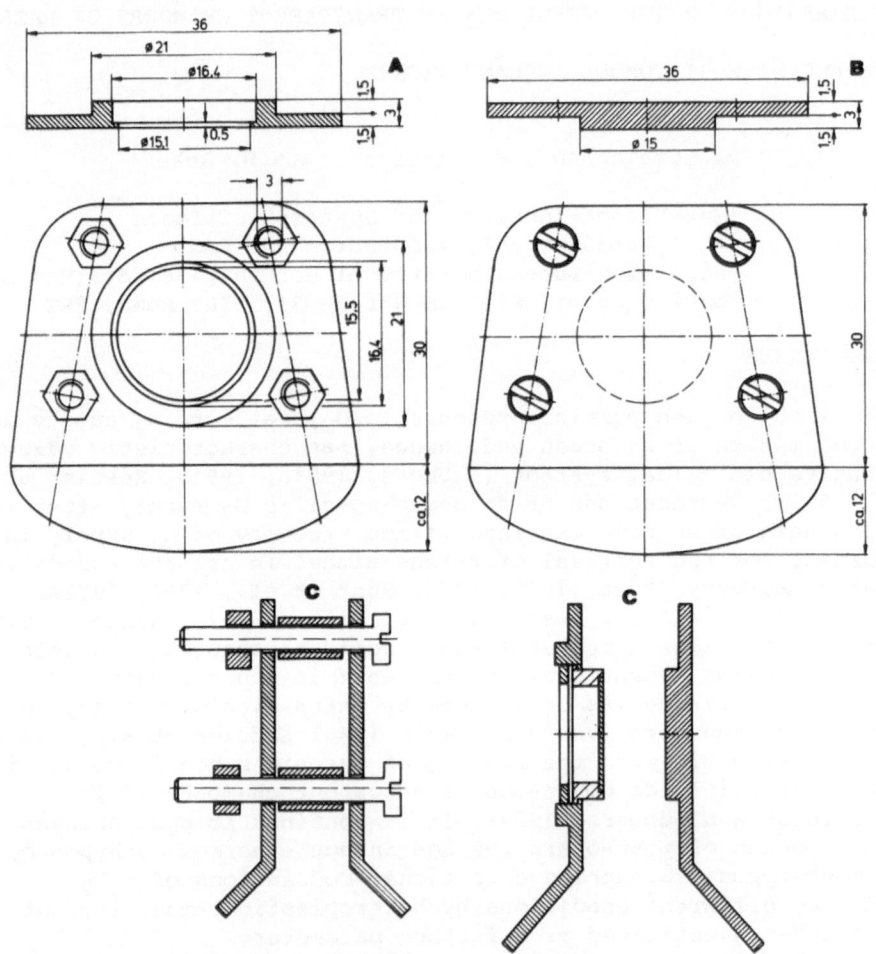

Fig. 1. Scheme of the transparent chamber (TK)
    A. 'window-side' (WS) with glass-covered insertion
       (top and longitudinal view)
    B. 'blind-window-side' (BWS), a projection cut out of a
       plexiglass base plate (top and longitudinal view)
    C. sections through different TK areas.

bital/kg). After operation, the animals lived in single cages at 30-31°C, about 50% rel. humidity, and natural light-dark cycles.

For p_tO_2 measurements the TKs were opened by removing the transparent inserts, which were fixed by dental cement and snap rings in the so-called 'window halves'. P_tO_2 was measured on an average of 10 different areas per wound with 4 wire surface electrodes (wire diameter: 15 μm, electrode surface area: 7 mm^2) according to Kessler and Lübbers (1966) in anaesthetized, spontaneously breathing rats. Tissue pO_2 of each area was tested within one minute for normoxia (N, air), within 30 seconds for hypoxia (H, 5% O_2 in N_2), and within one to two minutes for post-hypoxia (NR, air). The electrodes were calibrated in Ringer solution equilibrated with 5%, 10%, and 20% (air) O_2 and were recalibrated at regular intervals. In some animals arterial blood gas analysis was carried out at the end of the experiments, sampling blood from the common carotid artery.

In experiments with tumour implantation, spheroids of human anaplastic giant cell thyroid carcinoma (HTh7) were used (Carlsson et al., 1983). In vitro cultivation of the spheroids was done at 37°C in Ham's F10 medium containing 10% newborn calf-serum, 50 IU penicillin per 500 ml solution equilibrated with 95% O_2, and 5% CO_2 in agarose-coated culture dishes. Normally, two to three tumours (diameter: 300-600 μm) were implanted in the tissue pockets with very fine surface walls (Fig. 2). The vitality of the HTh7 spheroids was tested for about 24 h before the implantation by cell outgrowth kinetics in normal agarose-free culture dishes. The survival of tumour cells after implantation in rats was checked by comparing the outgrowth efficiency of original HTh7 spheroids with cell suspensions taken from the subcutis pocket at varying intervals. After 24 h in agarose-free dishes under above mentioned conditions, cells of non-transplanted spheroids formed small monolayers. Tumour cells which were transplanted for not longer than 4 days showed the same characteristic. After longer lasting implantations, the number of identifiable tumour cells forming monolayers was reduced remarkably.

RESULTS

Data of blood gas analysis are shown in Fig. 3. In tumour rats arterial pO_2 values (p_aO_2) were about 10% higher than in control animals and decreased in both experimental groups with post-operative age, whereas the arterial CO_2 data (p_aCO_2) increased only slightly without a significant difference between the test groups. The arterial pH curve (pH_a) rose gradually in tumour, while it fell in non-tumour groups. In general, the TK animals were hyperventilating and showed a mild alkalosis, which was somewhat more pronounced in tumour rats.

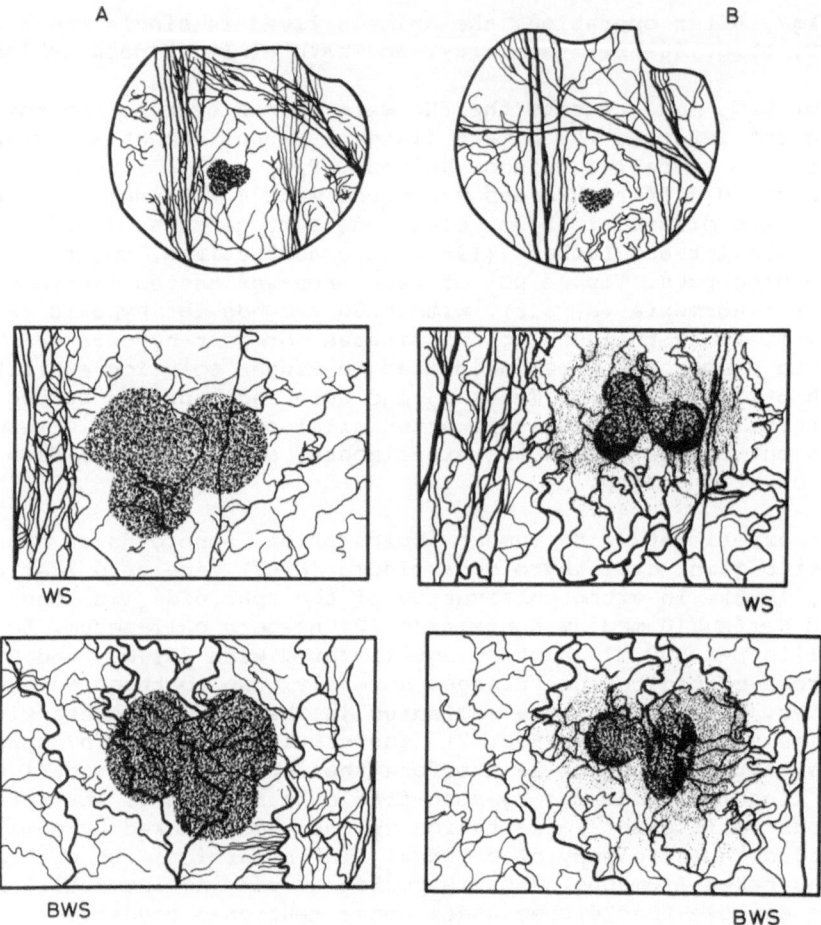

Fig. 2. Semi-schematic pictures of the subcutis tissue 1 hour (A) and 4 days (B) after surgery. Between the vertical blood vessel arcades of the thoraco-lumbal region, Th 12 and Th 13, three HTh7 tumour spheroids were implanted into a pocket.
A and B, views of the TK with a transparent area of origi- nally 12 mm Ø. WS and BWS, spheroid region and vessels of the thinner (WS) or thicker (BWS) pocket wall at a magnification of 32 X. Dark dotted areas are centers of HTh7 spheroid, light dotted areas are tumour peripheries.

With respect to successive post-operative age groups the mean p_tO_2 values (Fig. 4) had significantly higher levels in different breathing conditions in the edematous phase of wound healing (1st - 3rd day post-operative) than in the granulation phase (8th - ca. 20th day post-operative) and the differentiation phase (starting

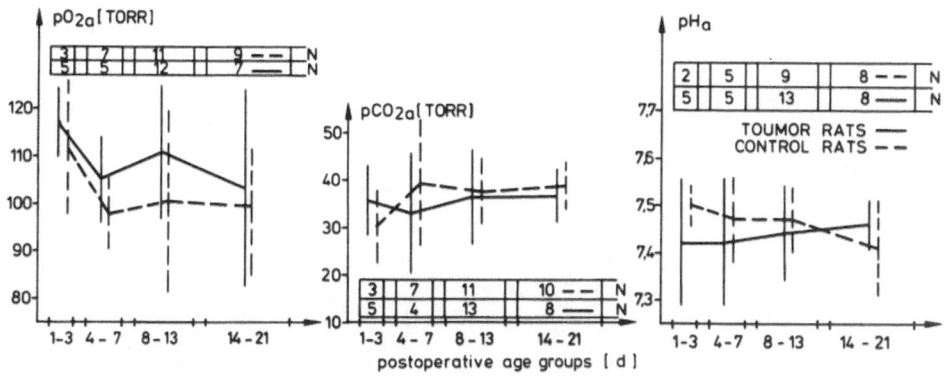

Fig. 3. Changes of p_aO_2, p_aCO_2, and p_aH in arterial blood samples taken from the carotid vessel. Mean values, their standard deviations, and the number (N) of animals per post-operative age group are shown.

from the 20th day post-operative onward). With regard to standard deviations individual differences were evident during the first seven days after TK implantations. Later age groups showed p_tO_2 values of about 25 Torr during normoxia and about 12 Torr after the hypoxic breathing period. The increase of standard deviations was a consequence of secondary inflammations as well as epidermations with regionally different intensities and patterns.

In HTh7 and non-tumour test groups the p_tO_2 values were similar, except the data during the edemation phase. In that phase of wound healing, spheroid-implanted rats had about 30% higher pO_2 levels. Within tumour TKs one could differentiate intra-vital-microscopically tumour-containing and tumour-free areas due to their colour and varying transparency in transilluminating light (Fig. 2). With regard to those regional differences HTh7 areas had higher p_tO_2 values. After subdivision of tumour regions into darker grey-coloured centres and light-grey peripheries, one could also observe p_tO_2 differences. The peripheral tumour regions have higher p_tO_2 values than the centres.

Changing breathing conditions had no influence on the p_tO_2 levels during the first phase of regeneration. From the 4th - 7th day post-operative onward, wound tissue reacted to hypoxic respiratory stimulation. With age progress, this reactivity improved. Differences in stimulus response behaviour to O_2 changes among tumour and non-tumour rats could hardly be seen. In tumour rats hypoxic stimulation induced reactions, which were, to some extent, more pronounced.

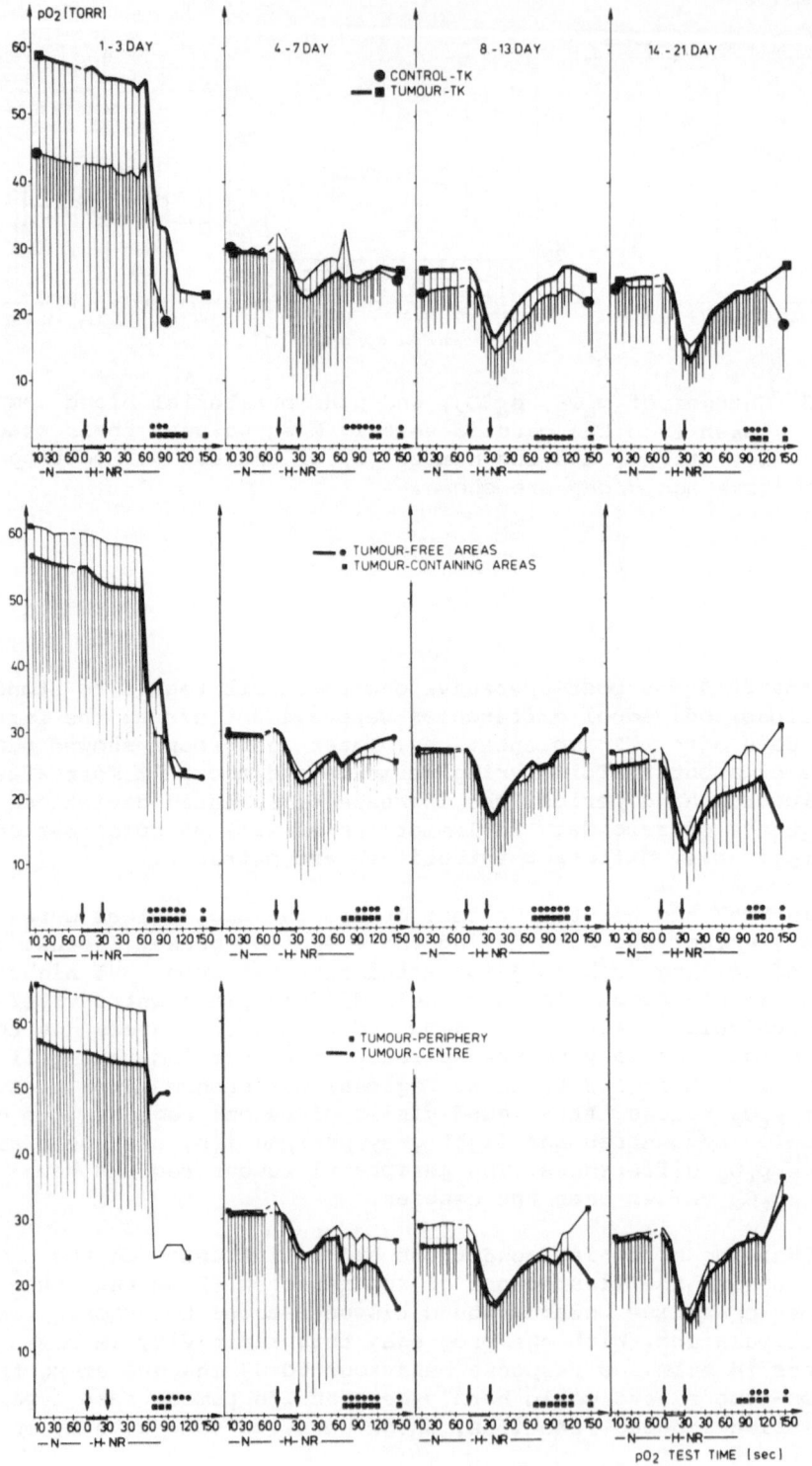

Fig. 4. Changes of tissue pO_2 values in TK covered subcutis wounds
of spontaneously breathing, Nembutal anesthetized female
Wistar rats with and without 2 spheroids of human thyreo-
idea anaplastic giant cell carcinoma in one minute normoxia
(N, air), 30 seconds hypoxia (H, 5 % O_2 in N_2, marked by
arrows), and one to two minutes post-hypoxia (NR, air) per
measured area with regard to post-operative age groups.
Mean values connected by lines and their standard deviations $\bar{x}$ - s in vertical lines in 10 seconds steps are
given. Reduced probe numbers are marked by square and
circle marks.

DISCUSSION

     The presented tissue pO_2 values measured during the first 10
days of wound healing differ substantially from pO_2 data measured
with other methods in different connective tissue. In experiments
with mesh cylinders Hunt and co-workers (1966, 1969, 1972a, 1972b)
found in wound fluids of animals kept in natural O_2 environment
pO_2 values of about 10 Torr during the first 10 days of regeneration. This discrepancy might be caused by non-airtight transparent
chambers resulting in an O_2 diffusion from the outside, which
could influence the pO_2 values of the tissue in the chamber. Influences of operation stress on the p_tO_2 levels must also be
taken into consideration, especially as in unilateral operated TK
subcutis wounds p_tO_2 had lower values than in bilateral ones
(Fischer et al., 1984). This finding might hint to the fact, that
cell numbers were reduced as a consequence of surgical manipulation
and the remaining probably had decreased O_2 consumption resulting
again in higher tissue pO_2 values. Other reasons, however, have to
be discussed, too. An increased microcirculation caused by disturbed thoraco-lumbal thermoregulation, its further enlargement by surgery, beginning wound healing, or infection defence processes must
be considered on the one hand; the hyperventilation of TK animals,
longer lasting vasodilations, which appeared 10 - 30 minutes after
finishing TK implantation, and higher pO_2 values in microbially
contaminated subcutis area (data not shown) on the other hand. Another aspect one has to regard in this context is the release of
histamine by mast cells, which became abundant in TK wounds just
after operation. This led to enhanced extravasates, by which the O_2
solubility coefficient of the tissue might become higher with
smaller pO_2 gradients (Vaupel, 1976).

     The decrease of tissue pO_2 values with progress in regenera-
tion was likely a consequence of reduced edema, intensified convection, normalized blood flow, increased vessel outgrowth, enlarged immigration of cells with enhanced activities, and higher oxygen
metabolism in general (compare Silver, 1978).

The additional increase of p_tO_2 levels in HTh7 rats 1 - 3 days after tumour implantation is hard to explain. One reason might be the higher arterial pO_2 in tumour rats. Beside this, one has to regard O_2 diffusion from the oxygen-equilibrated culture medium to the host tissue just after tumour transplantation, especially as by these procedures small quantities (ca. 1 ml) of in vitro medium were unavoidably transferred to the TK wound. Furthermore, the effect of intense extravasates induced by the immune response of the host tissue have to be discussed, too.

The differences between the tissue pO_2 levels of tumour-free areas in HTh7 rats and control animals may be based on a systematic error. As the borders of the pocket regions in HTh7 rats were hardly distinguishable from the non-disturbed connective tissue, it is reasonable to assume that the mean values of tumour-free areas were influenced by data already belonging to the tumour regions. Differences in p_tO_2 levels of peripheries and centres in HTh7 regions - the lower pO_2 values within the mid-portions - originated from higher cell numbers including living HTh7 and immigrating host defence cells, while the vessel number was unchanged. Indications for this were given by histological studies of the immune defence processes in TK rats with human glioma spheroid implantation (Streichhan and Wechsler, unpublished).

The compensation of the p_tO_2 differences in older tumour and non-tumour rats was not only a consequence of emigrating or dying tumour-cells but also the result of revascularization processes with varying intensities in both probes. This is clearly shown by the hypoxic reactivity of the tissue, which improved with post-operative age. As in wounds with heteroplastic tumour implantations non compatible proteins will be attached by the host immmune defence system, one should except - caused by higher cell numbers - lower p_tO_2 values in tumour peripheries and centres. However, as their p_tO_2 values were equal to those in tumour free regions of control animals, one has to assume an enhanced vessel growth in HTh7-influenced regions.

SUMMARY

Changes of tissue pO_2 levels in chronic subcutis wounds with and without heteroplastic tumour spheroid implants in thoraco-lumbal rat skinfolds covered by transparent chambers were followed in crosscut analysis by pO_2 surface electrodes as a function of post-operative age using constant normoxic, hypoxic, post-hypoxic breathing conditions and intervals for each measured area. The tissue pO_2 showed significantly higher values in the edematous phase of wound healing than in the granulation and differentiation phase. Tumour implantations induced even higher pO_2 values in the edematic phase. This difference vanished in later phases. The hypoxic reactivity of non-tumour and tumour tissue improved with post-operative age indicating a sufficient vessel outgrowth.

REFERENCES

van den Brenk, H. A. S., 1956, Studies in restorative growth processes in mammalian wound healing, Brit. J. Surg., 43:535-546.

Carlsson, J., Nilsson, K., Westermark, B., Ponten, J., Sundström, C., Larsson, E., Bergh, J., Påhlman, S., Busch, C., and Collins, V.P., 1983, Formation and growth of multicellular spheroids of human origin, Int. J. Cancer, 31:523-533.

Endrich, B., Goetz, A., and Messmer, K., 1982, Distribution of microflow and oxygen tension in hamster melanoma, Int. J. Microcirc. Clin. Exp., 1:81-99.

Fischer, M., Streichhan, P., and Acker, H., 1984, pO_2 histograms in subcutis tissues of chronical wounds in rats, Pflügers Arch., 400:R14.

Goodwin, C. W., and Heppenstall, R. B., 1978, The effect of chronic hypoxia on wound healing, in: "Oxygen Transport to Tissue - III", I. A. Silver, M. Erecińska, H. I. Bicher, eds., Adv. Exper. Med. Biol., Vol. 94, Plenum Press, New York and London, pp. 669-672.

Hunt, T. K., 1970, Current challenges for wound healing research J. Trauma, 10:1001-1009.

Hunt, T. K., 1973, Standards for wound healing research, Surgery, 73:153-154.

Hunt, T. K., and Hutchison, J. G. P., 1966, Studies on the oxygen tension in healing wound, in: "Wound Healing", C. Illingworth, ed., I. & A. Churchill Ltd., London, pp. 257-266.

Hunt, T. K., Linsey, M., Sonne, M., and Jawetz, E., 1972a, Oxygen tension and wound infection, Surg. Forum, 23:

Hunt, T. K., and Pai, M. P., 1972b, The effect of varying ambient oxygen tensions on wound metabolism and collagen synthesis, Surg. Gynecol. Obstet., 135:561-567.

Hunt, T. K., and Zederfeldt, B., 1969, Nutritional and environmental aspects of wound healing, in: "Repair and Regeneration", J. E. Dunphy, W. van Winkle, eds., McGraw-Hill, NY-Toronto-Sydney-London, pp. 217-228.

Kessler, M., Höper, J., Harrison, D. K., et al., 1984, Tissue O_2 supply under normal and pathological conditions, in: "Oxygen Transport to Tissue - V", D. W. Lübbers, H. Acker, E. Leniger-Follert, T. K. Goldstick, eds., Adv. Exper. Med. Biol., Vol. 169, Plenum Press, New York and London, pp. 69-80.

Kessler, M., and Lübbers, D.W., 1966, Aufbau und Anwendungsmöglichkeiten verschiedener pO_2-Elektroden, Pflügers Arch., 291:R82.

Lübbers, D. W., 1981a, Tissue oxygen supply and critical oxygen pressure, in: "Oxygen Transport to Tissue", Adv. Physiol. Sci., Vol. 25, A. G. B. Kovách, E. Dóra, M. Kessler, I.A. Silver, eds., Pergamon Press, Akadémiai Kiadó, Budapest, pp. 3-11.

Lübbers, D.W., 1981b, Grundlagen und Bedeutung der lokalen Sauer-stoffdruckmessung und des pO_2-Histogramms für die Beurtei-lung der Sauerstoffversorgung der Organe und des Organismus, in: "Messung des Gewebesauerstoffdruckes bei Patienten", A. M. Ehrly, ed., G. Witzstrock, Baden-Baden-Köln-NY, pp. 11-21.

Papenfuss, H. D., Gross, J. F., Intaglietta, M., and Treese, F. A., 1979, A transparent access chamber for the rat dorsal skinfold, Microvasc. Res., 18:311-318.

Silver, I. A., 1978, Tissue pO_2 changes in acute inflammation, in: "Oxygen Transport to Tissue - III", I. A. Silver, M. Erecińska, H. I. Bicher, eds., Adv. Exper. Med. Biol., Vol. 94, Plenum Press, New York and London, pp. 769-774.

Streichhan, P., and Lübbers, D. W., 1982, Transparent chamber technique in rat skinfold for neovascularization studies, Arzneimittelforsch. (Drug Res.), 32:1348-1349.

Vaupel, P., 1976, Effect of percentual water content in tissues and liquids on the diffusion coefficients of O_2, CO_2, N_2, and H_2, Pflügers Arch., 361:201-204.

Winter, G. D., 1978, Oxygen and dermal healing, in: "Oxygen Trans-port to Tissue - III", I. A. Silver, M. Erecińska, H. I. Bicher, eds., Adv. Exper. Med. Biol., Vol. 94, Plenum Press, New York and London, pp. 673-678.

METHODS

STOCHASTIC ANALYSIS OF TRANSPORT PHENOMENA

IN HETEROGENOUS TISSUE

Nathan A. Busch - University of Bristol
                  Bristol, U.K

Duane F. Bruley - California Polytechnic
                  San Luis Obispo, Cal., U.S.A.

INTRODUCTION

In the classical analysis of mass transport
phenomena, several basic assumptions must be made
before the mechanics of the transport analysis can be
implemented. The first is that the medium through
which the mass is being transported is homogenous.
Second is that the particle displacements in space from
a given point are normally distributed. The third
assumption is that each molecule or "particle" moves
independently of all the other particles and has zero
volume and mass. These conditions allow the formulation of the Green's function (which is used in the
solution of the mass transport equation) for the
respective geometry and boundary conditions. The last
basic assumption is that the classical transport process is Markov. This means that the events which occur
at some future time depend only upon the present state
of the system, and not on the past. This asumption
leads to the conclusion that for a diffusion process
the mean change in the velocity of a particle (the mean
acceleration) becomes infinitely great as the time
becomes infinitesimally small. Einstein (1905) indicated that the conclusion is a result of the hypotheses
of Brownian motion. He stated that for large times, a
process may become asymptotically Markov; that is, it
will "lose" memory of where it was, but the process
cannot be Markov for small time intervals.

In this paper, the formulation of the mathematics is presented for the Stochastic Analysis of Transport Phenomena in Heterogenous Media. The method is applied to two problems, both of which have been previously studied (Busch, 1984), to demonstrate that the Stochastic Analysis is a powerfull tool for analyzing the behavior of physiological systems. It is also demonstrated that the Stochastic Analysis is free of the constraints placed upon the analysis of transport phenomena under classical transport theory.

Definitions and Background

The method of Stochastic Analysis of Transport Phenomena in Heterogenous Media involves the determination of density functions for the behavior of individual particles and of an ensemble of particles within the defined system. The term "particle" as used here is a generic term for any single molecule of a catabolite species.

The density functions for three types of phenomena will be determined. The first is the density distribution function for the particle (or ensemble of particles) movement. The second is the density distribution function for the consumption of the particles. The third is the distribution function for the particles which enter or leave the environment. The first density function mentioned above is analogous to the particle random walk distribution function found in the study of Stochastic Processes. The second parallels the density distribution functions used in the study of birth and death processes. The third is analogous to the immigration and emigration processes referred to in the Theory of Stochastic Processes. As was demonstrated in Uhlenbeck and Wang (1945), and Busch (1984) (assuming that the acceleration of a particle is proportional to the sum of the forces on the particle) when the force on the particle is assumed to be normally distributed with mean zero and variance 2Dt (D is the diffusion coefficient, and t is time) then the particle movement density distribution function resulting from the use of Langevin's equation for performing

the random walk satisfies the diffusion equation. This
assumed form of the particle movement, that is,
normally distributed forcing function, results in the
basic equation of the field of classical transport
phenomena and of Brownian Motion. Since it is postulated that the actual particles in the system do not
behave according to the fundamental assumptions of
Brownian Motion nor is the movement process Markov,
then another form for the movement density function
must be found. The methodology presented here allows
for the determination of the movement density distribution functions for both single particles and an ensemble of particles. The methodology will be called Stochastic Analysis of Transport Phenomena in Heterogenous
Media. Definition of the parameters and variables in
Stochastic Analysis will lead to a better understanding
of the mechanics of the analysis.

     Let the transport of species occur in a convex and
bounded domain X=WxT, where T is the set of all time
points {t:t [O,T"]}, and W is the open set of all space
points which a particle may reach. Let W' be the boundary of W. The definition of W and the distinction
between W and W' are necessary and important in the
development of the Stochastic Analysis. A particle
which is wholly within the set W will behave as what is
labeled as an "internal" particle. While the particle
is not within W, that is to say in the region outside
W, it can no longer be called an internal particle and
thus is called an "external" particle. The two particles will behave differently and especially when an
external particle reaches the boundary of W.

     Define dw to be a small volume of the three-
dimensional Euclidian space, and dt to be a small
interval of time. Restrict both dw and dt to be
nonzero, and positive. The spacial position is denoted
by r, and time by t. The space-time point in the
domain X is denoted by the co-ordinate pair (r,t). The
point (r',t') is also a point in X, and represents the
point of origination of the particle, or the "source".
When an area of the surface W' of W is under consideration, it will be denoted by dv. A spacial point on the
surface W' is designated as s, and a "source" point on
the surface is designated as s'.

The probability is P(r,t|r',t')dwdt that given a
particle is at the point (r',t'), then it will reach
the volume dwdt which is situated around the point
(r,t). In specifying this functioin there is no need
to multiply by dw'dt' which is the volume situated
about the originating point (r't'); since we assume
that there is no uncertainty about the particles starting point. This conditional probability is only a
statement that if we know where the particle originates
(at (r',t')), then we will know approximately where it
will be some time later.

P(r,t)dwdt is the distribution of the particles in
the volume dwdt situated around the point (r,t). There
is a subtle difference between the density distribution
function P(r,t|r',t')dwdt and the distribution
P(r,t)dwdt. The first concerns the displacement
behavior of a single particle in the domain, (WxT); the
second reflects the total number of particles which
reach the volume dwdt about the point (r,t) from each
point (r',t') within the domain (W + W')xT. Each is
derivable from information about the other but they
cannot be used interchangeably. The function
P(r,t)dwdt is not necessarily uniformly continuous, and
in fact for analyses where the particles have a positive, nonzero volume, the function exhibits discontinu-
ties when the volume dwdt is shrunk to be less than the
volume of a single particle. Neither of the two distributions can exhibit the behavior of the Dirac delta
function as (r,t) approaches (r',t'); since that would
imply that any positive, nonzero number of particles
can be placed into a volume with zero measure.

The probability is F(r',0)dw'dt' of finding a particle in the volume dw'dt' situated about the point
(r',0). This serves as the initial condition for the
density distribution function P(r,t)dwdt. By the last
paragraph, for analyses involving particles with finite, nonzero, positive volumes this density cannot be
equal to the Dirac delta function. When the density
function P(r,t)dwdt is equal to the Dirac Delta function as time t approaches zero (as it is in the
Green's function formulation of the solution to the
diffusion equation) then the process will exhibit the

properties of a Markov process which is not what is desired.

The probability is g(r',t')dw'dt' that a particle initially in the volume dw'dt' situated about the point (r',t') will die, or, that a volume dw'dt' about (r',t') with no particle initially will experience a simple birth.

The probability is P"(r,t|s',t')dvdt that if a particle is in a small volume dv'dt' about the point (s',t') situated on the boundary W' of W, it will arrive in the volume dwdt situated about the point (r,t). This function is analogous to the function P(r,t|r',t)dwdt in that it defines the movement of a single particle given that its point of origin is known.

The probability is f"(s',t')dv'dt' that a particle will immigrate into or emigrate from the domain X through the volume dv'dt' situated about the point (s',t') on the boundary of X.

Theory

In order that a particle be found in the volume dwdt situated about the point (r,t) and thus contribute to the function P(r,t)dwdt, it must first have been in a volume dw'dt' about (r',t') and moved to dwdt about (r,t). There are three independent ways of originating in the volume dw'dt' about (r',t') and moving to the volume dwdt about (r,t). First,particles were originally in the volume dw'dt' about (r'0), and moved to the volume dwdt about (r,t) with probability P(r,t|r',t')dwdt[F(r',0)dw'dt']. Second,the particles were either in the volume dw'dt' about (r',t') and died, or did not exist and were born in the volume and moved to the volume dwdt about (r,t), with probability P(r,t|r',t')dwdt[g(r',t')dw'dt']. Third, the particles were in the volume dv'dt' about the point (s',t') on the boundary of X, (W'xT), and moved to the volume dwdt about the point (r,t) with probability P"(r,t|s',t')dwdt[f"(s',t')dv'dt'].

The volume dwdt about (r,t) will receive contributions from the volumes dw'dt' about all the points (r',t') in the domain X, and the volumes dv'dt' about all the points (s',t') on the boundary of X. Since the contributions are independent, they are additive to the amount

$$P(r,t) = \int_W P(r,t;r',t')_{t'=0} F(r',t') dw'$$

(1)

$$+ [\int_{t'=0}^{t} dt' \int_W P(r,t;r',t') g(r',t') dw'] + [\int_{t'=0}^{t} dt' \sum_{i=1}^{n} \int_{s_i} P''(r,t;r',t') f''(r',t') dv']$$

When the functions F(r',t'), and/or g(r',t'),and/or f''(r',t') are also dependent upon P(r,t), then Equation (1) is an integral equation and P(r,t|r',t') is its kernel.

When the motion of a particle is governed by Langevin's equation, then the function P(r,t|r',t') becomes the Green's function. For a defined geometry the functions F(r',t'), g(r',t'), and f''(s',t') may be specified to suit the case under consideration. The particle motion within the geometry is specified as P(r,t|r',t'). Once the geometry and P(r,t|r',t') are specified then P''(r,t|s',t') cannot be independently specified. The two functions P(r,t|r',t') and P''(r,t|s',t') are related, and in fact when P(r,t|r',t') is assumed to be equal to the Green's function the relationship between P(r,t|r',t') and P''(r,t|s',t') is completely known. In the case of an absorbing boundary, P''(r,t|s',t') is the differential of P(r,t|r',t') with respect to an outward directed normal evaluated on the respective boundary. When the boundary is reflecting, then P''(r,t|s',t') is identically P(r,t|r',t') evaluated on the boundary. Based on these observations, the following postulate is formulated:

Postulate 1.

    Let P(r,t|r',t')dwdt and P''(r,t|s',t') be density

distribution functions as previously defined.
Then for an absorbing boundary,

$$P''(r,t|r',t') = dP(r,t|r',t')/dn,$$

and for a reflecting boundary

$$P''(r,t|r',t') = P(r,t|r',t').$$

   With this postulate the formulation of the method
of Stochastic Analysis of Transport Phenomena in
Heterogenous Media is complete. Equation (1) for
$P(r,t)$ is the most general formulation for the solution. It is not restricted to any particular geometry
nor is it restricted by complexity of heterogeneity.
The nature of the particle movement in the domain X=W x
T is wholly contained in and explained by the two func-
tions $P(r,t|r',t')$ and $P''(r,t|s',t')$. The effect of the
initial behavior on all subsequent behavior is
reflected in the first integral. Birth and death of the
particle and its subsequent effect is accounted for by
the second integral. Boundary effects are handled by
the third integral on the right side. The analysis at
this point is still nonparametric, in that the forms
for $P(r,t|r',t')$ and $P''(r,t|s',t')$ have not been speci-
fied. Once they are specified, then the particle
motion behavior has been set and the analysis becomes
parametric for the motion of the particles. (Once
$F(r',t')$, $g(r',t')$, and $f''(r',t')$ have been specified
then the entire analysis is parametric.) Equation (1)
for $P(r,t)$ is a very powerful and broad statement concerning the behavior of heterogenous stochastic
processes. It will give the probability $P(r,t|r',t')$
for any specified geometry, boundary conditions, and
initial density. This function $P(r,t|r',t')$ is
appropriate for use in random walk simulations, since
it is a transition probability from point (r',t') to
(r,t). With $P(r,t|r',t')$, $F(r',t')$, $g(r',t')$, and
$f''(r',t')$ specified, the behavior of the heterogenous
stochastic process can be directly determined for any
point (r,t). Finally, with $P(r,t)$ determined from the
physical experiments, the inverse problem can be solved

to obtain P(r,t|r',t') and g(r',t'). F(r',t') and
P"(r,t|s',t') will be given directly from their experi-
mental interpretation.

Equation (1) for P(r,t) covers a myriad of cases
which cannot possibly be included in a single work.
Thus for demonstration purposes two cases will be
included, both of which have been studied by analytic
and Approximated Analytic methods in previous works
(Busch,1984). The first case is the one-dimensional diffusion - convection - reaction problem and the second
case is the three-dimensional diffusion - convection -
reaction problem.   In both cases the density function
P(r,t|r',t') in Equation (1) is the Green's function
for the respective geometry and boundary conditions.
For the one-dimensional case, with 1000 terms in the
Green's function and a Peclet number of 2, the result
is the surface plot in Figure 1. The geometry for the
three dimensional case is given in Figure 2.   The
capillary and neuron are assumed to be rectangulary for
simplicity. The solution to Equation 1 is obtained
for the (p,z) plane which is drawn in Figure 3.   The
(p,z) plane cuts both the capillary and the neuron
along their z-axes. The metabolic rate has a parabolic
profile in both time and space. The metabolic rate
starts to change at 0.2 time units and reaches a maximum at 0.5 time units. At 0.6 time units the metabolic rate is reduced to zero. The solution P(r,t) to
Equation 1 for time equal to 0.4 units, the solution is
drawn as a surface in Figure 4. The solution in the
neuron is represented by the deep depression in the
surface to the right of the figure. The capillary is
the rise in the surface along the left side of the figure. The solution P(r,t) along a line connecting the
center of the neuron with the z-axis of the capillary
is given in Figure 5. From the plot in Figure 5, it is
clear that with a zeroth order birth / death rate, the
density (P(r,t)) falls below zero within the neuron.
This indicates that a simple zeroth order birth / death
rate can lead to a physically meaningless solution.
The solution for time equal to 0.6 units, (the time at
which the metabolic rate is returned to zero) is given
in Figure 6. The solution along a line connecting the
neuron and capillary as described above is given in
Figure 7 for time equal to 0.6. The solution at time
0.6 units is very close to the soluton for time 0.4
which indicates that the system as defined tends to

reach the "steady - state" condition rapidly after a change in the metabolic rate. The surface in Figure 8 is for time 0.8 units. This solution is for time equal to 0.2 units after the metabolic rate has been returned to zero. It is clear on comparing Figure 6 with Figure 8 and Figure 7 with Figure 9, that the density within the neuron proceeds to a new steady state very rapidly after the onset of a change in metabolic rate.

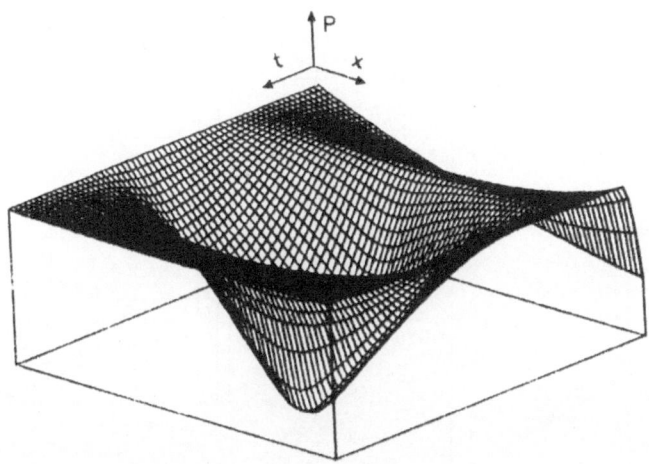

Figure 1. One dimensional Stochastic Analysis of the Diffusion - Convection - Reaction Model. $P(x,t)$ for Peclet number 0.0, $x \epsilon [0,1]$, $t \epsilon [0,1]$.

CONCLUSION

When the density function $P(r,t|r',t')$ in Equation (1) is the Green's function, the Stochastic Analysis results are identical to those obtained by both the analytical and Approximate Analytic solution methods (Busch, 1984). This is due solely to the fact that when $P(r,t|r',t')$ is the Green's function in the Stochastic Analysis method, then Equation (1) is exactly the solution to deterministic problems as investigated by Busch(1984). This emphasizes one of the primary points in this analysis, which is if random walks (Monte-

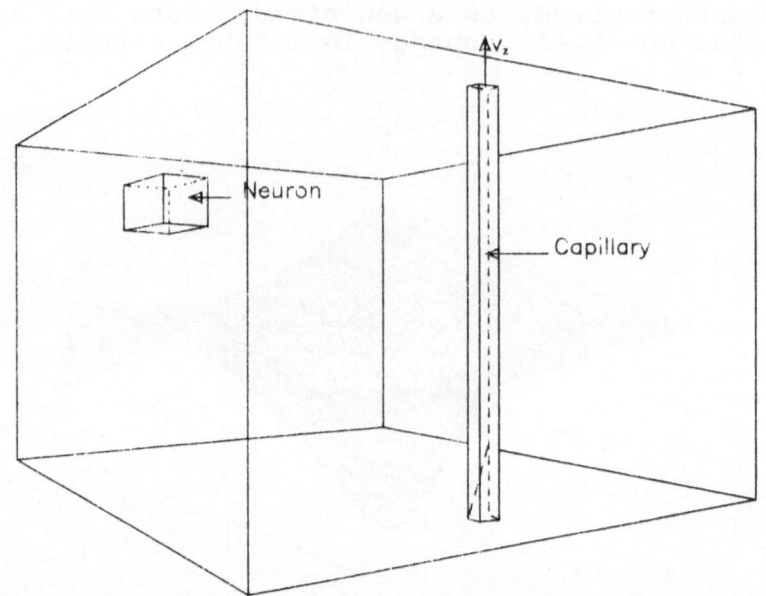

Figure 2.   Geometry for the Three Dimensional Diffusion, Convection, Reaction Medel.

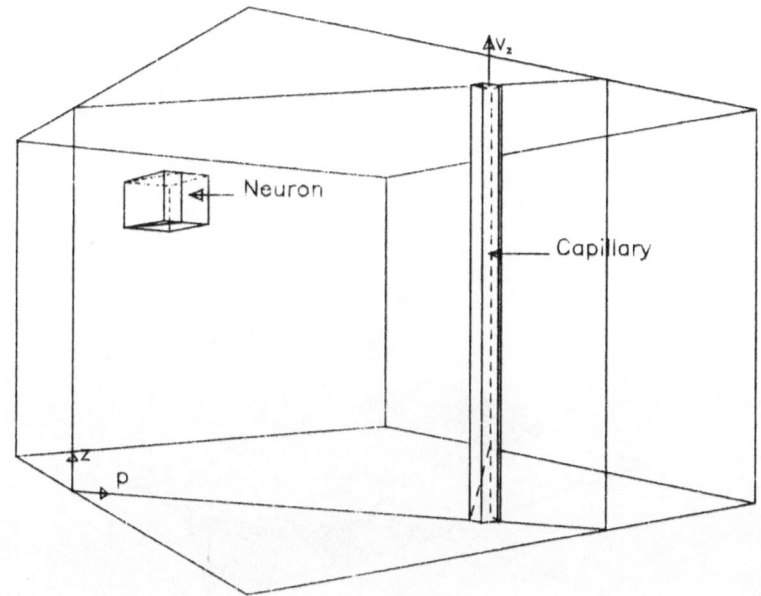

Figure 3.   Geometry for the Three Dimensional Diffusion,
Convection, Reaction Model.

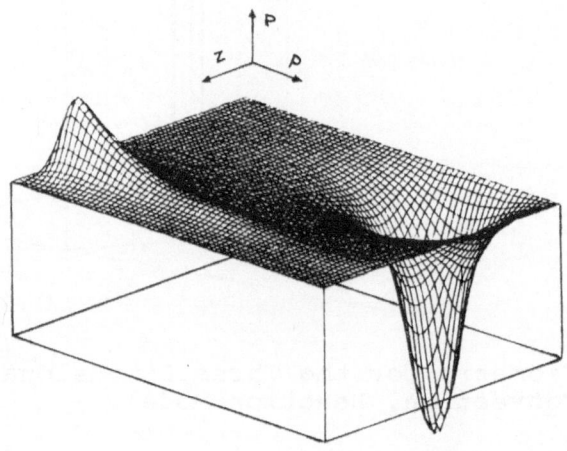

Figure 4. Three Dimensional Stochastic Analysis of the
            Diffusion - Convection - Reaction Model.
            p(p.z,0.4) for Peclet Number 2.0, pϵ[0,0.75]
            zϵ[0,1].

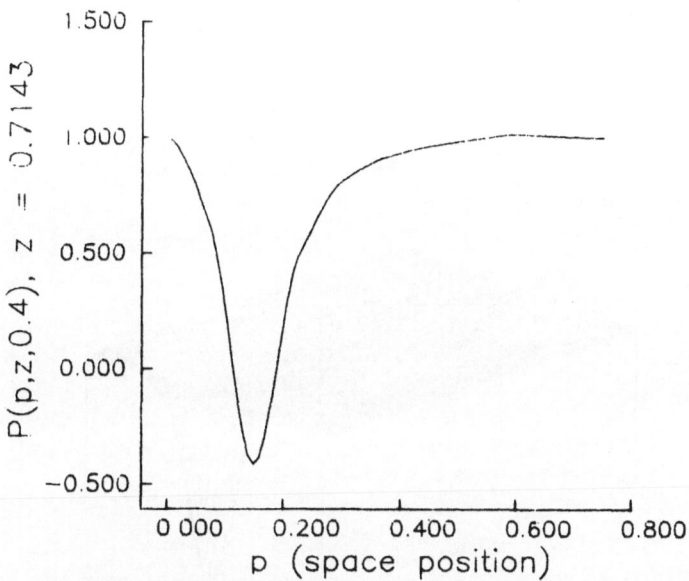

Figure 5. Three Dimensional Stochastic Analysis of the
DCR Model. P(p,z,0.4) vs. p, z = 0.7143, for
Peclet Number 2.0.

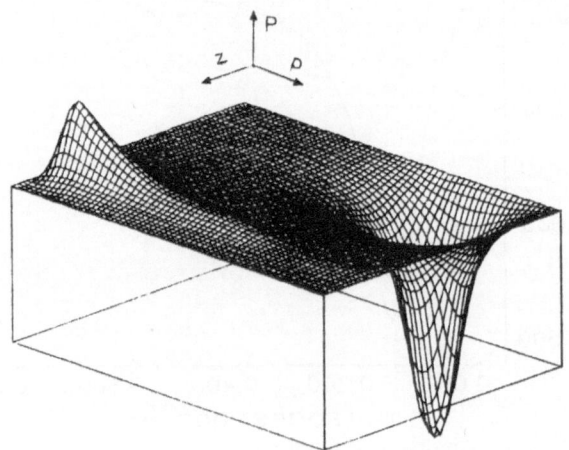

Figure 6.   Three Dimensional Stochastic Analysis of the
Diffusion - Convection - Reaction Model.
P(p.z.0.6) for Peclet Number 2.0, pε[0,0.75],
zε[0,1].

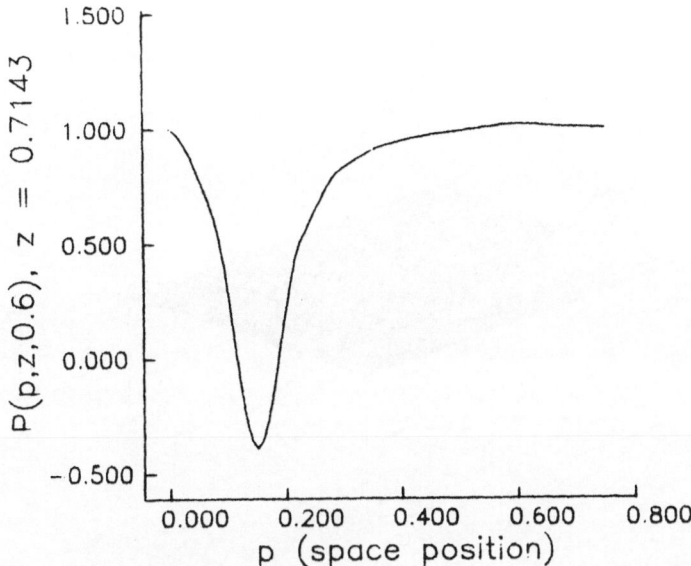

Figure 7. Three Dimensional Stochastic Analysis of the
DCR model. P(p,z,0.6) va. p, z = 0.7143, for
Peclet Number 2.0.

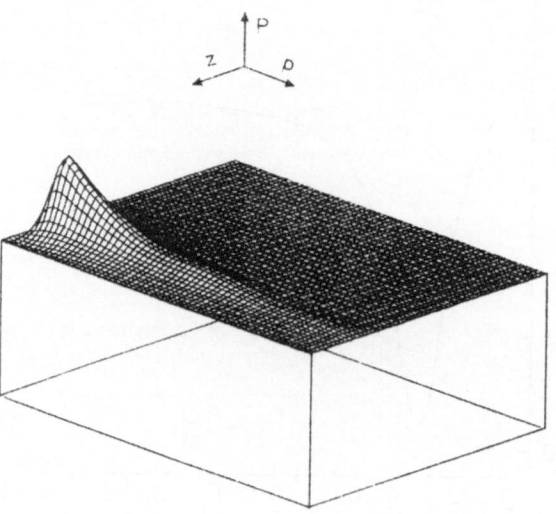

Figure 8. Three Dimensional Stochastic Analysis of the
Diffusion - Convection - Reaction Model.
P(p.z.0.8) for Peclet Number 2.0, pϵ[0,0.75],
zϵ[0,1].

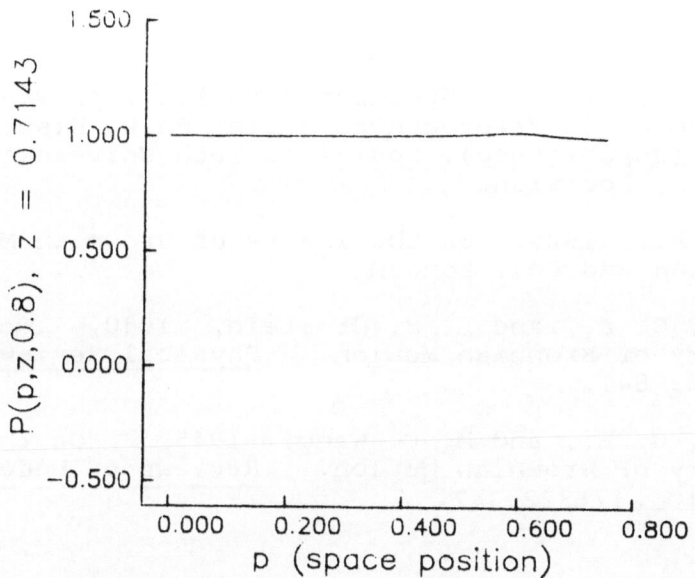

Figure 9. Three Dimensional Stochastic Analysis of the DCR Model. P(p.z.0.8) vs. p, z = 0.7143, for Peclet Number 2.0.

Carlo) are performed using Langevin's equation with a normally distributed forcing function, or if they are performed using the Green's function, then the resulting solution is identical to the solution which is obtained using the deterministic diffusion equation.

In the paper the foundation was presented for the Stochastic Analysis of transport phenomena in heterogeneous media. Two problems solved in previous works were discussed.

REFERENCES

Busch, N. A., 1984 , "Stochastic Analysis of Transport Phenomena in Heterogenous Media", Ph.D. Dissertation (unpublished), Louisiana Tech University, Ruston, Louisiana.

Einstein, A., 1926, "On the Theory of Brownian Motion", Methuen and Co., London.

Uhlenbeck, G. E., and L. S. Ornstein, 1930, On the Theory of Brownian Motion, Physical Review, 36:823-841.

Uhlenbeck, G. E., and M. C. Wang, 1945, On the Theory of Brownian Motion, Reviews of Modern Physics, 17:322-342.

CEREBRAL BIOENERGETICS AND IN VIVO CYTOCHROME c OXIDASE

REDOX RELATIONSHIPS

A.L. Sylvia, C.A. Piantadosi, and F.F. Jöbsis-Vander Vliet

Department of Physiology and Medicine
Duke University Medical Center, Durham, N.C.   27710

INTRODUCTION

Cytochrome c oxidase (cytochrome a,a_3) is almost completely oxidized in isolated mitochondria[1] which essentially respire at a maximal rate. The reduction level of cytochrome $\underline{a},a_3$ measured in intact brain and other mammalian organs, however, is much higher[2,3]. The in vivo oxidation-reduction level of this enzyme is also greatly affected by variations in tissue oxygenation[4]. Cytochrome $\underline{a},a_3$ becomes progressively more reduced by pathophysiological conditions which decrease cellular oxygen availability[5]. Thus, in situ changes in the oxidation level of cytochrome $\underline{a},a_3$ should provide an early sensitive means for determining intracellular levels of oxygen insufficiency which adversely affect tissue bioenergetics. We test this possibility in the present study. The effect of acute oxygen insufficiency on in situ changes in the oxidation level of cytochrome $\underline{a},a_3$ in the parietal cortex of skull intact normal blood circulated rat brain was directly compared with in vitro measured changes in the concentration of metabolites known to reflect limitations in cellular energy production.

METHODS

Studies were conducted using male Sprague Dawley rats weighing 150-200g. Animals were anesthetized with urethane (1.3gm/kg i.p.). Tracheotomies were performed and both femoral arteries and one femoral vein were cannulated. After paralysis with tubocurarine chloride (1.5mg/kg i.v.), the animal was placed on a positive pressure rodent respirator using $30\%O_2 + 70\%N_2$ as control breathing gas mixture. Tidal volume and respiratory rate were adjusted to maintain P_aCO_2 between 35-40mm Hg and a P_aO_2 above 100mm Hg. No attempt was made to maintain the P_aCO_2 constant during subsequent changes in the fractional content of inspired oxygen (FiO_2). Core body temperature, blood pressure, arterial P_aCO_2, P_aO_2, pHa (I.L. Model 513 pH/Blood Gas Analyzer), and EEG activity were monitored throughout experimentation. The head of the animal was positioned in a stereotaxic unit and the dorsal scalp was reflected. Reflectance spectrophotometry, in the visible region, was performed continuously through the translucent skull using a four wavelength differential spectrophotomer similar to that described by Jöbsis et al.[6] Absorption changes in cortical cytochrome a,a3 oxidation-reduction levels were measured at sample (s) minus reference (r) wavelength pairs of 605-(612+597)nm/2. Concurrent measurements of hemoglobin saturation and relative changes in cerebrocortical blood volume were measured at 597-586nm and negative feedback at 568nm, respectively. Cytochrome oxidation-reduction changes are expressed as a percentage of the total labile optical signal (%TLS) for each wavelength pair, i.e. (s) minus (r) wavelength signal difference obtained by ventilation with 85%O_2 + 15% CO_2 (maximal oxidation) and 100% nitrogen (maximal reduction). Absorbance measurements were recorded during sequential decreases in the fractional content of inspired oxygen. In vivo changes in the redox state of cytochrome a,a3 were compared directly with in vitro measured changes in cortical metabolites obtained by conventional techniques of freezing[7], extraction, and enzymatic analysis[8].

RESULTS AND DISCUSSION

Acute cerebral oxygen insufficiency, produced by sequentially lowering the fractional content of inspired oxygen, caused immediate and continuous increases in the level of reduced cortical cytochrome a,a3. This occurred concurrently with decreases in hemoglobin saturation and compensatory increases in cerebrocortical blood volume. Arterial blood pressure declined as the P_aO_2 was lowered: a response to hypoxia characteristically observed in anesthetized rats. Brain electrical silence, i.e. EEG isoelectricity, occurred approximately 60 seconds after subjecting animals to 100% nitrogen. Anoxia caused cerebrocortical blood volume to fall precipitously as cytochrome a,a3 attained maximal reduction and hemoglobin fully desaturated. A recording typical of the changes discussed above is shown in Fig. 1.

In vitro bioassay of cortical metabolites revealed that graded hypoxia caused an increase in lactic acid and a continuous rise in the lactate/pyruvate ratio. Both changes are considered to reflect increases in tissue glycolytic activity (Table 1). Throughout the hypoxia protocol, cortical ATP concentration was maintained while phosphocreatine content continuously decreased. A five minute period of anoxia caused marked depletion of phosphocreatine reserves, at which time cortical ATP significantly decreased (Fig. 2).

Table 1. Influence of hypoxia and anoxia on pyruvate, lactate, and the lactate/pyruvate ratio in the parietal cortex.

EXPERIMENTAL GROUP	PYRUVATE	LACTATE	L/P
Control 30%O_2	0.090±0.011 (6)	0.72±0.09 (6)	8.50±1.32 (6)
Hypoxia 18%O_2	0.080±0.004 (6)	1.43±0.19 (6)	17.67±1.68 (6)
Hypoxia 12%O_2	0.150±0.020 (9)	2.07±0.49 (10)	17.60±4.50 (9)
Hypoxia 9%O_2	0.200±0.030 (11)	7.22±0.43 (11)	39.20±5.90 (10)
Anoxia 100%N_2	0.210±0.013 (4)	26.00±0.48 (4)	129.10±9.64 (4)

Each value is the mean ± S.E.M. for the number of animals indicated within brackets.

Comparison of the high-energy metabolite profile with spectral changes in the oxidation-reduction state of the enzyme revealed that decreases in cortical cytochrome a,a3 oxidation sensitively tracked decreases in phosphocreatine as opposed to ATP concentration. Based on the percent total labile signal (%TLS) of cytochrome a,a3, determined at maximum oxidation (85%O_2 + 15%CO_2) and maximum reduction (100% nitrogen), the level of oxidation in the parietal cortex of rats breathing 30, 18, 12, 9, and 7% O_2 was determined to be 54, 48, 33, 24, and 16%, respectively.

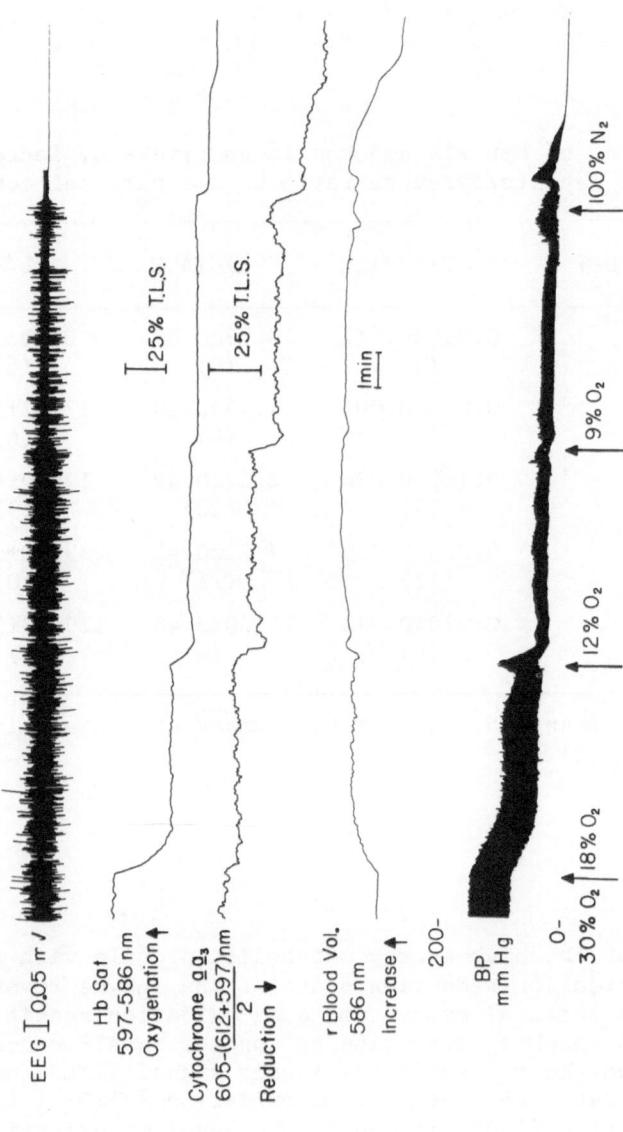

Fig. 1. Representative trace of the effects of acute decreases in the fractional content of inspired oxygen on cytochrome a,a3 redox state, hemoglobin saturation, and blood volume obtained in the parietal cortex of skull intact rat brain.

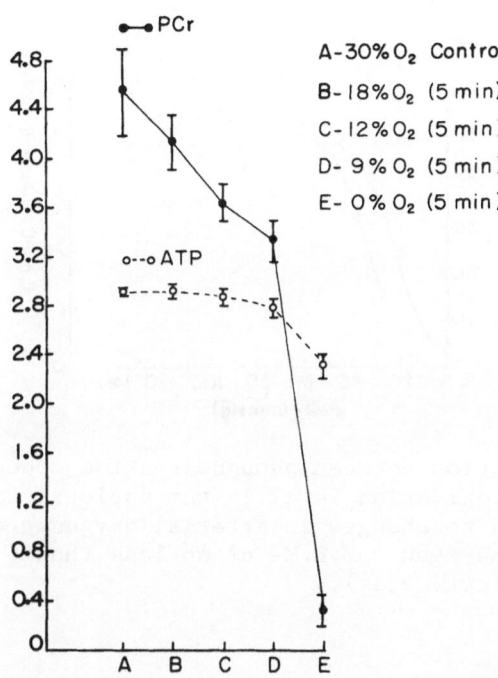

Fig. 2. Influence of five minute periods of graded hypoxia and anoxia on phosphocreatine and ATP concentrations in rat parietal cortex. Each data point is the mean ± S.E.M. of no less than 6 animals. Concentrations in μmole/g wet wt.

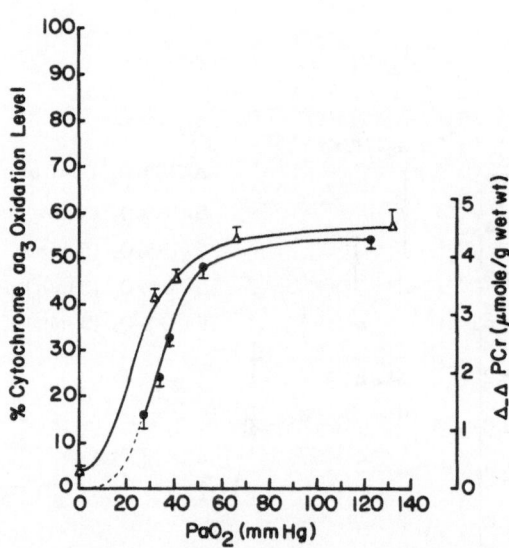

Fig. 3. Correlation between phosphocreatine concentration and cytochrome a̲,a̲3 oxidation level in the parietal cortex of rat brain as related to changes in arterial oxygen tension. Each data point is the mean ± S.E.M. of no less than 6 animals (PCr) and 10 animals (cyt. a̲,a̲3).

CONCLUSIONS

The data show that the _in vivo_ cytochrome a,a_3 redox state correlates sensitively with phosphocreatine, the most labile fraction of high-energy phosphate stores in the cerebral cortex. Thus, _in situ_ optical monitoring of changes in the oxidation-reduction signal of cytochrome a,a_3 provides a continuous, noninvasive, and reliable index of oxygen-limited cellular energy production.

REFERENCES

1. Chance, B. and Williams, G.R. Respiratory enzymes in oxidative phosphorylation. III. The steady state. J. Biol. Chem. 217:409-427, 1955
2. Jöbsis, F.F. and LaManna, J.C. Kinetic aspects of intracellular redox reactions. In Extrapulmonary Manifestations of Respiratory Disease, Marcel Dekker, New York, N.Y., pp. 63-108, 1978
3. Snow, T.R., Kleinman, L.H., LaManna, J.C., Wechsler, A.S. and Jöbsis, F.F. Response of cyt a,a_3 in the in situ canine heart to transient ischemic episodes. Basic Res. Cardiol. 76:289-304, 1981
4. Rosenthal, M., LaManna, J.C., Jöbsis, F.F., Levasseur, J.E., Kontos, H.A. and Patterson, J.L. Effects of respiratory gases on cytochrome a in intact cerebral cortex: Is there a critical PO_2? Brain Res. 108:143-154, 1976
5. Sylvia, A.L. and Rosenthal, M. The effect of age and lung pathology on cytochrome a,a_3 redox levels in the rat cerebral cortex. Brain Res. 146:109-122, 1978
6. Jöbsis, F.F., Keizer, J.H., LaManna, J.C. and Rosenthal, M. Reflectance spectrophotometry of cytochrome a,a3 in vivo. J. appl. Physiol. 43:858-872, 1977
7. Pontèn, U., Ratcherson, R.A., Salford, L.G. and Siesjö, B.K. Optimal freezing conditions for cerebral metabolites in rats. J. Neurochem. 21:1127-1138, 1973
8. Lowry, O.H. and Passonneau, J.V. A Flexible System of Enzymatic Analysis, New York: Academic Press, 1972

THE NEAR INFRARED (NIR) ABSORPTION BAND OF CYTOCHROME $\underline{aa}_3$ IN
PURIFIED ENZYME, ISOLATED MITOCHONDRIA AND IN THE INTACT BRAIN
IN SITU

H.H. Keizer, F.F. Jöbsis-Vander Vliet, S.S. Lucas,
C.A. Piantadosi, and A.L. Sylvia

Departments of Physiology and Medicine
Duke University Medical Center, Durham, N.C. 27710

The potential value of monitoring the redox state of cyto-
chrome $\underline{c}$ oxidase (cytochrome $\underline{aa}_3$ or cyt $\underline{aa}_3$) as an index to cerebral energetics was highlighted in the preceding contribution
(Sylvia et al., 1985). Hypoxically induced changes in the redox
state of cyt $\underline{aa}_3$ correlated well with creatine phosphate fluctuations. That study was performed using the well described absorption peak of reduced heme $\underline{a}$ in the visible part of the spectrum
as the marker (Jöbsis et al., 1977). Even as successful as that
effort has proved to be, a considerable drawback exists in the
fact that, except for very thin skulled animals such as rats and
birds, the cerebral cortex must be exposed to obtain the optical
signals. In order to be maximally useful, a totally non-invasive
approach should be provided for observations on larger species
including humans. Not only would this provide a greater range of
applicability, including routine monitoring of patients, but the
importance of preserving normal intra-cranial pressure relations
can hardly be overstressed.

In the near infra-red (NIR) range of the spectrum an absorption band exists which is assigned to the copper moieties of cytochrome $\underline{aa}_3$ (Wharton and Tzagoloff, 1964). These copper atoms, two
per cytochrome $\underline{c}$ oxidase complex, participate in the redox reactions according to the following diagram (in which the arrows
indicate the flow of electrons):

$$\text{cyt c} \xrightarrow{\quad} \text{heme } \underline{a} \xrightarrow{\quad} \text{heme } \underline{a}_3 \xrightarrow{\quad} O_2$$

with Cu above heme $\underline{a}$ and Cu above heme $\underline{a}_3$

The exact role of the copper atoms is not clear at this point. However, it has been established that they parallel the redox conditions of the hemes. They generate a broad absorption band (830 nm peak) in the NIR when in the oxidized condition, but not when in the reduced form. Thus monitoring of the sufficiency of the cerebral oxygen supply for normal function of the enzyme within the brain cells would also appear feasible using this absorption band. What appeared particularly attractive to us was the possibility that the well-known penetrating power of NIR radiation might make it possible to observe the behavior of the enzyme complex non-invasively through skin and bone tissue. To a first degree this possibility was demonstrated in early observations (Jöbsis, 1977). Considerable effort has been expended since towards proof of identity and source of derivation of these signals. This brief report is a first, preliminary account of the studies trying to ascertain whether the 830 nm band of the enzyme can be identified spectrophotometrically when monitoring the brain through the intact scalp and skull.

Because the visually inaccessible NIR absorption band was described much more recently than the visible ones and because it is much weaker, broader, and therefore, spectrophotometrically not as easily studied, the only published spectra have been derived from relatively concentrated preparations of the purified enzyme taken out of its mitochondrial environment and stripped of the remainder of the respiratory chain. It was therefore necessary to obtain spectra from the enzyme in functioning suspensions of isolated mitochondria before reasonable comparisons with in situ data could be made.

Mitochondria were isolated from liver, brain and kidney of rats and pigs by the usual methods of homogenization and differential centrifugation.* A differential wavelength scanning spectrophotometer was constructed for optimal performance in the NIR region. The mitochondrial suspension needed to be extremely concentrated, because of the low intensity of the NIR band, resulting in highly light scattering samples. The data were recorded at 0-4°C approximately as oxidized minus reduced spectra. Even at this low temperature either H_2O_2 or 100% O_2 were required as oxidants because of the tendency of the samples to become anoxic. In Figure 1 two spectra are shown and compared to two purified enzyme spectra which are representative of the published record. For this purpose the published spectra were photographically enlarged for more precise comparison. The spectra shown in Figure 1 are matched and normalized at 730 and 820 nm to facilitate comparison. Quite clearly, although similar, the two sets differ somewhat in the

---

* For the complete description of all methods the reader is referred to the article by Jöbsis-Vander Vliet (1985).

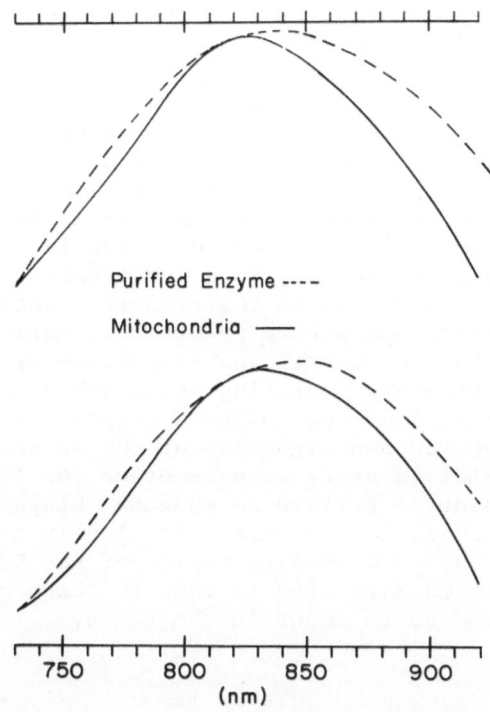

Fig.1. Comparison of NIR spectra recorded from purified enzyme
preparations with those derived from isolated mitochondria.
The set of curves at the top is from Griffiths and Wharton,
1961 (broken line) and our data from mitochondria isolated
from rat liver. The botton set is from Greenwood et al. 1974
(broken line) and our data from mitochondria isolated from
porcine kidney. For better comparison they have been normalized for 730 to 820 nm.

wavelength of the peak, but more significantly in bandwidth as will
be discussed shortly below.

The cyt aa_3 spectra of the intact preparations, i.e. rat's
and cat's heads, in the oxidized vs reduced mode would be obscured
by the hemoglobin absorption. For this reason we removed all blood
by exchange perfusion with blood substitutes until a hematocrit of
<0.1% was reached. Most commonly we used a fluorocarbon suspension
(FC43) with the animal ventilated on 100% oxygen or an O_2/CO_2 mix,
for instance 95/5 or 90/10 percent. In a smaller set of experiments
Krebs-Henseleit-Albumen solution (KHA) was used as a blood substitute. Because of the low O_2-carrying capacity of the latter, these
experiments were performed at 3 to 4 atmospheres of pressure (ATA)
in a hyperbaric chamber with the animal breathing a gas mixture of
98/2, 97/3 or 95/5 percent O_2/CO_2. For the sake of completeness we
also performed some experiments at 3 ATA using FC43. In rats the
head was transilluminated from temple to temple. In cats this
arrangement yielded too low a signal for a servicable signal to
noise ratio. For this reason we resorted to a reflectance mode in
which the light entry and pickup points were more or less lateral
to each other, 2 to 4 cm apart. Spectrophotometry was performed by
a single beam instrument, featuring an ultrahigh intensity, pre-
focused incandescent lamp and built-in compensation for signal
attenuation at the low and high ends of the wavelength scale.
Spectra in the oxidized state were recorded for later subtraction
of the reduced spectra. Difference spectra obtained in this manner
are shown in Figure 2. They adhere more closely to the values of
the half bandwidths and intensity ratios of the 605 nm to 830 nm
peaks of the isolated mitochondria than to those of the purified
enzyme preparations as is shown in the table.

Table 1.

	λmax	1/2 band-width	VIS/NIR ratio
Purified enzyme	843 nm	148 nm	39.6
Isolated mitochondria	833 nm	117 nm	13.0
Cat brain in situ	827 nm	102 nm	13.0
Rat brain in situ	830 nm	100 nm	13.4

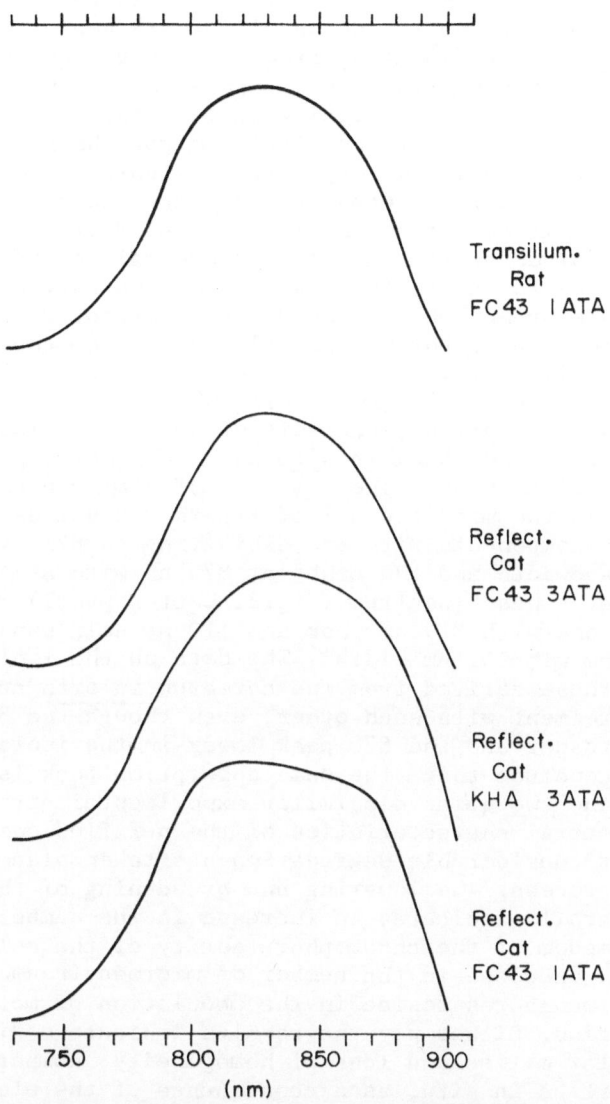

Fig.2. Spectra from rat's and cat's heads in the oxidized minus
reduced conditions. Variations related to means of blood exchange and to optical mode of recording transillumination
vs. reflectance were small. All data were normalized for
730 to 820 nm.

In addition to the numerically obvious discrepancies in bandwidth and VIS/NIR ratios, the shape of our NIR peaks, especially
of the in situ cerebral spectra, frequently gave the impression as
if they were composed of two closely spaced bands. We tested this
notion by performing a curve fitting test on the basis of two
Lorentzian line shapes using the fitting algorithm Praxis as
adapted to our DEC PDP 11/44 computer. In Figure 3 the analysis of
a mitochondrial and a rat's head spectrum are shown in contrast to
the purified enzyme data from the literature. Whereas the former
were easily resolved as the sum of two Lorentzians, satisfactory
fits could not be found for the NIR data of the enzyme preparations.
Instead a single broad band in the NIR was fitted. Peak and half
bandwidth of the single Lorentzian calculated from the Griffiths
and Wharton (1961) data were 830 nm and 312 nm respectively and of
those from Greenwood et al. (1974) were 839 nm peak and 248 nm
half bandwidth. In contrast, analysis of spectra of isolated mitochondria and of the cerebrum in situ shows a clear separation into
two Lorentzian line shapes. The analysis of a mitochrondrial suspension shown in the middle panel of Figure 3 resolves the overall
curve into two components with one exhibiting an 821 nm peak and
156 nm half bandwidth and the other at 875 nm with a 74 nm width.
A bloodless cat's head spectrum (Fig.3, bottom panel) was resolved
in two bands: one with 819 nm peak and 113 nm half bandwidth, the
other at 878 nm with 61 nm width*. The data on the isolated mitochondria and those derived from the cerebrum in situ are in
reasonable agreement with each other, even though the 820 nm peak
is somewhat broader and the 870 peak lower in the isolated mitochondria. We conclude that the same absorption peak is being
monitored in the two quite dissimilar experimental circumstances.
As for the spectral characteristics of the purified enzyme, we
postulate that considerable degradation has taken place in the
purification process. The lowering and broadening of the absorption peak generally indicates an increase in the number of
degrees of freedom of the chromophore entity of the molecule. Or
it may mean an increase in the number of microenvironments in which
individual chromophores reside in the population of molecules
under observation. Either way the results indicate a disturbance
of the molecular milieu and loss of homogeneity, compared to the
virginal condition in situ, as a consequence of the biochemist's
manipulations.

---

* Analysis of a number of different mitochondrial and intact preparations and of all published spectra show that the data of Figure
3 are representative, as will be published in detail in a forthcoming article (Jöbsis–Vander Vliet, in preparation).

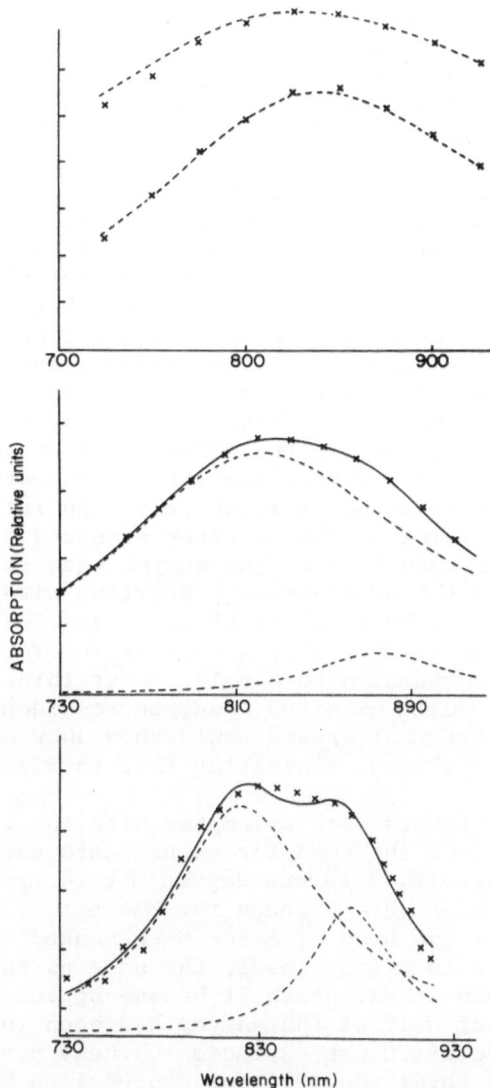

Fig. 3. Results of Lorentzian analysis of the NIR bands of various
preparations. Top panel: The tope curve shows the fit to
the Griffiths and Wharton spectrum (1961), the lower curve
to Greenwood et al. 1974. The computer fit the data by postu-
lating that a second Lorentzian must have occurred at a
much lower wavelength i.e. off the present scale. This produced also a somewhat artifically wide halfbandwidth reading. Middle panel: Spectral analysis of data from porcine
kidney mitochondria. The solid line is the computed sum of
the two Lorentzians identified by the computer program
(broken curves). Bottom panel: Double Lorentzian analysis
of a cat's head spectrum; blood replaced by FC 43.

For conclusive assignment of the NIR band to the cytochrome c oxidase complex or at least to the respiratory chain we used the inhibitors cyanide and carbon monoxide. The first of these, CN^-, combines directly with heme a_3 and inhibits transfer of electrons to oxygen. Carbon monoxide (CO) acts by competitively binding to the locus that otherwise binds O_2 for the electron transfer reaction. In both cases oxidation of the enzyme complex is interdicted and all redox components of the respiratory chain become reduced. In our in vitro experiments, titration of well oxygenated mitochondrial suspensions with CN^- resulted in the abolition of the NIR absorption band, in agreement with the idea that the erstwhile oxidized components absorbing in the NIR would become reduced. Chemical reduction of the CN^- treated aliquot had no further effect on the NIR spectrum. In Figure 4 we have plotted the results as the oxidized minus CN^- reduced difference spectrum in accordance with the previous figures. Clearly the NIR band shown is closely similar to the oxidized-anoxic spectra. Similar experiments with CO were complicated by the fact that a relatively high ratio of CO/O_2 was required. This lowering of the O_2 titer produced a tendency toward creating an anoxic reduction of the enzyme when the uninhibited fraction exhausted the available O_2. Starting with reduced suspensions as baseline, we bubbled one aliquot with 50% O_2 and 50% CO for several minutes at $0° - 1°C$. A rapidly recorded spectrum (Fig.4) showed a definite oxidation to a value about three quarters of that recorded with the fully oxidized spectrum recorded before. A second spectrum taken shortly afterward would then show a return to the totally reduced condition, indicating that anoxia had set in again.

Similar experiments were attempted with the intact, bloodless preparations. However the need for an adequate cardiac output precluded experiments with a severe degree of cytochrome aa_3 inhibition. The bottom panel of Figure 4 shows the NIR effect of $10^{-5}M$ CN^- on the spectrum of the head of a FC-43 exchanged rat breathing 100% O_2. The band shown is again closely the same as the anoxic ones shown earlier. Upon anoxic death it became approximately twice as intense, i.e. about half of the enzyme had been inhibited by the procedure. The use of CO was excluded in these preparations because of the low oxygen level required for appropriate CO/O_2 ratios. It is hoped that recourse to hyperbaric pressure may resolve the problem and these experiments will be performed as soon as the opportunity arises again.

So far these results indicate that the NIR band is sensitive to inhibitors of the terminal reaction of the respiratory chain. The only known components with an 830 nm absorption band are the

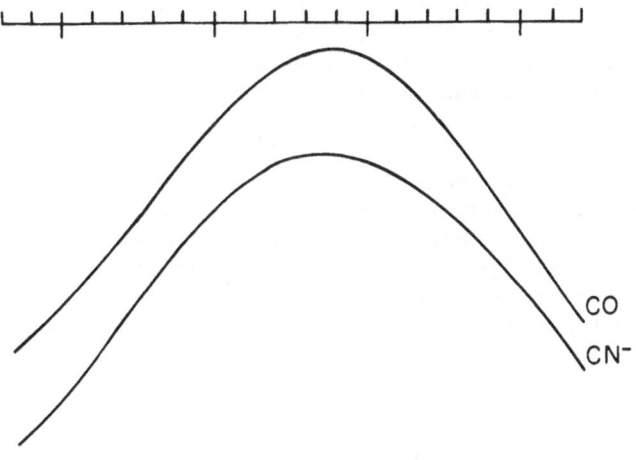

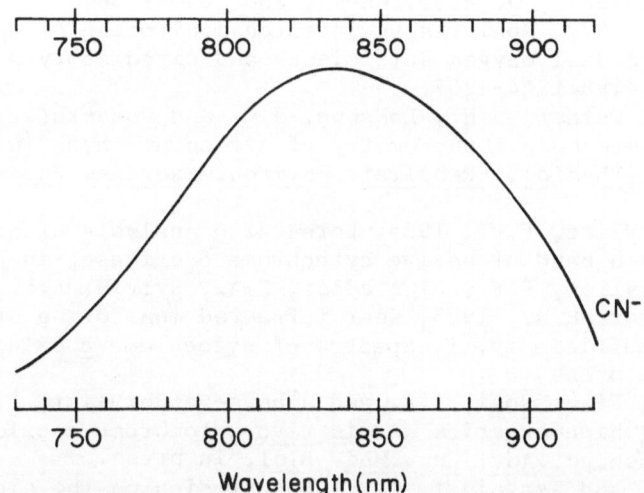

Fig.4. Effects of the terminal respiratory chain inhibitors carbon monoxide (CO) and cyanide (CN⁻) on mitochrondrial preparations (top two curves) and on an intact bloodless preparation. These spectra are displayed as oxidized minus inhibited and normalized for 730 to 820 nm.

copper moieties of cytochrome c oxidase. This point is strengthened
by other observations such as the fact that titration of mitochondrial preparations with inhibitors such as Antimycin A and rotenone,
which act at the cytochrome b level, does not influence the 830 nm
region. This narrows the candidates down to cytochromes c and c_1 and
cytochrome c oxidase. Since only the latter shows any optical activity around 830 nm, we tentatively conclude that the 830 nm band
is a redox dependent characteristic of cytochrome c oxidase. The
ability to demonstrate this in situ, with intact preparations monitored through the scalp and skull, suggest that it may be possible
to construct instrumentation for monitoring cerebral oxygen sufficiency on a continuous basis in the laboratory and possibly in the
clinical setting.

REFERENCES

Greenwood, C., Wilson, M.T. and Brunori, M., 1974, Studies on
    partially reduced mammalian cytochrome oxidase: reactions with
    carbon monoxide and oxygen, Biochem. J., 137:205-215.
Griffiths, D.E. and Wharton, D.C., 1961, Studies of the electron
    transport system XXXV. Purification and properties of cyto-
    chrome oxidase, J. Biol. Chem., 236:1850-1856.
Jöbsis, F.F., 1977, Noninvasive infrared monitoring of cerebral
    and myocardial oxygen sufficiency and circulatory parameters,
    Science, 198:1264-1267.
Jöbsis, F.F., Keizer, J.H., LaManna, J.C. and Rosenthal, M., 1977,
    Reflectance spectrophotometry of cytochrome a,a_3 in vivo,
    J. Appl. Physiol.: Respirat. Environ. Exercise Physiol. 43:
    858-872.
Jöbsis-VanderVliet, F.F., 1985, Lorentzian analysis of near infrared
    absorption band of native cytochrome c oxidase, in preparation.
Jöbsis-VanderVliet, F.F., Piantadosi, C.A., Sylvia, A.L., Lucas, S.K.
    and Keizer, H.H., 1985, Near infra red monitoring of cerebral
    oxygen sufficienty, 1. Spectra of sytochrome c oxidase, Neurol.
    Res., in press.
Sylvia, A.L., Piantadosi, C.A. and Jöbsis-VanderVliet, F.F., 1985,
    Cerebral bioenergetics and in vivo cytochrome c oxidase redox
    relationships, Adv. Exp. Med. Biol, in press.
Wharton, D.C. and Tzagoloff, A., 1964, Studies on the electron
    transfer system LVII. The near infrared absorption band of
    cytochrome oxidase, J. Biol. Chem. 239:2036-2041.

NON-INVASIVE, NEAR INFRARED MONITORING OF CELLULAR OXYGEN SUFFICIENCY IN VIVO

F.F. Jöbsis-Vander Vliet

Department of Physiology
Duke University Medical Center
Durham, N.C. 27710

Since soft tissues, skin and bone are relatively translucent to near infrared (NIR) light and since cytochrome c oxidase possesses a redox dependent absorption band in that region, it appeared important to exploit these two co-incident properties in the development of a non-invasive technique to monitor sufficiency of O_2 delivery to tissues in a variety of experimental and clinical situations. Aside from the enzyme and hemoglobin, in both the oxygenated (HbO_2) and the deoxygenated (Hb) form, very few if any other tissue components possess absorption properties in the NIR and we found none that exhibited O_2-dependent absorption changes. In order to correct the cyt a,a_3 signals for interference by changing perfusion, O_2 saturation and O_2 utilization conditions, means had to be found to strip out the contributions of HbO_2 and Hb to the overall absorbance properties of the tissue or organ being monitored. Towards this purpose we designed and constructed a multiwavelength differential spectrophotometer for the monitoring of intact, normally circulated tissues, such as brain and muscle, through skin and bone. An outline of the biological and design principles, proof of method and a brief consideration of the data format and significance is given in this first preliminary report.

PRINCIPLE

The methodology rests on the circumstances that: (1) light in the near infra-red (NIR) range of the spectrum penetrates skin and bone much more readily than other wavelengths; (2) that very few biological compounds absorb in the NIR; (3) that among these, hemoglobin and cytochrome c oxidase (a.k.a. cytochrome a,a_3 or cyt a,a_3) are the only absorbers detectably reacting to situations of hypoxia/anoxia and oligemia/ischemia; (4) that it has

833

proved possible to separately assess the blood and cytochrome reactions providing thereby some redundancy as well as greater insight in the causative factors leading to a deficient O_2 supply for cytochrome function; and (5) that laser diode light sources are available in the 750 to 905 nm range to provide narrow-banded light pulses for the purposes of multiwavelength, differential, near infrared spectrophotometry (NIRS).

The value of the technique hinges on the ability to obtain optical signals of NIR light absorbing activity related to the oxidative metabolic status of the brain or other tissue being monitored. Although monitoring of other organs has been performed successfully most of our efforts to date have been concentrated on the brain because of its vital dependence on oxidative metabolism and its easy accessibility through scalp and skull.

Cytochrome $\underline{a},\underline{a}_3$ is the indicator of its own functional state since curtailment of oxygen results in a shift toward more reduction and finally to a totally reduced state. This shift in the redox state results in characteristic absorption changes in the 800 to 900 nm region. Since skin and bone contain undetectably low titers of the enzyme, not a surprising finding in view of their very low O_2 uptake rates, the cyt $\underline{a},\underline{a}_3$ signal is derived only from tissue with strong oxidative metabolic capacity such as the neuronal cell bodies. In view of the much higher concentration of the enzyme in the cortex and because of the optical geometry used (see below) the cortical cells provide the much greater part of the signal compared to the white matter. Experiments with elimination of the skin or of the brain below the region of observation (by suction and introduction of an inert light scattering paste) showed trivial and minor contributions to the blood signals by skin and bone. Perhaps because of the pressure of the optic fiber bundles, no fraction of the blood signal could be assigned to the skin. The bone of the skull, however, did contribute in a minor way-maximally about 5%-to the blood signals, both in terms of oxygenated (HbO$_2$) and de-oxygenated (Hb) blood. The resulting signals, although not exclusively derived from brain tissue, do provide therefore excellent corroboration and indication of possible causes of cerebral oxygen insufficiency observed in the redox behavior of cytochrome $\underline{c}$ oxidase.

INSTRUMENTATION

The basis system consists of four laser diodes and fiber-optic means of monitoring one area of the head, or other organ, using a reflectance mode. Future instruments, now in the construction stage, will have dual monitoring capabilities for comparing left and right hemispheres, frontal vs occipital cortex, two different organs simultaneously (such as brain and muscle tissue), etc.

The light from the Ga-Al-As laser diodes is captured in fiber-optic bundles (2 mm diameter approx.) which together with a fifth bundle are intermixed to form a common, larger bundle that carries the light to the preparation. The bundle can be mechanically placed against the scalp of the animal immobilized in a head holder or can be held against the skin of the patient with adhesives. Another bundle picks up a fraction of the scattered light emanating from the skull some 3 to 5 cm lateral to the point of entry and conveys it back to the chassis for measurement.

The laser diodes are pulsed in sequence (200 nanosec pulses at 1 KHz) and the detectors are similarly modulated to provide for better ambient light rejection. In addition the fifth leg of each input bundle is used to detect light directly reflected from the skin at the point of input. This information is used as a reference for correction against fluctuations in laser brightness and for further elimination of ambient light interference. This approach has been sufficiently successful to allow monitoring of patients under normal illumination in a variety of settings, such as intensive care units, premature baby nurseries and in operating rooms (cf. Brazy et al. and Fox et al. in this volume). After demodulation, signal and reference detector outputs are ratio-ed and the logarithm is taken. The resulting signals at the different wavelengths are used to calculate, on line, the variations in amounts of Hb, HbO_2 and in the redox state of cyt $\underline{a},\underline{a}_3$. Since the former relate to conditions of the blood in the microcirculation, i.e. within the tissue, we have chosen to designate these signals tHb and $tHbO_2$. The cytochrome signal is, of course, derived from the cells of the tissue. For the calculation of these parameters alogrithms are used which were derived from experiments in which the hematocrit in the cerebral circulation was changed under totally reduced conditions of cyt $\underline{a},\underline{a}_3$ (artificial perfusion with completely anoxic RBC suspensions differing in hematocrit) or totally oxygenated conditions (hemodilution while respiring the preparation with 3 to 4 atmospheres of a 95% O_2, 5% CO_2 mix in a hyperbaric chamber). Since the wavelengths of the laser diodes can not be specified exactly in the manufacturing process the essential characteristics of our instrument vary each time a new diode is installed and new algorithms must be derived. So far no generalized solution has been obtained.

Read-out of changes in the tHb, $tHbO_2$, their sum i.e. change in microcirculatory blood volume (tBV) and in cyt $\underline{a},\underline{a}_3$ traces is available both by a pen and ink chart recorder and digitally. Although signal update occurs every 200 msec, the chart recorder usually works through a 1 or 2.5 second passive time constant.

DESCRIPTION OF DATA FORMAT

The information obtained by NIRS monitoring is mainly in relative terms or trends. At this stage of the development it has not been possible to provide data in absolute, quantitative units or to make them directly referrable to standard parameters such as blood gases, cardiac output, regional bloodflow etc. There are two reasons for this. For an analytic approach toward quantitative definitions in terms of concentrations the task is handicapped by the absence of information concerning the length of the optical path through the tissue. Thus the Beer-Lambert law for determining concentrations is not applicable. Secondly, the most crucially significant signal, the redox state of cytochrome a,a_3, is totally without precedent and is therefore not directly referrable to other, better known parameters. So, in fact, are the blood signals, since information concerning the O_2 saturation within the nutritive circulation is not available. All presently employed blood monitoring techniques relate to blood in the large vessels or at the organ level, i.e. on the macro-scale. Therefore the applications thus far have been limited to trend monitoring. Even then the point concerning the units in which the results are expressed should be considered. In order to distinguish our data from those obtained by spectrophotometry of samples in cuvettes, which are expressed in units of Absorbance (Abs) or of Optical Density (OD), we have chosen to call our results variations in density, abbreviated as v/d. The units are such that a tenfold change in the value computed through the algorithm is given a value of one v/d. (In daily laboratory jargon the units are referred to as "vanders".)

To demonstrate by a simple example:

if ΔtHb= 2.5 x (Δ intensity of the 765 nm signal) − 1.7 x (Δ800 nm intensity) −0.4 x (Δ870 nm intensity) −0.8 x (Δ904 nm intensity)

then the ΔtHb signal will have changed 1.0 v/d when the right side of the equation has changed 10-fold.

PROOF OF METHOD

In order to verify whether the blood and the cyt a,a_3 signals were sufficiently free from "cross-talk" we performed several series of experiments. The task was basically to devise manipulations by which ideally one but not the other two parameters could be expected to vary; or conversely two but not the third. Results obtained with two of the more incisive ones are shown in the way of proof that the separation of the signals has been achieved sufficiently well to merit confidence in the methodology (Figs. 1 and 2).

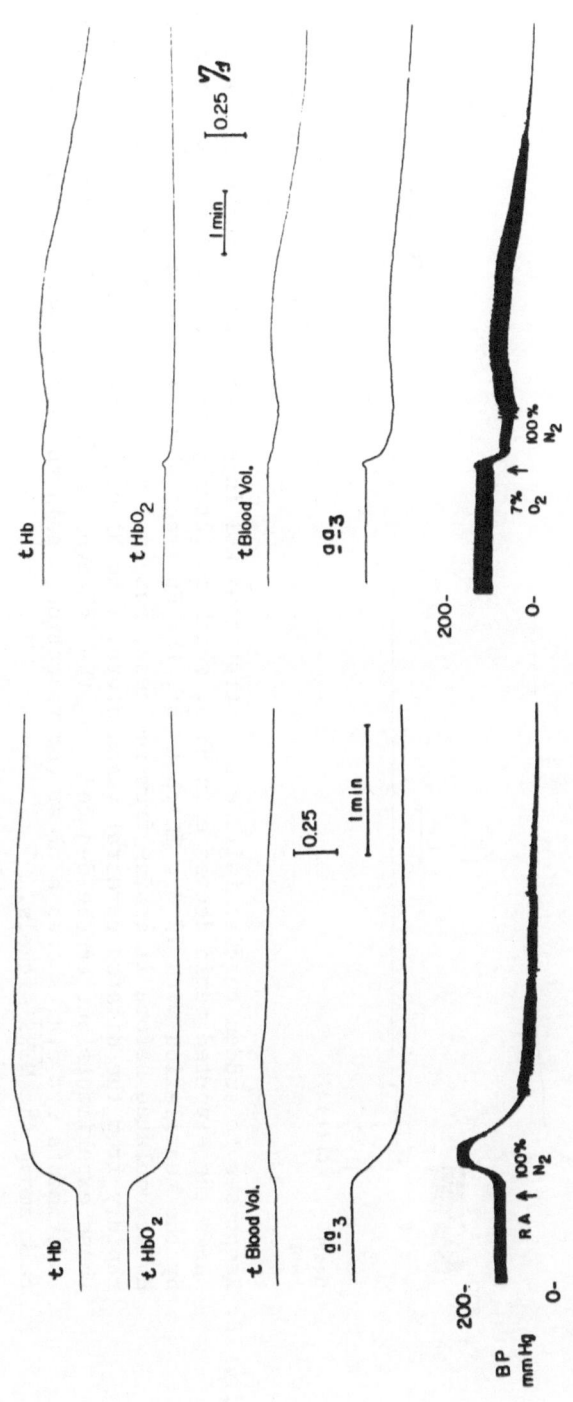

Fig. 1. Cerebral NIRS responses to anoxic death (this set of traces) and to ischemia (next page) starting from normoxia (breathing room air), P_aO_2 approx. 95 torr on the left; starting from hypoxia (breathing 7% O_2), P_aO_2 approx. 25 torr on the right (cats; pentobarbital; gallamine; positive pressure ventilation). Fig. 1A. Anoxic death at the low P_aO_2 shows that practically no arterially colored blood is present in the cerebral vasculature under observation and vasodilation was maximal. The waning trend of the tHb and tB.V. traces is ascribed to the draining of blood from the head in cardiac failure. Note that cyt a,a_3, although considerably more reduced at the low P_aO_2, still responds to anoxia whereas the blood traces do not. Thus it is shown that very little cross-talk exists between the signals.

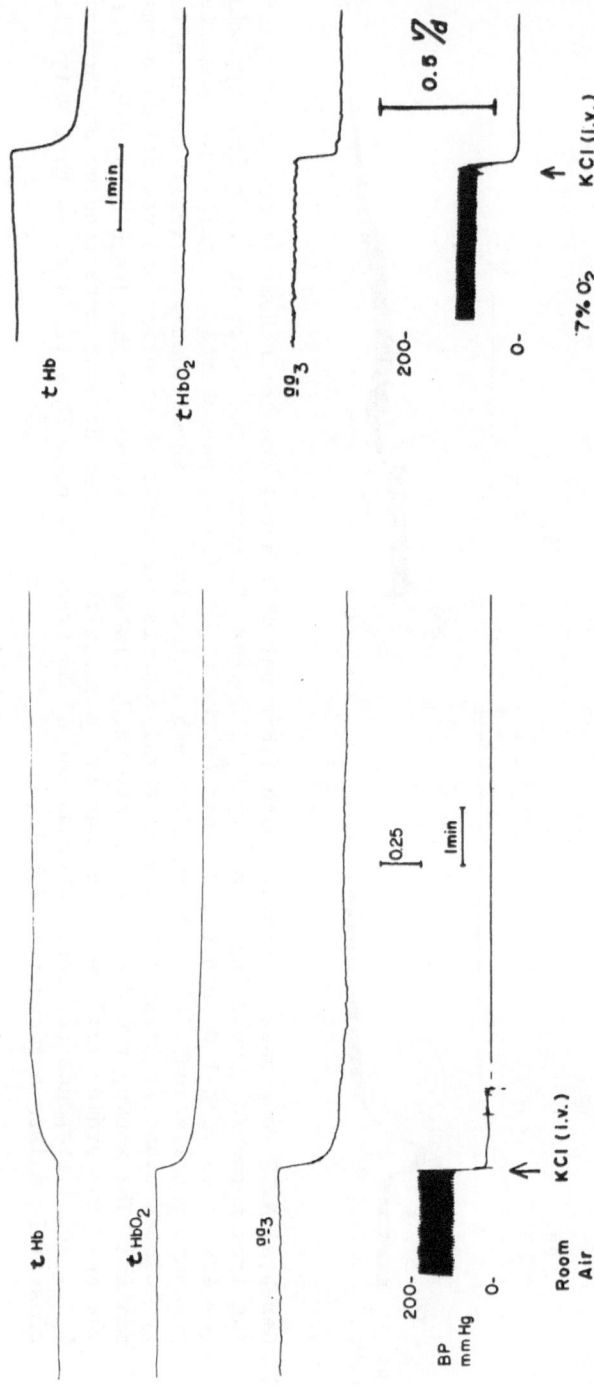

Fig. 1B. Responses to sudden cardiac failure by intravenous KCl injection. The response from normoxia shows the expected rapid decrease in HbO$_2$, which is totally absent at the low P$_a$O$_2$ produced by the ventilation with 7% O$_2$. In contrast, the Hb trace shows in the normoxic case that some Hb accumulates before it drains from the head, but in the low P$_a$O$_2$ case venous blood drains rapidly from the dilated cerebral vasculature. (The blood volume signal was not recorded in these experiments but can be deduced from the changes in the tHb and tHbO$_2$ traces). In both experiments cyt a,a$_3$ showed a clear cut reduction, again showing a lack of significant cross-talk among the NIRS signals.

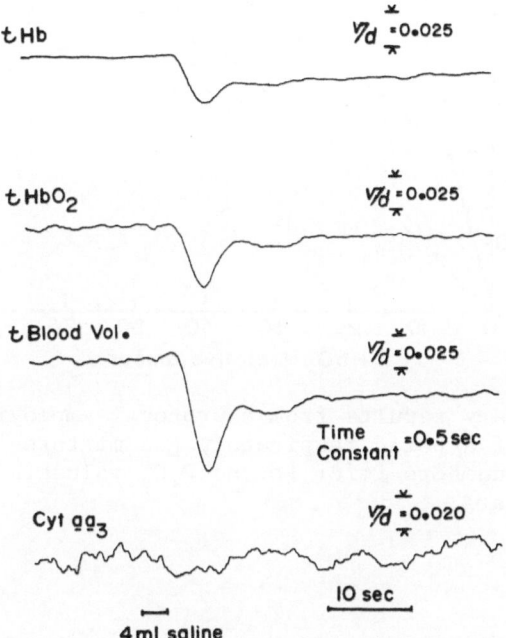

Fig. 2. Response of the NIRS system to the injection of 4 ml saline into the vena cava of an anesthetized cat. Note that as the bolus passes through the cerebral vasculature the hemodilution is recorded in the blood traces whereas the cyt $\underline{a},\underline{a}_3$ trace is not disturbed.

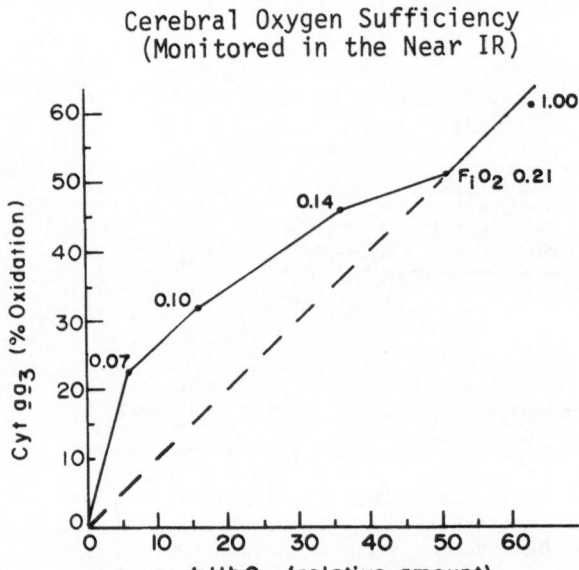

Cerebral Oxygen Sufficiency
(Monitored in the Near IR)

Fig. 3. Preliminary results from a protocol employing various
levels of hypoxic respiratory gas mixtures as well as 100%
O_2. The numbers refer to the F_iO_2 values. Results averaged
from 4 cats.

EXAMPLE OF PHYSIOLOGICAL DATA

The question of units of presentation caused us some concern and, at this point, the problem is not yet settled firmly. Since in each animal preparation the v/d units depend somewhat on the distance between and/or the angle of placement of the "optrodes" (the end assemblies of the fiber-optics bundles) they are not directly comparable in absolute units between preparations. For this reason we prefer to compare data in terms of "total labile signal" (TLS). The range from a nearly maximal hyperoxygenation, say by ventilating the animal with 5 or 10% CO_2 in O_2, to total anoxia at the end of the experiment is determined in each animal of an experimental series and given the value 100 TLS. The effects of other manipulations can be expressed in percent of TLS. Figure 3 shows the correlation of cyt $\underline{a},\underline{a}_3$ and oxyhemoglobin signals from a protocol of variations in F_iO_2 from 0.07 to 1.00. It should be remembered that for cyt $\underline{a},\underline{a}_3$ the total concentration of the enzyme is of course constant and the TLS units translate therefore into percent oxidation or reduction. The amount of hemoglobin, however, varies with the vasodilation in the brain. Thus it seems wiser to think of the amount of HbO_2 observed in the tissue rather than express it as the percentage of the total amount of blood. More experience with this type of monitoring will probably show the way towards the most informative form of data analysis and presentation.

The results shown in Figure 3 emphasize the value of the cyt $\underline{a},\underline{a}_3$ over the hemoglobin signal in terms of tissue viability. When ventilated with 7% O_2 + 93% N_2, which produced in our hands a P_aO_2 of about 25 torr, $tHbO_2$ was about 5% TLS whereas cyt $\underline{a},\underline{a}_3$ remained about 23% oxidized. These kinds of observations may increase our understanding of the interrelations between source and sink in the realm of oxygen transport to tissues.

MONITORING OF CEREBRAL OXYGENATION IN

THE INTENSIVE CARE NURSERY

Jane E. Brazy, D. V. Lewis, M. H. Mitnick,
F. F. Jöbsis-Vander Vliet

Departments of Pediatrics and Physiology
Duke University Medical Center
Durham, North Carolina

Prime objectives in neonatal intensive care include prevention of brain injury and maintanance of normal neurologic function. Since brain function is dependent upon adequate oxygen delivery, various techniques for oxygen monitoring have become integral parts of neonatal intensive care. However, most monitoring techniques currently in use determine oxygenation at sites distant from the brain (i.e. aorta, skin) and do not directly assess either cerebral oxygen delivery or oxygen utilization by the brain. Thus, an instrument which can provide continuous information on hemoglobin oxygenation and on cerebral oxidative metabolism may have marked advantages over current monitoring capabilities and offer the opportunity to observe the specific effects of medical therapies and nursing care on the infant's cerebral oxygenation.

In this paper we report the first observations regarding the impact of routine nursing care procedures on the cerebral oxygenation of small preterm infants using a non-invasive optical method for determining cerebral oxygen sufficiency. With this technique, light in the near infrared region is generated by 3-4 laser diodes and transmitted by a fiber optic bundle to an "optrode" placed on the infant's scalp in the fronto-temporal region. Another optrode, placed over the opposite fronto-temporal region detects the transmitted light (see Figure 1). The instrument uses differential absorbance of photons of selected wavelengths to assess changes in the oxygenation state of hemoglobin ($tHbO_2$ and tHb), in tissue blood volume (tBV) and in the oxidation – reduction of cytochrome aa_3 (cyt aa_3) in the transilluminated field.[1,2] Since scattering of light in the cranium prevents a definition of the optical path length, results are expressed in relative terms using units of variation in density (v/d) rather than absolute absorbance or

843

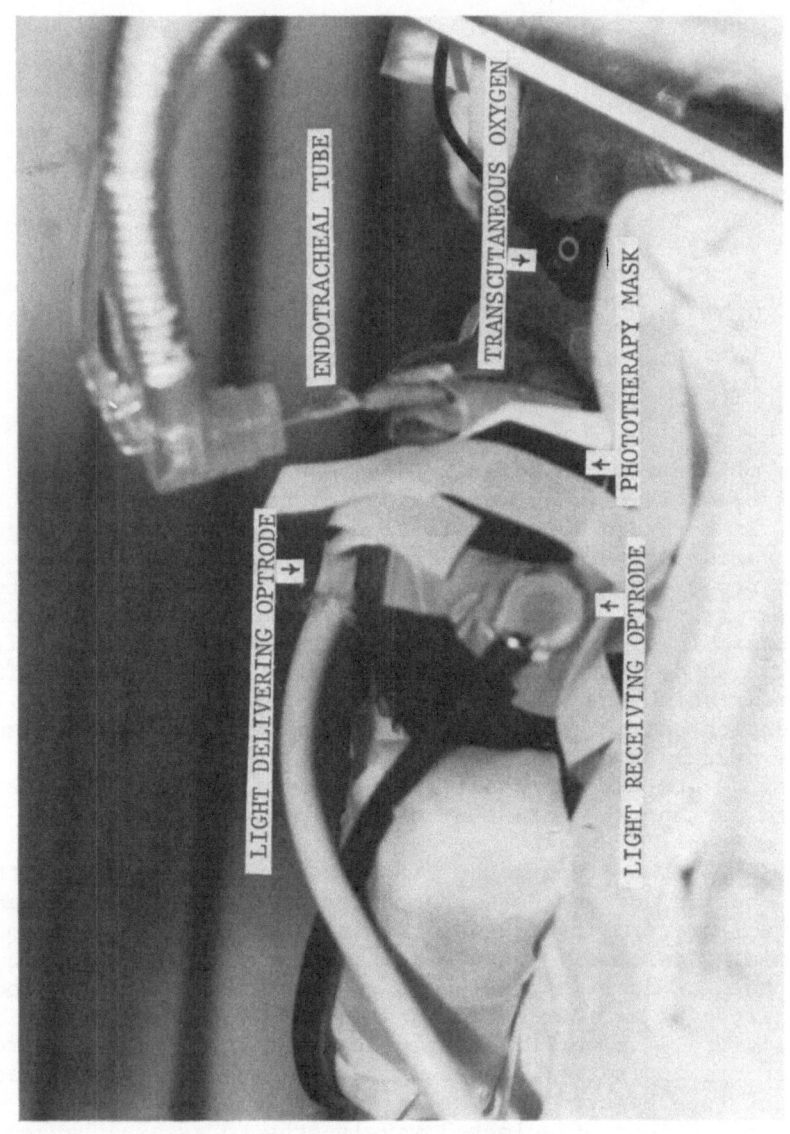

Figure 1: Close up of head of infant with optrodes and bilimask in place.

Optical Density units. Continuous measurements of both oxygenated
and deoxygenated hemoglobin provide information about oxygen supply
to the tissue in the optical field, and the sum of the two, i.e.
total hemoglobin, indicates relative blood volume. Cytochrome
aa_3 (cytochrome c oxidase) serves as the indicator of cerebral
oxygen utilization since it is the terminal member of the mitochondrial election transport chain and has photon absorption characteristics which change with the redox state of the enzyme.

In our study, small preterm infants were monitored at the
bedside within the Intensive Care Nursery. The sides of the
infant's head were supported by a foam rubber cushion to decrease
head motion and the eyes were shielded with a phototherapy mask
to prevent possible retinal exposure to the near infrared light
should the optrode dislodge. Infants were monitored for four to
six hours while receiving routine nursing and medical care. In
addition to tHb, $tHbO_2$, tBV and cyt aa_3, signals from the infant's
cardiorespiratory and transcutaneous oxygen monitors were displayed
on the instrument's chart recorder. Infant manipulations were
noted manually on the tracing.

Undisturbed infants who were healthy or who were clinically
stable demonstrated little or no variation in their cerebral oxygen
delivery or oxygen utilization as reflected in the $tHbO_2$ and cyt
aa_3 respectively. Slight fluctuations did occur in synchrony with
deep (sigh) respirations, especially during sleep. Nursing care
manipulations such as diaper change, temperature taking and gavage
feeding generally caused either a small transient decrease in
hemoglobin oxygenation or no change at all. Cytochrome aa_3 was
often unaffected, but if it became reduced, it would return rapidly
to the more oxidized state with the recovery of hemoglobin
oxygenation.

More dramatic changes in cerebral oxygenation occurred with
routine care in infants who were clinically less stable and had
more significant illness. A representative response is shown in
Figure 2 on the next page. At point 1 the nurse assessed the
infant's axillary temperature. During this procedure there was
a gradual decrease in cutaneous oxygenation ($TcPO_2$ from 70 to 50
torr). However, with the onset of body manipulation, a more
significant and rapid change occurred in cerebral oxygenation with
a shift to hemoglobin deoxygenation and a simultaneous abrupt
reduction of cyt aa_3. Tissue blood volume in the optical field
increased slightly showing some attempt by the infant to auto-
regulate cerebral oxygen delivery. During the two minutes following
the procedure, $tHbO_2$, tBV, cyt aa_3 and $TcPO_2$ concurrently returned
to their respective baselines. Shortly thereafter, point 2, the
nurse gavage fed the infant through an indwelling oral-gastric
tube. This caused an immediate shift in hemoglobin to deoxygenation and in the cytochrome to reduction. Again, a small increase

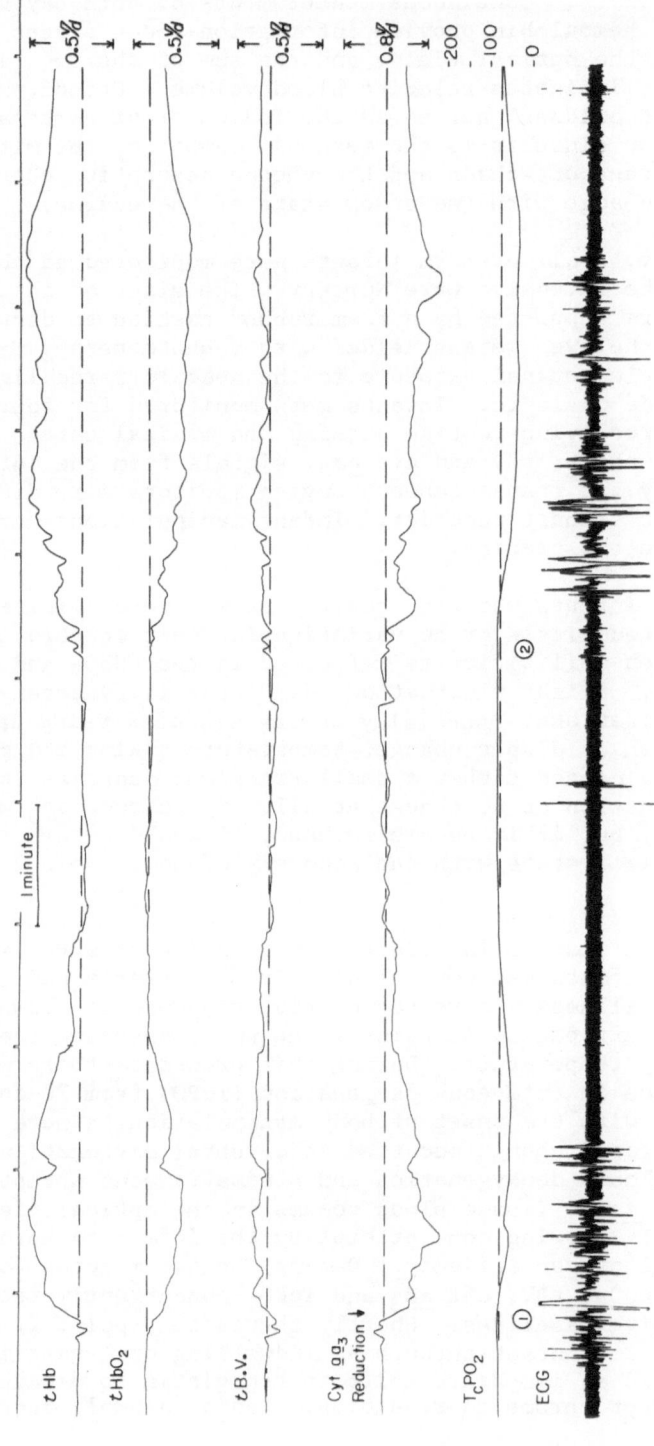

Figure 2: Tracing from a one Kilogram infant during routine nursing care. At point 1 the nurse took the infant's axillary temperature. Point 2 designates the onset of gavage feeding by an indwelling oral-gastric tube.

in tBV was recorded suggesting blood flow to the tissue in the transilluminated field was not only preserved but slightly augmented. Although the magnitudes of change in $tHbO_2$ and cyt $\underline{aa_3}$ were similar to those in the preceding event, the change in transcutaneous oxygenation was much greater. Presumably the marked fall in $TcPO_2$ represented, in part, a redistribution of blood from the skin to the gastrointestinal tract. In addition, acute gastric distention could have transiently compromised pulmonary gas exchange. By five minutes after the feeding (end of tracing) the $TcPO_2$ had returned to prefeeding levels, but cerebral oxygenation had not fully recovered. Blood volume remained elevated and $tHbO_2$ and cyt $\underline{aa_3}$ remained below their respective baselines. Tracings such as these demonstrate the limitations of using only transcutaneous oxygenation to assess the impact of hypoxic events upon the central nervous system.

Responses to nursing care or disease-precipitated events varied betweeen infants and within a single infant over time. Some responses were not easily predictable. One of these was the ability of the infant to demonstrate increased tBV with hypoxia. With intact cerebral autoregulation one would expect a response of cerebral vasodilation to decreased oxygenation. This would lead to greater hemoglobin volume (tBV) in the transilluminated field. Although the episode shown in Figure 2 demonstrated a compensatory increase in tBV with hypoxia, monitored events in other infants showed no change in blood volume with changes in hemoglobin oxygenation and cyt $\underline{aa_3}$ oxidation. Impaired autoregulation of cerebral blood flow in distressed newborns has been documented by Lou and others.[3] Use of the near infrared technique may help to identify this group of high risk infants.

The response of the cyt $\underline{aa_3}$ to episodes of hypoxia was more consistent. In general cyt $\underline{aa_3}$ reduced with hemoglobin deoxygenation and oxidized with hemoglobin reoxygenation; however, the temporal response was often influenced by the prior state of oxygenation. If preceded by a long period of apparently normal oxygenation, the reduction response of cyt $\underline{aa_3}$ to a transient period of hemoglobin deoxygenation was delayed or blunted and recovery occurred simultaneous with reoxygenation. If, however, the preceding period was one of inadequate blood flow, low oxygenation, or sequential hypoxic events, the response of the cytochrome was immediate reduction. In these circumstances recovery of cyt $\underline{aa_3}$ frequently lagged behind the return of $tHbO_2$ and $TcPO_2$ to their baselines.

Our observations on small preterm infants in an intensive care setting demonstrate that non-invasive continuous monitoring of cerebral oxygenation is possible at the bedside and can provide immediate information on the impact of everyday events upon the central nervous system.

REFERENCES

1. F. F. Jobsis, Noninvasive infrared monitoring of cerebral and
    myocardial oxygen sufficiency and circulatory parameters,
    Science 198:1264 (1977).
2. F. F. Jobsis, J. H. Keizer, J. C. LaManna, and M. Rosenthal,
    Reflectance spectrophotometry of cytochrome aa_3 in vivo,
    J. Appl . Physiol: Respirat. Environ. Exercise Physiol.
    43(5):858 (1977).
3   H. C. Lou, N. A. Lassen, and B. Friis-Hansen, Impaired
    autoregulation of cerebral blood flow in the distressed
    newborn infant. J. Pediatr. 94:118 (1979).

MONITORING CEREBRAL OXYGEN SUFFICIENCY IN ANESTHESIA AND SURGERY

Elisabeth Fox, Frans F. Jöbsis-VanderVliet and
Michael H. Mitnick

Departments of Anesthesiology and Physiology
Duke University Medical Center
Durham, N.C., 27710

Our ultimate concern in anesthesia is preserving the integrity of the brain, which is the target to which our anesthetic agents are directed and the organ most vunerable to hypoxia. Yet, so far, we have had no means of directly monitoring either the effects of anesthetic agents on the brain or its state of oxygenation.

In order to take one step towards the monitoring of cerebral oxygen sufficiency a methodology should be applied that would derive signals directly from components of the central nervous system. In addition these signals should indicate incipient oxygen deficiency at a low level, well below, and before the occurrence of, neuronal injury. For this purpose we have developed an optical method to monitor, continuously and in real time, the redox state oc cytochrome c oxidase (also known as cytochrome aa_3) in the cerebral cortex. In this technique we apply differential, multiwavelength laser spectrophotometry to the oxygen-sensitive absorption band of cytochrome c oxidase in the near infra-red, making use of the semi-transparant qualities of skin and bone in this region of the spectrum.

Cytochrome c oxidase (abbreviated cyt aa_3) is the terminal member of the mitochondrial respiratory chain and catalyzes approximately 95% of all O_2 utilization. In the parallel process of oxidative phosphorylation free energy is conserved in the form of high energy phosphate bonds and stored primarily as adenosine triphosphate (ATP) and creatine phosphate (CrP). These are utilized in the processes subserving cell maintenance and physiological function. Monitoring of this enzyme for gauging the adequacy of oxygen delivery for its normal functioning provides therefore the most direct information about cerebral oxygen sufficiency.

849

In the oxidized state the enzyme exhibits an absorption band
in the 800 to 870 nm region of the near infra-red spectrum, which
disappears upon reduction, i.e. when O_2 delivery is compromised.
However, hemoglobin (Hb) and oxyhemoglobin (HbO_2) also absorb light
in the near IR region. Thus the optical signals are affected by the
amounts of arterial-and venous-colored blood in the field of observation. Multiple, monochromatic light sources are required to
determine the Hb and HbO_2 contributions to the overall signal and
eliminate their interference with the cytochrome signal. However,
in the process of correcting for this interference, signals are
obtained from the blood in the brain tissue which provide some
diagnostic capability concerning the possible causes of an observed
occurrence of oxygen insufficiency for normal enzyme function.

In the instruments constructed for our brain monitoring purposes we used near infra-red light generated by several laser diodes
tuned to various wavelengths in the 700 to 950 nm range. Devices with
exact wavelength specifications are difficult to produce reliably
and therefore the wavelengths used in our applications have varied.
These variations are, however, corrected for by adjusting the algorithms used to strip the Hb and HbO_2 contributions from the cyt aa_3
signal. Light from the lasers is captured by glass fiber-optics
bundles to be guided to the patient's head. The strands of the individual bundles are combined and fixed in a terminal assembly, the
"optrode", that can be applied and fastened to the forehead. Light
passes through skin and skull to the brain and is scattered back by
the white matter. A second, "receiving" optrode is placed 4 to 6 cm
lateral to the point of entry and conducts the scattered photons
emanating at this point back to the instrument for measurement. Thus
an ovalshaped portion of cerebral cortex 4 to 6 cm in length consti-
tutes the field of observation.

Using appropriate detection, demodulation and amplification
techniques the three biological signals are derived and displayed
in logarithmic form in conformation with the Beer-Lambert Law.
Cytochrome aa_3 is present in measurable quantities only in the
cerebral cortex, skin and bone being practically devoid of the
enzymes as could be expected from the very low oxygen uptake rates
of the latter two tissues. Thus the cytochrome c oxidase signal is
confidently assigned to the frontal cortex of the brain. From animal
experiments (thus far unpublished) it was concluded that the skin
did not contribute significantly to the blood signals. We suspect
that the pressure of the optrodes, although light, is sufficient to
expel the blood from the skin in the optical path. The skull, however, was found to contribute a small fraction to the overall blood
signals, typically about 5%. In the figures the cytochrome c oxidase
signal is labelled cyt aa_3 and the blood signals $tHbO_2$ and tHb in
order emphasize that they refer to amounts of arterial- and venous-
colored blood in the tissue under observation. Sometimes the tHb
and $tHbO_2$ signals are summed and this sum is displayed separetly to

indicate changes in the total amount of blood, or the blood volume in the tissue being monitored (tB.V.).

At this point in the development of the technology, the instrumentation performs trend monitoring only. The signals are tuned and balanced with the patient awake and breathing room air before induction. These levels of cytochrome $\underline{aa_3}$ redox state and hemoglobin oxygenation are defined as baseline. Changes toward more oxidized cytochrome $\underline{aa_3}$ and more arterially colored blood should be interpreted as satisfactory. The technique was used in addition to all conventional monitoring in 50 patients undergoing general anesthesia for a variety of surgical procedures. In this account of our first somewhat preliminary observations we emphasize the events occurring during the induction.

Anesthesia was induced with sodium thiopental (3-4mg/kg) using a test dose of 50 mg followed by the sleep dose. Administration of the test dose resulted in a small, sometimes transient oxidation of cyt $\underline{aa_3}$ (Fig. 1) and a shift towards more arterially colored blood in the tissue ($tHbO_2\uparrow;tHb\downarrow$). The sleep dose invariably produced further oxidation and shifts to more arterially colored blood. Ventilation with $F_1O_21.00$ produced a further increase in cyt $\underline{aa_3}$ oxidation and $tHbO_2$ increase in all cases. These observations show that during the standard practices of inducing pentothal anesthesia the oxygenation of cerebral-cortical tissue is improved. These first results are perhaps indicative of a decreased $CMRO_2$ with a resetting of cerebrovascular autoregulation towards a higher ratio between flow and oxygen consumption.

On two occasions in this first set of cases the cyt $\underline{aa_3}$ signal rapidly decreased below the calibration baseline during the surgical procedure. Both instances were related to sudden hypotensive episodes and the trends were reversed as appropriate measures were taken to increase the blood pressure (Fig.2). Importantly, in both cases the change in the cytochrome signal was noted before any changes in blood pressure had been observed because of the intermittent nature (every two minutes) of the blood pressure measurements. Similar but less dramatic observations were occasionally noted during changes in respiratory regimen such as during weaning from the respirator.

The oxygenation state of the brain is a steady state resulting from the balance between O_2 supply and O_2 utilization. Under normal physiological conditions this balance is sensitively maintained by macro- as well as micro-circulatory adjustments of flow to metabolic needs. The system guards against hypo-perfusion, and hyper-perfusion as well, by various adjustments from the fine regulation of peri-

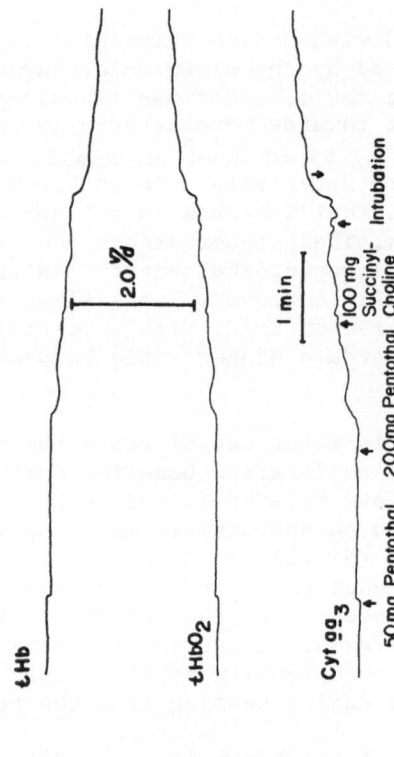

Fig.1. Induction of anesthesia with pentothal.
After the 50 mg. test dose, the sleepdose (200 mg) produces a marked oxidation of cytochrome c oxidase and a shift toward more arterially colored blood within the regional, cerebral circulation. Intubation and ventilation with 100% O_2 produced a further oxidation of cyt a,a_3 and a shift of the microcirculation toward greater oxygenation.

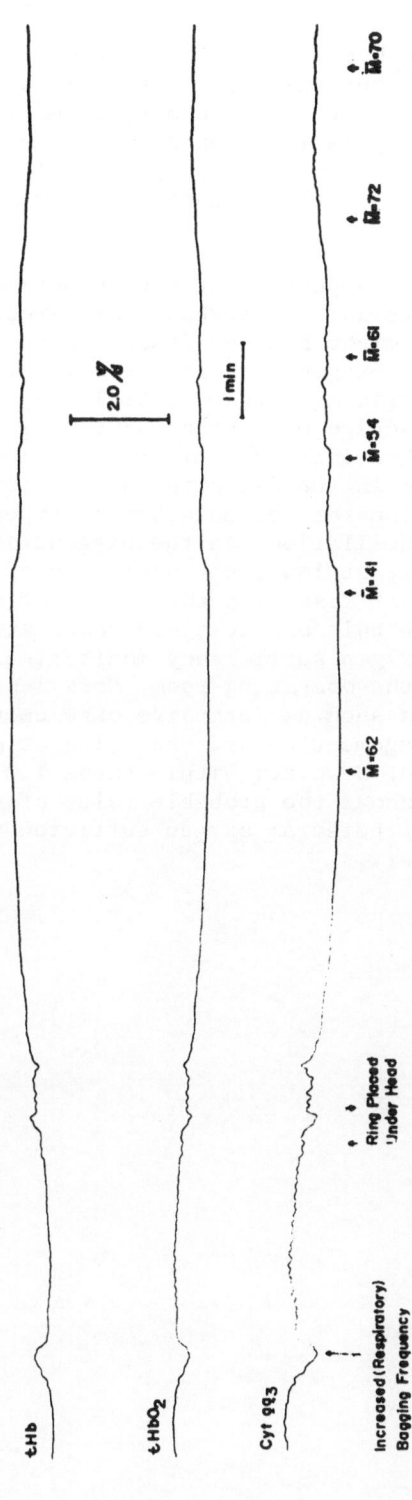

Fig. 2.   Occurrence of two incipient hypoxic episodes.
At left the rate of temporary manual ventilation was apparently not quite adequate to maintain the redox level of the brain constant as is corroborated by the increase in venous and decrease in arterial blood in the tissue. The problem was relieved by increasing the frequency of the manual ventilation. About three minutes later a slower reduction of cyt a,a_3 was recognized and then found to be related to a momentarily unrecognized drop in mean blood pressure. Restoration of blood pressure was accompanied by a return of the NIRS traces to their baselines.

pheral resistance by vaso-dilation or -constriction in the process called autoregulation, to major increases in central pressure and pulmonary ventilation during hypoxic stress. Most of the current methodology attempting to measure cerebral metabolic activity focuses on measuring regional cerebral blood flow and relies on the autoregulatory link for extrapolation toward oxidative metabolism. It is generally known, however, that during pathologic conditions this link is disturbed and blood flow ceases to be an index to metabolic needs or conditions.

From our observations it appears that the induction of anesthesia with pentothal results in a disturbance of cerebral autoregulation in a manner that might best be described as a resetting of the set-point at a higher oxygenation level. Aside from this direct effect of the anesthetic agent on cerebral oxygenation, the common anesthesiological practice of increasing the F_1O_2 to 0.30 or even 1.00 results in a further increased oxygenation level. Both these effects produce change in the direction of greater O_2 delivery, thus providing a buffer region for adequate brain oxygenation during the period of anesthesia. Oscillations in the oxygenation level are therefore no cause for alarm, at least not until the original baseline is crossed. The degree of risk with the extent of a fall below the baseline is not known at this point, since observations at the lower end of the scale of oxygen sufficiency monitoring have not occurred in the setting of the operating room. More insight must be obtained from other settings such as intensive care units. Until such time, conservative management toward exceeding or maintaining baseline levels is indicated. However, within these limits, our preliminary observations have shown the probable value of continuous, near infra-red monitoring of cerebral oxygen sufficiency during general anesthesia and surgery.

NEAR INFRARED OPTICAL MONITORING OF INTACT SKELETAL MUSCLE DURING HYPOXIA AND HEMORRHAGIC HYPOTENSION IN CATS

C. A. Piantadosi and F. F. Jöbsis-Vander Vliet

Departments of Medicine and Physiology
Duke University Medical Center, Durham, N.C. 27710

INTRODUCTION

Pathophysiologic states associated with decreased arterial oxygen delivery are often accompanied by fractional redistribution of cardiac output (1,2). Such responses, mediated in part by chemo or baroreceptor reflexes, divert oxygen flow away from resting tissues such as splanchnic viscera or skeletal muscle and towards more hypoxia-ischemia sensitive tissues such as brain. The feasibility of using non-invasive, near infrared (NIR) multiple wavelength optical assessment of skeletal muscle metabolism as a sensitive and early indicator of progressive O_2 insufficiency during physiological conditions associated with blood flow redistribution was investigated in anesthetized, paralyzed cats. Optically derived NIR cytochrome a,a_3 oxidation-reduction responses were recorded continuously and together with combined oxygen-labile optical density changes in capillary blood and myoglobin saturation during controlled protocols of hypoxic hypoxia or hemorrhagic hypotension and recovery.

METHODS

Adult cats of either sex were anesthetized with intraperitoneal injections of sodium pentobarbital (38 mg/kg). A tracheal tube was inserted and a thin polyethylene cannula was placed into the inferior vena cava near the right atrium. A second double lumen catheter was placed in the right femoral artery to allow continuous arterial blood pressure monitoring (Statham P23 DC pressure transducer) and arterial blood sampling for Pao_2, $Paco_2$ and pH measurements (Instrumentation Laboratories, Model 513 pH/blood gas analyzer). After surgery, the animals were paralyzed with gallamine

855

triethiodide (5 mg/kg i.v.) and ventilated with room air using a positive pressure respirator at a frequency of 20 breaths/min. Tidal volume was adjusted to provide a $Paco_2$ value of 30±2 mm Hg. Rectal temperature was maintained near 37°C with external heating. Sodium heparin (500 u/kg) was administered intravenously to animals used in hemorrhagic hypotension protocols.

Spectrophotometric measurements were obtained using a multiwavelength differential spectrophotometer. The intact, left hindlimb skeletal muscles (biceps plus gracilis) after removal of hair but including skin, were transilluminated with pulses of near infrared light at three wavelengths sequentially conducted to the tissue from separate light sources by means of a glass fiber optics bundle applied gently to the skin. Transmitted light, collected in a second fiber-optic bundle located on the opposite side of the muscle from the first, was conducted to a photomultiplier tube (Hammamatsu R936) for photoprocessing and NIROS-SCOPIC derivation of the blood and cytochrome $\underline{a,a_3}$ copper signals as described earlier in this symposium (3). Because myoglobin (Mb) and oxymyoglobin (MbO_2) have NIR absorbance bands similar to hemoglobin (Hb) and oxyhemoglobin (HbO_2), like optical species were treated as single compartments (Hb+Mb and HbO_2 + MbO_2) to obtain comprehensive signals.

Animal protocols were of two varieties. Animals were exposed either to graded alveolar hypoxia (15%, 12%, 9% or 7% O_2 balance N_2) with normoxic recovery or to arterial hemorrhage at approximately 2.5 mg/kg/min to below 50% circulating blood volume followed by reinfusion of shed blood. In some animals, optical signal interpretation was qualitatively validated by serial injections of indocyanine green (Cardio-green, Becton-Dickinson), a non-diffusible dye that absorbs near infrared light at 805 nm. Boluses of 0.4 ml of dye (0.5 mg/ml in saline) were injected rapidly into the inferior vena cava at steady state conditions and the muscle clearance curves recorded. This technique has been used previously to measure cerebral blood flow in the transilluminated brains of ducks (4).

RESULTS AND DISCUSSION

The NIR optical signals derived from the intact hindlimb were attributable almost exclusively to muscle tissue. Care was taken to exclude bone from within the optical field and the skin overlying the muscle was lightly compressed until it blanched. Figure 1 shows skeletal muscle NIR optical responses during hypoxia. As Pao_2 decreased, the relative amount of Hb+Mb increased, HbO_2+MbO_2 decreased, and the reduction level of the cytochrome $\underline{a,a_3}$ copper moieties increased. Abrupt cytochrome reduction responses usually occurred as Pao_2 decreased below 25 mmHg (Figure 1B). After brief hypoxic episodes (<5 min.), restoration of normoxia resulted in an "overshoot" of the optical signals consistent with reactive

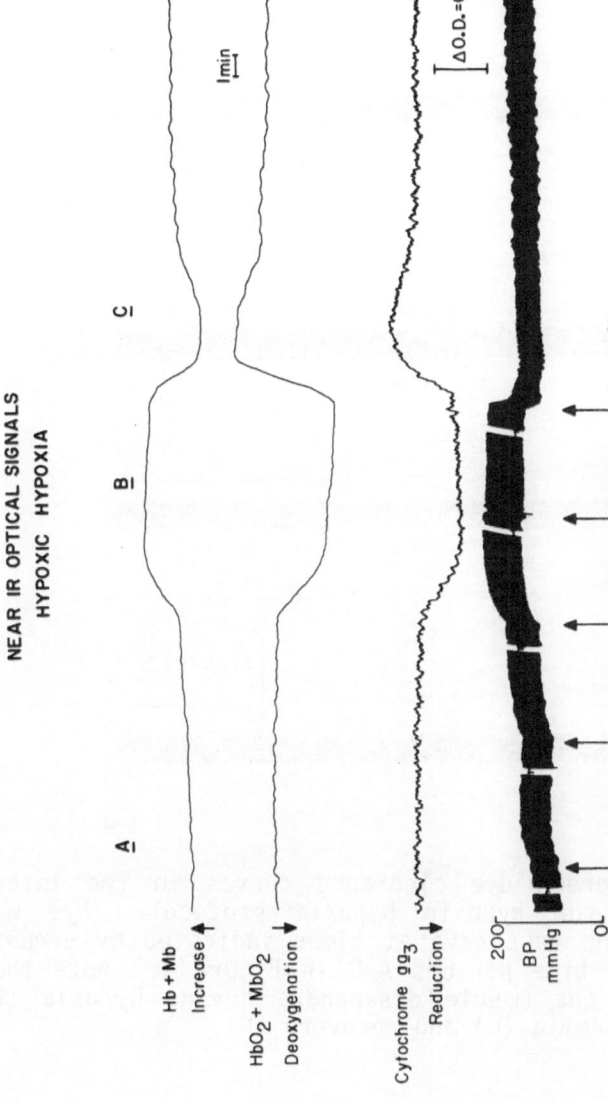

Figure 1. Near infrared optical responses to alveolar hypoxia in the intact hindlimb of the anesthetized cat (A,B). Hypoxia produces an increased reduction level of cytochrome a,a_3, an increased amount of deoxyhemoglobin plus deoxymyoglobin (Hb+Mb) and a decreased amount of oxyhemoglobin plus oxymyoglobin (HbO$_2$+MbO$_2$). Note that the gas change from 9% O$_2$ to 7% O$_2$ was not associated with further optical signal changes. After restoration of normoxia, there was a hyperemic phase (C) followed by return to baseline conditions (D).

857

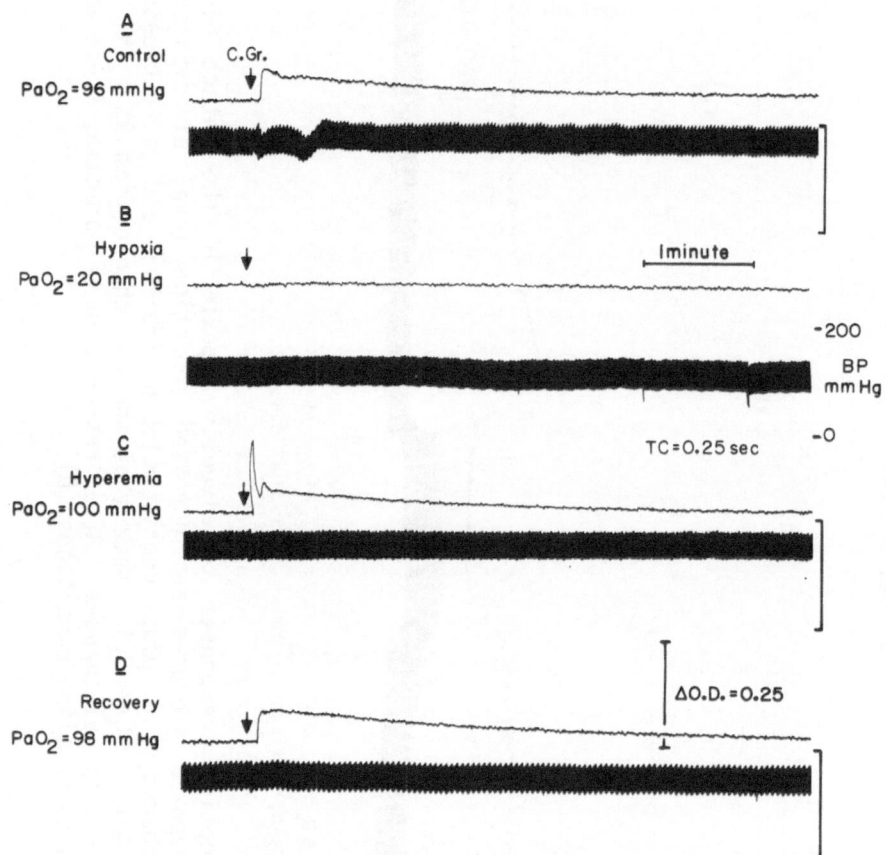

Figure 2. Indocyanine green dye clearance curves in the intact hindlimb muscle during the hypoxic hypoxia protocol. Dye was injected into the inferior vena cava at times indicated by arrows. Panels A-D correspond to time periods A-D in Figure 1. Note that dye circulation through the muscle disappears during hypoxia (B) and reappears during hyperemia (C) and recovery (D).

858

hyperemia (Figure 1 C). This hyperemic period was followed by gradual return of the optical signals to baseline levels (Figure 1 D).

The possibility that the muscle metabolic responses to hypoxia were mediated by decreases in nutritive blood flow was qualitatively confirmed by serial Cardio-green dye injections during A-control, B-hypoxic, C-hyperemic, and D-recovery conditions (Figure 2A-D). During control conditions, muscle dye clearance curves showed a large recirculation effect characteristic of low blood flow rates (Figure 2A). Dye injection during steady state hypoxia (Figure 2B) showed no circulation of the dye through the optical field consistent with an absence of nutritive blood flow. Injections of very high concentrations of Cardio-green (2.5 mg/ml) did show some dye circulation in the muscle, possibly indicating shunt flow. The hyperemic phase (Figure 2 C) was associated with greatly increased blood flow as shown by a marked increase in the height to area ratio of the clearance curve (4). After the hyperemic period, the Cardio-green clearance curve returned to the pre-hypoxia configuration (Figure 2 D).

Muscle NIR optical responses to hemorrhagic hypotension were similar to those responses observed during hypoxic hypoxia (Figure 3). During hemorrhage, muscle cytochrome $\underline{a,a_3}$ became reduced and did not recover during autonomic blood pressure compensation after cessation of bleeding. No further increase in the muscle cytochrome $\underline{a,a_3}$ reduction level could be produced even with ventilation on $\overline{100\%}$ N_2. Reinfusion of shed blood was often associated with a hyperemic response (not shown). Blood flow relationships during hemorrhagic hypotension correlated with the optical metabolic signals in a manner similar to hypoxic hypoxia. Figures 4 A and B show Cardio-green clearance curves obtained under optical conditions analogous to Figures 3 A and B respectively. Figure 4 C was obtained during post reinfusion hyperemia and tracing 4 D was obtained after recovery from the hemorrhagic episode. These latter two curves are interpreted in the same way as the post-hypoxia Cardio-green curves shown in Figures 2 C and 2 D.

CONCLUSIONS

1. The feasibility of using NIR-derived metabolic signals to non-invasively assess O_2 sufficiency in resting skeletal muscle has been demonstrated.
2. Interpretation of the optical data has been qualitatively confirmed using indocyanine green dye clearance curves.

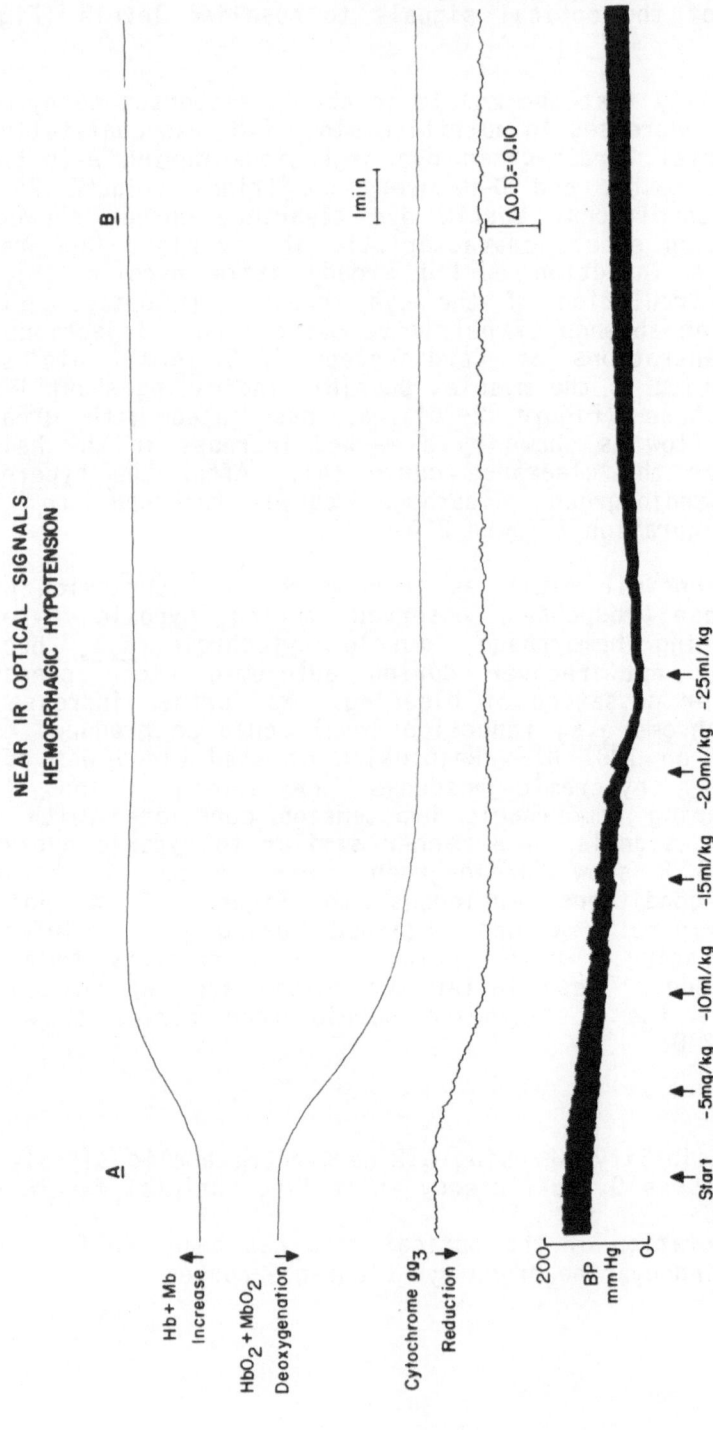

NEAR IR OPTICAL SIGNALS
HEMORRHAGIC HYPOTENSION

Figure 3. Near infrared optical responses to hemorrhagic hypotension in the intact hindlimb musculature of the anesthetized cat (A,B). These responses are qualitatively and quantitatively similar to those observed during hypoxia (Figure 1). No recovery of signals was seen during autonomic blood pressure compensation after bleeding stops (B). After reinfusion of shed blood, a hyperemic response occurred as in hypoxia, followed by return of signals to baseline (neither shown).

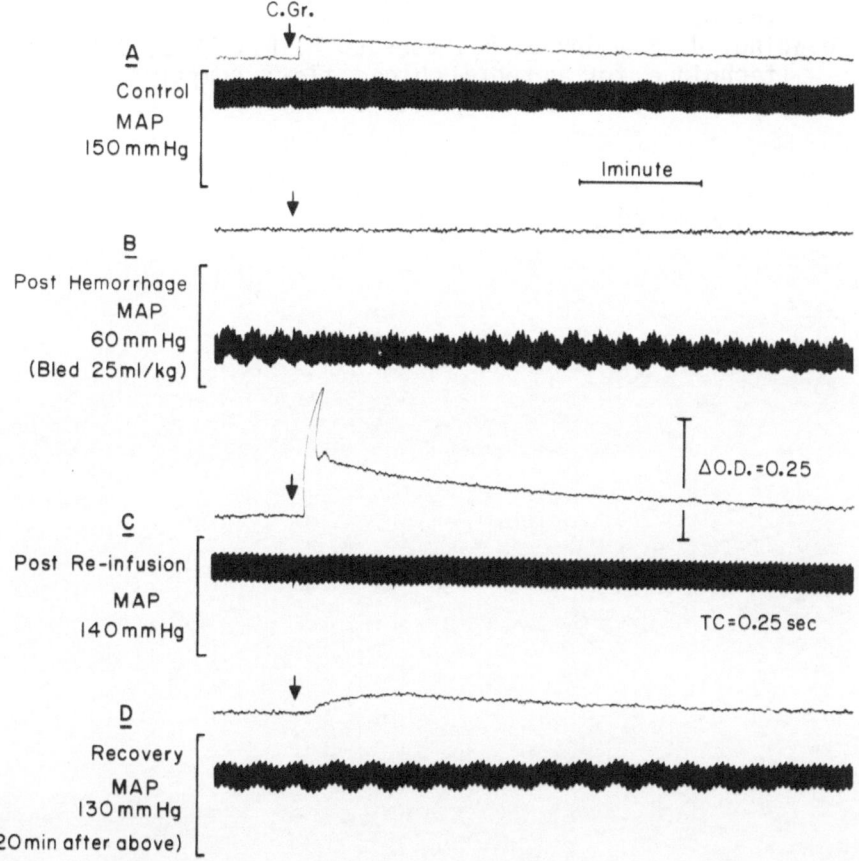

Figure 4. Indocyanine green dye clearance curves in the intact hindlimb muscles of the anesthetized cat during hemorragic hypotension. MAP is mean arterial blood pressure. Dye was injected into the inferior vena cava at times indicated by arrows. Dye curve interpretations are the same as those in Figure 2.

REFERENCES

1. Heistad, D. D., Abboud, F. M., 1980, Circulatory adjustments to hypoxia, Circulation, 61:463-470.
2. Kaihara, S., Rutherford, R. B., Schwentker, E. P. and Wagner, H.N., 1969, Distribution of cardiac output in experimental hemorrhagic shock in dogs, J Appl Physiol, 27:218-222.
3. Jöbsis, F. F., NIROS-SCOPY: Non-invasive, near infrared monitoring of cellular oxygen sufficiency in vivo, this volume.
4. Colacino, J. M., Grubb, B., Jöbsis, F. F., 1981, Infra-red technique for cerebral blood flow: comparison with xenon clearance, Neurol Res, 3:17-31.

NEAR INFRARED SPECTROPHOTOMETRY: POTENTIAL ROLE DURING INCREASED INTRACRANIAL PRESSURE

H. J. Proctor*, C. Cairns*, D. Fillipo*, and
F. F. Jöbsis-Vander Vliet[+]

*Trauma Section, Dept. of Surgery, Univ. of N. Carolina
 Chapel Hill, N.C. 27514
[+]Dept. of Physiology, Duke University
 Durham, N. Carolina 27710

INTRODUCTION

Miller et al.[1] noted that when the initial intracranial pressure was greater than 40 mm Hg in head injured patients with mass lesions, the eventual neurological outcome was poor. They further noted that in patients without mass lesions presenting initially with a normal intracranial pressure, a subsequent rise greater than 20 mm Hg was associated with increased morbidity. These observations illustrate that, at the present time, the widespread practice of monitoring intracranial pressure serves two functions, that of providing a prognostic index for future outcome, and a means of continuously monitoring the progress of a hospitalized patient, allowing rapid intervention at times of increasing intracranial pressure.

The multiplicity of devices for the monitoring of intracranial pressure[2] serves as testimony to the lack of satisfaction with any one method. All currently employed methods are invasive with approximately a 7% incidence of hemorrhage, ventriculitis, meningitis, or infection associated with their use[3]. Furthermore, a measurement of intracranial pressure does not directly measure the blood flow and the metabolic state of the brain.

Described herein are a series of experiments designed to establish the usefulness of near infrared spectrophotometry as a noninvasive monitor of brain oxygenation during increased intracranial pressure.

MATERIALS AND METHODS

Twenty female cats, 2-3 Kg, were anesthetized with pentobarbital sodium, 35 mg/Kg, injected intraperitoneally. A femoral artery and vein were cannulated to allow the injection of drugs, the monitoring of arterial pressure, and the withdrawal of arterial blood for pO_2, pCO_2, and pH determination. A lightly anesthetized state was maintained by intermittent administration of pentobarbital sodium intravenously. A tracheostromy was performed, the animals were paralyzed (Tubocurare, 2 mg/Kg, IV), and the connected to a Harvard ventilator. The cats were ventilated with room air and the ventilator was adjusted to achieve an arterial pCO_2 of 30-35 mm Hg, pH 7.30-7.35, and an arterial pO_2 of at least 100 mm Hg. The cats' heads were then mounted in a stereotactic holder and a sagittal incision was made through the scalp to allow reflection of the extracranial muscles to expose the skull. The fiberoptic bundle used to deliver light in the near infrared range (see below) was positioned against the parieto-occipital skull on one side and the photomultiplier detector positioned (through a burr hole) over the opposite parieto-occipital region. Dental compound was utilized to insure a rigid, water tight seal around the photomultiplier tube even though the tube was extradural.

The principles of niroscopy are explained elsewhere in this volume. Briefly, light at 813 nm, an absorption band of oxidized cytochrome a,a_3, is utilized to detect the quantity of oxidized cytochrome a,a_3 in the illuminated field. Since the spectra of reduced and oxidized hemoglobin overlap that of cytochrome a,a_3, additional reference wavelengths of 770 and 905 nm are used and by appropriate algorithms the artifactual contribution of hemoglobin to the cytochrome signal is subtracted. At the same time, these signals provide information regarding the quantity of reduced and oxidized hemoglobin. Summation of the two hemoglobin signals results in the total hemoglobin which, by inference, represents the total intracranial blood volume in the illuminated field.

Prior to the start of an experiment, the cats were ventilated for ten minutes with a mixture of 95% O_2 - 5% CO_2. The resulting optical signals were arbitrarily defined as 100% oxidation. At the conclusion of each experiment the cats were ventilated with 100% N_2, and the resulting optical signals defined as 100% reduction (0% oxidation). All experimental data are expressed as percent oxidation based upon this full scale oxidation-reduction range.

Experiment I

After positioning of the optics, two cannulas were inserted into the cisterna magna, one to instill "mock" CSF (38°C saline

864

buffered to pH 7.4) and the second to measure intracranial pressure. Correct positioning of the cannulas was judged by the appearance of a drop of CSF at the cannula hub and the recording of CSF pulsations when the cannula was connected to a transducer.

ICP was sequentially increased in 40 mm Hg increments by infusing "mock" CSF until it exceeded systolic blood pressure. The ICP was maintained at each increment until blood pressure, cytochrome a,a3 redox state, HbO_2 Hb, and HbT reached stable values usually after about five minutes. ICP was then sequentially decreased by withdrawing CSF until ICP returned to the original baseline value. Cerebral perfusion pressure (CPP), derived by noting the difference between mean arterial pressure and ICP, was then correlated with Hb, HbO_2, HbT and cytochrome a,a3 using linear regression.

Experiment II

Cardiogreen dye has an absorption peak at 800 nm. Using a modification of the technique of Colacino[4], injection of 0.1 mg/Kg IV through a central venous catheter allows the measurement of blood flow in the illuminated field by integration under the resulting curve using the method of Hamilton[5].

After a 15-30 minute period during which the stability of the optical signals, intracranial pressure and arterial blood gases was confirmed, two cardiogreen dye curves were obtained and averaged to measured baseline blood flow. "Mock" CSF was then infused to increase the intracranial pressure to 20 mm Hg. Since it was possible to accomplish this without a change in the arterial pressure, the result was a reduction in cerebral perfusion pressure. A second period of 15 minutes then ensued to allow stabilization of all parameters as described above. The animals were then hyperventilated to produce respiratory alkalosis with arterial pCO_2's in the 20-25 mm Hg range. The animals were again allowed to stabilize and data were recorded when the maximum reduction in intracranial pressure was achieved. Statistical significance was tested by analysis of variance.

RESULTS

Experiment I

The optically derived data correlated well with the direct measurement of the CPP. A typical record is shown in Figure 1. Note the covariation among the optically derived data and directly measured ICP. Table I lists the mean levels observed in Experiment I for CPP, cytochrome a,a3 redox state, HbO_2, and HbT. With each increment in ICP, significant (N=10, $p < 0.01$) reduction in cytochrome a,a3 redox state and the quantity of HbO_2 were observed.

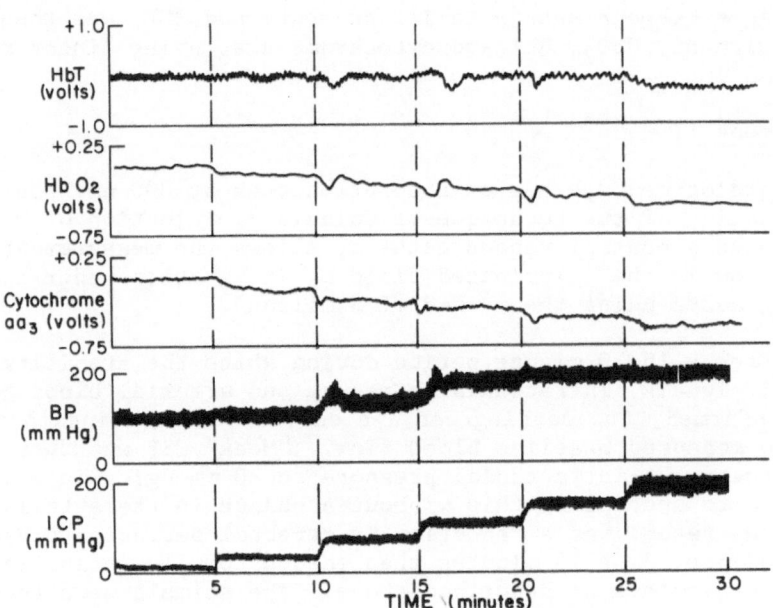

Fig. 1. Stepwise 40 mm Hg increments in intracranial pressure.
Note the progressive de-oxygenation of the hemoglobin in the
cerebral vasculature and the reduction of cytochrome a,a₃.

cerebral vasculature and the reduction of cytochrome a,a$_3$.

866

TABLE I - NIROSCOPE VALUES AS ICP IS INCREASING

CPP (nm Hg)	HbO$_2$ (%)	Hb (%)	Cyt. a,a$_3$ (% O$_2$)	HbT %[*]
90	53.59	13.7	80.73	100.00
70	44.33	22.21	77.66	98.88
15	33.69	35.19	67.11	102.36
0	14.16	21.70	50.45	53.29
p	<.01	<.01	<.01	

*Original Baseline is arbitrarily set as 100% for HbT.

TABLE II - NIROSCOPE VALUES AS ICP IS DECREASING

CPP (nm Hg)	HbO$_2$ (%)	Hb (%)	Cyt. a,a$_3$ (% O$_2$)	HbT %[*]
15	59.14	36.93	61.17	142.72
50	96.92	24.42	92.97	180.32
70	106.87	16.30	97.81	183.04
90	130.41	14.98	100.22	215.94

*Original Baseline is arbitrarily set as 100% for HbT.

The quantity of HbT remained relatively stable until the peak intracranial pressure was obtained, at which point HbT decreased. As intracranial pressure was reduced, the quantities of oxidized cytochrome a,a$_3$ and of the HbO$_2$ became elevated with respect to their original baseline (Table II). The substantially higher HbT indicates the occurrence of hyperemia.

Experiment II

Technical problems precluded collection of complete data from three cats, and they were eliminated from further consideration. A typical record from one of the seven cats from whom data were collected is shown in Figure 2. The alterations in mean arterial pressure, intracranial pressure, cerebral perfusion pressure and arterial blood gases for all seven cats are shown in Table III. By increasing the intracranial pressure gradually over ten minutes and not exceeding 20 mm Hg, the preparation proved stable and increases in arterial pressure response and plateau waves were avoided. Hyperventilation caused a predictable and significant reduction in intracranial pressure but little or no change in cerebral perfusion pressure since there was a decrease in arterial pressure concomitant with hyperventilation. The optically obtained data are summarized in Table IV. The expected reduction in cytochrome a,a$_3$ and HbO$_2$ was noted at the time of increased intracranial pressure (p<0.01). Flow, expressed as percent change from baseline, was also decreased by 7%. Hyperventilation, although decreasing intracranial pressure, was accompanied by a significant (p<0.001) further reduction in cytochrome a,a_3 redox state and quantity of HbO_2, an increase in Hb, and no significant change in HbT. There was no further reduction in blood flow, however, neither was there an improvement.

DISCUSSION

In Experiment I, there was an excellent correlation between changes in intracranial pressure and changes in the optical signals derived by niroscopy. An increase in ICP was associated uniformly with a reduction in brain oxygenation manifested by decreases in HbO_2 and cytochrome a,a_3. Conversely, a decrease in ICP was uniformly associated with an increase in brain oxygenation.

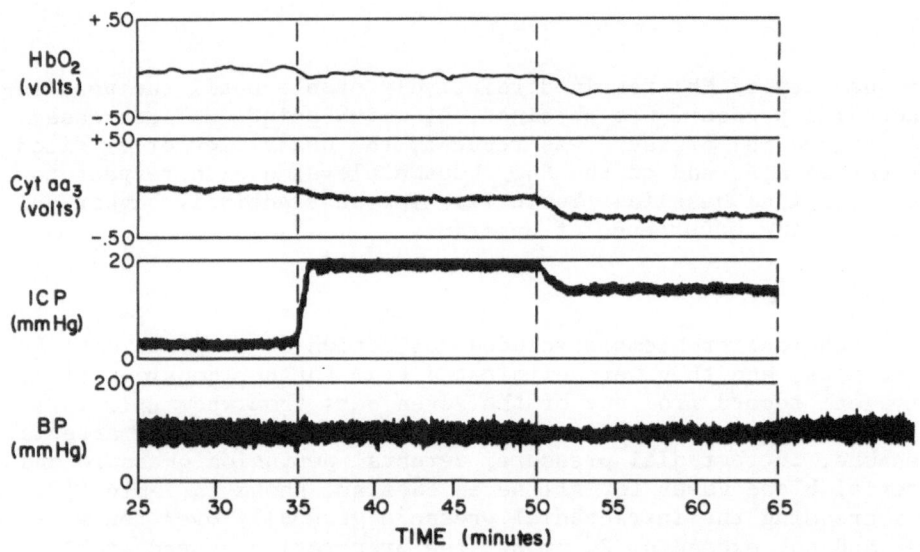

Fig. 2. Representative recording from one cat (redrawn) illustrating the overall findings of Experiment II. Note the reduction of cytochorme a,a_3 concomitant with the rise in intracranial pressure and a further reduction as well as a decrease in HbO_2 with hyperventilation. Not shown on this tracing are the flow signal or Hb signal.

TABLE III

	Baseline	Increased ICP	Hyperventilation
MAP	98.6	97.1	87.1
s.e.m.	(±5.084)	(±5.3)	(±7.47)
ICP	3.1	18.4	15.3
s.e.m.	(±1.0)	(±0.4)	(±0.9)
CPP	94.7	79.0	72.2
s.e.m.	(±5.3)	(±5.2)	(±4.3)
pCO_2	33.2	34.4	24.2
s.e.m.	(±0.8)	(±0.5)	(±0.1)
pH	7.3	7.29	7.66
s.e.m.	(±0.03)	(±0.01)	(±0.03)

Mean (± standard error (s.e.) and number of observation (n) for mean arterial pressure (MAP), intracranial pressure (ICP), cerebral perfusion pressure (CPP), arterial pH and pCO_2.

TABLE IV

	Baseline	Increased ICP	Post Hyperventilation
Total Hemoglobin	100 ± 4.8	99.4 ± 5.1	96.4 ± 6.1
Deoxyhemoglobin	19.4 ± 4.9	23.6 ± 3.7	32.5 ± 2.1
Oxyhemoglobin	44.9 ± 3.6	43.1 ± 2.2	27.0 ± 3.4
Cytochrome a,a_3	76.0 ± 2.9	73.2 ± 0.6	53.4 ± 1.4
Cerebral Flow	100 ± 2.0	93.0 ± 1.7	88.2 ± 2.2

It should be emphasized that our initial study (Exp. I) employed extreme levels (up to 200 mm Hg) of intracranial hypertension in order to demonstrate the relationship between the optically derived data and direct measurement of ICP over a wide range of perfusion pressures. Miller et al[1] have noted that such levels of ICP are associated in humans with severe neurological damage and, if sustained, are inevitably fatal. The second study (Exp. II) limited the increased ICP to levels more relevant to the clinical setting, notetheless, this level of intracranial pressure is also associated, according to Miller[1], with increased morbidity in humans.

The data collected in Experiment II in which intracranial pressure was varied between 0 and 20 mm Hg, values frequently encountered clinically, and then "treated" by hyperventilation, illustrate the shortcomings of intracranial pressure measurement as a reflection of brain metabolism.

Although mortality and morbidity from head injury have been reduced in our Trauma Unit with the advent of routine intracranial pressure monitoring, significant numbers of patients continue to die despite control of intracranial pressure by hyperventilation. The present data further illustrate that hyperventilation might not necessarily be in the best interests of the patient. Although intracranial pressure is decreased, it leads to a false sense of complacency since the decrease in intracranial pressure is accomplished by vasoconstriction with a further reduction in oxygen availability as evidenced by the increased reduction in HbO_2 and cytochrome a,a_3 redox state. This was matched by a reciprocal increase in Hb.

SUMMARY

Two experiments were conducted to assess the feasibility of near infrared spectrophotometry (niroscopy) to directly monitor the effects of increased intracranial pressure on brain metabolism. Intracranial pressure (ICP) was increased in cats by subarachnoid infusion of a "mock" CSF solution. Cytochrome a,a_3 redox state, oxyhemoglobin, deoxyhemoglobin and cerebral blood flow were non-invasively and continuously monitored by niroscopy. The results of both experiments indicated that untreated increases in ICP correlated with a reduction in cytochrome a,a_3 redox state ($p<0.01$), a decrease in the quantity of oxyhemoglobin and cerebral blood flow ($p<0.01$), and an increase in deoxyhemoglobin. This study suggests that niroscopy has the potential for providing non-invasively and continuously data assessing brain metabolic activity. The excellent correlations obtained with simultaneous direct measurements of intracranial pressure make this an attractive method for eventual application to humans at risk for increased intracranial pressure. The value of niroscopy is even more evident in Exp. II where it can be seen that knowledge only of ICP would give the physician a false sense of security, whereas direct, non-invasive, continuous assessment of brain perfusion and oxygenation may well prove to be more appropriate parameters to monitor.

REFERENCES

1. Miller, J. P., Becker, D. P., Ward, J. P., Sullivan, H. G., Adams, W. E., and Rosner, M. J., 1977, Significance of intracranial hypertension in severe head injury, J. Neurosurg., 47:503-516.
2. McGraw, P. C., 1976, Continuous intracranial pressure monitoring: review of techniques and presentation of method, Surg. Neurol., 6:149-155.
3. Narayan, R. K., Kishore, P. R. S., Becker, D. P., Ward, J. P., Enos, G. G., Greenberg, R. P., DaSilva, A. P., Lipper, M. H.,

Chor, S. C., Mayhall, C. G., Lutz, H. A., and Young, H. F., 1982, Intracranial pressure: to monitor or not to monitor, J. Neurosurg., 56:650-659.
4. Colacino, J., Grubb, B., and Jobsis, F. F., 1981, Infrared technique for cerebral blood flow: comparison with 133 xenon clearance, Neurol. Res., 3:17-31.
5. Hamilton, W. F., Riley, R. L., Attyah, A. M. Cournand, A., Fowell, D. M., Himmelitein, A., Noble, R. P., Remington, J. W., Richards, D. W., Wheeler, N. C., and Witham, A. C., 1948, Comparison of the Fick and dye injection methods of measuring cardiac output in man, Am. J. Physiol., 153:309-321.

CONTINUOUS NON INVASIVE MONITORING OF HUMAN BRAIN BY NEAR

INFRARED SPECTROSCOPY

M. Ferrari[+], I. Giannini[*], G. Sideri° and E. Zanette°

[+]Laboratorio di Fisiopatologia di Organo e di Sistema
Istituto Superiore di Sanità, Viale Regina Elena 299
00161 Roma, Italia
*ASSORENI, Monterotondo, Roma
°Dipartimento di Scienze Neurologiche, Università "La
Sapienza" Roma

INTRODUCTION

Precise time-and space-resolved measurement of brain energy metabolism and circulation in vivo would provide important information on the cerebral physiology and pathophysiology. Consequently different optoelectronic techniques based on spectroscopic signals of the normoxic-anoxic transition of pyridine nucleotide (NADH), flavoprotein (Fp) and cytochrome-c-oxidase (cyt a,a_3) have been developed (Tab. 1). Cyt a,a_3 which catalyzes more than 90% of cellular oxygen consumption,[3,4] has a greater visible absorption in the reduced than in oxidized form; it is characterized by a broad band in the near infrared (I.R.) centered at 830 nm and attributable to the copper component of oxidized enzyme.

Jöbsis (1977) first described near I.R. spectroscopy as non invasive diagnostic tool for analysis of in vivo brain metabolism underscoring the potential of this non-destructive/non-invasive approach based on brain tissue transparency to near I.R. light. This effect varies with wavelength and depends on the absorption of the most abundant chromophores, i.e. the heme of hemoglobin (Hb) and the above mentioned cyt a,a_3 absorption band. Consequently, near I.R. spectroscopy may be used for on line continuous monitoring of cerebral a) cyt a,a_3 redox state, b) Hb content, which is strictly correlated with blood volume and, c) oxygen saturation level.

Since 1980 we have been concerned with the assessment of in

873

Table 1. <u>In vivo</u> spectroscopic techniques for monitoring of biochemistry of brain function.

	Absorbing species	Examples of experimental uses	Clinical applications
Near UV fluorescence	NADH	Heart (Franke, 1976) Brain (Mayevsky, 1984) Kidney (Franke, 1980) Cornea (Masters, 1984) Liver (Ji, 1980)	Cortex monitoring during neuro-surgery (Fein,1982)
Visible reflectance	Hemoglobin Cyt a,a$_3$ Myoglobin	Brain (Jöbsis, 1977) Heart (Makino, 1983; Hassinen, 1981) Liver (Kimura, 1984)	
Visible fluorescence	Flavoprotein	Brain (Mayevsky, 1983) Kidney (Franke, 1980) Cornea (Masters, 1981)	
Near IR (700-900 nm) absorption and/or reflectance	Cyt a,a$_3$ Hemoglobin Myoglobin	Brain (Jöbsis, 1977; Giannini, 1982)	Brain monitoring on volunteers (Jöbsis, 1977), newborns and during surgical anesthesia (Fox,1982)

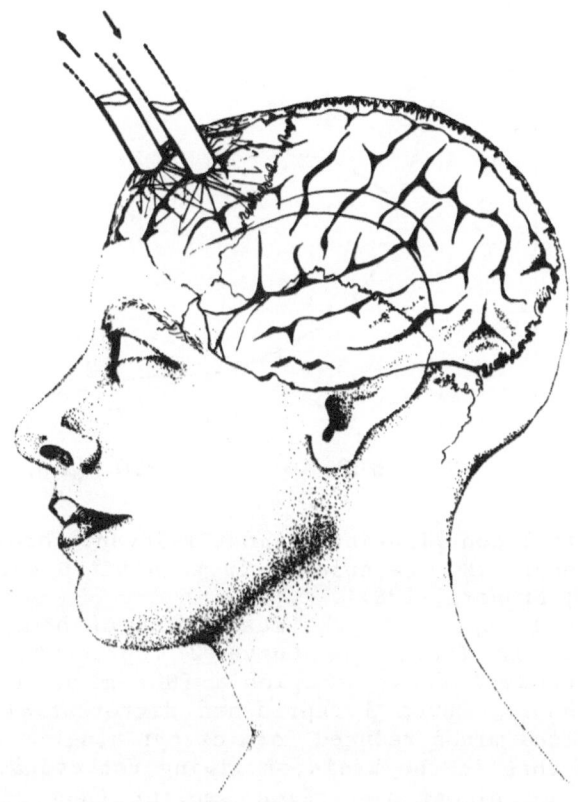

Fig. 1.   Standard arrangement of optic fibers for near I.R. brain
           monitoring.

vivo near I.R. spectroscopy as a diagnostic tool. Brain I.R.
spectra were recorded in normal and perfluorocarbon substituted
rats in order to clarify the biological meaning of the spectral
changes produced by altering the experimental conditions
(Giannini, 1982; Ferrari, 1983, 1984).

     From these data we got the algorithm straightened out to
evaluate the spectral contributions of the different chromophores.
On this basis, a 4 wavelengths instrument suitable for near I.R.
measurements on newborn and adult brain has been realized.

     In this paper, the first results obtained in normal volunteers
and in cerebrovascular patients are reported.

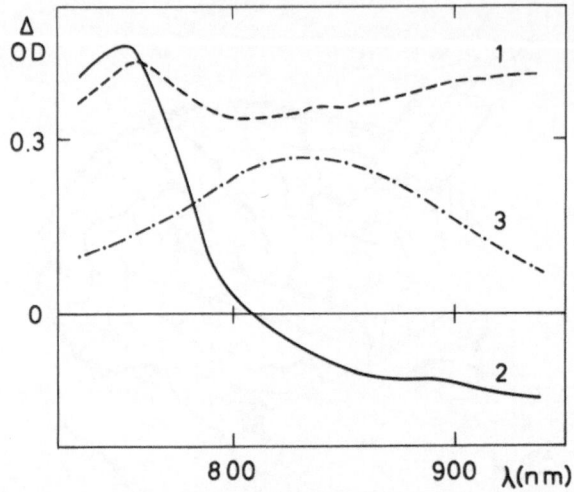

Fig. 2.   Spectral contribution of most relevant chromophores in
the near I.R.   calculated from in vitro data (Takatani,
1980; Brunori, 1981).
Curve 1 represents the mean value of hemoglobin absorption 1/2 (Hb+HbO$_2$); Curve 2 represents differential
spectrum of deoxy-hemoglobin (Hb) minus oxy-hemoglobin
(Hb-HbO$_2$); Curve 3 represents differential spectrum of
oxidized minus reduced form of cyt a,a$_3$.
Note that in the brain of living rat cyt a,a$_3$ contribution is almost two times smaller than represented in
curve 3.

METHODS

The instrument consists of optical, computing and display
sections. A Xenon flash lamp was used as the light source. The
emitted light was filtered with a broad band red filter. The light
was then carried by a glass-fiber optic 2 m in lenght to the
monitored area. Another optic fiber collected the emerging light
which entered an analyzer measuring the light at 4 wavelengths
using interference filters and photomultipliers. Near I.R. signals
and other physiological measurements were processed using a small
acquisition system based on 6502 microprocessor. Optic fibers were

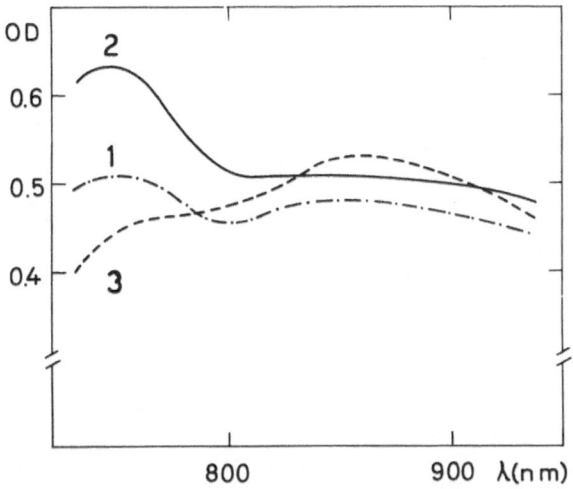

Fig. 3.   Calculated spectra of brain in different physiological
conditions.
Apparent optical densities calculated following Wodick
(1974) and data of Fig. 2. Curves fit experiments on rat
brain (Giannini, 1982). Curve 1 represents normoxia;
Curve 2 represents an hypoxic state, in which both
volume and Hb saturation level are changed; Curve 3
represents hypercapnic–hyperoxic state in which cyt a,a$_3$
is fully oxidized and Hb saturation level is high.

firmly applied to monitored area as in Fig. 1.

Adults volunteered for physiological experiments; the supine
subject breathed different gas mixtures (5% CO_2 in O_2; 10% O_2
90% N_2; 100% O_2; air) through a low dead space anesthesia mask
equipped with retainer. After 10 min of stabilization under air
breathing, near I.R. control recordings were performed for 5 min.
Then the different gas mixtures were inhaled in random order under
continuous I.R. recording.

In some experiments voluntary hyperventilation with room air
was maintained for 2–5 minutes, followed by apnea.

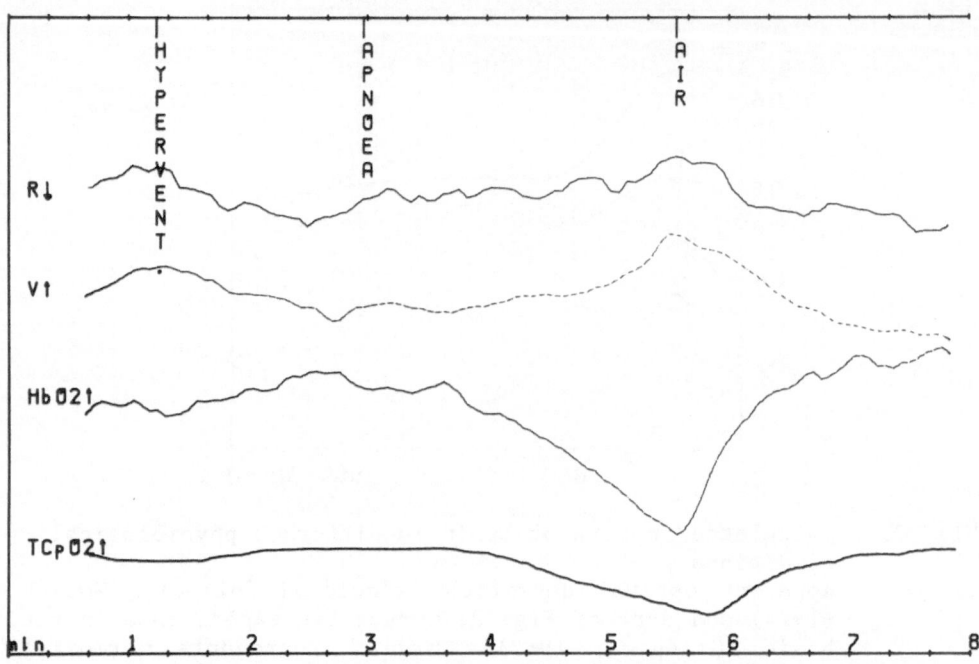

Fig. 4.   Near I.R. absorption signals recorded during a rapid
hyperventilation followed by apnoea. Fibers are firmly
applied to frontal area. Hb oxygen saturation (HbO_2)
follows the related trace of transcutaneous pO_2 measured
on the forearm ($TCpO_2$). After about two minutes of
apnoea an increase of blood volume content (V) and a
decrease of redox level (R) of cyt a, a_3 were recorded.

Transcutaneous pO_2 and pCO_2 ($TCpO_2$ and $TCpCO_2$) were
measured with the system TCM 220 (Radiometer, Copenhagen). The
electrodes were attached to the skin of the forearm by self-
adhesive rings; measurements were made at 44°C. $TCpO_2$ and $TCCO_2$
electrodes are now widely used as an indicator of arterial pO_2 and
pCO_2 in newborn infant; in adults they are more dependent on
cutaneous oxygen consumption and blood flow (Wimberley, 1983).
However, these semiquantitative data were extremely useful in the
evaluation of near I.R. signals over a wide range of pCO_2 and pO_2
values.

In cerebrovascular patients the polygraphic EEG and EKG
recordings were done using a 12 channel Elther machine. Blood
pressure was taken before, during and after carotid compression
which was carried out according to the classical procedure.
Cortical ischemia was demonstrated by appearance on the tracing of
localized or diffuse slow EEG activity with or without clinical
signs.

878

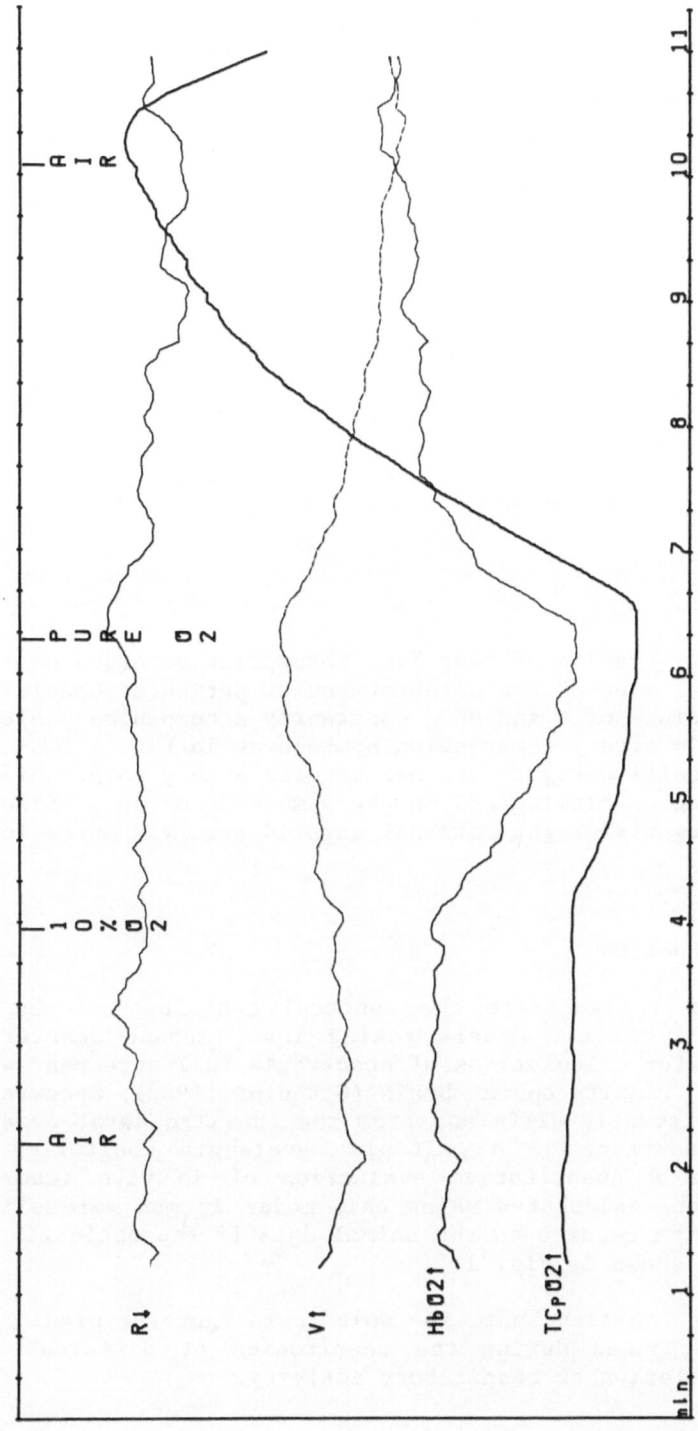

Fig. 5. Effects of different gas mixtures on the parameters reported in Fig. 4. Fibers are applied to frontal area. HbO_2 recording. During hypoxia blood volume increased while redox state of cyt a,a_3 is nearly unchanged.

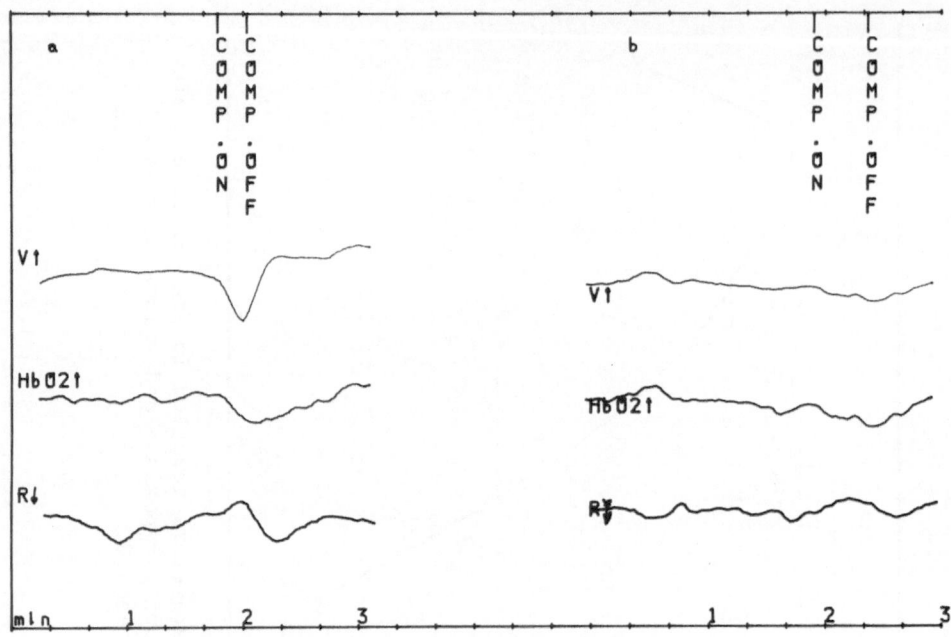

Fig. 6. Typical tracing of near I.R. absorption recorded on
frontal area of two cerebrovascular patients. Consistent
variations of V and HbO_2 constantly accompanied positive
carotid artery compression.Symbols as in Fig. 4.
(a) positive right internal carotid artery compression
leading to slowing EEG on the same side of optic fibers;
(b) negative right internal carotid artery compression.

RESULTS AND DISCUSSION

Fig. 2 and 3 illustrate the spectral contributions due to
hemoglobin and cyt a,a_3. Models taking into account scattering
effects allowed for calculations of spectra in full agreement with
the experimental results on rat brain (Giannini, 1982). Spectra of
Fig. 3 are consistently different from the in vitro data, eviden-
tiating the importance of a multiple wavelength monitoring in
order to obtain a quantitative evaluation of in vivo recorded
parameters.Spectra calculated using this model in man were slightly different with respect to the animal data if the optic fibers
are disposed as shown in Fig. 1.

Experiments carried out in volunteers gave typical and
reproducible responses during the respiration of different gas
mixtures and variation of respiratory activity.

880

As shown by Fig. 4 hyperventilation produced a slight increase in $TCpO_2$. This was followed, in the subsequent apneic period, by a marked fall in $TCpCO_2$ which reached a minimum at the end of the apnoea. There was a close correlation between $TCpO_2$ and the near I.R. signal for HbO_2. After two minutes of apnoea an increase in blood volume content and a decrease of cyt a,a_3 redox level were recorded.

Fig. 5 shows the time course of near I.R. signals during respiration of different gas mixtures. Hypoxic mixtures didn't substantially affect the redox level of cyt a,a_3. Even in this case strictly parallel changes in HbO_2 signal and $TCpO_2$ were recorded.

It is thus evident that, in normal volunteers, the effects of changes in respiration on brain I.R. analysis can be accounted for by the physiological and spectral properties of Hb and cyt a,a_3 as well as by the responses of cerebral circulation to hypoxemia. On this basis, the reliability of brain near I.R. spectroscopy as a diagnostic tool was investigated in cerebrovascular patients subjected to routine test of compression of the internal and/or external carotid arteries.

Fig. 6 gives the tracings recorded in two cases in which EEG slowing was present (a) or absent (b), following carotid compression. In the first case, a sharp reduction in Hb content and Hb oxygenation occurred within few seconds after the beginning of the compression whereas variations in cyt a,a_3 redox state took place after some delay. In general the initial changes preceded by 10-20 seconds the slowing of EEG. In the second case (b) these changes were absent.

According to the data thus far obtained, the Hb-dependent spectral changes here described have a well established physiological and physiopathological meaning. The redox fluctuations, frequently observed during changes in respiratory conditions as well as following carotid compression, are compatible with the fact that the redox level of Cu atom in cyt a,a_3 behaves as expected for a regulatory parameter and in this sense cannot be used as a singular probe of oxygen sufficiency (Dora, 1984). In our opinion, a better understanding of changes connected with oxygen availability in brain is necessary before a widespread use of near I.R. spectroscopy for monitoring of cerebral metabolism.

AKNOWLEGMENTS
This work was supported in part by C.N.R. P.F. Tecnologie Biomediche Grant N. 83.00526.57.
The authors are grateful to Piero Antonucci for software assistance and for his genuine interest in our work and wish to thank all members of our research group for helpful discussions.

REFERENCES

1. Brunori, M., Antonini, E. and Wilson, M.T. In "Metal ions in biological systems" Ed. H. Siegel 13, p. 187, 1981.
2. Dora, E. J. Neurochem. 42, 101, 1984.
3. Fein, J.M. and Olinger, R. Neurosurgery 10, 428, 1982.
4. Ferrari, M., Giannini, I., Carpi, A. and Fasella, P. Physiol. Chem. Phys. and medical NMR 15, 107, 1983.
5. Ferrari, M., Giannini, I., Carpi, A., Fasella, P., Fieschi, C. and Zanette, E. In "Angiology" p. 299, Ed. P. Balas, Plenum Publishing Co, London, 1984.
6. Fox, E.J., Harmel, M.H., Mitnick, M.H. and Jöbsis, F.F. Anesthesiology, 57, A160, 1982.
7. Franke, H., Barlow, C.H. and Chance, B. Am. J. Physiol. 231, 1082, 1976.
8. Franke, H., Barlow, C.H. and Chance, B. Int. J. Biochem. 12, 269, 1980.
9. Giannini, I., Ferrari, M., Carpi, A. and Fasella, P. Physiol. Chem. Phys. 14, 295, 1982.
10. Hassinen, I.E., Hiltunen, J.K. and Takala, T.E.S. Cardiovas. Res. 15, 86, 1981.
11. Ji, S., Lemaster, J.J. and Thurman, R.G. FEBS Letters 113, 37, 1980.
12. Jöbsis, F.F., Keizer, J.H., La Manna, J.C. and Rosenthal, M. J. App. Physiol. 43, 858, 1977.
13. Jöbsis, F.F. Science 198, 1264, 1977.
14. Kimura, S., Suzaki, T., Kobayaski, S., Abe, K. and Ogata, E. Biochem. Biophys. Res. Com. 119, 212, 1984.
15. Masters, B.R., Chance, B. and Fischbarg, J. TIBS 6, 282, 1981.
16. Masters, B.R. Curr. Eye Res. 3, 23, 1984.
17. Mayevsky, A., Zarchin, N., Kaplan, H., Haveri, J., Haselgroove, J. and Change, B. Brain Res. 267, 95, 1983.
18. Mayevsky, A. Brain Res. Rew. 7, 49, 1984.
19. Makino, N., Kanaide, H., Yoshimura, R. and Nakamura, M. Am. J. Physiol. 245, H237, 1983.
20. Takatani, S., Cheung, P.W. and Ernst, E.A. Annals Biomed. Eng. 8, 1, 1980.
21. Wimberley, P.D., Pedersen, K.G., Thode, J., Fogh-Andersen, N., Sørensen, A.M. and Siggaard-Andersen, N. Clin. Chem. 29, 1471, 1983.
22. Wodick, R.,and Lübbers, D.W. Hoppe-Seyler's Z. Physiol. Chem. 355, 583, 1974.

SIMULATION OF THE OPTICAL PROPERTIES OF AN ABSORBING AND SCATTERING MEDIUM USING THE MONTE-CARLO TECHNIQUE COMPARED WITH TWO- AND SIX-FLUX THEORIES

J. Hoffmann[1], F. Hannebauer[2], and D.W. Lübbers[1]

[1]Max-Planck-Institut für Systemphysiologie
Rheinlanddamm 201, 4600 Dortmund 1, FRG
[2]AEG, 6000 Frankfurt, FRG

INTRODUCTION

To describe an optical system in which light absorption and light scattering occurs, the two-flux theory of Kubelka and Munk (1931) is most widely used. In this theory absorption is described by a homogeneous absorption coefficient ($a(\lambda)$), dependent on the wavelength, and light scattering by a single scattering coefficient ($s(\lambda)$), which only takes into account backscattering (Kubelka, 1948, 1954). To study the effects of these simplifications we developed a Monte-Carlo model in which two scattering coefficients are introduced - backscattering ($s_B(\lambda)$) and transverse scattering ($s_T(\lambda)$) - and compared the numerical results with the predictions of the Kubelka-Munk theory.

THEORY

1) The Monte-Carlo Model

The free path length of a photon travelling inside the optical system is assumed to be

$$z = \frac{1}{e_{total}} \ln(r) \qquad (1)$$

with $e_{total} = a + s_B + 4s_T$ and r an uniformly distributed random number between 0+ and 1. Here the scattering coefficient is divided into backscattering s_B and transverse scattering s_T. Note that the scattering coefficients are defined with respect to the actual travelling direction of the photon.

After this path length the photon is absorbed or scattered with the probability a/e_{total}, s_B/e_{total}, and s_T/e_{total}, respectively. Suppose the optical system is a three-dimensional region with given boundaries. All photons travelling into the system start at the same entrance point, the outgoing (non-absorbed) photons can be classified by the direction of their leaving the optical system. As a result the Monte-Carlo experiment gives a light path distribution of the non-absorbed photons, and a local distribution of the absorbed photons, dependent on the modelling parameters.

Since absorption and scattering coefficients are independent from each other, the optical properties of the system can be deduced from the light path distribution:

$$(I/I_o)_i = \int w_i(s_B, s_T, z) \exp(-az) \, dz \qquad (2)$$

The subscript (i) characterizes the direction in which the photons leave the optical system ("reflection" or "transmission"), $w_i(s_B, s_T, z)$ is the density of the corresponding light path probability, dependent on the set of scattering coefficients in absence of absorption, I the light intensity.

2) Kubelka-Munk Theory

Transmittance and reflectance (i.e. the ratios of the transmitted or reflected light intensities to the incident light intensity) of an absorbing and scattering layer of thickness (d) is, according to the two-flux theory of Kubelka and Munk

$$T = \frac{\sinh(y)}{\sinh(kd + y)} \quad ; \quad R = \frac{\sinh(kd)}{\sinh(kd + y)} \qquad (3)$$

with
$$k^2 = a(a + 2s_B) \quad ; \quad y = \ln((a + s_B + k)/s_B) \qquad (4)$$

In case of a semi-infinite plane homogeneous medium reflection is

$$R_\infty = \exp(-y) = (a + s_B - k)/s_B \qquad (5)$$

Eq. (5) yields the light path distribution

$$R_\infty = \int w_{R_\infty}(s_B, z) \exp(-az) \, dz$$

with

$$w_{R_\infty}(s_B, z) = (1/z) \, I_1 (\, s_B z) \, \exp(\, -s_B z) \qquad (6)$$

(I_1: modified Bessel function). w_{R_∞} is a nonnegative decreasing function, $w_{R_\infty}(s_B, 0) = s_B/2$.

CALCULATION OF THE LIGHT PATH DISTRIBUTION

To test the Monte-Carlo model we calculate the light path distribution for different values of s_B, setting $s_T = 0$. For finite and infinite thicknesses of the optical medium we found the same numerical results as compared to the Kubelka-Munk theory. In the case of infinite thickness the photon is assumed to be lost if it is scattered more than 50 times . The Monte-Carlo calculations were performed sampling over 20,000 events.

For nonzero s_T we conclude that the Monte-Carlo calculation will yield the results of a "six-flux theory". We compute the "transformation" transmittance versus absorption and reflectance versus absorption (eq. (2)). Comparing these transformation curves with the predictions of the Kubelka-Munk theory we observe that the transformation curves are shifted with considerable accuracy. Setting $s_T = s_B$ the Monte-Carlo calculation yields the Kubelka-Munk results as well.

APPLICATION TO TISSUE REFLECTION PHOTOMETRY

Reflection spectra obtained from the surface of tissues can be regarded as reflection spectra of a semi-inifinite plane medium. The following plots show the transformation reflectance versus absorption and -log (reflectance) versus absorption for different ratios s_T/s_B. Note that $s_T = s_B$ yields the same transformation as $s_T = 0$. If s_T is less than s_B, the transformation reflectance versus absorption is shifted to lower values.

To quantify reflectance spectra obtained from an absorbing and scattering medium it is necessary to know the transformation between reflectance and absorption coefficient of the medium. We proposed the evaluation formula (Hoffmann et al., 1984)

$$a + s = s \cdot \cosh(\, y(\lambda) + y_0) \qquad (7)$$

where $y(\lambda)$ denotes the measured $-\ln$(reflectance). The evaluation method is constructed to be invariant to a linear scaling of the absorption and scattering coefficient. The offset y_0 to the measured spectra should identify that no absolute values of the spectra can be obtained and therefore, the correction term is

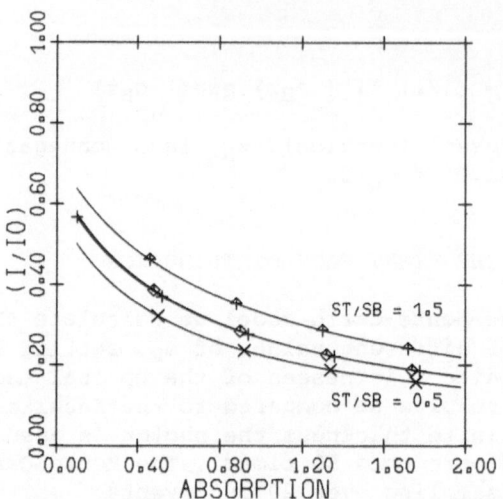

Fig. 1   Dependence of the reflectance (I/I_0) of a layer of in-
         finite thickness on the absorption coefficient for various
         values of the scattering coefficient, calculated according to
         the Monte-Carlo model. The middle trace ($s_T = s_B$) yields
         the Kubelka-Munk theory ($s_T = 0$).

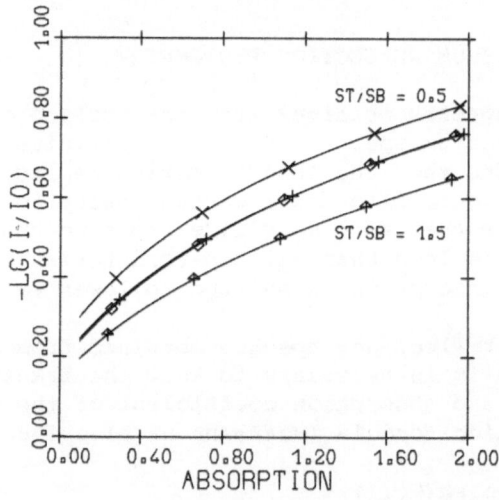

Fig. 2   Dependence of -lg(reflectance) of a layer of infinite
         thickness. The traces calculated by the Monte-Carlo method
         can be sufficiently well approximated in terms of
         $C_1 \cosh(y+y_0) + C_2$.

necessary. We can show, that the transformation between $y = -\ln$ (reflectance) and absorption coefficient obtained from the Monte-Carlo calculations can be sufficiently well approximated in terms of $c_1 \cdot \cosh(\, y + y_o) + C_2$ (c_1, c_2, y_o constants). Within the range of the absorption coefficient and the scattering coefficient found in the physiological measurements the evaluation method based on eq. (7) is valid even in the case of anisotropic scattering.

DISCUSSION

The aim of this paper is twofold: 1) We have evolved a Monte-Carlo model to describe the optical properties of an absorbing and scattering medium. This model gives (if we treat the one-dimensional case) the same numerical results as the one dimensional Kubelka-Munk theory. The simple formulation of the Monte-Carlo model easily allows three-dimensional treatment. We conclude that this Monte-Carlo model will yield the numerical results of a "six-flux theory". We are now able to study the effects of anisotropic light scattering. By knowing the transformation between reflectance and absorption we are able to quantify reflection spectra according to a given set of basic absorptions. The Kubelka-Munk theory predicts a special form of this transformation curve. If we modify this special form to be invariant to a) a linear scaling of the basic absorption spectra, and b) to be invariant of a shift of the measured $-\log$(reflectance), then the Kubelka-Munk theory is a sufficiently good approximation to describe tissue reflection spectra even in the case of anisotripic scattering. Kortüm (1969) stated, that under certain assumptions the resulting scattering coefficient of a many body scattering system is expected to be isotropic (i.e. $s_B = s_T$), and under certain conditions the Kubelka-Munk theory yields the exact optical properties.

2) To describe the effects of light scattering in an optical system there are several approaches: a) by definition of a scattering coefficient and b) by the introduction of the concept of a statistical light path distribution. We showed that both scattering coefficient and light path distribution can be transformed into each other. Which approach should be used depends on the problem. The light path distribution theory has the great advantage that it enables us to study the effect of inhomogeneous absorption. Further simulations have to be performed to study the problems of inhomogeneous absorption and/or inhomogenous scattering coefficients with respect to tissue reflection photometry.

REFERENCES

Dahlquist, G., and Bjorck, A., 1974, "Numerical Methods, Prentice

Hall, Englewood Cliffs, New York.

Hoffmann, J., Wodick, R., Hannebauer, F., and Lübbers D. W., Quantitative analysis of reflection spectra of the surface of the guinea pig brain, in: "Oxygen Transport to Tissue V," D. W. Lübbers, H. Acker, T. K. Goldstick, E. Leniger-Follert, eds., Plenum Press, New York (1983), pp. 831-839.

Hoffmann, J., Heinrich, U., Ahmad, H. R., and Lübbers, D. W., Analysis of tissue reflection spectra obtained from brain or heart, using the two-flux theory for non-constant light scattering, in: "Oxygen Transport to Tissue VI," D. F. Bruley et al., eds., Plenum Press, New York (1984), in print.

Kortüm, G., 1969, "Reflexionsspektroskopie," Springer, Berlin-Heidelberg-New York.

Kubelka, P., and Munk, F., 1931, Ein Beitrag zur Optik der Farbanstriche, Z. Techn. Phys., 11a:593-603.

Kubelka, F., 1948, New contributions to the optics of intensely light-scattering materials, part I, J. Opt. Soc. Am., 38:448-457.

Kubelka, F., 1954, New contributions to the optics of intensely light-scattering materials, part II, J. Opt. Soc. Am., 44:330-335.

QUANTITATIVE ANALYSIS OF REFLECTION SPECTRA: EVALUATION

OF SIMULATED REFLECTION SPECTRA

J. Hoffmann and D. W. Lübbers

Max-Planck-Institut für Systemhysiologie
Rheinlanddamm 201, 4600 Dortmund 1, FRG

INTRODUCTION

Reflection photometry is a useful tool to study in vivo kinetic changes of hemoglobin, myoglobin, and the cytochromes. The problem of quantifying reflection spectra is still not satisfactorily solved. To compare the validity and the limits of different methods to analyze optical spectra (dual wavelength evaluation, reference spectra method, two-flux evaluation method of multicomponent systems), calculations were performed on simulated reflection spectra. The simulation of the reflection spectra was carried out, using the two-flux theory of Kubelka and Munk (1931), (Kubelka 1948, 1954).

THEORY

To describe the optical properties of an absorbing and scattering medium, the two-flux theory of Kubelka and Munk is a simple approach. According to this theory, the reflectance of a semi-infinite plane homogeneous medium is, dependent on its absorption coefficient ($a(\lambda)$) and on its scattering coefficient ($s(\lambda)$:

$$R_{\infty} = (a+s-k)/s \qquad (1)$$

or

$$-\ln R_{\infty} = y = \ln((a+s+k)/s) \qquad (2)$$

with $k^2 = a(a+2s)$.

Considering randomly distributed non-interacting absorption centres, total absorption ($a(\lambda)$) is a linear combination of n single absorptions ($a_i(\lambda)$) with respect to the concentration of the single absorption centre, i.e.

$$a(\lambda) \;=\; \sum_{i}^{n} \; c_i a_i(\lambda) \qquad\qquad (3)$$

For a given set of basic absorption spectra ($a_i(\lambda)$) and a given scattering coefficient ($s(\lambda)$) the reflection spectra $y = -\ln R_\infty$ easily can be calculated.

Simulation of Tissue Reflection Spectra Obtained From The Blood-Free Perfused Guinea-Pig Heart

The pigments which cause absorption within the wavelength range of 450 nm to 650 nm are myoglobin and the cytochromes a (=aa$_3$), (b), and c. The symbol (b) denotes that the cytochrome (b) consists of different substances but we do not distinguish between them. To match experimental reflection values the following "standard" concentrations according to their absorption differences are chosen (Table 1).

The oxidation state g_i of the i-th component is the ratio of the concentration of the oxidized component to the total concentration. To simulate a kinetic experiment we assume an exponential time course of the oxidation states while the total concentrations of each component remain constant. We simulate two different kinetics: 1) "ischemia" (time constants myo:cyt.a:cyt. (b):cyt.c = 1:2:3:2) and 2) "cyanide" (time constants = 0:2:3:2, myo oxygenated).

Table 1. Absorption differences of all components used in the simulation

Component:	absorption difference:	measuring wavelength	reference
cyt.a,ox	0.074	599 nm	649.5 nm
cyt.(b),ox	0.109	538.5 nm	
cyt.c,ox	0.126	531 nm	
myogl.,ox	0.465	544.5 nm	
	0.503	582.5 nm	
cyt.a,red	0.248	604 nm	
cyt.(b),red	0.109	532.5 nm	
	0.160	562.5 nm	
cyt.c,red	0.185	521 nm	
	0.360	551 nm	
myogl.,desox	0.399	558 nm	

EVALUATION METHODS

1) Dual Wavelength Evaluation (DWE)

It is to be assumed that a chromophoric substance causes a specific change in the optical signal at a certain wavelength while an unspecific change in the optical signal due to the change of the scattering coefficient can be cancelled out using the other wavelength. The dual wavelength evaluation therefore depends on the validity of the following presumptions:

a) The existence of a wavelength pair so that the measured reflection signals are only due to the investigated chromophoric substance.

b) The existance of a defined calibration curve to correlate the change of the optical signal to the chemical composition of the observed substance.

2) Reference Spectra Method (RSM)

If it is possible to produce spectra of (1) fully oxygenated myoglobin and oxidized cytochromes, (2) deoxygenated myoglobin and reduced cytochromes, and (3) oxygenated myoglobin and reduced cytochromes, these spectra can be used as basic spectra of a (linear) component analysis to calculate the intermediate O_2 saturation of myoglobin and the (mean) redox state of the cytochromes. Due to the basic spectra it is not possible to distinguish the redox states of each cytochrome, but if a proper wavelength range is chosen the mean redox state of the cytochromes can be dominated by a single cytochrome (see for more details: Figulla et al., 1983).

3) Two-Flux Evaluation Method of Multicomponent Systems (TEMMS)

This multi-component analysis uses the absorption spectra of the pure substances as basic spectra. According to the Kubelka-Munk theory there is

$$a(\lambda) + s(\lambda) \;=\; s(\lambda) \cosh (y(\lambda) + y_0) \qquad (4)$$

(for more details see: Hoffmann et al., (1985). The method can be improved if eq. (4) is solved for abdorption and scattering coefficient iteratively (Table 2).

Table 2. Improved two-flux evaluation method of multicomponent
systems by iteration (ITEMMS)

step 0: initial assumption $s(\lambda)$, y_0

step 1: calculate the absorption spectra, eq. (4),
analyze the absorption spectra according
to the set of basic spectra, calculate the
total absorption $\bar{a}(\lambda)$, eq. (2), define
the error $\sum(a(\lambda) - \bar{a}(\lambda))^2$.

step 2: calculate the scattering coefficient, eq. (4),
using $\bar{a}(\lambda)$. It will be convenient if $\bar{s}(\lambda)$ is
restricted to be a monotonic decreasing func-
tion. Calculate y_0 using $\min(\bar{a})$ and $\min(\bar{s})$,
eq. (3), set $s=\bar{s}$ and go to step 1.

RESULTS

1) Dual Wavelength Evaluation (DWE)

a) Isobestic wavelengths. Isobestic wavelengths are defined
for the oxidized-reduced state of a single component. It is assumed
that all components have always a common unchanged isobestic
wavelength at 650 nm (reference wavelength). Due to the different
kinetics of the components used in the simulation stable isobestic
wavelengths of the total system can generally not be found.

For example by superposition of the normoxic and anoxic spectra a set of isobestic points is obtained (Table 3). However, during the transition from normoxia to anoxia ("ischemia") a shift of
the isobestic wavelengths occurs; the same holds for cyanide poisoning.

Table. 3 Isobestic points and their shifts.

isobestic wavelength (total system, ox-re)	maximum shift due to the different kinetics	
	"ischemia"	"cyanide"
509.5 nm	+ 1.0 nm	+ 0.5 nm
526.0 nm	+ 0.5 nm	+ 1.0 nm
547.0 nm	− 1.0 nm	− 3.0 nm
572.5 nm	− 0.5 nm	− 2.0 nm
590.5 nm	− 0.5 nm	− 4.0 nm
650.0 nm reference wavelength		

b) Characteristic wavelengths. Characteristic wavelengths are defined for the oxidized-reduced state of the total system in absence of the investigated component.

By excluding the spectra of the investigated component wavelengths can be found the absorption of which does not change in the oxidized-reduced state: Characteristic wavelengths. In the complete system these characteristic wavelengths are suitable to measure changes of the investigated component. However, it has to be confirmed that the characteristic wavelengths are not influenced by changes of the system without the component to be investigated. The expected change of the intensity of the reflection during normoxic-anoxic transition is calculated with constant and wavelength dependant scattering coefficient (+).

component	characteristic wavelength	maximum change of -log(Reflection)	
cyt.a	592.5 nm	0.03	0.02 +
cyt.(b)	507.5 nm	0.01 (!)	0.01
cyt.c	515.5 nm	0.02	0.02
	522.5 nm	0.02	0.02
	552.5 nm	0.07	0.06
myoglobin	584.0 nm	0.08	0.07

+ scattering coefficient wavelength-dependent. The change
  of the scattering coefficient may cause a change of the
  optical signal (-log R_∞) in the magnitude of 0.01.
  (constant part of the scattering coefficient: s = 0.5, Δs = 0.1)

The following figures give an example of the quantitative analysis using DWE for optimal conditions: constant absolute concentrations of each component (but different time courses of the oxidation states), and constant scattering coefficient. Note that DWE gives sufficiently good results for myo. and cyt.c but fails otherwise. If the scattering coefficient changes during the experiment and/or the concentration of the components changes DWE gives erroneous results.

2) Reference Spectra Method (RSM)

RSM is a multi-wavelength evaluation. Due to the basic spectra RSM gives the O_2 saturation of myoglobin and the mean redox state of the cytochromes within acceptable accuracy. Furthermore, RSM can detect changes of the scattering coefficient and changes of the total concentration if 1) the basic spectra can be obtained with the same concentration and 2) the relative concentration ratio of all observed substances remains constant. In addition, RSM

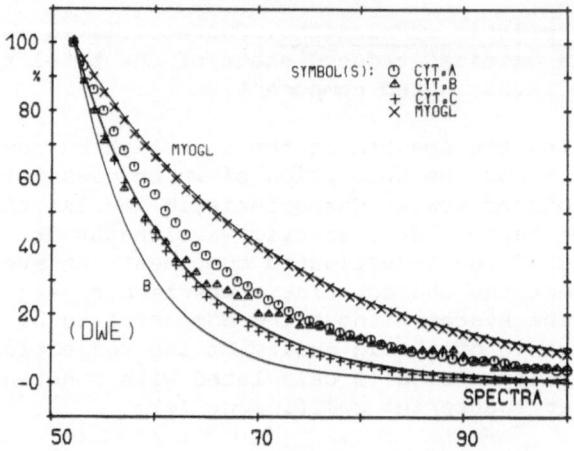

Fig. 1. DWE evaluation of simulated reflection spectra, ischemia.
Symbols: DWE, straight line: exact results. Characteristic wavelength: myo. 584 nm, cyt.a 592.5 nm, cyt.b
507.5 nm, cyt.c 552.5 nm

gives an error criterion to test the validity of initial assumptions. To obtain the absolute values of the oxidation states the
basic spectra are required to be in defined states.

   The following plot gives an example of the RSM analysis. Note
that the increasing error may indicate the splitted cytochrome
kinetic. If scattering coefficient is changed RSM will give
similar results.

3) Two-Flux Evaluation Method of Multicomponent Systems (TEMMS)

   The application of TEMMS on the simulated spectra tests the
validity of the practical calculation program. Starting the
iteration (Table 2) with wrong scattering coefficients and with a
wrong assumption y_0, ITEMMS yields the exact results within
considerable accuracy, too.

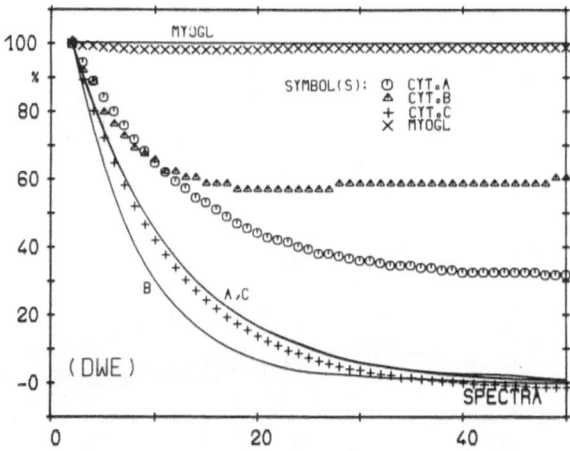

Fig. 2.   DWE evaluation of simulated reflection spectra, cyanide
experiment. Symbols: DWE, straight line: exact results

DISCUSSION

    Simulation of reflection spectra using the two-flux theory
gives spectra which are comparable to the experimentally measured
spectra of guinea pig heart. It was possible to simulate the
ischemia of the guinea pig heart by assuming an exponential
decrease of the oxidation states and by selecting proper time
constants.

    On simulated reflection spectra we have tested different
evaluation methods to quantify concentration ratios of the different spectral components. There are two difficulties which occur
during the evaluation: 1) the non-linear transformation between
absorption and reflection due to the scattering coefficient and 2)
the overlapping absorption peaks which makes the identification of
some components very difficult. If the over-all reflection peak
does not exceed a considerable magnitude, simulation experiments
show that linearizing the transformation 1) in the right way will
lead only to small errors. This is demonstrated with RSM and -
with assumptions here noticed - with DWE in case of myo. and
cyt.c, too.

    Although we have estimated the best pairs of wavelengths we
could not distinguish the redox-states of cyt.a (=aa$_3$) and cyt.b

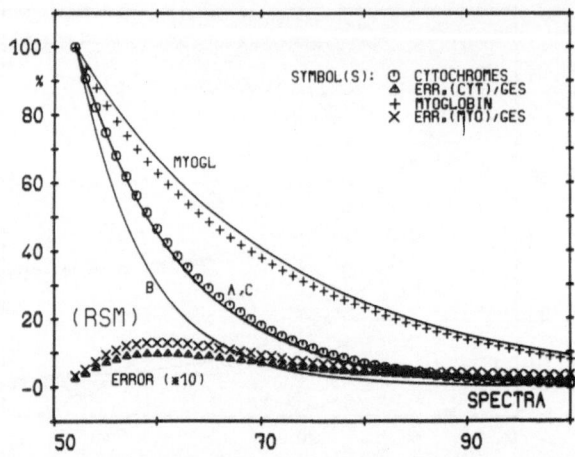

Fig. 3. RSM evaluation of simulated reflection spectra, ischemia.
Symbols: RSM, straight line: exact results. RSM cannot
separate the redox-states of the cytochromes. The increasing error (10 times enlarged) may indicate the splitted
cytochrome kinetic

sufficiently well using DWE because no stable characteristic
wavelength exist for these components. Due to the different time
courses the absorption signal of myoglobin disturbs the DWE
evaluation of cyt.a and cyt.b. Furthermore, DWE will give similar
time courses of the components.

REFERENCES

Figulla, H.R. Hoffmann, J., and Lubbers, D.W., Coronary conductivity
and tissue oxygenation as measured by the myoglobin O_2 saturation and the cytochrome aa3 redox state in the Langendorff
guinea pig heart preparation, in: "Oxygen Transport to Tissue
IV," H.I. Bicher, D.F. Bruley, eds., Plenum Press, New York
(1983), pp. 579-585.
Hoffmann, J., Heinrich, U., Ahmad, H.R., and Lübbers, D.W., Analysis
of tissue reflection spectra obtained bfrom brain or heart,
using the two-flux theory for non-constant light scattering,
in: "Oxygen Transport to Tissue VI," D.F. Bruley et al., eds.,
Plenum Press, New York (1985), in print.

Kortüm, G., 1969, "Reflexionsspektroskopie," Springer, Berlin-Heidelberg-New York.

Kubelka, P., and Munk, F., 1931, Ein Beitrag zur Optik der Farbanstriche, Z. Techn. Phys., 11a:593-603.

Kubelka, F., 1948, New contributions to the optics of intensely light-scattering materials, part I, J. Opt. Soc. Am., 38:448-457.

Kubelka, F., 1954, New contributions to the optics of intensely light-scattering materials, part II, J. Opt. Soc. Am., 44:330-335.

THE CALCULATION OF HEMOGLOBIN SATURATION IN SINGLE ERYTHROCYTES

T.E.J. Gayeski[1], J. Hoffmann[2], H. Grisar[2], and D.W. Lübbers[2]

1. The University of Rochester, School of Medicine and Dentistry, Rochester, NY
2. Max Planck Institute für Systemphysiologie, 4600 Dortmund 1, FRG

Spectrophotometric measurement of pigments has been used to monitor biological systems since the 1930's.[1] Recent methodology separates myoglobin (Mb) and hemoglobin (Hb) spectra spatially and calculates Mb saturation in subcellular volumes of frozen tissue. Using this methodology, results suggest a large RBC to tissue oxygen gradient at the capillary.[2] To measure this gradient directly the Hb saturation of single erythrocytes in capillaries and Mb saturation in the adjacent cells must be determined simultaneously. Hb saturation in unfrozen whole blood can be measured using commercial equipment. Determination of the Hb half-saturation (P_{50}) in unfrozen single erythrocytes has been attempted using a two wavelength method based on the Lambert-Beer law.[3] Because of the potential difficulties related to light scattering in those experiments, we undertook to determine single-erythrocyte Hb saturation using the multicomponent wavelength analysis of Wodick and Lübbers[4] as modified by Hoffmann and Lubbers (personal communication). The principal question we sought to answer was: Is there a variation amongst erythrocytes in the half-saturation of Hb (P_{50})? Additionally, the sensitivity of this methodology to changes in measuring parameters was investigated.

METHODS

Venous blood was taken from one of the authors (TEG). Separation of red cells and plasma was accomplished by centrifugation. The plasma was divided into approximately 1 cc aliquots and stored in liquid nitrogen. The packed erythrocytes were washed three times in normal saline and then lysed by addition of an equal volume of distilled water. After removal of the cell "ghosts" via centrifugation, the Hb solution was stored under liquid nitrogen.

To measure light transmitted through a single erythrocyte, a freshly drawn drop of blood from a finger prick was diluted in approximately a 0.5 cc aliquot of thawed plasma. Creation of a "miniature cuvette" minimized the movement of cells and plasma. This cuvette was constructed in one of three ways. First a 15u wire was placed between two quartz glass slides (10 mm in diameter) and the two slides were glued together. This method provided a "cuvette" into which fluid could flow via capillary action. Second, a small hole was made in a parafilm sheet (6 cm x 6 cm) with a 20 gauge needle. The parafilm was then stretched over a quartz glass slide held in a brass holder. The hole in the parafilm enlarged during stretching to 2-3 mm and was centered on the glass. A diluted blood sample was placed in this hole. Cellophane was then moistened with the same diluted sample and stretched over the parafilm covered slide. The moistened cellophane adhered well to the parafilm surface. A second circular brass piece had a 6 mm hole in the center which was covered by a quartz glass slide. This second brass piece mated to the first forming a small air tight chamber. The gas between the cellophane and glass of the second brass piece could be changed via an input and output port. Third, a glass slide was sprayed with shellac. Small areas of shellac (2 - 3 mm in diameter) were removed after the shellac dried. The schellac-covered slide was placed on the aforementioned brass holder. A diluted blood sample was then placed in the bare areas and a plasma-moistened piece of cellophane again covered the assembly. The mating brass piece formed an air tight chamber. After waiting ten to twenty minutes for movement of cells to cease, a spectrum from a single erythrocyte could be recorded. Eight consecutive transmission spectra were recorded from a single erythrocyte. A total time of five minutes was required for a set of 8 spectra. For each set the mean Hb saturation and the inner quartile range were calculated. While the first cuvette provided a stationary erythrocyte, it did not allow for rapid changes in sample PO_2. The second and third chambers provided this additional capability. Using a UMSP-1 microscope, eight spectra were recorded for each erythrocyte. Single erythrocyte spectra were recorded with cells in equilibruim with four different gases. Gases used were 95% O_2 + 5% CO_2; air, 0.15% O_2 + 94.25% N_2 + 5% CO_2; 100% N_2.

All spectra were measured in transmission with a Zeiss microscope (UMSP-1). The spectral analyses were carried out according to the method of Wodick and Lubbers,[4] as modified by Hoffmann and Lubbers (personal communication). This method is based on the reconstruction of the measured spectrum from three basic spectra: 1) a fully oxygenated Hb spectrum, 2) a fully deoxygenated Hb spectrum, 3) a straight line with varying slope. The Hb basic spectra must be made under identical conditions, i.e. same path length of light, same Hb concentration, same light scattering conditions. The calculation of the unknown Hb saturation consists of reconstructing the measured spectrum with these three basic spectra so that the least mean square error between the measured curve and its reconstruction are minimized over the entire wavelength range. In these experiments the range was 510 to 610 nm with 0.2 nm intervals for a total of 500 points. The "concentration" of the Hb in the measured spectrum is calculated by adding the fraction of each of the oxygenated and deoxygenated basic spectra used to reconstruct the measured spectrum. Thus, it represents the per cent of the product of the concentration times the path length of the basic spectra required to reconstruct that spectrum, i.e. it is a relative concentration and not an absolute one. The basic spectra for fully oxygenated and deoxygenated Hb were recorded from the same red cell rouleaux. Comparisons of spectra from Hb equilibrated with 95% O_2 plus 5% CO_2 and air-equilibrated Hb were made.

RESULTS

Selection of Diaphragms

To determine the optimal relationship amongst cell size, measuring diaphragm, and Hb saturation variability, erythrocytes were measured with 5 different pairs of illumination-field diaphragms. For each pair the ratio of measuring diaphragm to illumination diaphragm was maintained at 1 to 2 (Kohler illumination). For measuring diaphragms smaller than the size of the erythrocyte (0.8 and 2.5 microns) large inner quartile range (IQR) in saturation (30 to 50 percent) for individual erythrocytes were found. For measuring diaphragms larger than the erythrocyte (15.7 and 25 microns) the IQR was similar to that of the 8 micron measuring diaghragm. For the smaller measuring diaphragms the calculated Hb concentration was approximately 50 percent greater than for the 8 micron diaphragm. The Hb concentration calculated with the 8 micron diaphragm was approximately 20 percent higher than the 15.7 and 25 micron diaphragms. The reason for this difference in Hb concentration is thought to be related to the influence of scattering on the calculation. The Hb saturations calculated were comparable. Thus, the 8 micron measuring diaphragm was selected to maximize the Hb concentration and minimize the IQR.

Effect of plasma

Each spectral measurement for Hb-free plasma was made after refocusing the illumination diaphragm in the plane of focus. Note that the mean relative concentration was -0.01. Because this method of curve-fitting allows apparent concentrations less than zero, saturations can be greater than 100 per cent. In fact, the ranges of apparent concentrations for Hb-free plasma vary from -0.02 to +0.02. This apparent concentration in the absence of Hb represents approximately 15 percent of that of a single erythrocyte. Similar errors are found for normal saline.

Focal Plane

The focal plane was established for a single erythrocyte by visualizing the typical erythrocyte form. Eight individual spectra were then measured at this location and at +3 and -3 microns from the focal plane. For ten cells, there were no systematic differences amongst saturations, concentrations or IQR's for the three focuses. However, for large deviations from the focal plan (i.e. 10 microns), differences in saturation and concentration were appreciable (greater than 10% for saturation and concentration). Thus, variations in the plane of focus may affect the calculated saturation significantly but only for large deviation from the plane of focus.

RBC Location

The effect of erythrocyte location within the measuring diaphragm on the estimate of saturation was studied by choosing a large measuring diaphragm (25u diameter). Measurements with the cell at the edge of a 50 um illumination diaphragm, half-way between this edge and center, and at the center revealed a 15% and 10% difference between the edge and center saturations and the half-way point and center, respectively. Hence, location of the object within the field is important.

Intracellular Variation

Table 1 demonstrates the variation in saturation for each erythrocyte. For air-equilibrated erythrocytes the mean IQR of Hb saturation was 0.05; for N_2 equilibrated erythrocytes, 0.05; for partially saturated Hb, 0.05. Thus, the variation in saturation for the same cell was small and not saturation dependent.

Table 1. The mean variation in saturation from 8 spectra for each single cell under three conditions.

Within Single Erythrocytes

Equilibration with	N	Mean IQR of Saturation
Air	46	0.05
0.75% O_2	48	0.05
N_2	44	0.05

Intercellular Variation

The variation amongst cells brought into equilibrium with the respective gases is seen in Table 2. There are no differences amongst the groups with respect to concentration or least mean square error. However, a greater IQR was observed for both the air equilibrated and 0.15% O_2 equilibrated groups.

Table 2. The mean saturation and concentration of the population of erythrocytes. The IQR represents the variation of saturation within the population of measured cells.

Among Single Erythrocytes

Equilibration with	N	Mean Saturation	IQR (%)	Mean Concentration
Air	46	100	9	0.16
0.75% O_2	48	28	9	0.15
N_2	44	-1	5	0.18

Representative spectra and error signals for oxygenated and deoxygenated single erythrocytes are shown in Fig. 1. The scale on the error signal is 25 times that of the spectra. Thus, the

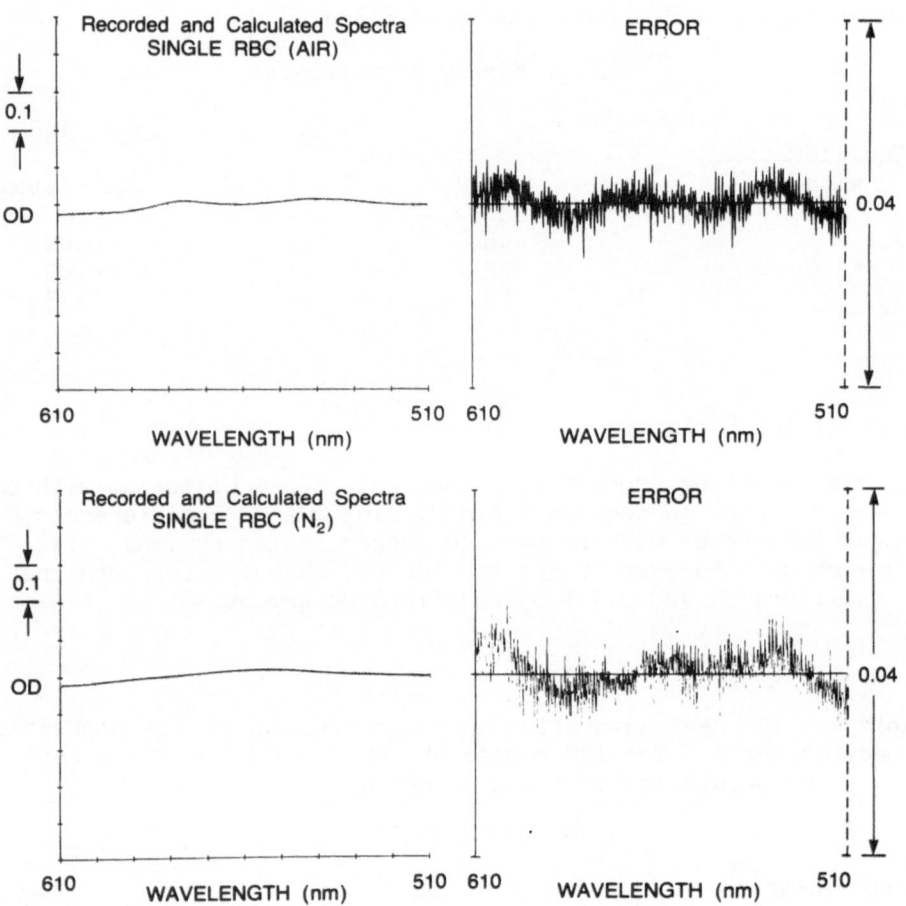

Fig. 1   The intervals of left and right hand curves' abscissas
are wavelength in nanometers (nm), those of the ordinates are
optical density (OD):   note scales.   The left hand curves are
representative of the   measured and calculated spectra for air-and
nitrogen-equilibrated erythrocytes.   The "error" curve is the
difference between the measured spectra and the calculated
spectra.

largest error is approximately 4% of the signal. Though the error is small, it may not be random. If the error signal is not systematic, a non-wavelength dependent error spectrum with a mean of zero should result when all error spectra are averaged. The resulting error spectra are shown in Fig. 2. The wavelength-dependent error spectra suggest that there remains a small systematic error in our measurements.

To demonstrate the effect of using an incorrect basic spectrum on the calculated saturation, we used a basic spectrum for frozen blood recorded on another spectrophotometer to calculate the saturations of air-equilibrated and N_2-equilibrated erythrocytes. The analysis of the spectra from air-equilibrated cells produced a saturation of 76% and the deoxygenated cells exhibited no significant change in the calculated saturation. Hence, the method appears to be more sensitive to differences in the oxygenated basic spectrum as might be expected, since there is a greater spectral variation for this condition. Despite these differences, the reconstructed spectra based on the incorrect basic spectra had no greater least mean square error than those spectra reconstructed with the correct basic spectra. Hence, the least mean square error is not an absolute measure of the correctness of the saturation calculation. It is only a measure of the fit of the basic spectra to the measured spectra.

DISCUSSION

Sources of Experimental Error

A source of error in the hemoglobin saturation calculation is inherent within the cuvette chamber. The careful measurement of a spectrum from 510 to 610 mm in the absence of any object in the object path results in a spectrum whose wavelength dependence is small relative to a tenth of an optical density. However, if one introduces the aforementioned cuvette chamber containing saline or plasma in the object path, the resulting spectrum has a wavelength dependence. This wavelength dependence results in a calculated hemoglobin concentration of approximately 10% of that resulting from a single erythrocyte. Furthermore, the saturation of this cuvette chamber varies over a very large range. The mean apparent Hb concentration of this non-Hb containing chamber is approximately a negative 10% of the Hb concentration resulting from a single erythrocyte. These results suggest that the UMSP-1 system in single erythrocyte experiments can bias the hemoglobin saturation in the direction of a higher saturation by 10%. Additionally these results explain in part at least the variation in the saturation for single erythrocytes at a given oxygen

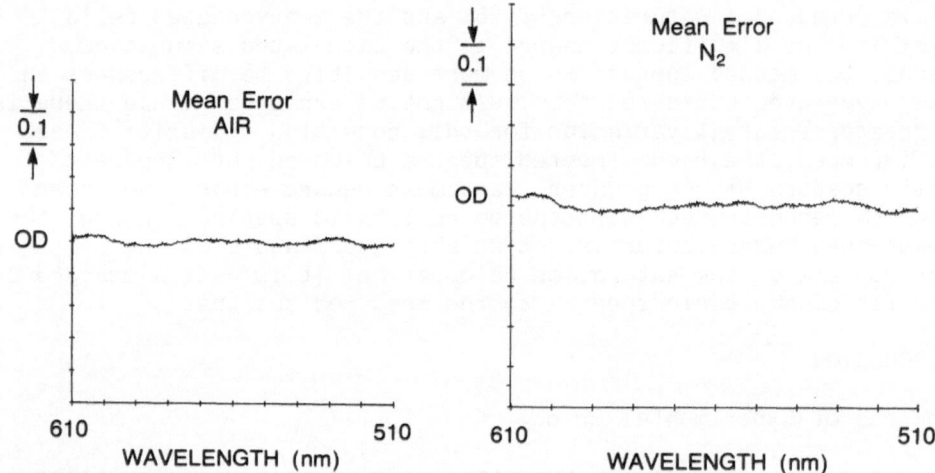

Fig. 2   The left and right hand curves are the error spectra
resulting from averaging all the individual error curves for air-
and nitrogen-equilibrated cells.   The abscissa is linear.   The
zero point is at line 5 on the ordinate.   Note the small scale
difference and the similarity between the two mean error spectra.

tension. Whether modern microspectrophotometer design will solve this problem must be explored.

In addition to the aforementioned problems, difficulties resulting from the erythrocytes must be considered. First, if the measuring spot is small with respect to the size of the erythrocyte, submicron movement of the erythrocyte in the measuring field during a spectral scan can result in large alterations in light absorption due to the erythrocyte's shape. The reasons for these spectral shifts are thought to be changes in path length through the erythrocyte and possible changes in scattering. Second, the effect of variations in the focal plane can be significant. We find that changes of three microns do not significantly influence the calculated saturation. However, larger changes lead to deviations in saturation of greater than 10%. Third, the influence of cell location within the illumination diaphragm is important. Variations of approximately 15% saturation can occur for the same cell when located at the edge of a large illumination diaphragm as compared to a central location. If location within the two diaphragms becomes more critical as diaphragm and erythrocyte size approach each other, small variations in the location of the object with respect to the field and measuring diaphragms could explain the variations in our results.

POSSIBLE METHODOLOGIC ERRORS

As seen in figure 2, a wavelength dependent averaged error curve results from averaging all error spectra of single, isolated cells. Furthermore, the averaged error curves for the fully oxygenated and fully deoxygenated cells are strikingly similar. The explanation of this finding could lie in the inapplicability of the linear multi-component analysis or the utilization of basic spectra recorded from rouleaux for single erythrocytes. At present, with the existing signal to noise ratio we cannot distinguish between these possibilities.

HEMOGLOBIN P_{50}

These experiments were designed to measure the reproducibility of calculating Hb saturation amongst erythrocytes. Cell shape and signal size present potential difficulties. Cell shape raises the question of the applicability of the multicomponent wavelength analysis and sets stringent requirements on acceptable cell motion during measurement. Signal size is less than 0.1 optical density units. The effect of system errors results in a range of variation in calculated Hb saturation of $\pm15\%$. Newer microspectrophotometer design may reduce this error.

Nevertheless, at room temperature, Hb saturation was reproducible to within $\pm$ 5%. There was no difference in variability amongst cells equilibrated with room air and those equilibrated with 0.75% O_2 gas mixture. Comparing our results to those of Waldeck[3], we find that the results are comparable. The difference between the papers is that Waldeck interprets the variation in saturation he observed as actual variation in the P_{50} value. We interpret our variations as errors in the determination. Thus, these results suggest: 1) It is possible to calculate Hb saturation from single erythrocytes at room temperature. 2) The variation in P_{50} from cell to cell is within experimental error. Hence, efforts to attempt to measure the capillary to tissue O_2 gradient remain feasible.

REFERENCES

1. Millikan G.A.: 1937, Experiments in muscle haemoglobin in vivo; the instantaneous measurement of muscle metabolism. Proc. Roy. Soc. B 123:218-241.

2. Honig C.R., Gayeski T.E.J., Federspiel W., Clark A., Jr., Clark, P: 1984, Muscle O_2 gradients from hemoglobin to cytochrome: new concepts, new complexities. In: Oxygen Transport to Tissue-V, eds. D.W. Lubbers, H. Acker, E. Leniger-Follert, and T.K. Goldstick. Ad. Exp. Med. Biol., Vol. 169, Plenum Press, New York and London, 23-38.

3. Waldeck F: 1966, Ein mikrophotometrisches Verfahren zur Aufnahme der Sauerstoffbindungskurve von einzelnen Erythrocyten. Pflugers Arch. 295:1-14.

4. Wodick R., Lübbers D.W.: 1973, A new method for determining the degree of oxygenation of hemoglobin spectra of inhomogeneous light paths, explained with the analysis of spectra of the human skin. Pflugers Arch. 342:41-60.

MEASUREMENTS AND PROCESSING OF INTRACAPILLARY HEMOGLOBIN SPECTRA BY USING A MICRO-LIGHTGUIDE SPECTROPHOTOMETER IN CONNECTION WITH A MICROCOMPUTER

M. Brunner, R. Ellermann, K.H. Frank, and M. Kessler

Institut für Physiologie und Kardiologie der Universität
Erlangen-Nürnberg, Waldstr.6, D-8520 Erlangen

INTRODUCTION

The degree of oxygenation of the oxygen carrier hemoglobin
plays an important role for the oxygen supply situation in the
capillary network of body tissue.
Because of the different absorption characteristics of
oxygenated and deoxygenated hemoglobin, it is in principle possible
to provide information concerning the instantaneous degree of
oxygenation in surface capillaries by means of reflection spectroscopy without destroying or even affecting sensitive structures.

MEASURING UNIT

The micro-lightguide spectrophotometer we used is a further
development of the spectrophotometer described several times in the
past (Brunner, 1980; Brunner et al., 1981).
A schematic drawing of the spectrophotometer is shown in Fig.1.
From the light source the light is guided through a lens system via
an emitting optical fiber to the tissue. The reflected light is
conducted via six fibers which are arranged annulary around the
emitting fiber to a wavelength selector. The selector consists of
an interference filter disc, which is rotated by a motor and serves
as a monochromator at which light of different wavelengths between
502 and 628 nm is selected as a function of the angle of rotation.
The intensity of the transmitted light is measured in a photomultiplier and an analog voltage signal $x(t)$, dependent on the intensity,
is generated. With every revolution of the interference filter disc
trigger pulses tr and ts can be derived from the trigger unit.

DATA ACQUISITION

The data acquisition is performed by a microcomputer (Fig.2) and is synchronized by trigger pulses derived from the trigger unit. The trigger tr functions as a start- and reset-command and is generated once for each revolution of the interference filter disc. The trigger ts directly drives the digitalization of the voltage

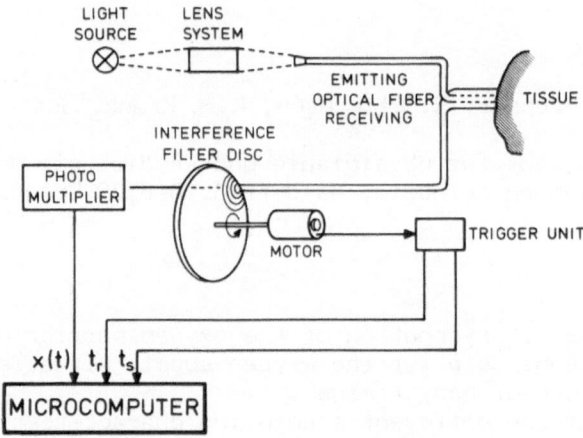

Fig. 1. Block-diagram of the micro-lightguide spectrophotometer.

signal x(t) by the analog-digital converter.

The time-courses of the signal produced by the spectrophotometer are shown in Fig.3. The voltage signal x(t) is superimposed by considerable noise which can easily be filtered by applying an anti-aliasing filter.

The digitalization-trigger ts are not equidistant because the wavelength characteristic of the interference filter is not linear.

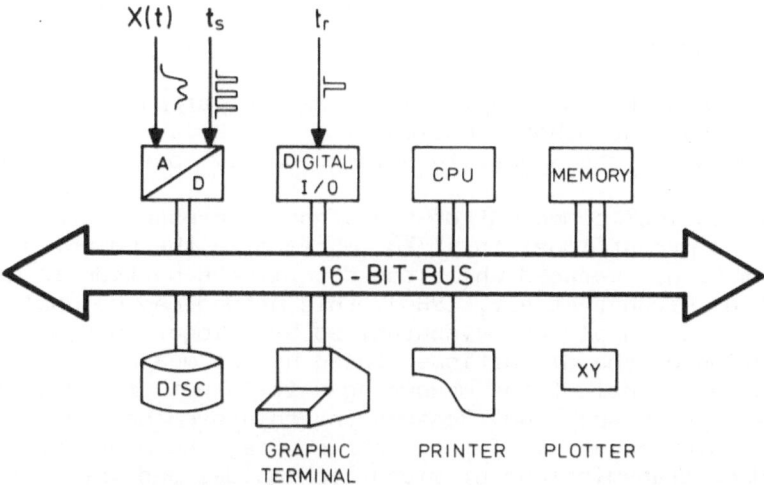

Fig. 2.   Block-diagram of the microcomputer (LSI 11/2, Digital
          Equipment Corp.).

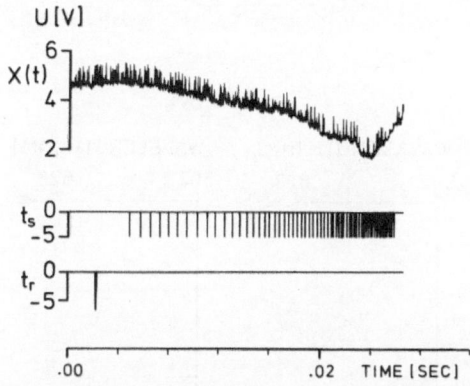

Fig. 3.   Output signals from the micro-lightguide spectrophotometer:
          x(t): voltage signal (reflection-spectrum)
          ts: digitalization-trigger
          tr: start- and reset-trigger.

PREPROCESSING

The purpose of the preprocessing ist the preparation for the measured signal for quantification.

1. Improvement of the signal-to-noise ratio by correlated signal averaging:
   The statistical component of the signal decreases with arithmetic averaging proportional to $1/\sqrt{n}$ where n is the number of spectra to be averaged while the determinate portion is not affected (Brunner et al., 1984). this method can be applied because the signals are synchronized by trigger pulses.

2. Correction of the distortions caused by the measuring unit:
   The output signal of the measuring unit is not proportional to the reflection spectrum. Reasons for this are the nonlinearity of the emission-spectrum of the light source, the wavelength-dependent transmissions of micro-lightguides and interference filter disc, and the wavelength-dependent sensitivity of the photomultiplier.The resulting distortions are shown clearly in Fig. 4 on the left side. Points of equal reflection are connected by dashed lines. One reflection spectrum is drawn to point out the effects of the distortions.

The result of the computational correction of the apparative distortions is shown in Fig.4 on the right side. The wavelength at maximum reflection is chosen as a reference point in the scale.

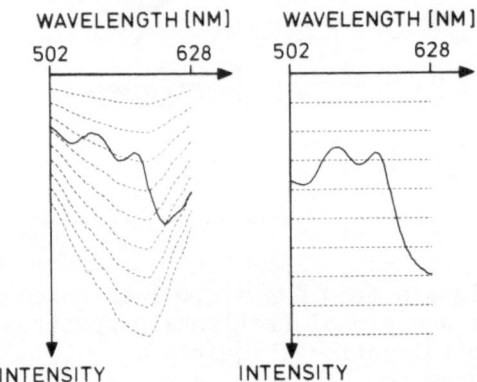

Fig. 4.   Distorted (left) and corrected (right) wavelength-intensity diagrams.

FEATURE EXTRACTION

It was our intention to use the entire information contained in the spectrum for the quantitative analysis in order to obtain an exact and robust method.

In the physiological range of hemoglobin concentration the spectrum is primarily determined by its shape, which mathematically can exactly be described in the frequency domain (Ellermann et al., 1983; Brunner et al., 1984). Fig.5 shows intensity-wavelength diagrams and their corresponding amplitude-frequency diagrams.

The measured spectrum is not a pure hemoglobin spectrum but a composition of many components (Lübbers, 1973; Wodick, 1973), in which hemoglobin plays the most important role.

Transformation into the frequency domain, suppressing those components, which give no significant contribution to the

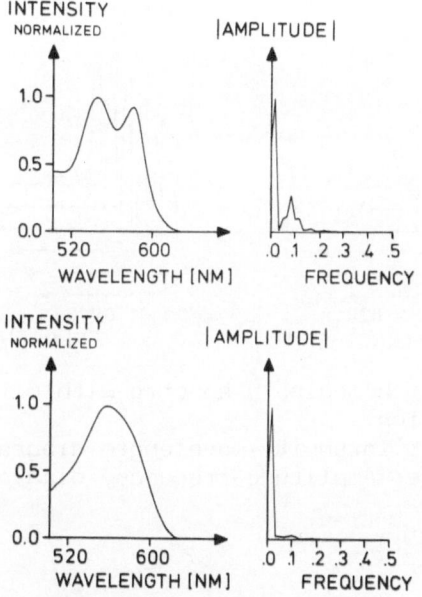

Fig. 5.   Intensity-wavelength diagrams (left) and amplitude-frequency diagrams (right) of oxygenated (upper part) and deoxygenated hemoglobin (lower part).

hemoglobin spectrum, and inverse transformation result in a nearly
pure hemoglobin spectrum whose shape is determined by the degree of
oxygenation (Fig.5).

Obviously the frequency domain representation consists of fewer
parameters than the wavelength domain spectra.

Thus only few features remain which completely decribe the
spectra.

QUANTIFICATION

Changes in hemoglobin oxygenation bring about a definable
variation of the corresponding amplitude-frequency diagrams. The
proportion of the high frequencies varies in a characteristic
manner with oxygenation levels and can therefore be regarded as a
quantitative measure of the degree of oxygenation (Fig.6).

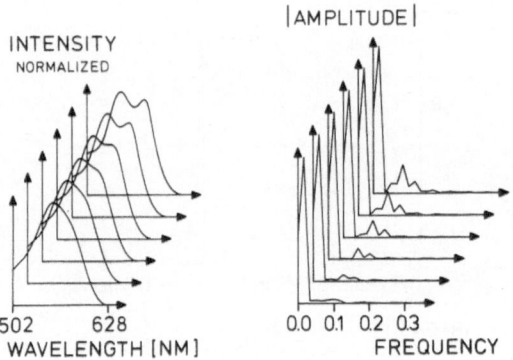

Fig. 6. Series of hemoglobin spectra with different degree of
         oxygenation.
         Left side: Intensity-wavelength diagram
         Right side: Amplitude-frequency diagram.

As mentioned above, the described algorithm is applicable in
cases where the influence of the hemoglobin concentration on the
amplitude-frequency diagram is higher than that of other components. This precondition is true for the physiological concentration range.

We measured the correctness of the method in the rat liver
down to a limit of 3.5 g% Hb.

914

APPLICATIONS

Fig.7 shows a typical application of our system. The spectra were measured on the human skin before, during, and after tourniquet ischemia. In the upper part of the picture the spectra are plotted pseudo-three-dimensionally as a function of wavelength, normalized intensity, and time. Corresponding wavelength of succesive spectra are connected by lines. During the occlusion the transition from oxygenatad to deoxygenated hemoglobin is clearly visible.

In the lower part of Fig.7 the corresponding course of the oxygenation is plotted, evaluated with the method described above.

The described system was applied to different tissues such as beating heart, lung, liver, skeletal muscle, skin and eye. The quantification method produced good results even from spectra of the beating heart in the dogs.

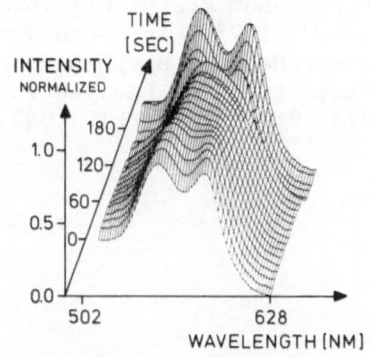

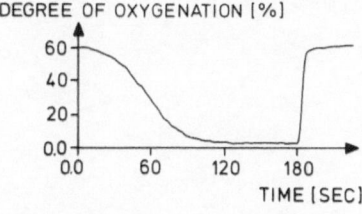

Fig. 7. Upper part: Series of hemoglobin spectra from the human skin.
Lower part: Corresponding degree of oxygenation.

REFERENCES

Brunner, M., 1980,On-line Verarbeitung von Hämoglobin-
    Reflexionsspektren mit einem Mikro-Lichtleiter-Spektro-
    photometer hoher Repetitionsrate, Diplomarbeit,Universität
    Erlangen-Nürnberg, Erlangen.
Brunner, M., Kastner, N., Schabert, A., Höper, J., Kessler, M.,
    1981, On-line Verarbeitung von Hämoglobin-Reflexionsspektren
    hoher Repetitionsraten, in: "Medizinische Informatik und
    Statistik", 28, S.Koller, P.L.Reichertz, K.Überla, eds.,
    Springer, Berlin-Heidelberg-New York.
Brunner, M., Ellermann, R., Kessler, M., 1984, Some aspects of
    signal analysis applied to intracapillary hemoglobin spectra,
    in: "Oxygen transport to tissue", D.W.Lübbers, H.A.Acker,
    E.Leniger-Follert, T.K.Goldstick, eds., Plenum Press, New
    York and London.
Brunner, M., Ellermann, R., Kessler,M., 1984, Online-processing of
    intracapillary hemoglobin spectra with a microcomputer, Pflü-
    gers Archiv, 400, Suppl., R 55, 220.
Ellermann, R., Brunner, M., Kessler, M., 1983, Quantification of
    intracapillary hemoglobin spectra by transformation into the
    frequency domain, Proc. Deutsche Gesellschaft für Mikrozir-
    kulation, Erlangen, Jahrestagung 25.-26.11.1983.
Lübbers, D.W., 1973, Spectrophotometric examination of tissue
    oxygenation, in: "Oxygen transport to tissue", H.I.Bicher,
    D.F.Bruley, eds., Plenum Press, New York and London.
Wodick, R., Lübbers, D.W.,1973, Ein neues Verfahren zur Bestimmung
    des Oxygenierungsgrades von Hämoglobinspektren bei inhomogenen
    Lichtwegen, erläutert an der Analyse von Spektren der mensch-
    lichen Haut, 1973, Pflügers Archiv, 342, 41.

916

CAPILLARY RED CELL RESIDENCE AS A MEASURE OF TISSUE OXYGEN DELIVERY

Ian S. Longmuir, James A. Knopp, and Philip Weinbrecht

Department of Biochemistry
Box 7622
North Carolina State University
Raleigh, North Carolina 27695-7622

Experimental measurements of changes in the fluorescence intensity of endogenous and exogenous indicators of tissue oxygen tension must be corrected for changes in red cell mass in the observed volume of tissue. In our presentation last year (Longmuir et al. 1984) we assumed that localized increased oxygen consumption in the sensory cortex on peripheral stimulation would result in increases only in red cell mass. Thus any observed increases in fluorescence of pyrenebutyric acid would be equal to or less than the actual change in fluorescence quenching by oxygen: that there was a real fall in local tissue oxygen tension. However, subsequent studies have shown that following sensory stimulation, some areas of the cortex show reduced red cell mass. These reductions in microregional blood flow do not appear to be a direct consequence of sensory stimulation, but are part of the normal pattern of fluctuations in the distribution of red cells which occur continuously in the brain, giving rise to the oscillations in local Po_2 described by Manil et al. (1984). When large areas of cortex are studied, these fluctuations average out and the problem of correction is simplified. However, to study changes in small areas, less than $(100_\mu)^2$, requires some understanding of these changes. In addition, since the oxygen content of red cells is about two hundred times that of the same volume of plasma, their transit through capillaries is a much more important parameter of tissue oxygen delivery than blood flow. Krogh (1919) recorded the observation that red cells are never stationary in muscle capillaries. If this is true in all tissues and the red cells do not fully discharge their oxygen, then a measurement of the number of red cells in a given volume of tissue at any instant of time is a measure of oxygen supply.

METHOD

The apparatus (Fig. 1) we use to measure red cell mass has been described (Longmuir et al., 1984). A window is sealed into an anaesthetized cat's skull. The cortex is illuminated with visible light at a wavelength isosbestic to haemoglobin and oxyhaemoglobin. The cortex is observed by the microscope in either of two modes, direct observation at an optical magnification of 40x (4x objective and 10x eyepiece) or at a similar magnification with the SIT television camera (4x objective and the rest of the magnification electronically). Both of these systems resolve to about 8μ horizontally; thus capillaries are just perceptible with the eyepiece. Because of some degradation of the image by the SIT camera, we cannot see the capillaries on the television screen. Although the resolution in the horizontal plane is approximately the same with the two systems of observation, the resolution in the vertical axis, the depth of focus, is dramatically different. The axial resolution is a function of the optical magnification and the numerical aperture. In the case of the television system it is 3.0 mm, while with the eyepiece it is 0.16 mm. Epiillumination of the brain penetrates to 650μ (Benson and Knopp, 1984). Thus, in the case of the television system, all observable structures are in focus. If an area of brain is selected where no vessels can be resolved, it will contain no vessels greater than 8.0μ. Changes in light reflection in this area can only be due to changes in the number of red cells in capillaries. The change in light reflection by the addition or subtraction of a single red cell in a small pixel is considerably greater than the known range of optical properties of tissue which would be necessary to produce the same change (Benson and Knopp, 1984).

We conducted experiments in order to confirm Krogh's observation that red cells are never stationary in capillaries in the brain. Cats were anaesthetized with pentobarbital or chloralose, both lightly and deeply. Windows were placed over the parietal cortex and the brain illuminated with visible light. The image from the television camera was projected on the screen, and areas free of observable vessels were selected for digitization. When steady readings were obtained, the heart was stopped with KCl and shortly afterwards the brain perfused with saline. In some experiments the cortex was observed through the eyepiece during these manoeuvers.

RESULTS

In all experiments, stopping the heart resulted in an increase in reflected light (Fig. 2). In the lightly anaesthetized animals the increase was large and there was no further increase on perfusion. In the more deeply anaesthetized cats the rise was not so

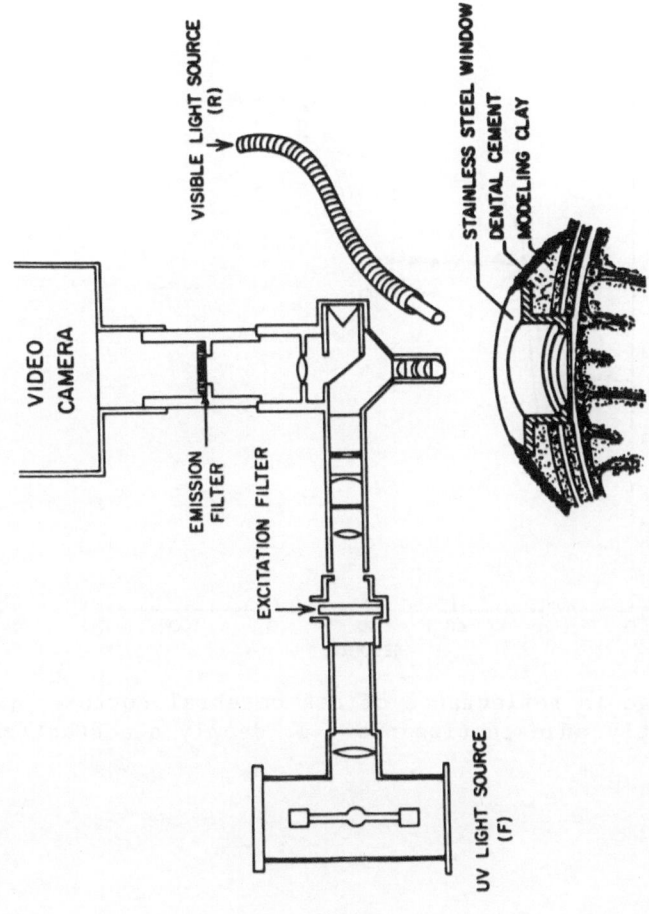

VISIBLE LIGHT SOURCE (R)

VIDEO CAMERA

EMISSION FILTER

EXCITATION FILTER

UV LIGHT SOURCE (F)

STAINLESS STEEL WINDOW

DENTAL CEMENT

MODELING CLAY

Surgical Window in Brain

Fig. 1. Diagram of apparatus

919

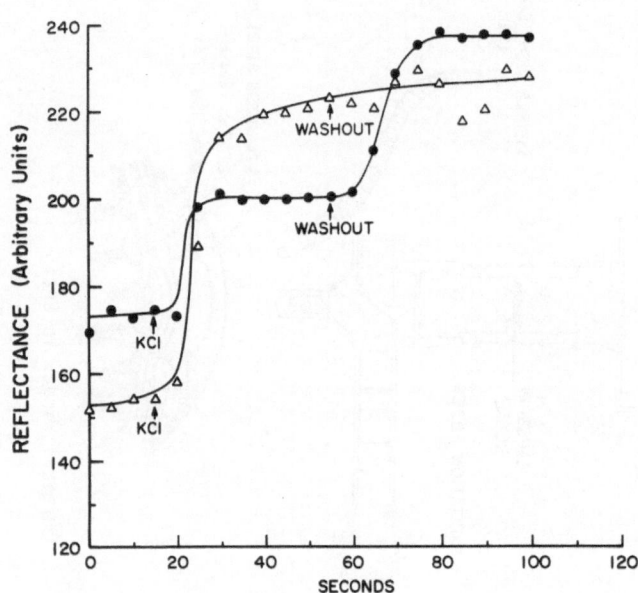

Fig. 2. Change in reflectance of cat cerebral cortex. Δ—Δ,
Lightly anaesthetized; ●—●, deeply anaesthetized.

great and there was a second increase following washout. Visual observation confirmed that all the capillaries emptied in the first group of experiments, but only about half in the second.

DISCUSSION

Tissue light reflection with the appropriate conditions, a depth of focus greater than the depth of illumination, appears to offer a method of measuring capillary red cells, provided the level of anaesthesia is not so deep that red cells stop in capillaries. If the red cells do not become completely deoxygenated during capillary transit, then this method gives a measure of tissue oxygen delivery which may be more appropriate than capillary blood flow.

Acknowledgement—This work was supported in part by NIH grant HL16828.

REFERENCES

Benson, D. M., and Knopp, J. A., 1984, Effect of tissue absorption and microscope optical parameters on the depth of penetration for fluorescence and reflectance measurements of tissue samples, Photochem. Photobiol. 39:495-502.
Krogh, A., 1919, The supply of oxygen to the tissues and the regulation of the capillary circulation, J. Physiol. 52:457-474.
Longmuir, I. S., Knopp, J. A., and Pittman, J. L., 1984, Changes in cerebral oxygen tension and red cell content on sensory stimulation, in: "Oxygen Transport to Tissue – V, Advances in Experimental Medicine and Biology," Vol. 169, D. W. Lübbers, H. Acker, E. Leniger-Follert, and T. K. Goldstick, eds., Plenum Publishing Corp., New York.
Manil, J., Bourgain, R. H., Van Waeyenberge, M., Colin, F., Blockeel, E., De Mey, B., Coremans, J., and Paternoster, R., 1984, Properties of spontaneous fluctuations in cortical oxygen pressure, ibid.

DEVELOPMENT OF AN IN-VITRO METHOD FOR

SIMULATION OF OXYGEN TRANSPORT IN THE MICROCIRCULATION

E. J. Boland[1] J. S. Olson[2] and J. D. Hellums[1]

Biomedical Engineering Laboratory[1] and
Department of Biochemistry[2]
Rice University, Houston, TX 77251

INTRODUCTION

Measurement of oxygen transport rates in the microcirculation has been the subject of numerous in vivo investigations and considerable progress has been made. However, there are experimental difficulties in exact determination of several important parameters including the capillary wall boundary conditions and the capillary dimensions. These difficulties have constituted the incentive for our continuing development of an in vitro system in which the capillary dimensions are determined precisely by light and electron microscopy; the flow rate is carefully regulated; the inlet concentration of red cells or hemoglobin is controlled independently; the fractional saturation of hemoglobin is measured spectrophotometrically; and the boundary conditions in the silicone rubber capillary bed can be computed by established mathematical techniques. Accurate measurement of these variables should prove to be useful in testing and validating the several mathematical models which have been used in simulation of microcirculatory oxygen transport. A preliminary report on the project has described the basic features of the method (Boland, et al, 1984). Here we will briefly outline the approach used, describe several improvements in methodology, and present some of the results on both erythrocyte suspensions and hemoglobin solutions.

Artificial capillaries are fabricated of silicone rubber, and placed on the stage of a microscope. Erythrocyte suspensions or hemoglobin solutions are oxygenated or deoxygenated while flowing through the capillary, and dual wavelength microspectrophotometry is used to determine oxygen saturation at various axial positions.

923

THE CAPILLARY SYSTEM

The capillary system is indicated schematically in Figure 1. The reservoir of liquid feeding the capillary is exposed to the gas which is present in the external gas space. A different gas is blown through the capillary gas space. Thus, the oxygen saturation of the incoming red cell suspension or hemoglobin solution and the rates of oxygen transport in the capillary are controlled independently. The capillaries used in most of the preliminary studies to date are 27 μm in diameter, 5mm in transport length, and imbedded in a silicone rubber film of 150-230 μm thickness.

A new design of the capillary casting system was made using stainless steel instead of plexiglass except for the coverplates which must be transparent. The new design permits much more accurate determination of dimensions, and much better reproducibility in casting capillaries. Furthermore, in the new design we were able to reduce the thickness of the silicone rubber film to 120 μm. This thinner film yields an improvement in accuracy in determining resistance to oxygen transport in the blood, because blood resistance is determined by subtraction of the silicone resistance from the total resistance. The new design has stainless steel sleeves extending from the tubing connection through the silicone rubber to a depth even with the edges of the gas space. These sleeves eliminate a rather ill-defined transport "end effect," and reduce the "hold up" of unstirred fluid volume in the end pieces.

In preliminary experiments we examined the possibility that the pressure changes required to change flow rate might cause significant variations in the luminal diameter of the capillaries. The microspectrophotometer serves as a sensitive indicator of changes in luminal diameter when hemoglobin solutions are used. In the infusion mode at high flow rates, the positive pressure generated by the pump caused a significant swelling of the capillary (a 5-10% increase in diameter). In contrast, there were no detectable changes in luminal diameter over the range of flow rates used when the perfusion pump was used in the withdrawal mode. Thus, the withdrawal arrangement is the mode of choice.

DETERMINATION OF OXYGEN SATURATIONS
Outline of the Method

A schematic drawing of the spectrophotometric system in given in Figure 2. In a typical experiment determinations of oxygen saturation are made at 4 to 8 different axial positions along the capillary. Extraneous light is minimized by passing the beam through a rectangular diaphragm which is adjusted to allow only light passing through the capillary to be incident upon the beam splitter. The diaphragm is closed down until a square (1 X 1) or rectangular (2 X 1)

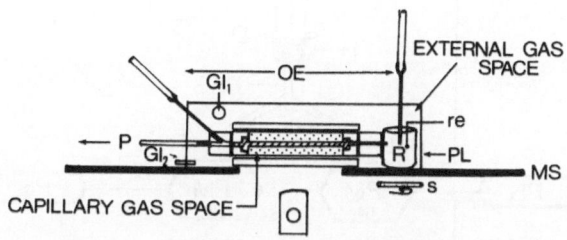

Figure 1. Capillary Infusion and Environment Control System
GI$_1$, gas inlet for external gas space; GI$_2$, gas inlet for
capillary gas space; O, objective lens; P, line to pump; PL,
plexiglas covering; OE, oxygen electrode; R, reservoir; re,
reference electrode; s, stirrer.

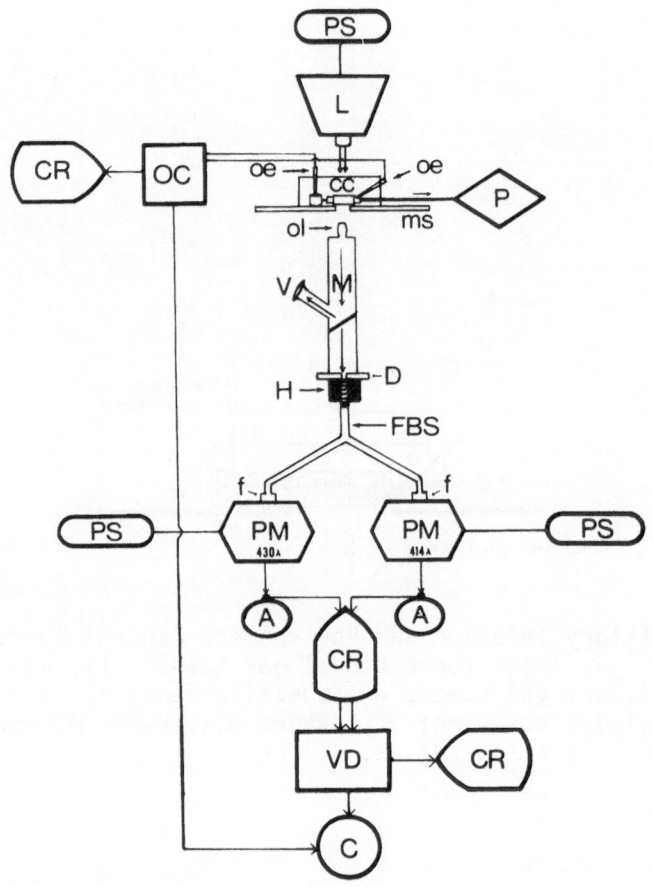

Figure 2: Schematic Diagram of Apparatus
A amplifier; C, microcomputer; cc, capillary chamber; CR, chart recorder; D, retangular diaphram; f, light filter; FBS, fiber optic beam splitter; H, light guide holder; L, light source; M, microscope; ms, microscope stage; oe, oxygen electrode; PM, photomultiplier tube; PS, DC power supply; V, viewing lens; VD, voltage divider.

measurement area is outlined. This area is observed through the viewing lens and reduced to exclude light external to the lumen of the capillary. For example, in measurements on the 27 μm diameter capillary, light is admitted from an area centered in the capillary which is about 25 μm (transverse) by 25 to 50 μm (axial). Thus, the oxygen saturation values obtained are space-averaged over an axial length of one to two capillary diameters.

Simultaneous measurements are made to light transmitted at two wavelengths (414 nm and 430 nm) in application of the technique described by Olson (1981). Determinations are made at the same flow rate for three conditions of oxygen saturation: (1) fully oxygenated (the capillary and external gas space are both flushed with pure O_2), (2) fully deoxygenated (the perfusate specimen is deoxygenated in a tonometer and the capillary and external gas spaces are flushed with N_2), and (3) the "measurement" condition of interest in the experiment (in the measurements discussed here the external gas space is flushed with pure O_2, and the capillary gas space with pure N_2). Then the oxygen saturation is given by

$$S = 1 - \frac{\Delta A_2 - \Delta A_1}{\Delta A_2^t - \Delta A_1^t} \tag{1}$$

ΔA denotes the change in absorbance from the absorbance from the "measurement" condition to the fully saturated condition. The superscripts "t" denote the total change in absorbance between the fully desaturated and fully saturated conditions. The subscripts "1" and "2" denote the two different wavelengths.

Deviations from the Lambert-Beer Law

The calculations of oxygen saturation described above are somewhat idealized. Scattering by erythrocytes is the most important mechanism for deviation from the Lambert-Beer Law, but there are several others which can be important in some circumstances. The "sieving effect" is related to the fact that in erythrocyte suspensions light passing through the specimen passes through variable amounts of hemoglobin solution at various positions in the field of view of the detector. "Glare" and "stray light" effects are associated with the fact that some light will reach the detector which has not passed through the specimen. Still other deviations from the Lambert-Beer Law are associated with the fact that optical filters do not yield purely monochromatic light. A good recent discussion of the "sieve" and "glare" effects has been given by Pries, et al (1983).

These deviations from the idealized Lambert-Beer Law are dealt with in the spectrophotometric method of this work in a way that is both practical and on a theoretically sound basis. Scattering effects are the most important. They are minimized by using differences between simultaneous absorption determinations at 414 and 430 nm. Since scattering is wavelength dependent in this range, there will be a small effect even after subtraction of the changes at 430 and 414nm. This residual scattering effect is compensated for by using absorption differences from the fully saturated condition at the same wavelength. Both of these differences are indicated in the expression for the hemoglobin oxygen saturation, Equation (1). Use of the later difference assumes that the hematocrit is the same for the two measurements. This assumption has caused little problems in our experiments because the transmittance is a sensitive indicator of hematocrit, thus any significant change in hematocrit is indicated.

The other deviations from the Lambert-Beer Law also are minimized by measuring absorption differences from the fully saturated condition. In fact, Equation (1) may be regarded as an interpolation formula between the two known conditions of complete oxygenation and complete deoxygenation. The theory of the "Glare" and "Sieve" effects admits the possibility that the relationship between oxygen saturation and the absorbance differences could deviate from the linear relationship of Equation 1. One of the important advantages of our in-vitro system is that we can easily manipulate the oxygen saturation of the suspension in the capillary to known, constant, intermediate levels. Thus we can directly test for this possible non-linearity and correct for it if necessary.

It is instructive to consider the advantages and disadvantages of the present method over that of Pittman and Duling (1975 a,b). The Pittman and Duling method has a number of important advantages (independence of hematocrit is among them), and it has certainly had a major impact on microcirculatory research. However, in the present context it must be emphasized that, as Pittman and Duling demonstrated clearly, their original method is not applicable to conduits less than about 15 μm in diameter. They found that their method of treating scattering caused problems in the Soret band wavelengths (those used in the present work). Use of the Soret wavelengths is of crucial importance in spectrophotmetry in thin layers of hemoglobin. Sinha (1969) has shown that 430 nm can be used to follow oxygen saturation changes in single erythrocytes. In our procedure we have accepted the disadvantage that to eliminate scattering error we need an approximately constant hematocrit while measurements are made at three oxygen saturation levels. In return we have gained accuracy in measurements in smaller vessels.

TREATMENT OF DATA
Addition of Voltage Divider and Computer System

It can be shown that in application of Equation (1), no indicator of incident light intensities were needed. We only need the ratio of the two photomultiplier readings. On this basis we have installed a voltage divider for the two signals as indicated in Figure 2. This relatively simple addition greatly improves accuracy by reducing noise (due for example to fluctuations in the light source or in hematocrit).

Another improvement is the addition of an IBM CS-9000 laboratory computer system dedicated to data collection and analysis. This high-speed data collection system is of great value in all our measurements and will be of particular importance in studies with smaller vessels. Sarelius and Duling (1982) have described a technique of using tracer amounts of fluorescently labeled erythrocytes as indicators of the behavior of the total cell population. By diluting the marker particles, this technique obviates the coincidence problems which would make difficult use of flourescence in the determination of axial red cell flux in larger capillaries. The red cell flux can be readily obtained by counting the number of fluorescence optical pulses, and our system is being modified to do this. A third optical fiber and photomultiplier will be introduced and a more intense xenon arc used as a light source. Thus, Sarelius and Duling's method will be used as an independent check on the determinations of erythrocyte axial flux made from measurement of hematocrit and volumetric flow rate.

TREATMENT OF EXPERIMENTAL DATA

All the experiments discussed below involved deoxygenation of hemoglobin solutions or red cell suspensions during flow through the capillary system. The capillary wall oxygen flux was calculated directly from an oxygen material balance between measurements made at two adjacent axial positions in the capillary. Material balance requires knowledge at each of the two positions of (1) the mixed-mean hemoglobin oxygen saturation, and (2) the axial flux of erythrocytes (or overall flow rate in the case of homogenous hemoglobin solutions). The total volumetric flow rate is established directly from the rate of displacement of the microsyringe which controls the flow. Furthermore the "discharge" hematocrit can be determined by direct sampling of the effluent. The microspectrophotometric method yields a space-averaged oxygen saturation, not the mixed-mean concentration. Conversion from a space-averaged to a mixed-mean concentration requires detailed knowledge of the concentration and velocity profiles. These profiles can be estimated with sufficient accuracy from our theoretical work. Our calculations indicate that the two types of average concentrations differ by only a few percent. In the oxygen material balance we use the change in oxygen saturation between adjacent axial positions. This change amplifies the difference and there is a significant correction.

TREATMENT OF BOUNDARY CONDITIONS

It is important that the data be analyzed and interpreted in a way that is device-independent. In this work we are focusing attention on the oxygen transport in the blood, and the mass transfer Nusselt number is the variable of main interest. The Nusselt number, defined below, is a dimensionless parameter inversely related to resistance to oxygen transport in the blood.

$$Nu = \frac{fR}{(\bar{C} - C_W)D} \qquad (2)$$

where Nu is the Nusselt number
   f is the capillary wall flux
   R is the capillary radius
   C is the mixed-mean oxygen concentration in the capillary
   C_W is the oxygen concentration at the capillary wall
   D is the diffusivity coefficient for oxygen

Calculation of the Nusselt number from the experimental data requires knowledge of the capillary wall oxygen tension. The capillary wall oxygen flux and the oxygen tension outside the silicone rubber are known. The silicone rubber film which contains the capillary is rectangular in cross-section. Thus, accurate determination of the boundary concentration requires solving the diffusion equation in the rectangular (in cross-section) film of silicone rubber which surrounds the capillary. A sketch is given below with the dimensions of a typical capillary. The problem is treated as a two-dimensional Dirichlet problem. In other words, Laplace's equation is solved in the rubber film treating the capillary wall as at a uniform concentration.

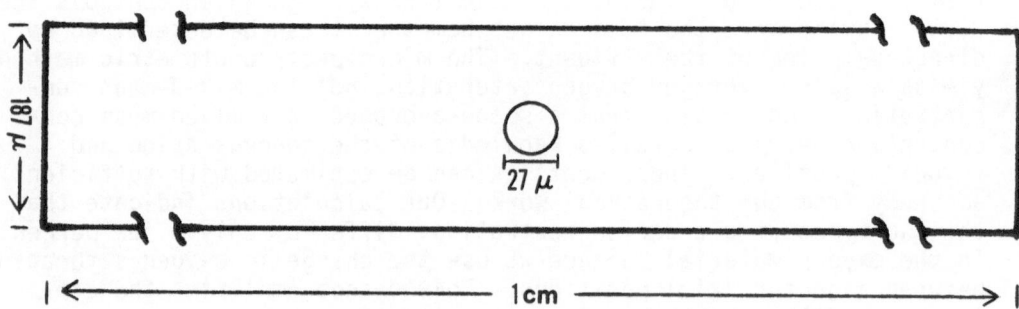

Figure 3. Typical Dimensions of Capillary Film Cross Section

Solutions to Laplace's equation for this configuration have been developed by several workers (Dugan, 1972, and Shih, 1970). A thorough treatment has been given by Balcerzak and Raynor (1961). From their work it is clear that the asymptotic solution for an infinitely wide strip is applicable. This solution can be expressed in a simple closed form:

$$\Delta P = \frac{1}{K}(fR\ln(2b/\pi R)) \qquad (3)$$

K is the permeability to oxygen
Δp is the overall drop in oxygen tension
b is the thickness of the silicone rubber film
R is the capillary radius
f is the capillary wall oxygen flux

Application of this formula indicates that the resistance to oxygen transport in the film is of the same order as that in the blood. This finding is important since if the resistance in the silicone film were dominant, it would not be possible to determine accurately the resistance in the blood.

We have found that there is surprisingly high degree of variability in values of the permeability of silicone rubber to oxygen reported in the literature. Values from 93×10^{-9} to 360×10^{-9} (ml O_2-cm)/(mm Hg-min-cm^2) (Heineken, et al, 1978; Stern, et al, 1978; Anon., 1968; Brondrup and Immergut, 1966) have been reported. Direct measurements with our films indicate a permeability higher than those indicated in the literature. We have concluded that the permeability depends heavily on the variables associated with casting technique, including extent of curing. Consequently, we measure the permeability of our films in the form in which they are cast.

RESULTS
Comparison with Theory

Oxygen transport in hemoglobin solutions during laminar flow in a cylindrical conduit can be posed as a system of second order non-linear partial differential equations. Analytical solution of this system is not possible. However, the system can be solved by numerical methods. Various simplifying assumptions in this mathematical model have been examined in our prior work, and a solution has been developed which appears to be on a firm basis (Yap, 1984). Thus, for the case of the hemoglobin solution the numerical solution can be looked upon as a method for testing and validating the experimental work.

TABLE I. OVERALL COMPARISON OF EXPERIMENTAL
AND THEORETICAL NUSSELT NUMBERS

Axial Distance from Entrance mm	Oxygen Saturation %	Wall Oxygen Flux X10^{10} g moles/(cm^2-sec)	Experimental Nusselt Number	Theoretical Nusselt Number
	Case I. 1.0 mM hemoglobin solution			
0	100			
1	93	6.38	3.2	2.5
2	85	6.55	3.7	2.7
3	82	3.37	2.0	2.9
4	78	3.70	2.6	3.1
Overall Average		$\overline{5.00}$	$\overline{2.9}$	$\overline{2.8}$
	Case II. 0.5 mM hemoglobin solution			
0	100			
1	90	4.92	1.5	2.3
2	80	4.80	2.9	2.4
3	75	3.03	2.1	2.4
4	67	4.17	3.9	2.5
Overall Average		$\overline{4.23}$	$\overline{2.6}$	$\overline{2.4}$

A preliminary comparison is given in Table I in terms of the Nusselt number at several axial positions These results are for a 27 μm diameter capillary with a flow of a hemoglobin solution as a rate of 9.4 μl/hr.

It should be noted that the variability in the experimental values is almost certainly due, at least in part, to nonspecific experimental errors. It should also be noted that the theory and experiment are not on exactly the same basis: The theory is for a uniform capillary wall oxygen flux, whereas the actual capillary wall oxygen flux varies with axial position in the experiment. It should also be noted that expressing results in terms of the Nusselt number tends to amplify errors in concentration determination, because the difference in capillary concentrations appears in the denominator as shown in Equation 2. Despite these factors the agreement between theory and experiment is gratifying. Thus, we gain confidence in our results on red cell suspensions in which case no theoretical results are possible without rather drastic simplifying assumptions.

Comparisons of Erythrocyte Suspensions with Hemoglobin Solutions

Figure 4 presents a direct comparison between oxygen saturation changes for an erythrocyte suspension and those for a hemoglobin solution. The difference is marked. Near the entrance to the capillary the rates of deoxygenation for the two cases differ by a factor of three. Since the flow rates, total hemoglobin concentration and other conditions of the two experiments were essentially the same, the marked differences in oxygen flux shown in Figure 4 represent a strong confirmation of two principal theses which were derived from our theoretical work (Hellums, 1977; Baxley and Hellums, 1984) (1) the resistance to oxygen transport in the blood is a significant fraction of the total resistance to oxygen transport in the microcirculation, and much higher than previously estimated. Most prior workers have neglected this resistance entirely. (2) The continuum approach seriously underestimates the resistance to oxygen transport in the microvascular system. Almost all workers who have taken the resistance into account in simulation of the microcirculation have used the continuum approach. The two curves of Figure 4 are a direct indication of difference between the transport properties of continuum (hemoglobin solution) and those of a suspension of erythrocytes.

The results of Figure 4 also confirm that O_2 diffusion through the silicone rubber bed cannot be limiting markedly the observed rates of gas exchange in the 27 μm capillary. If the permeability of the rubber were extremely small, no difference between the cell suspension and the hemoglobin solution would be observed. The high resistance to oxygen transport by the erythrocytes is due to both intra- and extracellular factors. The protein concentration inside

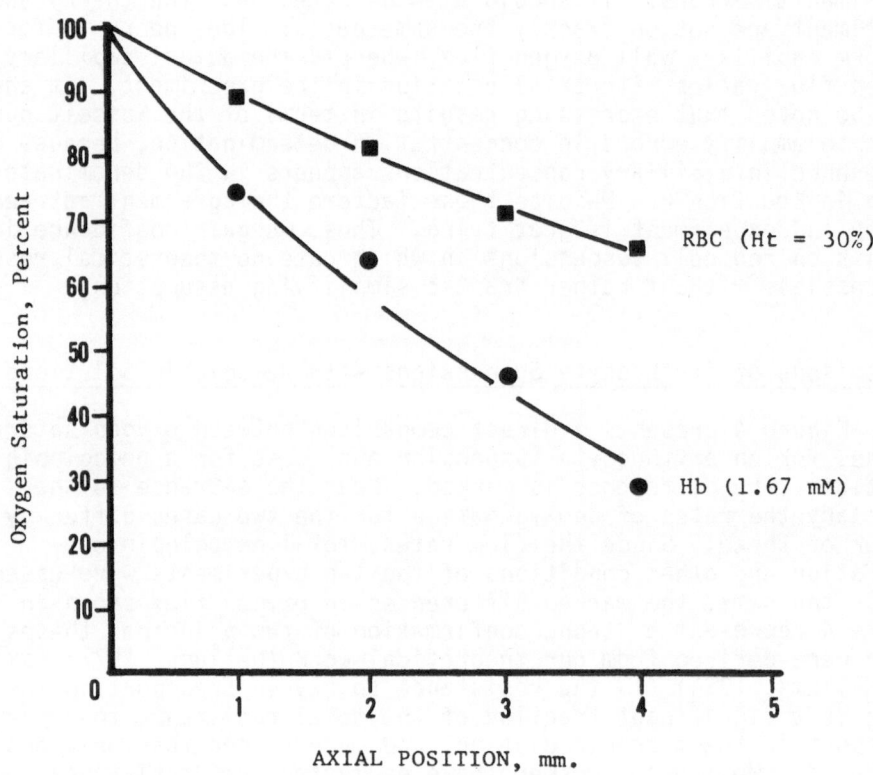

Figure 4. Comparison of Oxygen Release by Red Blood Cells with a
Hemoglobin Solution
Parameters are (1) Capillary diameter, 27 m; (1) flow,
11.5 l/hr; Capillary film thickness, 187 m; temperature,
27ºC; pH, 7.36; osmolarity, 275 mOsm.

the red cells is roughly 10 times greater than that in the hemoglobin solution. As a result, the intracellular O_2 diffusion constant is 2-3 times smaller than that in plasma or the 2 mM hemoglobin solution. Substantial resistance is also associated with external diffusion sublayers (diffusion boundary layers) which surround the red cells. In large capillaries, O_2 diffusion through these unstirred plasma layers will greatly decrease the apparent rates of oxygen uptake and release. This latter effect has been studied thoroughly by one of us in conventional stopped-flow, rapid mixing experiments and analyzed quantitatively using three-dimensional models and detailed hydrodynamic considerations (Coin and Olson, 1979; Vandegriff and Olson, 1984). In one sense, the results in Figure 4 represent an extension of these studies to the more physiological flowing capillary situation.

ACKNOWLEDGMENT

This work was supported by the National Institutes of Health under grant RO1 HL 19824, and by IBM under an equipment grant.

REFERENCES

Anon., 1968, Encyclopedia of Polymer Science and Technology 8: 630, J. Wiley and Sons.
Balcerzak, M.J., and Raynor, S., 1961, Steady state temperature distribution and heat flow in prismatic bars with isothermal boundary conditions,Int. J. Heat Transfer 3: 113-125.
Baxley, P. T., and Hellums, J. D., 1984, Simulation of oxygen transport in the microcirculation, Ann. Biomed. Eng., in press.
Boland, E. J., Unno, H., Olson, J. S., and Hellums, J. D., 1984, An in-vitro method for simulation of oxygen transport in the microcirculation, Proceedings of International Society on Oxygen Transport to Tissues Meeting, Plenum Publishing Corp., in press.
Coin,, J. T., and Olson, J. S., 1979, The rate of oxygen uptake by human red blood cells, J. Bio. Chem., 254, 1178-1190.
Dugan, J. F., 1972, On the shape factor for a hollow, square cylinder, Am. Inst. Chem. Engrs. J. 18: 1082-1083.
Hellums, J. D., 1977, The resistance to oxygen transport in the capillaries relative to that in the surrounding tissue, Microvascular Res., 13, 131-136.
Olson, J. S., 1981, Rapid mixing measurements of ligand binding data, Methods in Enzymology, 76: 631-651.
Pittman, R. N., and Duling, B. R., 1975a, A new method for the measurement of percent oxyhemoglobin, J. Appl. Physiol. 38: 315-320.

Pittman, R. N., and Duling, B. R., 1975b, Measurement of percent oxy-hemoglobin in the microvasculature, J. Appl. Physiol. 38: 321-327.

Pries, A. R., Kanzow, G., and Gaehtgens, P., 1983, Microphotometric determination of hematocrit in small vessels, Am. J. Physiol., 245 (Heart Circ. Physiol. 14): H167-H177.

Sarelius, I. H. and Duling, B., 1982, Direct measurement of micro-vessel hematocrit, red cell flux, velocity, and transit time, Am. J. Physiol.,243 (Heart Circ. Physiol. 12): H1018-H1026.

Shih, F. S., 1970, On the temperature field of a square column embedding a heating cyclinder, Am. Inst. Chem. Engrs. J. 16: 134-138. See also a correction, Ibid, 16, 1109.

Sinha, A. K., 1969, O_2 uptake and release by red cells through capillary wall and plasma layer, Ph.D. Thesis in Physiology, University of California, San Francisco, CA.

Vandegriff, K. and Olson, J. S., 1984, A quantitative description in three dimensions of oxygen uptake by human red blood cells, Biophys, J., 45, 825-835.

Yap, E., 1984, Mathematical Modeling of oxygen transport in the microcirculation , M.S. Thesis in Chemical Engineering, Rice University.

936

ASSESSMENT OF CEREBRAL OXYGENATION VIA THE CONJUNCTIVA

S. Faithfull*, H. vd Zee**, W. Erdmann*, T. Kuypers***,
M. Dhasmana* and P. Kimmich****

Departments of Anaesthesia, Erasmus University
Rotterdam, The Netherlands* and Albany Medical College
New York, USA**; Honeywell Medical Electronics, Best
The Netherlands*** and Department of Physiology
University of Nijmegen, The Netherlands****

The first membrane-covered polarographic cell was introduced
by Clark (1956) and since that time many refinements in oxygen
polarography have occurred. As a result accurate measurements can
now be made in a great variety of situations. Nevertheless,
continuous on line assessment of arterial oxygen partial pressure
(PaO_2) has not yet been realised. A method of performing this is
particularly needed in the operating theatre or in situations,
such as the intensive care unit, where the critically ill patient
is being treated. The technique should preferably be non-invasive
and apparatus should be simple and robust enough to be used by
technicians and nursing staff alike.

An early electrode for on line estimation of oxygen tension in
the capillary bed of the palpebral conjunctiva ($PconO_2$) was
developed by Kwan and Fatt (1971), but this had a response time of
up to 2 minutes and was therefore not suitable for detection of
sudden changes in the physiological state of the patient. The
clinical use of a conjunctival PO_2 electrode has recently been
described by Yelderman (1983) but no mention of response speed was
made. It was stated that PaO_2 was always higher than conjunctival
oxygen tension $PconO_2$. Doubt exists as to whether $PconO_2$ and
PaO_2 are in fact closely related (Andriano et al.1984) and this
paper reports our own experimental results using a recently
produced microchip PO_2 conjunctival sensor (Honeywell Medical
Electronics).

937

METHODS

Studies were performed on anaesthestised Wistar rats in which unconsciousness had been produced using a gas mixture of 33 per cent oxygen in nitrous oxide and to which 0.5 percent halothane vapour had been added from a Cyprane Fluotec Mark III vapouriser. After a tracheostomy had been performed, the animals were ventilated to normal end expiratory carbon dioxide tensions (as measured on a Godart Type 1467 capnograph) using a Loosco Amsterdam infant ventilator. Muscular relaxation was achieved by the administration of pancuronium bromide, at a rate of 0.4 mg per hour; this was delivered by a Braun Melsungen Perfusor apparatus.

Arterial blood pressure was monitored using a 1 mm diameter catheter that had been introduced into the femoral artery. The pressure signals were transduced by a Gould P23 pressure transducer and, after amplification through a Grass 7B polygraph, were displayed on an inkwriting oscillograph. Blood gas and acid/base values were regularly estimated using a Radiometer ABL 1 acid/base laboratory. The oxygen sensor was applied between the upper eyelid and cornea, the chip facing the palpebral conjunctiva, and the eyelids were sewn closed.

Inspiratory oxygen concentration (FIO_2) was measured using an Instrumentation Laboratory Oxygen Monitor 404 and was varied between 0.2 and 0.5. Arterial blood samples were taken for blood gas estimation at the end of a 15 minute period of ventilation at each FIO_2. In some animals hypotension was induced to further investigate the responses of the sensor. Other rats were hyper-ventilated, or hypoventilated, to ascertain if changes in cerebral circulation which would be produced by changes in partial pressure of carbon dioxide would be reflected in the oxygenation of the palpebral conjunctival capillary bed.

The conjunctival oxygen sensor

The sensor is constructed using the principle of the ring-shaped cathode system as described by Kimmich and Kreuzer (1969) and was incorporated by constructing two rectangular spirals (Kimmich,1978). In this manner it was possible to combine the small width of the cathode, which determines the sensitivity of the polarographic cell to oxygen flux, with a relatively large total cathode area, and thus stronger electrode current. This has several advantages, such as small zero current and improved stability - two factors which are difficult to achieve in miniaturized microelectrodes.

The gold cathode and the silver anode are vapor-deposited on a silicon substrate, while a silicon-oxide layer is used for insulation between the electrodes. A porous cross-linked polymer

938

matrix between the cathode/ anode system and the rubber membrane
serves as carrier for the electrolyte. The polymer matrix, the
electrolyte and the membrane were all applied by spin coating.
The electrode is activated just prior to use by equilibrating in
saline. This procedure has several advantages, but it obviously
restricts applicability of the cell for the measurement of oxygen
in a completely fluid medium.

The cable is only 140 microns in diameter, protected by a
teflon tube, and fastened to the chip by ultrasonic bonding
techniques. The dimensions of the chip are 0.7 mm x 3.7 mm and it
has a thickness of 0.4 mm. The whole is embedded in a flap of
silicon rubber in such a way that the membrane of the chip is in
direct contact with the inner surface of the eyelid. This flap is
45 mm long, 4 mm wide and 0.5 mm thick, thus enabling it to be
fixed directly onto the skin adjacent to the eye. The soft
surface of the pliable rubber is in contact with the eyeball so
there is no danger of damaging the surface of the eyeball.

Prior to application, the O_2 sensor was calibrated in 0.9
NaCl equilibrated with air. The electrode current was fed into a
Philips XV 1506 amplifier system, and conjunctival oxygen tension
was continuously recorded using a Philips PM 822 pen recorder.

RESULTS

The responses of the subconjunctival oxygen sensor to stepwise
alterations in FIO_2 are shown in Fig 1. It can be seen that the
ouput from the sensor correlated reasonably well with expected
changes in PaO_2 and that a rapid response time was present. Fig. 2
demonstrates the relationship between PaO_2 and conjunctival
oxygen tension - the regression line is drawn in. Good correlation
exists between the two parameters and the correlation coefficient
is statistically significant at 0.93. However, the sensor appeared
to give better indications of PaO_2 in the normal and hypoxic
range than in the hyperoxic range. When figures were examined for
both of these ranges it was seen that the correlation coefficient
was 0.81 in each instance - this is statistically significant.
However, the slope was 0.93 in the lower range but only 0.55 in
the hyperoxic range.

Fig. 3 demonstrates response of the O_2 sensor to injection of
ketamine hydrochloride into the cisterna magna of rats. Also shown
are effects of withdrawal of blood and subsequent reinfusion of
either blood or 0.5 per cent saline solution. It can be seen that
the $PconO_2$ closely parallels ensuing changes in mean arterial
pressure. The effects of halothane induced hypotension on $PconO_2$
are illustrated in Fig 4. Also illustrated are subsequent changes

produced by intra-cisternal ketamine. The decrease in conjunctival PO_2 following halothane was clearly less than that for ketamine induced hypotension. This would indicate that vasodilation produced by halothane was maintaining better microcirculatory perfusion during severe hypotension than during falls in systemic blood pressure produced by ketamine.

The effects of hyperventilation, hypoventilation and temporary apnoea are demonstrated in Fig 5. Hyperventilation was produced by increasing the tidal volume on the Loosco Ventilator and results in a rapid rise of $PconO_2$. Continued hyperventilation does not maintain this improvement in oxygenation of the conjunctival tissue and one can observe a slow decline below the original base-line level. This may be the result of a vaso-constrictor effect of low carbon dioxide tensions. It is interesting to note that this effect reached a maximum value and was followed by a slight increase in conjunctival PO_2 readings - this may indicate an altered vascular response to very low $PaCO_2$ (hypoxic vasodilation). Also shown in this figure is the occurrence of temporary apnoea which produces an immediate fall in the $PconO_2$ response. Following hyperventilation, the animal was hypoventilated and this resulted in a fall of PaO_2 to 39 mm Hg and a concomitant rise in $PaCO_2$ to 60 mm Hg. An immediate decrease of conjunctival PO_2 values was seen, followed by a slow increase which was probably due to the vasodilatory effects of the rising $PaCO_2$.

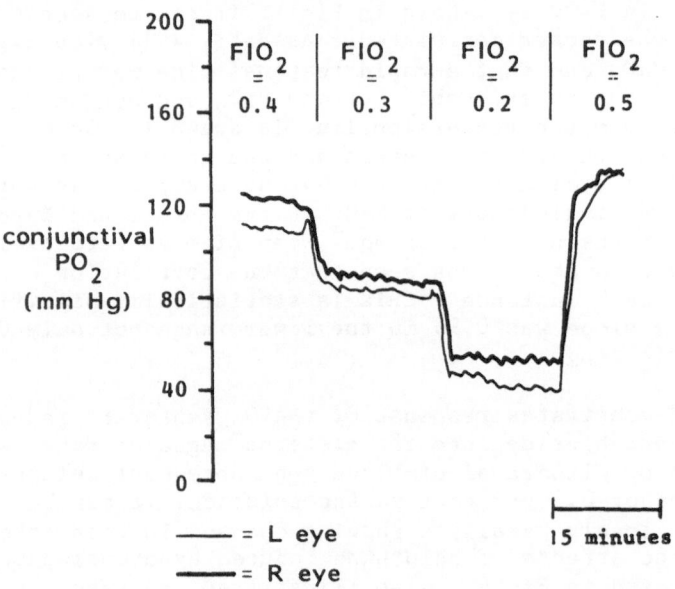

Figure 1. Responses of the subconjunctival oxygen sensor to stepwise alterations in fractional inspired oxygen concentrations (FIO_2).

940

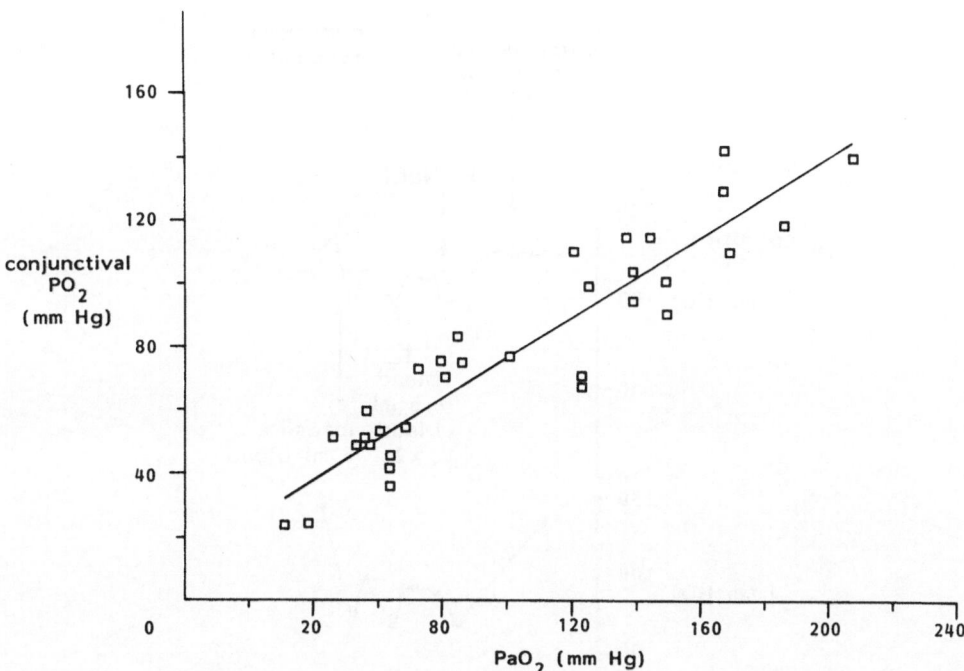

Figure 2. The relationship between arterial oxygen tension (PaO_2) and conjunctival oxygen tension. The regression line is drawn in, the correlation coefficient is 0.93.

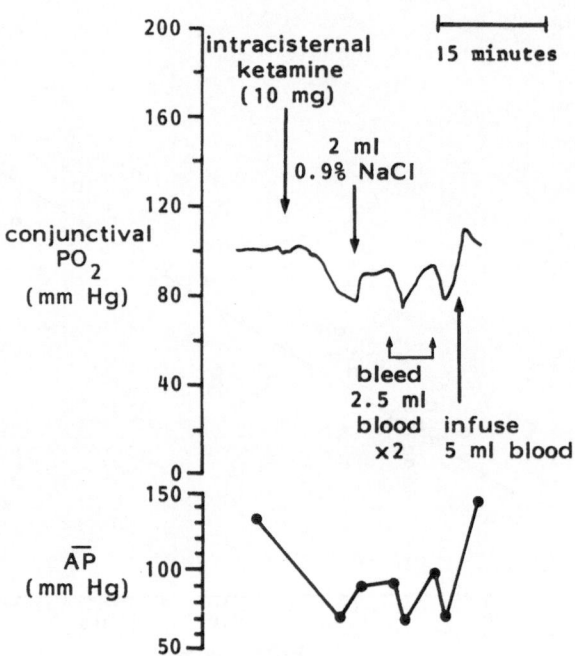

Figure 3. The influence of intracisternal ketamine, intravenous administration of 0.9 per cent NaCl, bleeding and reinfusion of blood on the mean systolic pressure (AP) and on conjunctical (PO_2).

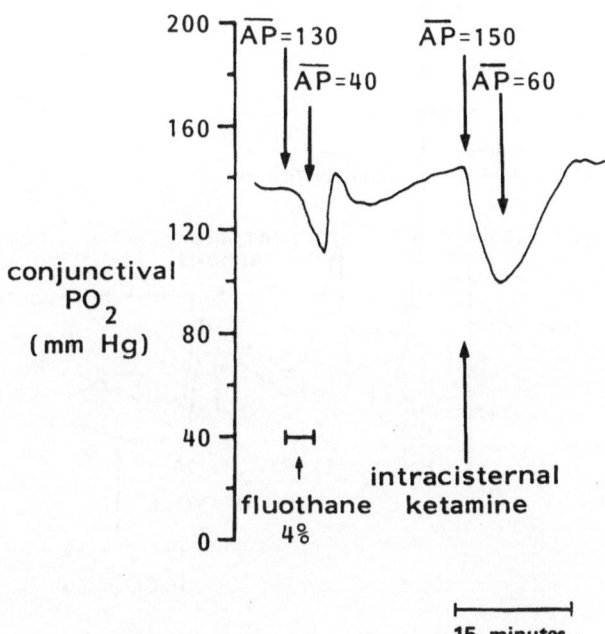

Figure 4. The effects of halothane induced hypotension on $P_{con}O_2$.

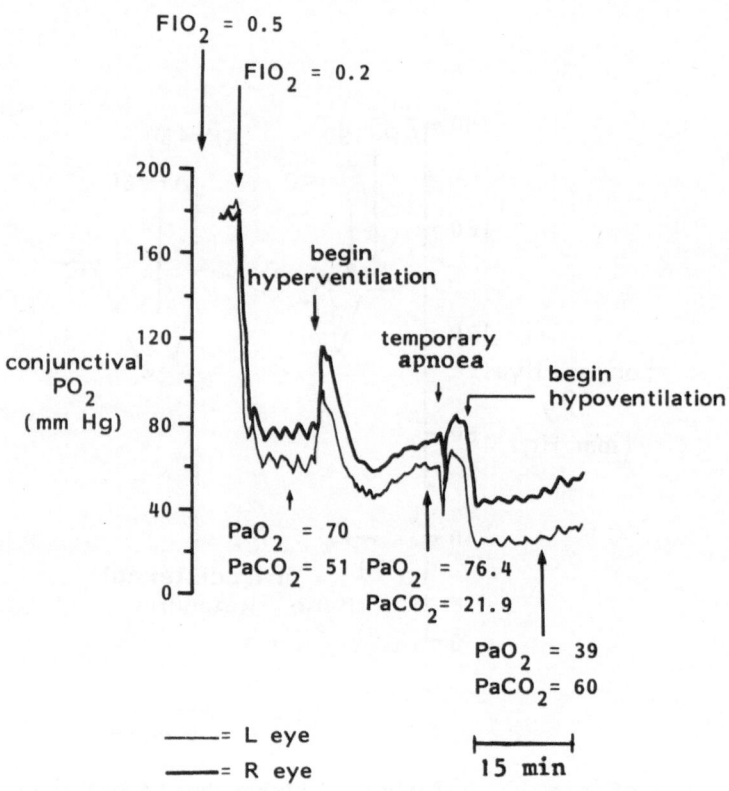

Figure 5. The effects of hyperventialtion, apnoea and hypoventilation on subconjunctival oxygen tension.

DISCUSSION

The solid state O_2 sensor used in our experiments proved to be a reasonably accurate sensor of the state of conjunctival tissue oxygenation and there was a high correlation between $PconO_2$ and PaO_2. The question naturally arises as to why the response was observed to be less sensitive and the slope relationship between the two values was less when PaO_2 was in the hyperoxic range. The answers to this problem may lie in both the anatomical derivation and the physiological function of the capillary bed of the palpebral conjunctiva.

The internal carotid artery has as its first branch, the ophthalmic artery which provides the blood supply to the eyeball, developmentally an integral part of the brain, and other intraorbital structures. It also supplies the palpebral conjunctiva with blood, via the medial palpebral artery and the lateral palpebral branch of the lacrimal artery (Gray,1958).

The conjunctiva possesses a dense vascular bed with the conjunctival capillaries located very close to the surface layers, hence minimising the distance over which oxygen must diffuse to oxygenate the cornea when the eyelids are closed and the cornea is no longer able to obtain its oxygen directly from the ambient air. It is tempting to suggest that the blood vessels in the conjunctiva will react to various physiological conditions in the same way as do blood vessels in the cerebral circulation. Hence vasoconstriction will be caused by hyperoxia and by hyperventilation; this would explain the reactions of the oxygen sensor that were observed under these conditions. Similarly, hypoventilation and carbon dioxide retention would result in release of vasoconstrictive tone and improved microcirculation and oxygenation of both the cerebral and conjunctival vessels. It might also be postulated that the relatively low PO_2 in the conjunctiva in the presence of hyperoxic PaO_2's should be considered as a protective mechanism that defends the cornea against the effects of oxygen toxicity.

From the manner and degree to which the sensor responds to alterations in PaO_2 and haemodynamic conditions, it is suggested that the electrode is reflecting changes in cerebral oxygen flux. Kwan and Hunt (1973) have maintained that a change in the oxygen carrying capacity of the blood has no effect on the $PconO_2$. However, it is quite possible that, in their studies employing

haemodilution with low molecular weight dextran,the cardiac output
of the experimental animals (rabbits) was, due to the decrease in
blood viscosity, increased to the extent that total cerebral
oxygen flux was unchanged.

Further experiments are of course required in order to prove
or disprove the above hypothesis and work is underway to this end.
Radioactive microspheres are being used to estimate regional
perfusion in rats. Measurements of PaO_2 and oxyhaemoglobin
saturation then enable cerebral oxygen flux to be calculated.
Early results suggest that a relationship may well exist between
this flux and $PconO_2$ within the individual animal, but sample
numbers are not yet of a magnitude to permit statistical analysis.

REFERENCES

Andriano KP, Pace NL, Wilbrink J, Zwanikken P, Stanley TH, 1984,
    Intraoperative transcutaneous PO_2 ($TcPO_2$) monitoring quanti-
    tates PaO_2. Fact or fiction? Anesth Analg, 63: 178.
Clark LC Jr, 1956, Monitor and control of blood and tissue oxygen
    tension, Trans Am Soc Artif Intern Organs, 2: 41-48.
Gray, H, 1958, in: "Gray's Anatomy", 32nd edition, T.B. Johnson
    et al., eds., Longmans, Green and Co, London, New York and
    Toronto.
Kimmich HP and Kreuzer F, 1969, Catheter PO_2 electrode with low
    flow dependency and fast response, in: Oxygen Pressure Recor-
    ding in Gases, Fluids, and Tissues, F. Kreuzer, ed., Progress
    in Respiration Research, Vol. 3, H. Herzog, Series Editor,
    S. Karger, Basel and New York, 100-110.
Kimmich HP, 1978, Oxygen monitoring in blood and gases, in:
    International Workshop on Biomedical Transducers and
    Measurements, Madrid, 17.
Kwan M and Fatt I, 1971, A noninvasive method of continuous
    arterial oxygen tension estimation from measured palpebral
    conjunctival oxygen tension, Anesthesiology, 35: 309-314.
Kwan MR and Hunt TK, 1973, Continuous tissue oxygen tension
    measurements during acute blood loss, J Surg Res, 14: 420-425.
Yelderman M, 1983, Transconjunctival oxygen measurements in
    critical care medicine, Anesthesiology, 59: 266-267.

INFLUENCE OF CO_2 ON POLAROGRAPHIC OXYGEN SENSORS

H.P. Kimmich, F. Kreuzer and J. Spaan

Department of Physiology, University of Nijmegen
P.O. Box 9101
NL-6500 HB Nijmegen, The Netherlands

INTRODUCTION

For the assessment of oxygen transport to tissue, both for physiological research and clinical routine monitoring, continuous measurement of PO_2 is essential. Both during in vitro and in vivo experiments oxygen is generally not present alone but is in close relation to other blood gases, especially CO_2. It is thus important to know and understand the effects of variable CO_2 concentrations on the oxygen measurement.

Polarographic oxygen cells are well known to be sensitive, besides to oxygen itself, also to a number of other variables like temperature, flow of the medium, acceleration, CO_2 and anesthetic gases. The influence of most of these variables on the polarographic reduction of oxygen is typical for the polarographic process and can be well described both qualitatively and quantitatively (temperature, flow, acceleration). In spite of this fact only 4 out of 42 publications (Kreuzer et al., 1980), describing catheter O_2 electrodes between 1953 and 1979, also give details on CO_2 sensitivity. Three electrodes (Soutter et al., 1975; De Haas, 1977; Parker et al., 1978) claim no CO_2 sensitivity of their oxygen cells. Kimmich et al. (1975) found a CO_2 effect corresponding to about 2 mm Hg of PO_2 for physiological concentrations of CO_2.

CO_2 sensitivity of polarographic cells is not a characteristic of polarography itself but, especially in miniaturized versions, is typical for individual types of electrodes and, more importantly, may even differ substantially for a single transducer, particularly if it is frequently used over prolonged periods of time. So far two basically different mechanisms of influence of CO_2 on polarographic

947

oxygen electrodes have been found, namely a direct influence on the pH of the electrolyte, and an indirect influence on the oxygen reduction.

CHANGE OF pH OF THE ELECTROLYTE BY CO_2

When CO_2 diffuses into the electrolyte of polarographic oxygen cells it shifts the pH of the electrolyte to lower values, resulting in a horizontal shift of the diffusion-limited (flat) part of the polarogram, the so-called "plateau", to lower voltages. The slope, mean current and extension over the voltage range of the polarographic "plateau" remain practically unchanged.

By using buffer solutions as electrolytes this effect can be substantially reduced, especially in oxygen electrodes with wide and flat polarographic "plateaus". In miniaturized versions, e.g. in catheter oxygen cells, the amount of electrolyte in the vicinity of the cathode is generally very small and thus only able to buffer a small amount of diffused CO_2. The buffer solution involved at the cathode is then renewed by solution from the main buffer reservoir at slow rates typical of the type of electrode. This leads to an equilibrium situation for each constant CO_2 flux with a pH drop from the main electrolyte reservoir to the site of the oxygen reduction. The magnitude of this drop depends (non-linearly) on the amount of CO_2 diffusing into the oxygen cell.

A small pH shift, resulting in a small horizontal shift of the polarogram, has little influence on the electrode current. A small influence (less than 1% of the reading) may be found because of the not quite horizontal current–voltage curves of polarographic cells at the polarization point. This small effect is often negligible and may have been considered as no CO_2 effect by most electrode designers (Soutter et al., 1975; De Haas, 1977; and Parker et al., 1978). Larger influences may be found as soon as the amount of CO_2 diffusing into the system exceeds a certain critical level, resulting in a shift of the polarographic plateau to values outside the polarization region. This means practically no influence of CO_2 up to a certain concentration of CO_2 in the measuring medium and a strong influence at higher concentrations. It should be noted that the maximum acceptable amount of CO_2 in the medium also depends on variables such as membrane thickness and temperature. In a critical situation the CO_2 sensitivity may easily become ten times as high when decreasing the membrane thickness by a factor of two (in order to improve the transient response of the oxygen cell), e.g. from a 6 μ Teflon membrane to a 3 μ Teflon membrane (Küchler et al., 1978). Possible CO_2 effects thus show more clearly in fast oxygen cells. In spite of the more complex behavior in miniaturized oxygen cells, the effect of CO_2 on the pH of the electrolyte is well understood and can generally be reduced to a level influencing the electrode current only slightly.

CHANGE OF OXYGEN REDUCTION PROPERTIES BY CO_2

When CO_2 diffuses into the electrolyte of polarographic oxygen electrodes, it may alter also the chemistry of oxygen reduction at the cathode.

In miniaturized versions of polarographic oxygen electrodes, the reduction process is still not entirely understood. All basic studies on the polarographic reduction of oxygen have been done in open systems with relatively thick electrolyte layers, either on the dropping mercury electrode or on solid electrodes. The chemical reactions are quite complex, and different possible solutions have been described by different authors (e.g. Delahay, 1950; Vielstich, 1958; and Vetter, 1961). They have in common a full four-electron reduction for each reduced O_2 molecule with an overall reaction as:

$$O_2 + H_2O + 4e^- \rightleftharpoons 4OH^- \tag{1}$$

In miniaturized electrodes this simple reaction is complicated by a partial lack of reversibility and by the presence of partial react-ions. The partial reactions, depending on many factors such as cathode surface composition and smoothness (adsorption of species, oxide formation), temperature, bacteriological contamination, pH, composition of the electrolyte, and polarization voltage, prevent a full four-electron reaction, as may be easily checked by comparing cathode size, membrane, and current of the major catheter oxygen electrodes. The main reason for the deviation from a four-electron reduction is the intermediary occurrence of H_2O_2 or HO_2^-:

$$O_2 + H_2O + 2e^- \rightleftharpoons HO_2^- + OH^- \tag{2}$$

HO_2^- may be further reduced according to:

$$HO_2^- + H_2O + 2e^- \rightleftharpoons 3OH^- \tag{3}$$

leading again to an overall reaction with a four-electron reduction, or may be decomposed according to:

$$HO_2^- \longrightarrow \tfrac{1}{2} O_2 + OH^- \tag{4}$$

The half oxygen molecule produced according to equation (4) is ge-nerally lost for further reduction at the cathode, leading to an overall reaction with a two-electron reduction. Practically both types of oxygen reduction occur simultaneously in miniaturized electrodes, leading to consumption of two to four electrons for each oxygen molecule.

A direct influence of CO_2 on the oxygen reduction process may be avoided by choosing appropriate electrolyte compositions. Un-changed composition is guaranteed by oxidizing the anode (rather than chloridizing it) and/or frequent renewal of the electrolyte solution. Management of the influence of CO_2 on the cathode condition is more difficult, especially in aged cathodes, if the electrodes are used over prolonged periods of time. It is likely that the presence of CO_2 contributes to the ageing of the cathode. The vertical shift of the polarogram due to the shift of the cathode reaction from four- to two-electron reduction is most significant with small (1 to 4%) values of CO_2 whereas higher values do not add much more to this shift.

This shift from a four- to two-electron reduction depends on many factors and is also catalyzed by components produced during the four-electron reduction. This means that with high concentrations of oxygen a two-electron reduction is more likely. Practically, this may not only lead to a non-linear calibration line at high oxygen values but also to a much stronger influence of CO_2 at high oxygen concentrations. Lackermann et al. (1983) have demonstrated that electrodes with marked CO_2 sensitivity at 21% oxygen show almost no sensitivity to CO_2 at 5% oxygen.

PRACTICAL TESTING

To get more insight into the behavior of miniaturized oxygen electrodes concerning their sensitivity to CO_2, a number of electrodes (Kimmich and Kreuzer, 1969) have been tested three times over a period of 13 years, namely after production in 1971/1972, ten years later and finally in 1984. The electrodes showed only sensitivity to CO_2 due to the change in pH of the electrolyte in 1971, with a maximum reversible error of up to 1% for physiological values of CO_2 (up to approx. 5% CO_2) as shown in figure 1.

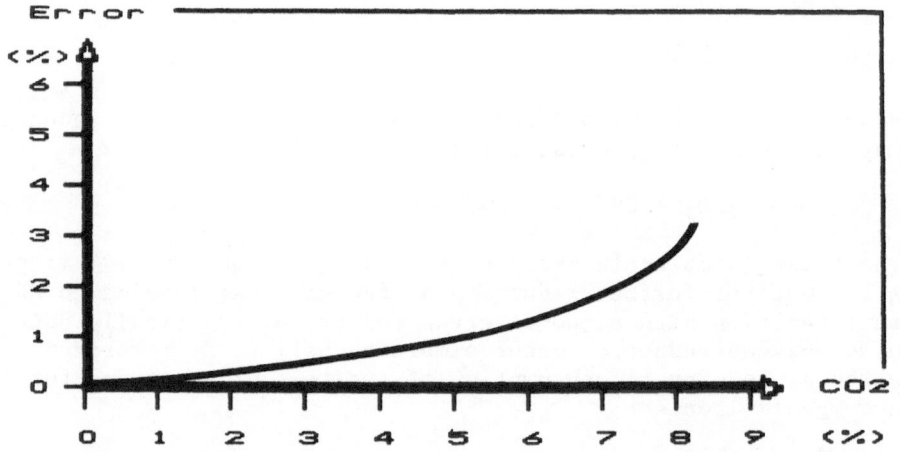

Fig. 1: CO_2 sensitivity of a miniaturized polarographic oxygen cell measured in 1971, shortly after its production.

950

For the practical testing, gases from cylinders were mixed with the aid of one or two Wösthoff gas pumps. In 1971 gases from different cylinders were used and in 1984 only one Wösthoff pump was available. This did lead to slight variations in oxygen supply (20 ± 1%). This slight variation in oxygen concentration was obviously compensated for, and should not have had any qualitative influence on the measured effect and only a negligible quantitative influence.

In 1979/1980 incorrect measurements with electrodes from the 1971 serie were detected, leading eventually to an extensive testing for CO_2 sensitivity in 1981 (Lackermann et al., 1983). The result showed a clear sensitivity to CO_2 according to the oxygen reduction mechanism (fig. 2). The figure gives the mean of several measurements with a representative transducer. The other oxygen electrodes showed qualitatively identical CO_2 effects of similar magnitudes.

The CO_2 effect on the oxygen electrodes was also tested for other concentrations than 21%. With lower concentrations the effect gradually decreased, reaching virtually zero at 5% oxygen.

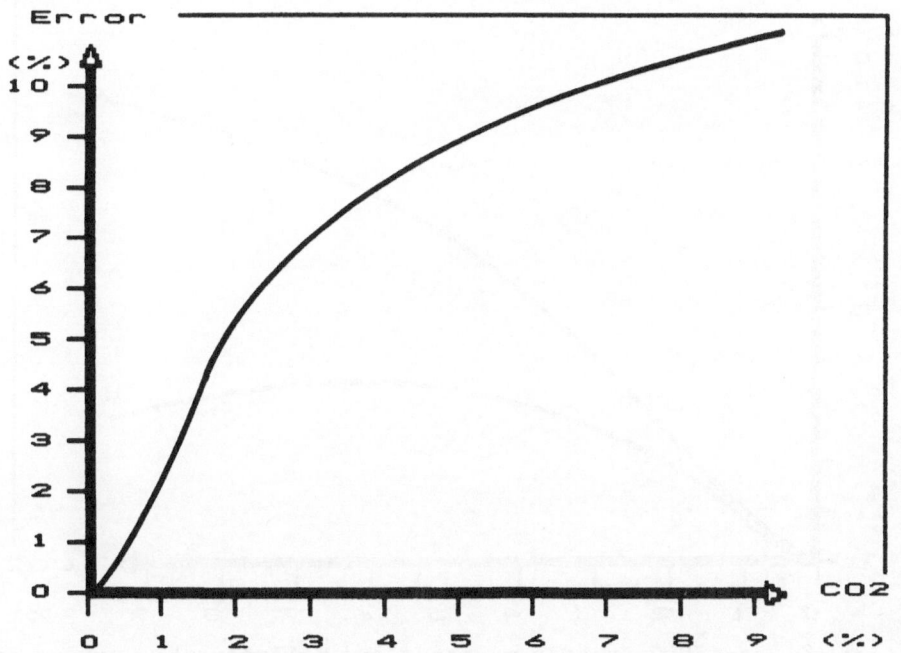

Fig. 2: CO_2 sensitivity of a miniaturized polarographic oxygen cell measured in 1981 (10 years after production) after extensive use in vitro and in vivo. Note the qualitative and quantitative difference as compared to the measurement in 1971 (fig. 1).

At higher concentrations of oxygen the CO_2 effect was not markedly increased. At even higher concentrations of CO_2, up to 100%, which are not found physiologically and clinically, the CO_2 effect was slightly different from that in the discussed standard conditions but the effect tended to decrease with increasing CO_2 concentrations. At these high concentrations the left shift of the polarogram, due to pH change of the electrolyte, may partly cancel the effect of the oxygen reduction mechanism which, on its own, leads to a downward and left shift. There is no influence of CO_2 on the "nitrogen current" of polarographic cells.

In 1984 the electrodes showed a similar CO_2 effect as in 1981 (fig. 3). At the same time the influence of cathode treatment is shown (curve B, fig. 3).

Unfortunately it is not known when the electrodes first started to show CO_2 sensitivity according to the second mechanism. It is likely that this occurred only after several years, because incorrect measurements of oxygen were detected only in 1979/1980.

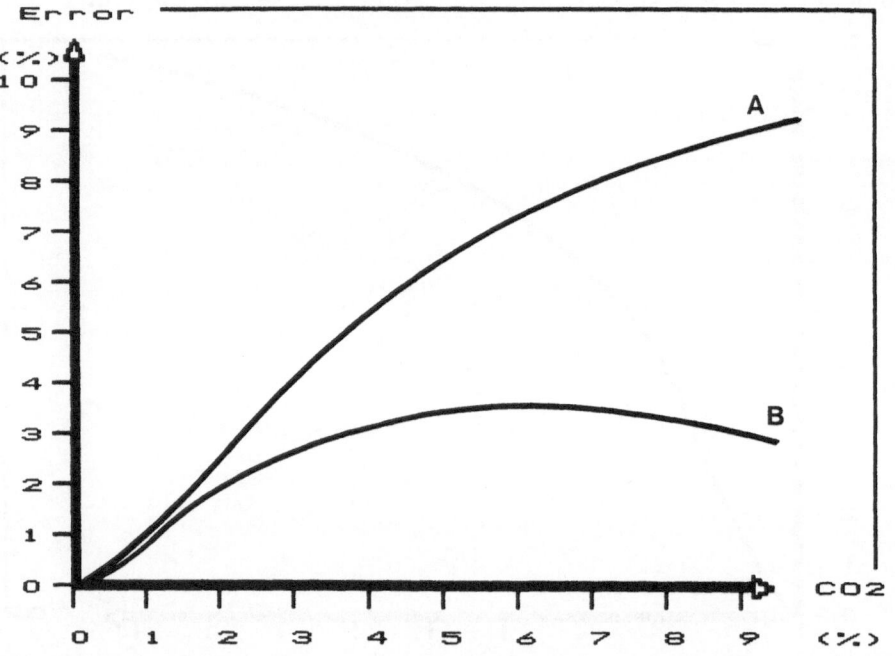

Fig. 3: CO_2 sensitivity of a miniaturized polarographic oxygen cell measured in 1984, 13 years after production (curve A). A marked quantitative improvement may be achieved by polishing the cathode surface (curve B) without, however, approaching the curve obtained shortly after production of the electrode (fig. 1).

DISCUSSION

The buffer solution was identical in all trials, i.e., a phosphate buffer adjusted to pH 8. It is therefore most likely that the change in the response to CO_2 was mainly due to the ageing of the cathodes. Therefore it was tried to improve the properties of the electrodes by exposing the cathode surface to positive polarization voltage, chemical agents and repolishing. All these interventions had only a quantitative but not qualitative effect. In some cases reduction of the CO_2 sensitivity to less than half its value was possible (fig. 3, curve B). It should be noted that repolishing of these electrodes with PVC insulation is difficult and can never be performed perfectly.

It is also astonishing that the polarogram did not show any significant changes in the period from 1971 to 1981, when the changes in CO_2 behavior occurred. From the polarograms measured before the 1981 testing, a clean single-metal cathode could be predicted. It is thus likely that the impaired "smoothness" of the platinum cathode acts, in the presence of CO_2, as a catalyzer for the two-electron reduction of oxygen.

CONCLUSIONS

The behavior of miniaturized polarographic cells concerning their sensitivity to CO_2 depends on many factors and may be substantially different with various types of electrodes, especially in miniaturized versions. In addition, these properties may change with time, either due to a change in composition of the electrolyte, which can be avoided with proper sensor design, or due to the change in cathode surface conditions. The CO_2 sensitivity of polarographic cells should therefore be tested frequently, or the electrode should be calibrated in gases or solutions containing CO_2 in a concentration similar to that expected in the experimental situation.

Reaction to CO_2 occurs with a delay of several seconds compared to the fast transient response of the sensor to oxygen. Fast changes of CO_2 are thus not detected, whereas changes of oxygen at the same rate can easily be detected. A shift of the calibration line can be avoided by in vivo calibration which is possible because CO_2 does not affect the nitrogen current. Future composition of electrolytes for polarographic cells should aim at preventing a derangement of the ratio of four- and two-electron reduction due to effects of CO_2, which obviously is not easy.

Measuring systems containing an automatic gain control, such as in continuous assessment of respiratory PO_2 with readjustment of the gain during the inspiratory phase (Kimmich and Kandelaars, 1980), also correct properly for any CO_2 effect.

REFERENCES

Delahay, P., 1950, A polarographic method for the indirect determination of polarization curves for oxygen reduction on various metals. I. Description of the method – Case of platinum. J. Electrochem. Soc. 97:198–212.

Haas, De, P.W., 1977, De ontwikkeling en toepassing van een zuurstofelectrode voor het continu meten van de intra-arteriële zuurstofspanning bij pasgeborenen met ademhalingsproblemen. Thesis, Rotterdam, 128 pp.

Kimmich, H.P., and Kreuzer, F., 1969, Catheter PO_2 electrode with low flow dependency and fast response. in: Progr. Resp. Res. 3, F. Kreuzer, ed., H. Herzog, Series ed., Karger, Basel: pp 100–110.

Kimmich, H.P., Kreuzer, F., and Spaan, J.G., 1975, Rapid blood oxygen transducer, mounted on a 1.2 mm catheter. Biocapt. 75:307–312.

Kimmich, H.P., and Kandelaars, J.J., 1980, Calculation of oxygen uptake from continuously telemetered flow and PO_2 with the aid of a 8085 microprocessor, in: Biotelemetry V, G. Matsumoto and H.P. Kimmich, eds., Sapporo, pp 229–234.

Kreuzer, F., Kimmich, H.P., and Brezina, M., 1980, Polarographic determination of oxygen in biological materials, in: Medical and Biological Applications of Electrochemical Devices, J. Koryta, ed., John Wiley & Sons Ltd., Chichester – New York – Brisbane – Toronto, Chapter 6, pp 173–261.

Küchler, G., Wagner, W., and Wolburg, I., 1978, Experimental study on errors in dynamic measurement of oxygen intake, in: Biotelemetry IV, H.-J. Klewe and H.P. Kimmich, eds., Braunschweig, pp 109–112.

Lackermann, E.M., Kreuzer, F., Folk, G.E., Jr., and Kimmich, H.P., 1983, The measurement of pO_2 by O_2 electrode in the presence of changing pCO_2. Proc. Iowa Acad. Sci. 90:141–143.

Parker, D., Delpy, D., and Lewis, M., 1978, Catheter-tip electrode for continuous measurement of pO_2 and pCO_2. Med. Biol. Eng. Comput. 16:599–600.

Soutter, L.P., Conway, M.J., and Parker, D., 1975, A system for monitoring arterial oxygen tensions in sick newborn babies. Biomed. Eng. 10:257:260.

Vetter, K.J., 1961, Elektrochemische Kinetik. Springer-Verlag, Berlin.

Vielstich, W., 1958, Zum Mechanismus der Sauerstoffelektrode in alkalischem Elektrolyten. Z. physik. Chem. Neue Folge 15: 409–428.

OXYGEN TRANSFER FROM GAS BUBBLE INTO LIQUID

M. Riethues[+], H. Baumgärtl[*], R. Buchholz[+],
U. Onken[+], and D.W. Lübbers[*]

[+] Lehrstuhl Technische Chemie B, Abt. Chemietechnik
    Universität Dortmund, FRG
[*] Max-Planck-Institut für Systemphysiologie
    4600 Dortmund 1, FRG

SUMMARY

Oxygen transfer from a gas bubble into the surrounding liquid is examined by measuring oxygen pressure with Po_2-needle electrodes at different distances from the bubble. From there, the mass transfer coefficient can be calculated. First measurements yielded results in the range to be expected.

INTRODUCTION

Oxygen transfer from a gas bubble through a liquid to living cells is of high importance in biochemical engineering. According to the extended film theory the whole process can be divided into seven steps with different transport resistances (Fig. 1). At most conditions diffusion of oxygen through the liquid film of the bubble is the step that determines the velocity of the whole transport. Our investigation is therefore limited to this field.

Lee et al.[1] and Bungay et al.[2] carried out measurements at plane surfaces, but mass transfer from bubbles still has not been examined. The mass transfer coefficient β_L is defined by:

$$dc \, / \, dt = \beta_L * a * (c^+ - c)$$

and can be calculated by:

$$\beta_L = D \, / \, \delta .$$

The Sherwood-number (dimensionless mass transfer coefficient) is defined by:

$$Sh = d * \beta_L \, / \, D, \text{ therefore } Sh = d/ \, \delta .$$

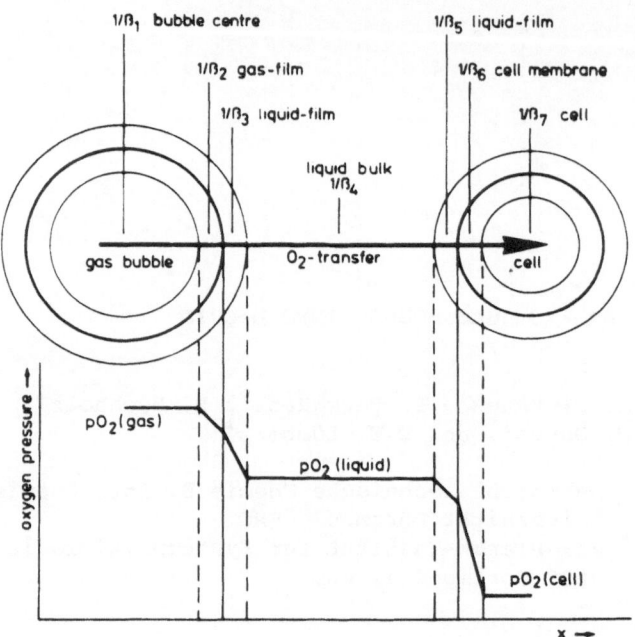

Fig. 1. possible transfer resistances during oxygen transfer from
a gas bubble to a living cell in an aerobic submers
fermentation

Symbols used:
dc/dt: change of concentration with time
β_L: liquidside mass transfer coefficient
a: bubble area per bubble volume
c^+: equilibrium oxygen concentration in liquid
c: actual oxygen concentration in liquid
D: oxygen diffusion coefficient in liquid
δ: thickness of diffusion boundary layer
d: bubble equivalent diameter

METHODS

The distribution of oxygen pressure near the bubble is
measured with oxygen microelectrodes developed by Baumgärtl and
Lübbers[3] and P_{O_2}-concentrations are calculated. The air bubble
is formed at the outlet of a capillary tube and caught with a
wire-spiral made of Pt-wire (Fig. 2). It is positioned in the
downstreamer of a small loop-reactor (column-diameter: 30 mm),
thus simulating the ascent of a bubble in quiet liquids (Fig. 3).
Distilled N_2-equilibrated water was used with a small quantity
of electrolyte added. The electrode can be moved relative to the
bubble in defined steps by means of a nanostepper (Bachofer,
Reutlingen). In this way it is possible to determine oxygen
concentrations at different distances from the bubble surface.

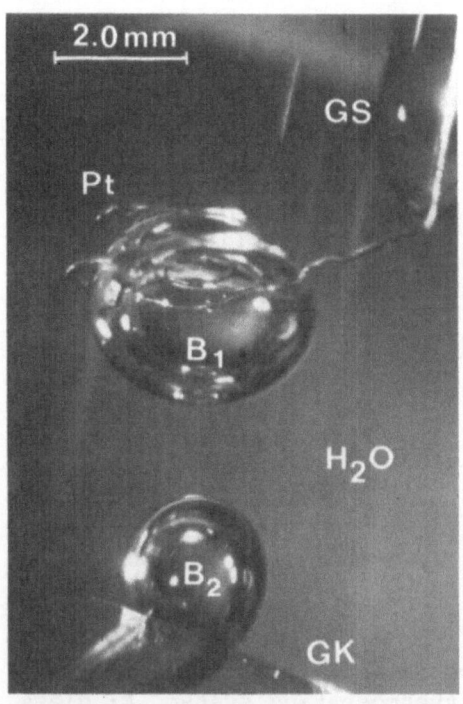

Fig. 2. air bubble (B1) captured in a holding device
         B2: gas bubble (just being produced)
         GK: glass capillary, GS: holding device (glass bar)
         M: medium, Pt: platinum wire-spiral

a) Measurements in Still Water

In the first experiments the loop-reactor was operated without liquid flow. Without convection there should be pure diffusion.
Concentration profiles obtained in these experiments are shown in
Fig. 4. The concentrations around smaller bubbles decrease faster
with distance than that of larger bubbles. To eliminate the
influence of the bubble size the distance from the bubble centre
was divided by the bubble equivalent radius. The resulting curves
(Fig. 5) are much lower than expected for pure diffusion. Furthermore, O_2-concentrations above the bubbles are lower than those
under the bubbles. Therefore it is supposed that liquid is still
not at rest, but slowly moving downwards. Ihme et al.[4] calculated
that a Peclet-number of about 100 would cause values like these
which means a downward liquid velocity of 70 µm/s. In the experimental arrangement used such a value seems to be plausible.
It can be seen in a microscope even after a long time of rest that
the liquid is not really stagnant.

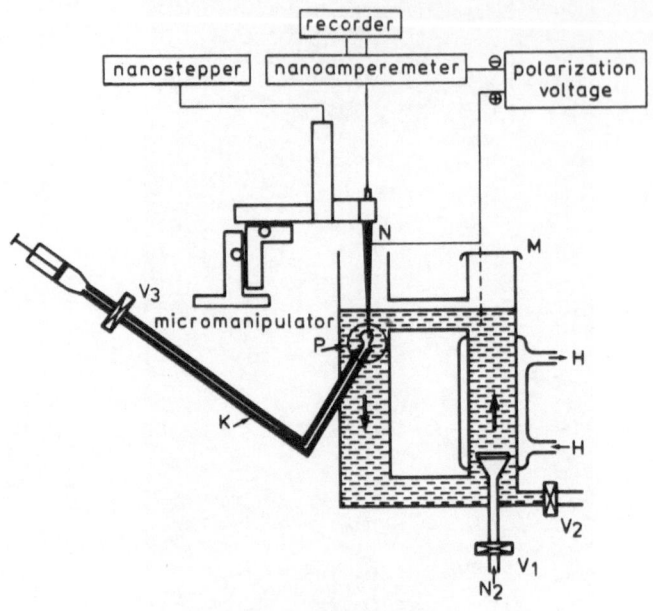

Fig. 3.   experimental arrangement
H: thermostating system, K: glass capillary
M: membrane, N: Po_2-needle electrode
V_1, V_2, V_3: valves

b) Measurements in Still Ethylene Glycol-Solutions

For reducing convection highly viscous ethylene-glycol solutions were used instead of water. All the values are larger than
the ones for water at a viscosity of 12 mPas (Fig. 6).

c) Measurements in Moved Water

In Fig. 7 results of loop-reactor runs (moved liquid) are
shown. As expected concentrations decrease with higher velocities.
Unfortunately liquid downward velocities could not be measured
yet. Therefore our results still cannot be compared with literature
data.

d) Determination of Response-Time

Another application of the experimental setup is to measure
the response-time of the electrodes to a sudden Po_2 step.
For measuring fast response-times there are two main problems 1)
generation of a fast Po_2-step, 2) fast data acquisition.

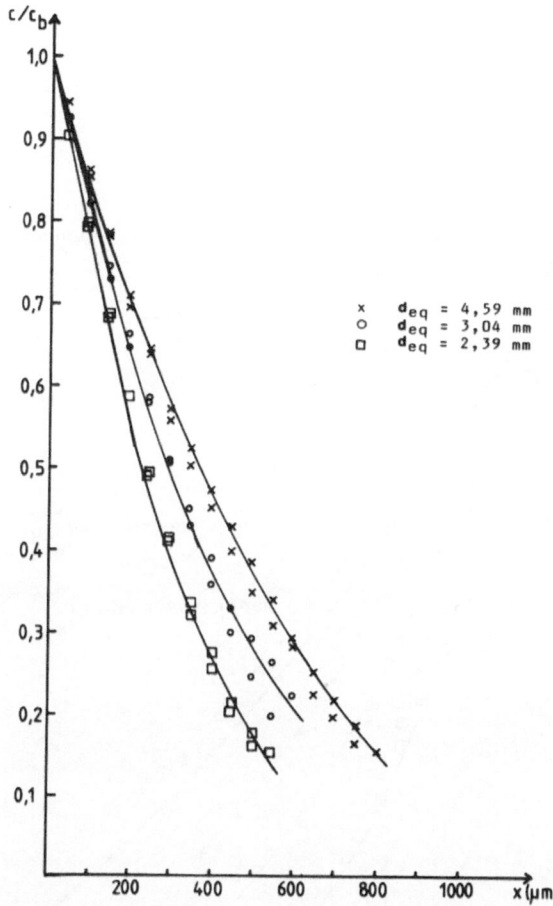

Fig. 4. profiles of oxygen concentration around single air
bubbles in still N_2-equilibrated water at different
bubble diameters
c/c_b: normalized oxygen concentration
x : distance from bubble surface

The Po_2-step is produced by moving the electrode up or down
in the concentration field of the bubble (Fig. 8) which takes less
than 1 ms by using the nanostepper. Thus a Po_2-step of about 100
torr is generated. A nanoamperemeter with a response-time of less
than 15 ms is used and measured values are transferred to a
storage-oscilloscope. Response-times (t_{90}) of the used electrodes
were in the range of 35-100 ms.

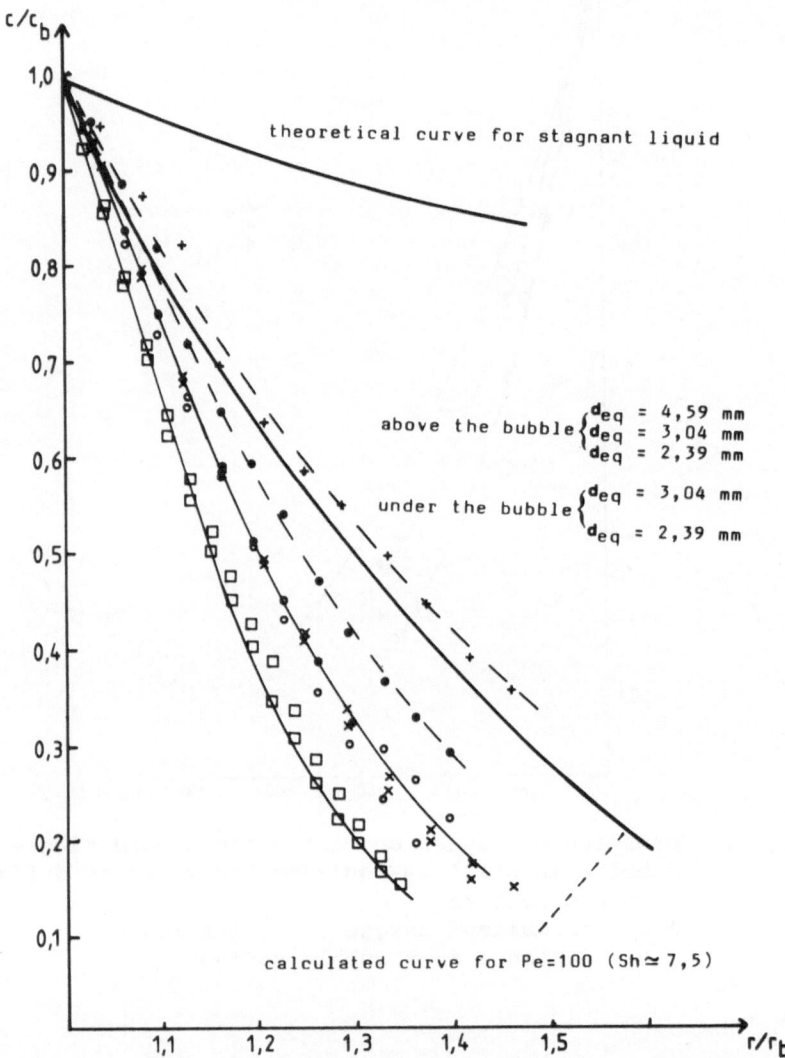

Fig. 5. profiles of oxygen concentration around single air
bubbles in N_2-equilibrated still water at different
bubble diameters
c/c_b: normalized oxygen concentration
r/r_b: distance from bubble centre/bubble radius

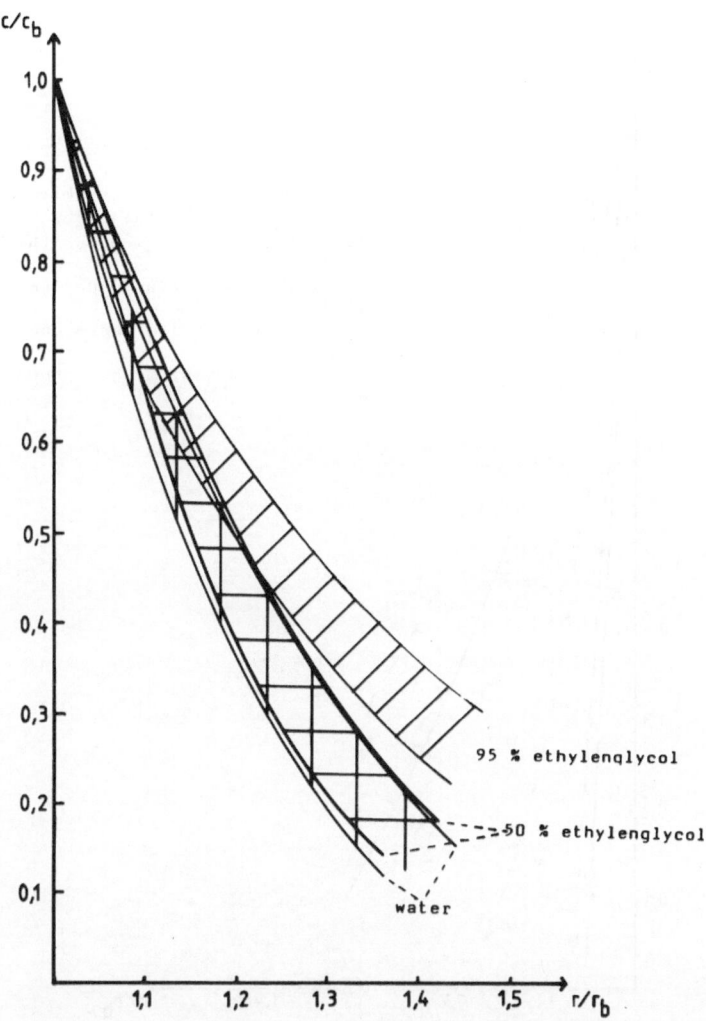

Fig. 6.   profiles of oxygen concentration around single air
bubbles in still N_2-equilibrated water, 50% ethylene
glycol and 95% ethylene glycol
c/c_b: normalized oxygen concentration
r/r_b: normalized distance from bubble

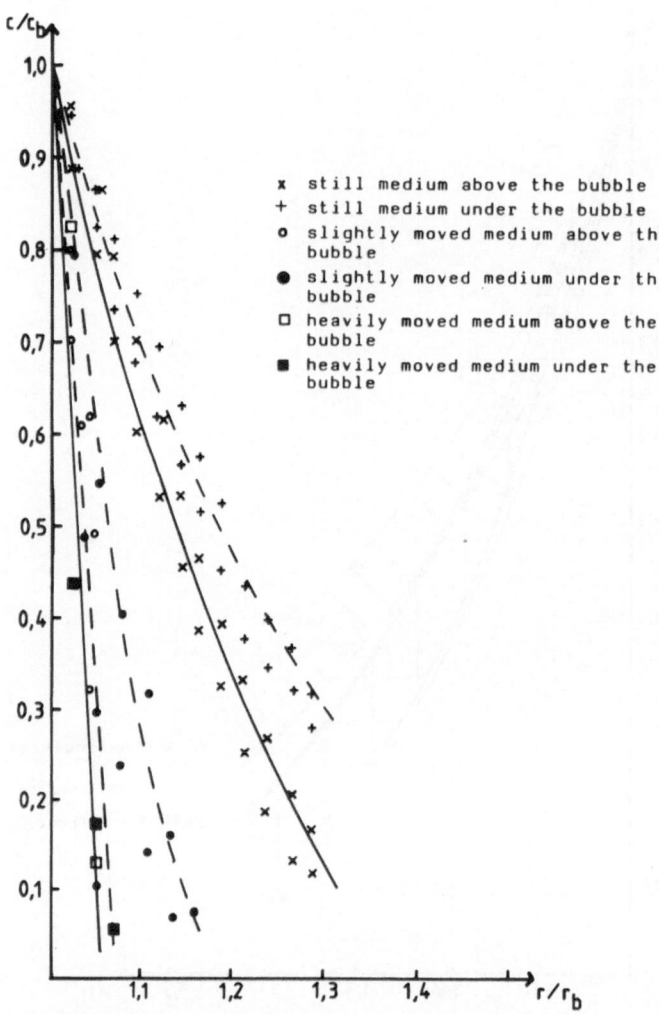

Fig. 7. profiles of oxygen concentration around single air
bubbles in N_2-equilibrated water
c/c_b: normalized oxygen concentration
r/r_b: normalized distance from bubble

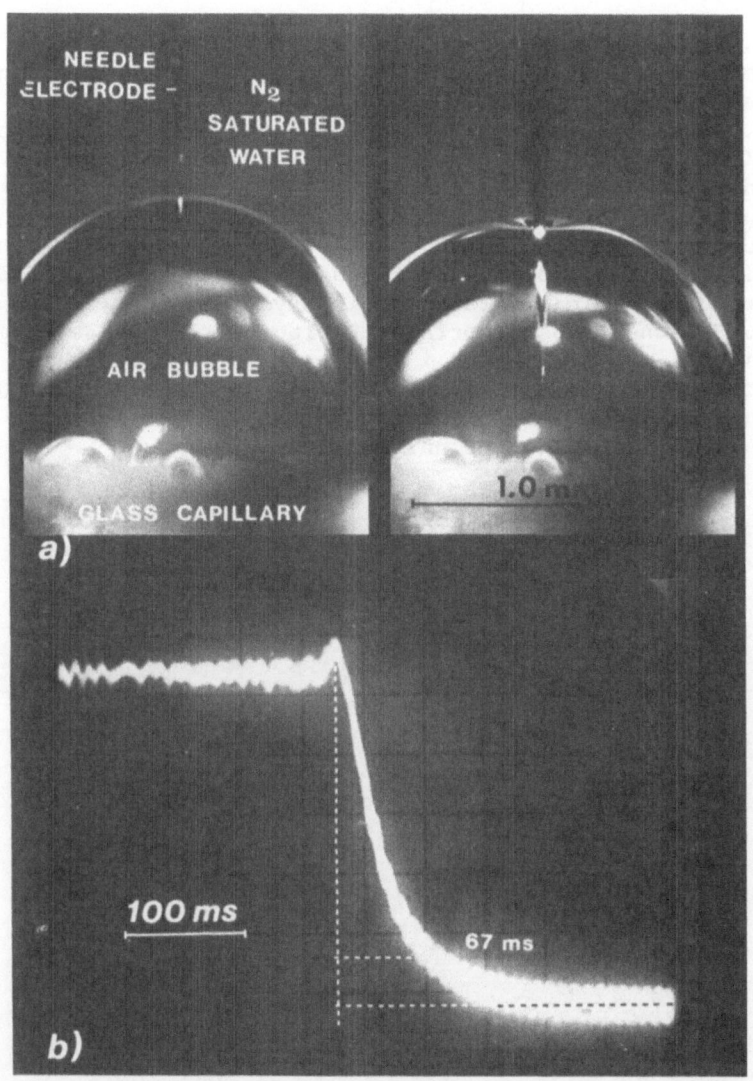

Fig. 8. experimental setup for measuring the response-time
a) air bubble with electrode at different distances
b) photo from a trace of the storage-oscilloscope

REFERENCES

1. Y. H. Lee, G. T. Tsao, and P.C. Wankat, Ultramicroprobe method
    for investigating mass transfer through gas-liquid inter-
    faces, Ind. Eng. Chem. Fundam. 17:59 (1978).
2. H. R. Bungay, W. M. Sanders, and W. J. Whalen, Microprobe tech-
    niques for determining diffusivities and respiration rates
    in microbial slime systems, Biotechn. Bioeng. 11:765 (1969).
3. H. Baumgärtl, and D. W. Lübbers, Microcoaxial needle sensor
    for polarographic measurement of local O_2 pressure in
    cellular range of living tissue. Its construction and
    properties, in: "Polarographic Oxygen Sensors," E. Gnaiger,
    H. Forstner, eds., Springer Verlag, Berlin-Heidelberg
    (1983), pp. 37.
4. F. Ihme, H. Schmidt-Traub, and H. Brauer, Theoretische Unter-
    suchung über die Umströmung und den Stoffübergang an
    Kugeln, Chem. Ing. Techn. 44:306 (1972).

PROPOSAL FOR USING A STANDARDIZED TERMINOLOGY ON OXYGEN TRANSPORT TO TISSUE

R. Zander[1] and P. Vaupel[2]

[1]Institute of Physuilogy
[2]DEpartment of Applied Physiology
University of Mainz, D-6500 Mainz

The aim of the present proposal is to recommend some definitions of important and frequently used terms in the field of oxygen transport to tissue. The latest glossary on this topic is dated 1973 and was published by the International Union of Physiological Sciences (J. Appl. Physiol. 34, 549 - 558, 1973). In the meantime, some of these definitions are either outdated or are used in another sense. Therefore, definitions are proposed for the following terms:

Oxygen partial pressure (P_{O_2})

The partial pressure of O_2 in the alveolar space, in blood or tissues, expressed as kPa or mmHg.
Synonym: O_2 tension.

Normoxia

A state in which the O_2 partial pressure in the alveolar space, in blood or tissues is normal compared to that of a healthy man at rest.

Hypoxia, Hyperoxia

A state in which the O_2 partial pressure in the alveolar space, in blood or tissues is lower or higher, resp., than in normoxia.

Oxygenation of hemoglobin

The bivalent iron of the heme group can form a loose coordinate bond with molecular O_2 (conversion of hemoglobin into oxyhemoglobin). To indicate that this binding occurs without change in valence of the iron, this reaction is called oxygenation; accordingly the splitting off of O_2 is designated as deoxygenation.

Oxidation of hemoglobin

Apart from the oxygenation of the heme group, oxidation can occur. Hereby, the result is a conversion of the bivalent iron to the trivalent state (hemiglobin or methemoglobin formation).

Hemoglobin derivatives

Hemoglobin (Hb): Deoxyhemoglobin, i.e., Hb in the deoxygenated state.
  Not recommended: reduced hemoglobin.
Oxyhemoglobin (HbO_2): Hemoglobin with reversibly bound O_2, i.e., Hb in the oxygenated state.
  Not recommended: oxidized hemoglobin.
Carboxyhemoglobin (HbCO): Hemoglobin with reversibly bound carbon monoxide.
Hemiglobin (Hb^+, HHb): Hemoglobin in the oxidized state, i.e., the iron is in the ferric state, and, therefore, incapable of O_2 binding.
  Synonym: methemoglobin (MetHb).

Hüfner factor

The maximum amount of O_2 bound by 1 g of hemoglobin with normal binding power. Assuming that 1 mole of hemoglobin (= 64,458 g) can bind 4 moles of O_2 (= $4 \cdot 22.394$ l) a theoretical value of 1.3897 ml O_2/g Hb is obtained; for practical use 1.39 ml O_2/g Hb is recommended.

Oxygen saturation (S_{O_2})

The amount of O_2 combined with hemoglobin expressed as the percentage or fraction of the O_2 capacity. Or: The concentration of oxyhemoglobin (HbO_2) expressed as the percentage or fraction of the total amount of hemoglobin, i.e., Hb, HbO_2, HbCO and Hb^+.
Note: The two definitions are the result of two different principles of measurement of the O_2 saturation, namely
(1) measurement of the O_2 concentration, or
(2) photometric determination of hemoglobin derivatives.
Not recommended: The concentration of oxyhemoglobin as a percentage or fraction of hemoglobin capable of reversible binding to O_2, i.e., Hb plus HbO_2.

Oxygen concentration (C_{O_2})

The concentration of O_2 in a blood sample, including both chemically bound and physically dissolved O_2. Expressed as ml O_2 (STPD)/dl, l/l, %(v/v), or mmol/l.
Synonym: O_2 content.

Normoxemia

A state in which the O_2 concentration in blood is normal compared to that of a healthy man at rest.

Hypoxemia

A state in which the O_2 concentration in blood is lower than in normoxemia.

Hypoxic hypoxemia

Hypoxemia caused by a decrease of the O_2 partial pressure in blood. P_{O_2}, S_{O_2} and C_{O_2} are lowered.

Anemic hypoxemia

Hypoxemia caused by a lowered hemoglobin concentration in blood. P_{O_2} and S_{O_2} are normal, C_{O_2} is lowered.

Toxemic hypoxemia

Hypoxemia caused by an altered O_2 binding power of hemoglobin (e.g. by carbon monoxide). P_{O_2} is normal, S_{O_2} and C_{O_2} are lowered.

Hyperoxemia

Any state in which the O_2 concentration in blood is higher than in normoxemia (caused by hyperoxia or an increase in the hemoglobin concentration).

Oxygen capacity

The maximum amount of O_2 bound by hemoglobin in a unit volume of blood. The O_2 capacity is a theoretical value, obtained by the product of the Hb concentration (g/dl) and the Hüfner factor (1.39 ml O_2/g Hb). Expressed as an O_2 concentration, ordinarily as ml O_2 (STPD)/dl.
Note: Until now, no experimental procedure is known for the measurement of this theoretical value because of the fact that traces of hemoglobin do not bind O_2 (e.g. HbCO, Hb^+) but are included during measurement of the total hemoglobin concentration.
Not recommended: O_2 combining capacity, O_2 transport capacity.

Oxygen binding curve of hemoglobin

Oxygen saturation as a function of O_2 partial pressure.
Synonym: O_2 dissociation curve of hemoglobin, O_2 hemoglobin equilibrium curve.

Oxygen equilibrium curve of blood

Oxygen concentration of blood (i.e., chemically bound plus physically dissolved O_2) as a function of the O_2 partial pressure.
Note: In many cases the O_2 equilibrium curve of blood is transformed into the O_2 binding curve of blood (expressed as O_2 saturation as a function of O_2 partial pressure) after the O_2 concentration is corrected for the physically dissolved O_2, and then given as a percentage of the (theoretical) O_2 capacity. In these cases the definition O_2 binding curve of blood (S_{O_2} vs. P_{O_2}) should be used instead of O_2 equilibrium curve of blood (C_{O_2} vs. P_{O_2}).
Not recommended: O_2 dissociation curve of blood.

Oxygen affinity of hemoglobin or blood

The degree of O_2 saturation of hemoglobin (Hb solution or whole blood) at a given O_2 partial pressure under defined conditions (e.g. temperature, pH value).
Generally the half saturation pressure (P_{50}, i.e., the O_2 partial pressure at 50% saturation) is used for the description of the affinity.
Note: O_2 affinity can only be used for the O_2 binding curve of hemoglobin or blood, but not for the O_2 equilibrium curve of blood.

Oxygen supply

The amount of O_2 transported within the arterial blood of the systemic circulation per unit time. It is the product of the cardiac output and the arterial O_2 concentration and is usually expressed as unit volume or amount of O_2 per unit time (e.g. ml O_2/min):

O_2 supply = cardiac output $\cdot$ $C_{a_{O_2}}$
Synonym: O_2 transport capacity.

Oxygen availability

The amount of O_2 transported within the blood into a given organ per unit time. It is the product of the absolute organ blood flow rate (perfusion rate) $\dot{Q}$ and the arterial O_2 concentration and is usually expressed as unit volume or amount of O_2 per unit time (e.g. ml O_2/min):

$$O_2 \text{ availability} = \dot{Q} \cdot C_{a_{O_2}}$$

Synonym: O_2 delivery.

Oxygen consumption rate ($\dot{Q}_{O_2}$)

The oxygen consumption rate of perfused organs or tissues is the amount of O_2 consumed by these organs or tissues per unit time. It is found according to Fick's principle from the absolute blood flow rate (or perfusion rate) $\dot{Q}$ multiplied by the arterio- venous O_2 concentration difference ($avD_{O_2} = C_{a_{O_2}} - C_{v_{O_2}}$):

$$\dot{Q}_{O_2} = \dot{Q} \cdot avD_{O_2}$$

The O_2 consumption rate is ordinarily expressed as unit volume or amount of O_2 per unit time (e.g. ml O_2/min). If the absolute organ blood flow is replaced by the specific (= weight- related) blood flow one refers to the specific O_2 consumption rate.The latter is expressed as unit volume or amount of O_2 per unit wet weight of the organ and unit time (e.g. ml $O_2 \cdot g^{-1} \cdot min^{-1}$).
Not recommended: O_2 usage, O_2 utilization, metabolic rate for O_2 (MRO_2).

Respiration rate ($\dot{Q}_{O_2}$)

In the case of isolated respiring cells or tissues in vitro the O_2 consumption rate is often referred to as respiration rate and is expressed as unit volume or amount of O_2 per unit dry weight and unit time (e.g. μl $O_2 \cdot mg^{-1}$ per h).

Oxygen uptake ($\dot{V}_{O_2}$)

This is the amount or the volume of O_2 taken up by the whole body or a whole organism from the environment and equals the O_2 amount taken up by the blood from the alveolar space. It is identical with the O_2 transport capacity and is generally expressed as volume or amount of O_2 per unit time (e.g. ml O_2/min).
The O_2 consumption rate of all tissues of the body is equal to the O_2 uptake only when the O_2 stores are constant.
Note: The term "O_2 consumption" instead of O_2 consumption rate, respiration rate or O_2 uptake should be avoided as it is too general.

Oxygen utilization

The O_2 utilization is a measure of the adequacy of the O_2 availability to an organ or tissue. It is defined as the ratio of the O_2 consumption rate to the respective

O_2 availability:

O_2 utilization = O_2 consumption rate/O_2 availability

$$= avD_{O_2}/C_{a_{O_2}}$$

It is generally expressed as percent(%) or fraction.
Synonyms: O_2 utilization ratio, O_2 extraction (ratio).
Not recommended: O_2 removal ratio, coefficient of O_2
utilization.

O_2 solubility coefficient (α_{O_2})

The O_2 solubility coefficient indicates the volume or the
amount of O_2 physically dissolved in a unit volume of
liquid at a given O_2 partial pressure. It is ordinarily
expressed as ml $O_2 \cdot$ ml$^{-1} \cdot$ atm^{-1} (type of liquid and temperature must be specified).
Synonyms: Bunsen's coefficient, O_2 solubility.

Krogh's O_2 diffusion coefficient (K_{O_2})

This coefficient indicates the volume or the amount of O_2
diffusing through a layer with a certain thickness and
surface area per unit time at a given partial pressure
difference. It can be expressed as ml $O_2 \cdot$ cm$\cdot$cm$^{-2} \cdot$min$^{-1} \cdot$atm^{-1}
or in a more simplified form: ml $O_2 \cdot$ cm$^{-1} \cdot$min$^{-1} \cdot$atm^{-1}
(material and temperature must be specified).
Synonyms: Krogh's diffusion constant, O_2 diffusion conductivity.
Not recommended: Krogh's constant; the use of the following unit should be avoided: cm$^2 \cdot$min$^{-1} \cdot$atm^{-1}.

Oxygen diffusion coefficient (D_{O_2})

This coefficient indicates the volume or the amount of O_2
diffusing through a layer with a certain thickness and
surface area per unit time at a given O_2 concentration
difference. Considering Henry- Dalton's law ($C_{O_2} = \alpha_{O_2}$
times P_{O_2}) and after reducing the fraction the unit
that results is as follows: cm^2/s (material and temperature must be specified).
If K_{O_2} and α_{O_2} are known, D_{O_2} can be calculated using
the following equation:

$$D_{O_2} = K_{O_2}/\alpha_{O_2}$$

Synonym: O_2 diffusion constant
Not recommended: diffusivity.

The authors would be most pleased to receive any additional comments or suggestions for further improvement of
this glossary.

Muscle (continued)
      399, 409, 419, 429, 703,
      855
   capillarity, 355
   PO_2, 419
Myocardial capillarity, 249
   ischemia, 281
   oxygenation, 257
   oxygen consumption, 193, 257
   oxygen diffusion, 271
   oxygen pressure, 21, 203, 211
Myoglobin, 263, 433

NADH laser fluorimetry, 229
Near infrared spectrophotometry,
      823, 833, 843, 849, 855,
      863, 873
Necrosis in multicellular
      spheroids, 775
Neuronal activity, 101, 163
Nude rats, 737, 753

Oxygen, 131, 543
   affinity, 473
   binding properties, 473, 485,
      505
   and carbon dioxide solubility in
      fluosol, 453
   consumption, 193, 257, 291, 365,
      409, 775
   consumption and blood flow
      mismatching, 257
   content difference, 553
   debt, 399
   deficit, 399
   diffusion, 271
   dissociation curve, 505, 619
   exchanges in muscle, 309
   permeability, 565
   pressure, 21, 429, 601, 719
      distribution, 183
      fields, 131
   saturation, 263, 899, 909
   supply, 3, 21, 77, 217, 445,
      523, 693, 753, 917
   tension, 173, 663
   toxicity, 655
   transfer, 523, 955
   transport, 323, 533, 611, 737,
      923

Oxygen (continued)
   transport to tissue, 965
Oxygenation, 37, 257

Pancreas, 693
Peptides, 121
Perfluorocarbon, 463
Perfusate oxygenation, 675
Peritoneal perfusion, 463
pH responses in carotid body, 709
Physically dissolved oxygen, 674
Pig, 203, 637
   heart, 203
Polarographic oxygen sensors, 947
Portocaval anastomosis, 419, 703
Post-exercise anemia, 579
Pyridine nucleotide, 375

Rabbit, 281, 333
Rat, 107, 111, 239, 249, 341, 419,
      571, 579, 703, 785
   heart, 239
   kidney, 675
   liver, 473
Reactive hyperaemia, 683
Red cells, 301, 485, 495, 899,
      917
Red cell oxygen transport, 495
   residence time, 917
   transit time, 301
Red muscle, 291
Redox relationships, 815
   state, 263
Reflection spectra, 85, 263, 883,
      889
Regional cerebral blood flow, 3,
      101, 107, 131
   cerebrovascular resistance, 111
Regulation of cerebral blood flow,
      91
Renal cortex, 703
   function, 675
Reticulocytosis, 571
Rheological factors, 523

Salicylate, 655
Shunt-sink hypothesis, 309
Simulation of oxygen transport in
      microcirculation, 923
Skeletal muscle, 37, 291, 309,